STANDARDS FOR
CRITICAL CARE

BRENDA CRISPELL JOHANSON, R.N., M.A., Ed.M., CCRN

Associate Nurse Epidemiologist, The New York Hospital–Cornell
University Medical Center, New York, New York;
formerly, Clinical Specialist, Surgical Anesthesia Intensive Care Unit,
Surgical Cardiac Intensive Care Unit,
Columbia-Presbyterian Medical Center, New York, New York

CONSUELO URTULA DUNGCA, R.N., M.A., Ed.M.

Medical Clinical Specialist,
Columbia-Presbyterian Medical Center, New York, New York

DENISE HOFFMEISTER, R.N., M.A., CNRN

Neurological Clinical Specialist,
Columbia-Presbyterian Medical Center, New York, New York

SARA JEANNE WELLS, B.S.N., M.N.

Cardiovascular Clinical Specialist,
Columbia-Presbyterian Medical Center, New York, New York

The C. V. Mosby Company

ST. LOUIS • TORONTO • LONDON   1981

Printed in the United States of America

The C. V. Mosby Company
11830 Westline Industrial Drive, St. Louis, Missouri 63141

Library of Congress Cataloging in Publication Data

Main entry under title:

Standards for critical care.

  Bibliography: p.
  Includes index.
    1. Intensive care nursing—Standards.
I. Johanson, Brenda Crispell, 1950-
[DNLM: 1. Critical care—Standards—Nursing texts.
WY154   S785]
RT120.I5S7   610.73′61   80-15476
ISBN 0-8016-2527-0

AC/CB/B 9 8 7 6 5 4 3   05/A/598

CONTRIBUTORS

JO ANNE BENNETT, R.N., M.A., CCRN

Assistant Executive Director, Maternal Child Care Services, Metropolitan Hospital, New York, New York; formerly, Associate Director for Patient Care and Staff Development, Pediatric Acute Care Project, International Rescue Committee, Saigon, Vietnam; Staff Nurse, Neonatal Intensive Care Unit, St. Vincent's Hospital, New York, New York

JOAN HOLTER GILDEA, R.N., M.A.

Administrative Supervisor, Pediatrics, New York University Medical Center University Hospital, New York, New York

MARY FRAN HAZINSKI, R.N., M.S.N.

Pediatric Clinical Specialist, Presbyterian Hospital of Pacific Medical Center, San Francisco, California

PAT LYBARGER, R.N., M.S.N.

Clinical Specialist, Pediatric Medical and Surgical Intensive Care, Babies Hospital, Columbia-Presbyterian Medical Center, New York, New York

CATHERINE MUTTART, R.N., M.S.

Staff Associate in Clinical Nursing, Department of Pediatrics, Columbia-Presbyterian Medical Center, New York, New York

ANN AURIGEMMA NUTT, R.N., M.A.

Inservice Instructor, Pediatrics, New York University Medical Center University Hospital, New York, New York

CAROL E. SHANIK, R.N., M.S.

Associate in Nursing, Graduate Program in Perinatal Nursing, Faculty of Medicine, Columbia University, New York, New York; formerly, Clinical Nurse Specialist, Perinatology Center, The New York Hospital–Cornell University Medical Center, New York, New York

FOREWORD

It is always a pleasure to read a text written by busy clinicians. *Standards for Critical Care* provides a lasting example of the clinician's concern for quality patient care and the education necessary to accomplish that goal. The dedication and discipline required to produce a book such as the one you are about to read can only be fully appreciated by other clinician authors.

Critical care nursing educational programs were developed at a staggering rate during the 1970s. Those programs were then and remain today unparalleled in quality and quantity. With the establishment of critical care educational programs in virtually every town and city in the United States, as well as in every acute care hospital, the expectations for critical care nursing practice were widely disseminated.

As the United States moves into the 1980s, critical care nursing practice is moving into a decade of aggressive professional development. Of primary concern to the profession is the establishment of standards for critical care nursing practice, which can be implemented and then tested and modified. This text is the first publication devoted to standards for critical care nursing; this achievement is indeed a milestone for our profession. I am sure the authors look forward to your experiences in implementing these standards. Let them hear from you.

Diane C. Adler, R.N., M.A., CCRN

Clinical Director of Critical Care,
Hospital of the University of Pennsylvania,
Philadelphia; Past President, American
Association of Critical-Care Nurses

PREFACE

The formidable challenge of caring for the acutely ill patient has been met by a rapidly expanding understanding of physiological and psychological interactions in multisystem diseases. Technological advancements have led to the development of more sophisticated procedures and equipment, which therefore facilitate heroic life-sustaining interventions and more subtle manipulations for altering the course of an illness. The level of sophistication necessary to carry out such large-scale intervention is indeed high.

The setting in which critical care occurs is unique in that continuous subjective and objective monitoring of labile parameters is essential to assure quality care. The critical care nurse, therefore, must integrate a knowledge of physiological principles involving multiple organ systems with a minute-by-minute monitoring of function. An accurate assessment followed by an appropriate activity is of utmost importance.

Educating new nurses and maintaining standards that guarantee high-quality care are two primary objectives in any nursing unit. In critical care, the difficulties encountered in realizing these objectives are intensified by the breadth of material to be mastered and the severely compromised, often unstable, state of the patients. A comprehensive, problem-oriented manual that describes common conditions encountered in a critical care setting, along with accepted therapeutic and preventive interventions and their indications, is needed to facilitate the training process.

Nursing care standards must be in writing and must be re-emphasized frequently. Standards are the basis for formulating plans for ongoing care as well as for evaluating the effectiveness with which it is delivered. The educational value of an inclusive collection of standards is obvious. A beginning critical care nurse will be able to refer to such a source for introductory reading in an orientation program as well as when preparing a daily care plan. Moreover, instructors, clinical specialists, and head nurses are provided with a tool for evaluating the quality of care delivered and the performance of staff members in many specific situations.

Standards of care can also form the basis of an audit program, an evaluation process that helps to assure the delivery of safe, high-quality care. In this age of closer public scrutiny of health care delivery, a written policy describing established procedures at every level of hospital function is mandatory to maintain institutional accreditation and public approval.

Standards for Critical Care is designed for use in the clinical setting, in the classroom, in administrative planning, and in evaluation. This book's clinical value is its problem-oriented approach to a wide variety of conditions and its efficient delivery of essential information.

Standards for Critical Care includes more than lists of objectives and procedures. Each standard includes an introduction, assessment parameters, goals of care, and a problem-oriented chart composed of nursing activities. The introduction to each topic summarizes the salient features of pathophysiology underlying each disease state and outlines various diagnostic and therapeutic modalities that may be used. Thus the introduction provides a rationale for the sections that follow. The nurse's assessment focuses attention on a selected set of parameters that should be monitored throughout a given patient's hospital course. It serves as a guide or "organizer" of parameters to be assessed. Each assessment factor takes on more or less significance depending on the specific case as well as the staff and equipment available for monitoring. By referring back to the introduction and ahead to the chart of nursing activities, the reader will be able to understand and formulate a priority for each assessment factor and integrate the information into an actual care plan. Moreover, a thorough, ongoing assessment provides for a precise definition of the patient's clinical status and permits early detection of abnormalities associated with the patient's primary health problem. For each of these "potential" problems, nursing activities that serve to prevent, detect, evaluate, and resolve the abnormality are described.

The patient and family must be adequately informed and supported during the hospital experience. Each standard outlines essential components of the teaching plan, including information about diagnostic tests, the disease process, and therapy. For surgical intervention, teaching guidelines regarding the surgery and perioperative experiences are enumerated. Special attention is given to follow-up care at the end of most standards. Finally, each standard cites comfort measures, which can make the hospital experience more pleasant.

The nursing activities in these standards form the basis for a plan of care that is tailored to the patient's illness and clinical presentation. As the nurse administers treatments to alter the patient's clinical course, nursing measures will be modified according to hospital policy and protocol. Thus the activities described in these standards serve as a guide for developing a plan of care that best supports the patient at any point in his/her acute illness.

To all who assisted in the preparation of this book, we extend our thanks. Special thanks goes to the contributing authors, whose standards form an essential component of the book. Because of the current paucity of literature on standards for neonatal-pediatric care, chapters in this area were invaluable to us. We extend our appreciation and gratitude to the following authors for their contributions: to Jo Anne Bennett for The Unstable Premature Infant, Neonatal Necrotizing Enterocolitis, Reye's Syndrome, and Diaphragmatic Hernia; to Joan Holter Gildea and Ann Aurigemma Nutt for Poisoning, Croup Syndrome, and Asthma/Status Asthmaticus; to Mary Fran Hazinski for Near Drowning, The Patient with a Tracheostomy, Cardiac Catheterization, Tracheoesophageal Fistula, and for developing the chart on congenital heart defects in the Cardiac Surgery chapter; to Carol E. Shanik for Growth Retardation, Neonatal Respiratory Distress, and Hemolytic Disease Due to Rh/ABO Incompatibility.

We also acknowledge the contribution of Pat Lybarger in laying the groundwork for The Patient with a Tracheostomy, Near Drowning, and Tracheoesophageal Fistula. Catherine Muttart lent her special expertise in nutrition in Total Parenteral Nutrition Through Central Venous Catheter, done jointly with Brenda Johanson. Finally, we are grateful for the thoughtful foreword prepared by Diane Adler.

The dedication and patience of our typists in completing this monumental task deserve special recognition. Thanks goes to Rosa de la Rosa Urtula, Charlotte Vetter, and Bessie Ibanez. The typing done by Annette Kirshner and Fran Rivera is also appreciated.

Brenda Crispell Johanson
Consuelo Urtula Dungca
Denise Hoffmeister
Sara Jeanne Wells

CONTENTS

Respiratory

1   Pulmonary edema of cardiac origin, 1

2   Acute respiratory failure, 6

3   Thoracic surgery, 17

4   Near drowning, 27

5   The patient with a tracheostomy, 36

6   Mechanical ventilation, 42

7   Positive end expiratory pressure, 48

8   Chest physiotherapy, 52

Cardiovascular

9   Angina pectoris, 55

10   Acute myocardial infarction, 60

11   Heart failure (low cardiac output), 74

12   Cardiogenic shock, 83

13   Shock, 92

14   Pericarditis, 97

15   Endocarditis, 102

16   Arrhythmias, 107

17   Pacemakers: temporary and permanent, 114

18   Intra-aortic balloon pumping (counterpulsation), 122

19   Hemodynamic monitoring, 132

20   Cardiac catheterization, 141

21   Cardiac surgery, 147

22   Vascular surgery: aneurysms, 171

23   Embolic phenomena, 181

Neurological

24   Increased intracranial pressure, 193

25   Head trauma, 203

26   Subarachnoid hemorrhage, 215

27   Subdural hematoma, 222

28   Supratentorial craniotomy, 229

29   Infratentorial craniotomy, 238

30   Internalized shunting procedures, 249

31   Carotid endarterectomy, 258

32   Transphenoidal hypophysectomy (pituitary tumors), 266

33   Seizures, 272

34   Meningitis/encephalitis, 281

35   Myasthenia gravis (including thymectomy), 292

36   Guillain Barré syndrome, 312

Gastrointestinal

37   Peritonitis, 321

38   Liver failure/decompressive portovenous shunting procedures, 326

39   Pancreatitis, 336

40   Pancreatic surgery, 341

41   Acute upper gastrointestinal bleeding, 347

42   Gastrointestinal surgery, 353

43   Jejunal-ileal bypass surgery, 365

Renal

44   Acute renal failure, 373

45   Peritoneal dialysis, 378

46   Hemodialysis, 388

47   Renal transplantation, 401

Metabolic

48   Diabetic ketoacidosis, 411

49   Total parenteral nutrition through central venous catheter, 417

General

50   Multiple trauma, 424

51   Burns, 441

52   Disseminated intravascular coagulation, 449

53   Poisoning, 453

Neonatal-pediatric

54   The unstable premature infant, 460

55   Growth retardation, 472

56   Neonatal respiratory distress, 475

57   Hemolytic disease due to Rh/ABO incompatibility, 481

58   Neonatal necrotizing enterocolitis, 486

59   Croup syndrome, 491

60   Asthma/status asthmaticus, 497

61   Reye's syndrome, 502

62   Diaphragmatic hernia, 507

63   Tracheoesophageal fistula, 510

Bibliography, 517

Appendices

A   Abbreviations, 523

B   Surgical procedures: assessment, 524

C   Neonatal-pediatric data, 526

STANDARDS FOR
CRITICAL CARE

RESPIRATORY

1 □ Pulmonary edema of cardiac origin

Acute pulmonary edema is a cardiac emergency that occurs when the hydrostatic pressure in the pulmonary capillaries (normally 7 to 10 mm Hg) exceeds the intravascular osmotic pressure (25 to 30 mm Hg), resulting in transudation of fluid into the alveoli. This reduces the amount of lung tissue available for gas exchange. It may develop suddenly or evolve slowly. The most common cause of pulmonary edema is acute left ventricular failure, usually secondary to acute myocardial infarction. Other causes include decompensating chronic heart failure, mitral valve disease, hypertension, circulatory overload, and central nervous system (CNS) injuries.

Management of pulmonary edema includes measures for decreasing venous return to the heart and, consequently, the pulmonary vasculature; improving gaseous exchange; improving cardiac output and the efficiency of left ventricular function; controlling anxiety; and treating complications that may evolve. The problems are interrelated; many of the approaches and medications used influence several of these management objectives.

For a discussion of the adult respiratory distress syndrome, or "shock lung," see Standard: *Acute respiratory failure*.

ASSESSMENT

1. History of recent myocardial infarction, left heart failure (acute or chronic), mitral valve disease, hypertension, CNS injury, and/or recent parenteral fluid administration to evaluate circulatory overload
2. Presence of
   a. Extreme restlessness
   b. Orthopnea
   c. Tachypnea
   d. Extreme dyspnea—air hunger
   e. Bubbling rales
   f. Wheezing
   g. Coughing
   h. Nature of secretions—blood-tinged, frothy sputum
3. Level of anxiety

4. Hemodynamic status
   a. Blood pressure (BP)
   b. Pulses
   c. Heart sounds
   d. Venous pressure
   e. Fluid balance
   f. Mental status
   g. General appearance
   h. Invasive monitoring if indicated
      (1) Intra-arterial pressure
      (2) Pulmonary artery pressure (PAP) and pulmonary capillary wedge pressure (PCWP)
      (3) Cardiac output
      (4) Central venous pressure (CVP)
5. Monitor electrocardiogram (ECG) for
   a. Arrhythmias
   b. Changes reflecting electrolyte imbalance, especially potassium
   c. Changes reflecting myocardial damage, for example, acute myocardial infarction
   d. Drug effects
6. Lab data results of
   a. Blood gases
   b. Electrolytes
   c. Blood urea nitrogen (BUN)/creatinine clearance
   d. Chest radiograph for pulmonary congestion and heart size
   e. Drug levels
   f. Any tests performed to evaluate precipitating or aggravating factors
7. Patient/family's perception of and reaction to disease process, symptoms, assessment, and treatment modalities

See Standard: *Heart failure*

GOALS

1. Absence of respiratory distress—adequate oxygenation and ventilation
2. Hemodynamic stability—adequate cardiac output
3. Electrophysiological stability

4. Patient verbalizes physical comfort
5. Decreased anxiety with resolution of symptoms and provision of information
6. Patient verbalizes fears and concerns
7. Maintenance goals—see Standard: *Heart failure*

Potential problems	Expected outcomes	Nursing activities
■ Respiratory distress related to excessive accumulation of fluid in alveoli, resulting in abnormal ventilation/perfusion ratios	■ Normal respiratory effort	■ Ongoing assessment of patient's respiratory effort Extreme dyspnea—air hunger Orthopnea Tachypnea Wheezing Cough—often producing copious, frothy blood-tinged sputum Check for and record nature of secretions, noting amount, color, and presence of blood
	Lungs clear to auscultation	Auscultate lungs q1 hr or more frequently if indicated for presence and distribution of adventitious sounds, often described as *bubbling*
	Arterial blood gas levels within patient's normal limits	Monitor blood gas results for evidence of hypoxia and hypercapnia that is not chronically present Intra-arterial line may be inserted because of frequent need for samples and to monitor BP
	Hemodynamic stability	Check BP and pulse (P) for hypertension or hypotension and tachycardia Evaluate changes in venous pressure, noting Amount of distention of neck veins Peripheral or sacral edema Engorgement of peripheral veins Hepatomegaly Ascites
	Adequate cerebral oxygenation	Assess mental status for indications of cerebral hypoxia Restlessness, extreme anxiety Confusion Stupor Coma
	Clear lung fields on radiograph	Obtain and review results of chest radiograph If problem occurs, record occurrence and responses to therapy and report to physician Maintain patent IV route using microdrip or infusion pump to regulate administration of fluid and drugs Implement measures to decrease venous return, decrease pulmonary congestion, and improve gaseous exchange as ordered Position patient in high Fowler's position with lower extremities dependent; if patient is hypotensive, this position may not be well tolerated and feet may need to be flat and head of bed lowered somewhat until corrected
	Absence and/or resolution of pain	Administer morphine sulfate IV as ordered to control pain, decrease anxiety, and decrease venous return and respiratory effort, thereby improving oxygen exchange Check respiration (R) for respiratory depression Check BP for hypotension Have morphine antagonist available Morphine contraindicated in presence of cardiogenic shock, history of chronic pulmonary disease, or recent cerebrovascular accident (CVA)

Potential problems	**Expected outcomes**	**Nursing activities**

	Electrolytes within normal limits
	Urine output 30 ml/hour or more; output increases with diuretics
		Administer diuretics IV as ordered to reduce blood volume and pulmonary congestion
		Insert Foley catheter as ordered and check urine output ql hr
		   Check specific gravity; with furosemide and ethacrynic acid, diuresis should occur within 15 to 30 minutes
		   Observe for indications of urinary tract obstruction in patients with prostatic hypertrophy
		   Check for hypotension, tachycardia, and decreased urine output, indicating circulatory intolerance
		Monitor lab report results, and observe for signs and symptoms of potassium and sodium depletion
		   Administer potassium supplements as ordered
		      Use caution and administer slowly to avoid cardiac complications
		      Never add to infusions that contain antiarrhythmics or cardiotonic agents that may be titrated
		Monitor lab report results for BUN and/or creatinine clearance
		Avoid local infiltration of IV ethacrynic acid, which is extremely irritating to tissues
		Apply rotating tourniquets if ordered
		   Connect to upper portions of three extremities (leave IV extremity free) with pressure settings midway between systolic and diastolic readings
		   Check for presence of peripheral pulses and check warmth and color of extremities; adjust pressures if necessary to maintain palpable pulse
		   Ensure that tourniquets rotate in sequence q15 min; rotate more frequently for patients with vascular insufficiency
		   Reposition tourniquet on extremity q2 hr (when rotates off)
		   Observe for edema, pain, and/or loss of function of extremity; the latter two indicate prolonged constriction
		   If edema develops, elevate limb and explain to patient that condition will resolve
		   When removing, rotate off one at a time at 15-minute intervals
		   Tourniquets are contraindicated with cardiogenic shock
		Prepare for and assist with a phlebotomy if ordered
		   May be indicated if the initiating problem is fluid overload
		   Rarely used with concomitant left heart failure because the procedure would aggravate shock
		Administer O_2 as ordered; pressure must be high enough to exceed pressure barrier of edema fluid without excessively reducing venous return, which would result in circulatory collapse; usual airway pressure necessary is 4 to 9 cm H_2O
		If positive pressure mask is ordered
		   Explain to patient that it is temporary, since it may be frightening to a patient who already feels he/she is suffocating
		   Adjust mask to fit snugly
		   Pad face straps for comfort if necessary
		   Set O_2 concentration at 100%
		   Begin at 0 and slowly increase sensitivity setting to patient's respiratory effort
		   When removing positive pressure mask, slowly decrease sensitivity to 0 before discontinuing
		If patient requires intubation, see Standards: *Mechanical ventilation; Positive end expiratory pressure*

Potential problems	**Expected outcomes**	**Nursing activities**
■ Decreased cardiac output related to left ventricular dysfunction	■ Hemodynamic stability	■ Assess for development and/or acceleration of left heart failure; early recognition allows intervention that may prevent onset of pulmonary edema See Standard: *Heart failure* If acute pulmonary edema has occurred Check BP q15-30 min or more frequently if indicated Initially, a normotensive patient may become hypertensive secondary to extreme anxiety and activation of the sympathetic nervous system; hypotension occurs as a result of deteriorating left ventricular function or secondary to therapeutic maneuvers indentified in Problem, Respiratory distress related to excessive accumulation of fluid in alveoli Check P q15-30 min or more frequently if indicated; decreasing tachycardia may be indication of resolution of pulmonary edema and anxiety Observe for presence and degree of Pallor Cyanosis Diaphoresis Weakness Lethargy Restlessness Auscultate or review chart for presence of S_3 gallop Participate with physician in the identification and treatment of conditions known to increase myocardial O_2 consumption such as Anxiety, fear Hypertension or hypotension Arrhythmias Tachycardia Electrolyte imbalance Hypoxia, hypercapnia Administer medications as ordered to improve cardiac function through alterations in preload, afterload, or contractility Digoxin IV frequently ordered 1. Determine if patient has been taking digoxin 2. Monitor lab results closely for hypoxia and hypokalemia, which promote digoxin toxicity 3. Monitor ECG continuously for development of arrhythmias Aminophylline IV 1. Administer slowly through IV soluset or infusion pump to avoid complications of syncope or sudden death 2. Assess effect on relieving bronchospasm and promoting diuresis in addition to inotropic effect 3. Observe for or ascertain presence of hypotension, ventricular tachyarrhythmias, palpitations, headache, dizziness, and nausea; inform physician if any of these occur Nitroprusside or other vasodilators IV may be ordered if pulmonary edema is accompanied by hypertension 1. Maintain patent intra-arterial line 2. Administer via infusion pump 3. Maintain patent pulmonary artery line if indicated 4. Monitor the effects of medication closely and for hypotension and arrhythmias Ensure emergency equipment available and functional; check every shift

Potential problems	Expected outcomes	Nursing activities

■ Acute anxiety related to
Fear of suffocation
Cerebral anoxia
Treatment modalities
	■ Reduction of anxiety with relief of symptoms and provision of information
	Patient verbalizes fears and concerns
	Patient cooperates with treatment regimen
		■ Ongoing assessment of level of anxiety; relate findings to psychological/physiological status
		Remain with patient, maintaining a calm, controlled appearance
		Provide emotional support and reassurance to patient/family that therapeutic measures will reduce symptoms
		Explain purpose and expectations of treatment modalities used; this is particularly important if positive pressure mask and rotating tourniquets are ordered; repeated explanations are necessary because of the high anxiety level
		Make patient as comfortable as possible
		  Positioning
		  Padding face mask
		  Mouth care
		  Tourniquet suggestions as noted in Problem, Respiratory distress related to excessive accumulation of fluid in alveoli
		  Prompt relief of pain
		Reduce environmental stimuli as much as possible
		Encourage patient/family to verbalize concerns and ask questions

■ Arrhythmias related to
Hypoxia
Hypokalemia
Medications
Concomitant disease
Anxiety
	■ Electrophysiological stability
	Optimum cardiac rhythm
		■ Maintain continuous ECG monitoring
		  Select lead best demonstrating atrial and ventricular complexes
		  Set rate alarms; avoid use of audio component if possible without compromising patient safety
		Participate with physician in identifying the etiology of arrhythmias, and treat as ordered
		  Review medications patient is receiving
		  Monitor lab results for
		    Hypoxia
		    Hypokalemia
		    Acidosis/alkalosis
		  Assess alterations in level of anxiety related to onset of arrhythmia
		  Assess status of underlying disease states, particularly left heart failure, hypertension, or acute myocardial infarction
		Assess effect of arrhythmia on cardiac output and pulmonary edema
		Check emergency equipment every shift, ensuring proper function and availability
		Treat arrhythmia as ordered
		
		SEE STANDARDS: *Arrhythmias*
		               Acute myocardial infarction
		               Heart failure

2 □ Acute respiratory failure

Respiratory failure is a condition wherein the respiratory system cannot supply adequate oxygen to maintain metabolism and/or cannot eliminate sufficient carbon dioxide to prevent respiratory acidosis.

Etiological factors for the development of pulmonary failure include the following (for management of etiological factors 1 and 3 to 7, refer to the appropriate standards of care):

1. Acute primary lung disease, such as aspiration pneumonia, near drowning, hyaline membrane disease, or pneumonitis
2. Secondary lung disease due to hypoxia, shock (adult respiratory distress syndrome, embolism, severe heart failure, or fluid overload)
3. Acute deterioration of chronic lung disease in which some stress such as superimposed infection or heart failure precipitates decompensation in patients with chronic obstructive lung disease
4. Depression of the respiratory center related to drugs, endocrine and metabolic disorders (e.g., encephalitis), stroke, tumors, trauma
5. Neuromuscular disorders such as myasthenia gravis, Guillain-Barré syndrome, tetanus
6. Chest trauma that may cause mediastinal emphysema, a flail chest, pneumothorax, etc., which may result in respiratory failure
7. Thoracic surgery produces pain and promotes hypoventilation; a pneumonectomy results in hyperperfusion of the remaining lung, which reduces capillary diffusion time and may result in perfusion of even poorly ventilated lung areas, thus promoting respiratory insufficiency and failure

Each of these etiological factors that promote pulmonary insufficiency may be associated with one or more of three pathological mechanisms.

Hypoventilation. This is defined as an arterial P_{CO_2} above 45 mm Hg, which results from reduced air reaching the alveoli with a reduced minute volume. It results in decreased Pa_{O_2} and an increased Pa_{CO_2} that is inversely proportional to the alveolar ventilation. This occurs in acute airway obstruction, restrictive defects, obstructive defects, neuromuscular defect, and respiratory depression.

Intrapulmonary shunting or ventilation/perfusion mismatch. Intrapulmonary shunting refers to blood that does not participate in oxygen transfer (from alveolar air to arterial blood). The mechanism may include absence of alveolar ventilation such as occurs in atelectasis and/or bronchospasm (normal amount of shunted blood is 5% to 6%). Ventilation/perfusion mismatch refers to:

1. Perfusion of unventilated alveoli (pneumonia, asthma, atelectasis, hyaline membrane disease, adult respiratory distress syndrome)
2. Ventilation of unperfused alveoli (e.g., pulmonary embolus)

Diffusion impairment. This occurs when the alveolar capillary membrane is thickened, impairing the diffusion of gases, as the result of interstitial fibrosis, interstitial pneumonia, or collagen diseases such as scleroderma or hyaline membrane disease. Hypoxemia is usually the primary effect and can often be relieved by the administration of 100% oxygen.

The clinical signs and symptoms of impending acute respiratory failure may be varied and nonspecific, resulting in delayed diagnosis and treatment. The most prominent features are related to hypoxia. Clinical manifestations usually include an altered level of consciousness, confusion, headache, asterixis, papilledema (due to increased P_{CO_2}), cyanosis, tachycardia, diaphoresis, and rapid shallow respirations. The onset may be either fulminant and acute or insidious in nature.

Arterial blood gas determination permits the confirmation of acute respiratory failure. Severe impairment of gas exchange and hypoxemia ($Pa_{O_2} < 60$ mm Hg) are seen. When the patient has generally healthy lungs, compensatory hyperventilation results in lowered arterial P_{CO_2}. When chronic lung disease or another impairment of respiratory function is present, acute respiratory failure and hypoxia are usually accompanied by hypercapnia ($Pa_{CO_2} > 75$ mm Hg). Acidosis is usually present. Once the diagnosis is established, the therapy will include treatment of the pathogenesis, maintenance of adequate oxygenation, removal of carbon dioxide, correction of acidemia, and prevention or treatment of respiratory infection.

ACUTE DETERIORATION OF CHRONIC OBSTRUCTIVE PULMONARY DISEASE

Chronic obstructive pulmonary disease (COPD) is a descriptive phrase that refers to airway obstruction, including chronic bronchitis, emphysema, and asthma.

Airway obstruction results from excessive secretions, bronchospasm, and mucosal swelling. Bronchospasm frequently occurs in patients with asthma, chronic bronchitis, and, to some extent, in patients with emphysema. In patients with asthma, immune reactions produce constriction of the airway. Irritants such as fumes, dust, smoke, and cold air can also promote bronchospasm, probably via neurogenic mechanisms; chemical substances such as serotonin and histamine may directly constrict the airway. Mucosal swelling from edema and the inflammatory process in the peripheral airways may result in bronchial and peribronchial fibrosis and kinking, narrowing, and occlusion of the air passages.

Bronchitis is inflammation and production of excessive mucous secretions in the bronchial structure with a chronic cough continuing for several months and recurring annually. The principal cause of bronchitis is prolonged irritation of the bronchial mucosa due to recurrent infections, smoking (more than 20 cigarettes daily), environmental pollutants, allergy, and autoimmune diseases. It is characterized by a generalized enlargement of goblet cells lining the wall of the trachea and bronchi. There is some loss of cilia with metaplasia of the epithelium. Functional findings show increased or normal functional residual capacity (FRC), decreased vital capacity (VC), increased residual volume (RV), and decreased forced expiratory volume, or volume exhaled in first second of the forced exhalation (FEVC). Alveolar hypoventilation causes ventilation/perfusion mismatch, which may result in severe hypoxemia and hypercapnia. The alveolar-arterial oxygen difference is always increased. Chronic hypoxemia produces compensatory polycythemia (increased hematocrit).

Emphysema is described as an anatomical alteration in the lungs characterized by overinflation of the distal air spaces beyond the terminal bronchioles with progressive destruction of the alveolar and capillary membranes. The destruction of the alveolar walls results in the loss of support of the surrounding lung and collapse of small airways during expiration. Sputum production is usually minimal. Emphysema may be caused by recurrent infections, allergy, autoimmunity, environmental pollutants, and smoking (more than 20 cigarettes daily). Functional findings include increased FRC, RV, and total lung capacity (TLC) and decreased VC and FEV. As a rule, the arterial blood gas sample shows hypoxemia from loss of alveolar surface and airway dysfunction and normal P_{CO_2} due to increased respiratory drive and resultant hyperventilation. The alveolar-arterial oxygen difference is

always increased. A majority of patients demonstrate signs and symptoms of both chronic bronchitis (marked by thickened secretions, recurrent infections, and bronchospasm) and emphysema (marked by pulmonary hyperinflation, collapse of airways, and dyspnea).

Asthma is defined as paroxysmal dyspnea caused by spasm of the bronchial tubes, hypersecretion of mucus, and edema of the mucous membrane. Due to airway compression it is often accompanied by adventitial sounds. Cough is usually the first symptom that the patient experiences; this is followed by dyspnea, tachycardia, and diaphoresis. Wheezing may or may not be present. Airway spasm results in increased work of breathing and the use of accessory muscles. Initial arterial blood gas analysis during an attack will show hypocapnia and hypoxemia as a result of increased respiratory drive and ventilation/perfusion mismatch. If the patient's respiratory status deteriorates, hypercapnia and acidosis will result. Asthma may be present in two forms. *Extrinsic* asthma usually occurs in individuals predisposed by heredity and can be induced by exogenous factors to which the patient is allergic. *Intrinsic* asthma is caused by endogenous factors such as a hypersensitivity response. Psychological factors (especially stress) play an important role in the development of asthma.

Status asthmaticus is the term used for severe asthmatic attacks that are not responsive to the patient's own maintenance regimen or parenteral sympathomimetic amines.

Prolonged severe COPD usually leads to cardiac compromise, called *cor pulmonale*. It is characterized by degenerative, fibrotic perivascular changes with increased pulmonary vascular resistance and ultimate right heart failure. Cor pulmonale is more commonly seen in patients with chronic severe hypoxia and compensatory pulmonary vasoconstriction. The ultimate result is a permanent increase in pulmonary vascular resistance and a severe increase in right ventricular afterload. The right heart eventually fails while attempting to generate extremely high pressure.

ADULT RESPIRATORY DISTRESS SYNDROME

For reasons that are not completely understood, hypoxic, septic, or traumatic injury to the lung causes massive pulmonary edema, atelectasis, and hyaline membrane deposits. Alveolar membranes are also injured, causing further loss of fluid into the alveoli and resulting in alveolar hypoventilation; the later development of pneumonitis and interstitial fibrosis causes a decrease in diffusion capabilities.

Lung compliance and FRC are tremendously reduced. Marked alveolar hypoventilation produces ventilation/ perfusion mismatch and severe hypoxemia. Hypocapnia may be present while compensatory hyperventilation occurs. Development of hypercapnia indicates severe patient deterioration. With progressive hypoxia, acidosis is unavoidable.

These patients often require mechanical ventilation with high inspiratory and end expiratory pressures. Plasma oncotic agents are usually administered to pull fluid back into the intravascular space (although administration of these was previously controversial). Some centers advocate the administration of corticosteroids in an effort to reduce inflammation and fibrosis of alveolar surfaces. Cardiac output must be maintained at a good level to avoid further pulmonary edema and patient deterioration.

The best approach to adult respiratory distress syndrome is prevention. Individuals at risk for the development of sepsis or shock must receive careful management to avoid acute hypoxic or hypotensive episodes. Once the predisposing crisis has occurred, strict fluid management with observation for early signs of respiratory distress must be performed.

ASSESSMENT

1. Baseline information regarding history, presence, and nature of
   a. Onset and length of illness
   b. Recent changes in character and amount of sputum
   c. Repeated colds
   d. Frequency of exacerbation of acute attacks and/or infections
   e. Decreased tolerance for physical activity
   f. Progressive dyspnea
   g. Chronic morning cough
   h. Complications—bronchopneumonia, pleurisy, bronchiectasis, abdominal hernia (due to cough), pulmonary embolism
   i. Any allergies to food, drugs, or adverse reactions to changes in weather
   j. Presence of related illness
      (1) Cor pulmonale
      (2) Hypertension
      (3) Renal disease
      (4) Diabetes
      (5) Peptic ulcer
   k. Family background—members of immediate family with pulmonary illnesses
   l. Place of residence
   m. Occupation
   n. Smoking habits (past and present)
2. Presence and extent of
   a. General abnormalities indicating evidence of hypoxemia such as
      (1) Muscle twitching, coarse tremor
      (2) Malodorous breath
      (3) Abnormalities in skin color, including pallor, cyanosis
         (a) Peripheral: note particularly appearance of extremities, tip of ears and/or nose
         (b) Central: note particularly appearance of tongue and lips
      (4) Alterations in central venous system function that may be associated with pulmonary failure, including presence of restlessness, confusion, visual defects; fatigue
   b. Pulmonary abnormalities indicating evidence of respiratory distress, including
      (1) Tachypnea, dyspnea, orthopnea, shortness of breath
      (2) Abnormal breath sounds; adventitious breath sounds, including rales, rhonchi, wheezing
      (3) Changes in voice sounds
      (4) Abnormal vocal fremitus, noting location— left and right apices, mid lung and lower lung
      (5) Abnormal resonance of underlying thoracic tissue
      (6) Pleural friction rub
      (7) Abnormalities in sputum—color, consistency, quantity, and odor
3. Signs and symptoms of chronic lung disease
   a. Abnormal posture
      (1) Short and stocky appearance
      (2) Thin and asthenic appearance
   b. Malnutrition and weight loss
   c. Abnormalities in the configuration of thorax and its movements, such as pigeon breast, funnel chest, barrel chest, scoliosis, kyphosis
   d. Use of neck muscles for quiet respirations
   e. Clubbing of fingers
   f. Abnormal rate, rhythm, and amplitude of respiratory excursions of upper, anterior, middle, and posterior lower chest
   g. Sputum—any increase in amount, color, and consistency
   h. Persistent cough; loose, rattling cough, which is

usually worse in the morning and evening and worse in damp and/or cold weather

   i. Cor pulmonale, including ankle edema, evidence of pulmonary hypertension, loud pulmonic closure sound, strain and enlargement of right ventricle, right ventricular gallop

   j. Cardiovascular dysfunction, including abnormal vital signs, hypotension or hypertension, tachycardia, arrhythmias and palpitations, chest pain, abnormal location of apical pulse, jugular venous distention, peripheral edema, cool skin temperature; oliguria

4. Baseline diagnostic and lab data

   a. Serial blood count for decreased hematocrit (Hct) and hemoglobin (Hgb); presence of polycythemia and leukocytosis

   b. Cultures

      (1) Urinalysis indicating bacteriuria

      (2) Sputum culture and sensitivity (C and S) results

   c. Electrolyte levels

   d. Sedimentation rate

   e. Arterial blood gas levels

   f. Pulmonary function tests

      (1) Lung volume

      (2) Lung capacity

      (3) FEV

   g. Chest radiographs

      (1) Anteroposterior diameter (may be increased with COPD)

      (2) Position of trachea

      (3) Density in both lung bases

      (4) Differences in lung size

      (5) Presence of any abnormalities such as atelectasis, right ventricular hypertrophy, flattened diaphragm, hyperinflation, and bullae

   h. ECG for any abnormalities, including signs and symptoms of cor pulmonale such as abnormal P wave and QRS complex

   i. Lung scan for any abnormalities

   j. Bronchoscopy

5. Level of anxiety related to signs and symptoms present and their effect on patient/family's behavior and life-style

6. Extent of patient/family's knowledge regarding disease process, diagnostic procedures, and planned therapy

GOALS

1. Optimal respiratory function and adequate pulmonary ventilation

2. Adequate functioning of regulatory mechanisms, that is, elimination of waste and acid-base balance within patient's normal limits

3. Absence of pneumonia and other infections

4. Absence of complications of respiratory failure—pleural effusion, pulmonary interstitial edema, pulmonary microemboli, abdominal hernia, stress ulcer, malnutrition, and anemia

5. Electrolytes and blood count results within normal limits

6. Intake of nutrients sufficient to prevent weight loss or, if needed, achieve weight gain and positive nitrogen balance

7. Reduction of patient/family's anxiety with provision of information and explanation of disease process, diagnostic procedures, and therapeutic plans

8. Before discharge patient/family is able to

   a. Explain relationship between disease process and therapy prescribed

   b. Describe dietary, medication, and activity regimen

   c. Identify signs and symptoms of respiratory infection requiring medical attention

   d. Verbalize influence of environmental factors on illness and perform necessary measures to control these factors

   e. Explain importance of follow-up

Potential problems	Expected outcomes	Nursing activities
■ Patient/family's anxiety related to dyspnea and fear of dying	■ Patient/family demonstrates decreased level of anxiety with provision of emotional support and information Patient uses pursed lip breathing effectively	■ Assess level of anxiety Prevent physiological factors that promote restlessness, anxiety Monitor vital signs and temperature Check that O_2 delivery device is functioning properly, i.e., patent tubing Observe for signs of hypoxia Position patient with head elevated Stay with the patient or reassure patient that nurse will be close at hand Encourage pursed lip breathing q1 hr

Potential problems	Expected outcomes	Nursing activities
		Encourage verbalization of anxiety or fear related to dyspnea and course of therapy Encourage pursed lip breathing every hour Encourage participation in care as tolerated Perform treatments in an unhurried manner, allowing rest periods between treatments Provide comfort measures Administer analgesics as needed if ordered
■ Patient/family's anxiety related to limited understanding of Diagnostic procedures	■ Patient/family's behavior demonstrates decreased level of anxiety with provision of information and explanations	■ Ongoing assessment of level of anxiety Describe the nature of the disease process and the signs and symptoms the patient is experiencing
Disease process and prognosis Therapy employed	Patient/family verbalizes understanding of disease process and its relationship to therapy employed	Explain the relationship of the disease process and the rationale for various therapeutic interventions at a level appropriate for patient/family's comprehension and degree of anxiety present
Separation from family Disruption of life-style	Patient/family participates actively in planning and implementing care	Explain the anticipated procedures involved in diagnostic process/plan of care and what patient will experience Assist in preparing patient for diagnostic procedures Encourage patient/family's questions and verbalization of fears and anxieties Involve patient/family in planning for care Communicate findings to physician on a continuing basis
■ Obstruction to gas exchange, which may be related to Thick viscous bronchial secretions Bronchial edema Bronchospasm Fibrosis and parenchymal destruction	■ Patent airway Both lungs fully aerated as visualized on chest radiograph Clear breath sounds in all areas Absence of signs and symptoms of hypoxia	■ Prevention Employ measures to prevent respiratory infection (see Problem, Pulmonary infection) Employ measures to remove secretions as needed Frequent postural drainage for large volume of secretions Chest physiotherapy Turn and position q2 hr Cough and deep breathe Administer bronchodilators as ordered for bronchial edema and bronchospasm Encourage pursed lip breathing by having patient purse lips or say ''F'' during exhalation, especially for patients with fibrosis and parenchymal destruction Provide humidification of upper airway structures by means of face mask or high humidity tent Monitor for Tachypnea Persistent cough; syncopal episodes related to sudden fit of coughing Increasing amount of sputum with changes in color, consistency, and odor Presence of abnormal breath sounds, rales, wheezing, stridor/snorting, and use of accessory muscles (retractions, nasal flaring, jaw tugging) Fever, sore throat Altered behavior; restlessness and/or changes in obtundation Onset of urticaria and/or hay fever Deterioration in arterial blood gas levels Serial blood count for leukocytosis Decreased breath sounds Increased respiratory effort and fatigue

Potential problems	Expected outcomes	Nursing activities

Notify physician for any of these abnormalities

If problem occurs

  Employ measures for removal of secretions as ordered

    Increase fluid intake (in the absence of heart failure)

    Liquefy sputum by steam inhalation

    Administer intermittent positive pressure with nebulizer therapy

    Administer vigorous chest physiotherapy unless contraindicated; breathing exercises q1 hr

    Frequent change of position in accordance with therapeutic regimen q2 hr

    Chest physiotherapy with postural drainage q2 hr

    Aseptic tracheal suctioning if patient unable to cough out secretions

    Administer medications such as iodides, detergents, and/or enzymes

  Administer antibiotic therapy as ordered

  Check vital signs including temperature q1 hr until stable; if fever occurs, notify physician and obtain needed cultures and then administer antipyretic agent or antibiotics as ordered to decrease fever and O_2 requirements

  Monitor serial arterial blood gas results q1 hr until stable

  Monitor serial chest radiograph, sputum, C and S; look for presence of any pathogenic organisms or infiltrates

  Monitor for abnormalities in fluid and electrolyte balance

  Maintain strict intake and output; daily weights

  Monitor for any increase or decrease of abnormal and/or adventitious breath sounds, rales, stridor/snorting, wheezing, rhonchi, and retractions

  Observe for any marked changes in level of consciousness such as confusion, restlessness, somnolence, and obtundation

  Observe for cyanosis and/or changes in skin color, including mucous membranes and nail beds

  Notify physician for any significant deterioration

  Allow rest periods between treatments

  Explain treatments before administration

  Provide for a quiet, restful environment

  Stay with the patient or reassure patient that nurse will be close at hand

  Prepare patient for therapies that may be employed

    Therapeutic bronchoscopy

    Intubation with mechanical ventilation (see Standard: *Mechanical ventilation*)

For COPD patients additional specific measures often include

  Monitoring for any changes in amount, color, viscosity, and odor of sputum; C and S result

  Monitoring for increasing tachypnea, dyspnea, cough, and fatigue

  Use of bronchodilators, i.e., theophylline, epinephrine, and corticosteroids; corticosteroids are specific for status asthmaticus patients

  Vigorous chest physiotherapy q1 hr

    Pursed lip breathing q30 min

    Postural drainage and chest physiotherapy q30 min

    Aseptic suctioning q30 min and prn; use of nebulized aerosols and/or intermittent positive pressure breathing (IPPB) machine

  Maintain position in accordance with therapeutic regimen

Potential problems	Expected outcomes	Nursing activities
		Teach breathing exercises, including pursed lip breathing
		Maintain environmental conditions to facilitate breathing
		Commonly used articles within reach
		Humidifiers in room
		Allow rest periods between treatments
		Maintain unhurried and calm demeanor when giving care
■ Pulmonary infections	■ Absence or resolution of pulmonary infection	■ Prevention
		Use strict aseptic technique in suctioning and in other nursing activities as appropriate
	Chest radiograph, sputum, and C and S results show no evidence of infection	Administer prophylactic antibiotic therapy if ordered
	No clinical manifestations of infection evident	Administer prophylactic measures such as postural drainage, inhalants, chest physiotherapy, and pursed lip breathing
		Monitor or observe for
		Sore throat
		Progressive dyspnea (respiratory distress)
		Fever
		Changes in amount, color, viscosity, and odor of sputum
		Lab results of
		Sputum C and S for any evidence of infection
		CBC for leukocytosis
		Chest radiograph for atelectasis or density
		Notify physician for any abnormalities
		If problem occurs
		Administer antibiotic therapy as ordered
		Monitor for abnormal breath sounds or presence of rales, rhonchi, or wheezing
		Check vital signs including temperature q1-2 hr until stable
		Administer antipyretic as ordered to reduce fever and decrease O_2 requirements
		Administer vigorous chest physiotherapy as tolerated
		Reposition patient q1-2 hr; postural drainage if indicated
		Aseptic tracheal suctioning if patient is unable to cough out secretions
		Observe for increasing cough and changes in color, consistency, and odor of sputum
		Monitor result of serial sputum C and S
		Monitor result of serial chest radiograph
■ Acid-base disturbance, hypoxia related to alveolar hypoventilation or right to left shunting	■ Arterial blood gas levels within patient's normal limits	■ See problem, Obstruction to gas exchange, for prevention activities
	Absence of signs of hypoxia including restlessness, lightheadedness, dizziness, and cyanosis	Monitor for
		Arterial blood gas results, indicating acidosis and/or hypoxemia
		Symptoms of fatigue, drowsiness, headache, apathy, inattentiveness, restlessness, confusion, and somnolence
		Signs of respiratory distress—air hunger, cyanosis, dyspnea, and tachypnea
		Sudden changes in vital signs and temperature
		Presence of arrhythmias
		Increase in blood lactate level
		Decrease in urine output
		If problem occurs
		Careful administration of O_2 as ordered
		Check that O_2 delivery device is functioning properly, i.e., patent

Potential problems	Expected outcomes	Nursing activities
		Monitor
		Serial arterial blood gas levels q1-2 hr until stabilized
		Level of consciousness
		Serial electrolytes, specifically K^+ and Cl^- levels
		Blood lactate levels
		TPR and BP q2 hr
		Heart rhythm and cardiac output
		Chest radiograph results
		Monitor for
		Abnormal breath sounds, rales, rhonchi, wheezing, and stridor/snorting
		Increase or decrease in dyspnea, tachypnea, cyanosis, restlessness, headache, and somnolence
		Cardiac activity
		Frequently change position for drainage of secretions q2 hr
		Administer vigorous chest physiotherapy as tolerated; aseptic tracheal suctioning if patient is unable to cough out secretions
		Administer antibiotics if ordered
		Careful administration of bicarbonate to decrease lactic acid level if ordered
		Promote effective chest expansion by positioning with pillows for comfort in accordance to therapy
		Decrease O_2 consumption by
		Limiting patient communication to necessary verbalization
		Limiting patient activities
		Providing uninterrupted rest periods
		Providing environment conducive to rest
		Limiting visitors
		Reducing anxiety (see Problem, Patient/family's anxiety)
		Notify physician for any abnormalities
		If these measures fail, mechanical ventilation may be instituted (see Standard: *Mechanical ventilation*)
■ Decreased appetite related to dyspnea and weakness Malnutrition related to prolonged debilitating lung disease	■ Appetite improved, weight maintained, or weight gain if appropriate Positive nitrogen balance Patient consumes most of required food on meal trays Absence and/or resolution of any signs of malnutrition Regular elimination	■ Prevention
		Gather baseline diet history data, including how dyspnea affects intake of nutrients
		Assess patient's baseline nutritional status and plan intervention accordingly
		Ensure intake of required fluids and nutrients
		Frequent small meals
		Monitor for
		Signs and symptoms of malnutrition
		Presence of swollen face with dark cheeks and circles under eyes
		Any enlargement of parotid glands
		Dull eyes with pale or red membranes, presence of bloodshot ring around corneas, gray spots on conjunctiva, red and fissured eyelid corners
		Swollen lips
		Spongy tender gums that bleed easily; presence of dental decay and missing teeth
		Flaky, dry skin with spots or bruises
		Brittle and split nails
		Poor skin turgor, swollen joints, muscle atrophy, decreased subcutaneous fat
		Altered mental status—restlessness, irritability, and confusion
		Presence of tingling and burning of hands and feet and decreased reflexes

Potential problems	Expected outcomes	Nursing activities
		Musculoskeletal hemorrhages
		Liver and spleen enlargement
		Weight loss
		Hypothermia
		Lethargy and decreased exercise tolerance
		If problem is present
		Set required caloric and fluid intake with physician and dietitian
		Monitor intake and output, daily weight
		Provide required nutritional intake with meals and snacks
		Ensure required caloric and fluid intake
		List foods and fluids taken during meals and snacks
		Note any abnormal eating patterns
		Provide frequent small feedings as necessary
		Encourage the patient to eat acid food first on meal trays
		Permit special food request as much as possible
		Allow home cooked foods within set limits
		Have dietitian plan meals and meal substitutes with patient
		Keep food as nearly ''regular'' as possible, soft rather than pureed, etc.
		Provide conditions conducive to eating
		Oral hygiene before and after meals and prn
		Assist with cleaning and/or clean dentures as needed
		Assist with eating, i.e., cutting foods, pouring liquids
		Position patient for comfort and easy reach of foods
		Provide equipment for eating, i.e., special device if necessary
		Remove evidence of sputum or anything that will hinder patient's appetite
		If patient is receiving tube feedings
		Ensure patency and proper location of tube
		Place patient in semi-Fowler's position
		Aspirate feeding tube before each feeding; test aspirate for heme; notify physician for abnormal amount and positive Hematest*
		Do not feed patient if amount of aspirate is more than 100 ml or an amount indicated by physician
		Check feeding for any change in consistency and odor
		Warm feedings before giving to patient
		Start with small amounts of feedings at frequent intervals with gradual increase in amount and decrease in frequency as tolerated
		Administer tube feedings at slow drip rate
		Check for bowel sounds every shift
		Notify physician for any vomiting, diarrhea, and/or constipation
		Initiate bowel regimen as appropriate
		Monitor for resolution or presence of any signs and symptoms of malnutrition
		Notify physician for any abnormalities
■ Emboli related to polycythemia and increased blood viscosity	■ Absence of emboli Normal pulmonary function	■ Monitor for signs and symptoms of thrombophlebitis, pulmonary emboli, and other types of emboli (see Standard: *Embolic phenomena*) If problem occurs, see Standard: *Embolic phenomena*

*Hematest, Ames Co., Elkhart, Ind.

Potential problems	Expected outcomes	Nursing activities

■ Cor pulmonale as a complication of long-standing severe chronic obstructive lung disease	■ Absence of signs and symptoms of cor pulmonale
	Normal cardiac output
	Pa_{O_2} within patient's normal limits
		■ Prevent by immediate medical therapy to alleviate problems (see Problems, Obstruction to gas exchange; Pulmonary infections; Acid-base disturbance and hypoxia; Decreased appetite related to dyspnea and weakness)
		Monitor for
		  Signs and symptoms of pulmonary hypertension and right ventricular strain
		    Gradual increasing edema of legs and ankles
		    Abnormal CVP, pulmonary pressures, PCWP, and cardiac output if available
		    Jugular venous distention, hepatomegaly, and puffy eyelids
		  Abnormalities in arterial blood gas levels
		  Chest radiograph evidence of cardiogmegaly
		  Tachycardia and presence of gallop rhythm
		  P wave and QRS complex abnormalities/changes in ECG
		  Any alterations in level of consciousness
		  If problem occurs, see Standard: *Pulmonary edema*

■ Gastrointestinal (GI) bleeding—ulcers and gastritis	■ Negative Hematest of emesis and/or NG aspirate and stool
	Absence of abdominal pain, hematemesis, or melena
	Hct and Hgb within normal limits
	Normal GI function
		■ Prevention
		  Administer all medications with meals or when stomach is full
		  Administer antacid prophylactically as ordered
		  Minimize activities and allow for uninterrupted rest periods
		  Maintain a calm and restful environment
		  Allow patient to verbalize fears and to ask questions
		  Explain all therapy before administering
		  Encourage patient to participate in care as tolerated
		  Encourage required nutrients and bland food
		Monitor for
		  Vital signs and temperature q4 hr; be aware of any sudden rise in pulse rate
		  Check all stools, emesis, and/or NG aspirate for Hematest
		  Any GI upsets—anorexia, vomiting, abdominal distention, pain, cramps, diarrhea, and/or constipation
		  Serial Hgb and Hct
		  Symptoms of sudden dizziness or syncope
		  Changes in size of abdominal girth
		Notify physician for an abnormality
		If problem occurs, see Standard: *Acute upper gastrointestinal bleeding*

■ Insufficient knowledge to comply with discharge regimen*	■ Patient/family has sufficient information to comply with discharge regimen
	Patient/family accurately describes dietary, medication, and activity regimen
	
	Patient/family identifies signs and symptoms of respiratory infection requiring medical attention
	Patient/family performs special therapeutic procedures correctly
		■ Assess patient/family's level of understanding, ability to comprehend, and any physical limitations regarding follow-up plan of care or discharge regimen
		
		Describe the discharge regimen, including
		  Medications—purpose, side effects, route, dose, and schedules
		  Dietary therapy regimen
		  Activity progression—avoid overfatigue; allow for rest and relaxation
		Identify signs and symptoms that would require medical attention, especially respiratory infections such as cold, sore throat, fever, and cough irritability
		
		Describe and demonstrate to patient/family special therapeutic measures and safety precautions for specific residual pulmonary disease

*If responsibility of the critical care nurse includes such follow-up care.

Potential problems	Expected outcomes	Nursing activities
		Specific therapeutic measures for patient with COPD
		Chest drainage and chest physiotherapy
		Assist in developing program for physical conditioning and bronchial hygiene
		Specify positions to be assumed to facilitate drainage of lung segments
		Emphasize that postural drainage mobilizes secretions not moved by normal air movement and brings secretions to areas where cough is effective
		Emphasize that if patient obtains no immediate relief, he/she may cough up secretions later in the day
		Breathing exercises
		Emphasize that breathing exercises strengthen muscles of expiration
		Instruct patient on breathing exercises, including diaphragmatic breathing by placing one hand on the stomach just below the ribs and the other hand on the middle of the chest; breathe in slowly and deeply through the nose allowing the abdomen to protrude as far as possible; then breathe out through pursed lips while contracting the abdominal muscles; while breathing the hands must press inward and upward on the abdomen
		Correct use of nebulizers and IPPB machine
		Allow patient/family to do return demonstration of therapeutic measures
		Encourage any questions and/or verbalization of anxiety regarding therapeutic procedures
	Patient/family verbalizes influence of environmental factors on illness and performs necessary preventive measures	Emphasize the importance of a calm, safe, and comfortable environment; specific measures for patients with COPD include
		Importance of congenial family attitude and avoidance of hostility and emotional and upsetting situations
		Avoid exposure to crowds, people with respiratory infections, and respiratory irritants (smoke, chemicals, dust fumes, etc.)
		Do not smoke
		Avoid excessively dry air and extremely cold weather
		Avoid sudden changes in temperature
		Organize daily activity to allow work activity with least amount of effort
		Avoid activities causing excessive dyspnea
		Perform work and activities at a slow pace
		Allow for specific rest periods
		Keep environment clean and free from dust
		When using air conditioner make sure filter is clean
		Avoid devices in which water can stand and become stagnant
		Maintain good eating and elimination habits
		Nonflowering house plants help provide relative humidity of 50%
		Encourage fluid intake to 2000 ml daily unless contraindicated
	Patient/family accurately describes plans for follow-up care	Describe the plan for follow-up visits, including the purpose for, when and where to come, who to see, and what specimens to bring

Potential problems	Expected outcomes	Nursing activities
		Provide opportunity for and encourage patient/family's questions and verbalization of anxiety regarding discharge regimen
		Assess patient/family's potential compliance with discharge regimen
		Provide information for use of community health agencies when necessary

3 □ Thoracic surgery

Thoracic surgery involves entry into the chest wall or cavity for the repair or resection of abnormalities associated with the chest wall, pleura, lungs, mediastinum, esophagus, trachea, or heart.

Indications for a thoracotomy include traumatic injury in which there is evidence of extensive intrathoracic damage. Various infectious processes such as empyema and refractory bronchiectasis require surgical drainage through thoracotomy incisions. Removal of a segment, lobe, or entire lung (pneumonectomy) becomes necessary in treating malignancies that have not metastasized.

Certain nonmalignant abnormalities of the lung such as large bullous formations require surgical resection. A bullectomy is performed when adjacent lung tissue becomes compromised by the growing size of bullae, thus making infection and/or oxygenation problems likely.

A thoractomy is useful for correcting various congenital or acquired deformities of the chest wall. Elevation of the sternum in pectus excavatum often improves chest wall mechanics and also provides a desirable cosmetic effect.

Postoperative goals are focused on providing adequate oxygenation and ventilation as well as hemodynamic stability. Because the integrity of the chest wall has been compromised, constant attention must be directed toward maintaining the lungs in a fully expanded state. The airway must be frequently cleared of secretions that build up quickly in the postoperative patient.

ASSESSMENT

1. History, presence, nature, and severity of
   a. Pulmonary problem; previous pulmonary surgery
   b. Medical management of pulmonary problem
   c. Result of laboratory tests to date
   d. Smoking—number of packs per day, number of years
   e. Secretions—color, amount, consistency, odor
   f. Chest discomfort and, if present, the pattern (duration, severity)
   g. Altered activity levels; toleration of various activities of daily living
   h. Esophageal reflux, heartburn
   i. Pain, paresthesia, and numbness in lower arms and hand when structures in shoulder and neck are compressed by certain body movements
2. Pulmonary status, particularly
   a. Quality of respirations
   b. Breathing pattern for presence of dyspnea
   c. Presence of abnormal or adventitious breath sounds
3. Results of lab and diagnostic procedures
   a. Pulmonary function studies
   b. Arterial blood gas levels
   c. Bronchoscopy
   d. Mediastinoscopy
   e. Tomography
   f. Scalene node biopsy
   g. Pleural biopsy
   h. Open lung biopsy
   i. Radiograph—anteroposterior and/or lateral
   j. For esophageal and esophagogastric problems
      (1) Fluoroscopic studies
      (2) Esophagoscopy
      (3) Esophageal motility studies
4. Patient/family's knowledge regarding operative therapy
   a. What they have been told

b. Their expectations

c. Previous experiences with surgery if any

5. Information and detail surgeon has provided about the need for surgery, the actual surgery to be done, and the expected outcomes

6. Patient/family's anxiety related to disease process, hospitalization, therapy planned, potential surgery, and expected outcome

GOALS

1. Reduction in patient/family's anxiety with provision of information and explanations

2. Patient/family complies with preoperative regimen (particularly with regard to not smoking)

3. Hemodynamic stability; absence of arrhythmias

4. Respiratory function sufficient to maintain Pa_{O_2} and Pa_{CO_2} within normal limits; absence of atelectasis, pulmonary infection

5. Infection free, afebrile; absence of empyema

6. For specific surgery

a. Pneumonectomy

(1) Bronchial stump intact

(2) Absence of pulmonary interstitial edema

(3) Adequate cardiac output; no heart failure

b. Esophagogastrectomy

(1) Absence of pulmonary aspiration of gastric contents

(2) Minimal to no reflux of gastric contents

(3) Food passes readily from mouth into stomach

(4) Patient complies with prescribed dietary alterations and chews food thoroughly

(5) Voice is unchanged; absence of hoarseness

c. Lobectomy; segmental resection

(1) Full expansion of remaining lung tissue

(2) Absence of a pneumothorax

(3) Minimal air leak in immediate postoperative period, which quickly progresses to no air leak

d. Tracheal resection (see goals 1 to 5)

(1) Patent airway

(2) Breathing without distress

(3) Tracheal anastomosis intact, without local tracheal or pulmonary infection

7. Patient has full range of motion (ROM) of arm and shoulder on the affected side

8. Coagulation studies within normal limits; absence of signs of thrombophlebitis, pulmonary embolism, or other types of emboli

9. Before discharge, patient/family verbalizes understanding of activity progression, dietary alterations, and medication regimen

10. Patient/family accurately describes signs and symptoms that require medical attention

11. Patient/family accurately describes plan for follow-up visits

Potential problems	Expected outcomes	Nursing activities
Preoperative		
■ Patient/family's anxiety related to Disease process Hospitalization Medical therapy employed Diagnostic tests planned Impending major surgery and associated risks Altered family roles Separation from family members Loss of job	■ Patient/family's behavior indicates reduction in anxiety with provision of information, explanations, and encouragement	■ Ongoing assessment of level of patient/family's anxiety Assess knowledge and understanding of patient/family of the disease process, medical therapy employed, anticipated diagnostic procedures, and anticipated surgery if planned Explain in simple terms the nature of patient's pulmonary/thoracic problem and the symptoms the patient is experiencing Explain in simple terms what patient will experience during diagnostic procedures; assist in preparing patient for procedures, which may include Radiograph, tomography Blood samples for arterial blood gas analysis Pulmonary function tests Bronchoscopy, mediastinoscopy Biopsy Other tests specific for the patient's pulmonary problem Collaborate with physician and other members of health team on necessary teaching When surgery is planned and the physician has discussed it with the patient and family, assess their understanding of the information Reinforce the purpose and nature of the surgery and the expected outcomes

Potential problems	**Expected outcomes**	**Nursing activities**

Describe the perioperative experience (adjust explanation according to patient's anxiety level and desire to know), including

Preoperative

  Refer to chest physiotherapist, if available, to orient patient to

1. Coughing and deep breathing
2. Incentive spirometry
3. Postural drainage

  Prep and shave

  Light dinner and NPO after midnight

  Medication for sleep if needed

  Morning bath/shower

  Preoperative medications

  Hospital gown

  Care of valuables

  To operating room on stretcher

  Scrub suits, masks, and caps worn by operating room staff

  Anesthesia

Postoperative

  Regaining consciousness in the recovery room/intensive care unit

1. Describe general environment (size of unit, room, etc.)
2. Nurse always nearby
3. Dull continuous noises
4. If anticipated, describe breathing tube in nose or mouth that will be in place to ease work of breathing and load on the heart; explain that talking will not be possible while tube in place, but other means of communication will be possible
5. NPO until "breathing tube" removed
6. Incision with bandage
7. Intravenous, arter
8. If anticipated, chest tubes and bloody drainage expected
9. ECG monitoring
10. Medicine for discomfort, pain
11. Policy for family visits

  Describe responsibility of patient for achieving a speedy recovery by taking an active role in coughing and deep breathing

Describe the process as patient progresses

  Tubes, lines out

  Allowed to eat

  Postural drainage, deep breathing, and coughing

  Getting stronger, ambulation

  Home again

Provide opportunity for and encourage questions and verbalization of anxiety

Reassure patient that nurse will be nearby at all times

Provide calm, quiet environment

Perform treatments in an unhurried manner, allowing rest periods between treatments

Involve patient/family in planning for care

Assess reduction in level of anxiety

Potential problems	Expected outcomes	Nursing activities

■ Respiratory insufficiency	■ Adequate oxygenation and ventilation	■ Encourage patient to stop smoking as soon as admitted to hospital with suspected pulmonary problem
		Implement chest physiotherapy as ordered to achieve optimal pulmonary function before surgery
		  Demonstrate coughing and deep breathing; have patient practice five deep slow breaths with an effective cough on the fifth breath
		  Demonstrate and have patient practice use of pillow
		  Teach proper diaphragmatic breathing exercises using abdominal muscles
		  Chest physiotherapy q2-4 hr and prn
		  Humidified, oxygenated air as needed
		  Incentive spirometry
		Monitor
		  Respirations for rate and quality; note tachypnea, dyspnea
		  Nature, amount, and consistency of sputum production
		  Breath sounds for decreased or absent breath sounds; presence of rales, rhonchi, or wheezes
		  Arterial blood gas results; note hypoxemia, hypercapnia
		  Chest radiograph results for atelectasis, fibrosis, and other abnormalities
		Notify physician of any of these abnormalities
		Administer therapies as ordered
		  Frequent chest physiotherapy to areas of atelectasis, collapse
		  Antibiotics
		  Bronchodilators
		  Expectorants, enzymes, and/or mucolytic agents
		  Incentive spirometry therapy
		Evaluate for improvement in respiratory function in response to these interventions

Postoperative		

■ Hemodynamic instability related to
  Pulmonary hypertension (particularly in pneumonectomy patients), resulting in heart failure
  Arrhythmias that may result from hypoxia, ventricular strain, acid-base imbalance
  Hemorrhage
	■ Patient hemodynamically stable
	ECG indicates absence of arrhythmias; all beats perfused
	Blood loss minimal (less than 800 ml in the first 24 hours)
		■ Prevent by
		  Administering fluid cautiously as ordered, particularly to the pneumonectomy patient (the remaining lung receives approximately twice its normal blood flow)
		  Administering therapy to prevent or to correct factors that predispose to arrhythmia formation, including acid-base imbalance and hypoxemia
		  Providing for a patent chest drainage system
		Monitor
		  BP, P q½-1 hr and prn until stable; note presence of hypotension and tachycardia
		  CVP and PAP q1 hr and prn until stable
		  Urine output with specific gravity q1 hr; note oliguria
		  Indices of adequate peripheral circulation and mentation
		  Amount and character of drainage in chest bottles (most pneumonectomy patients do not have chest tubes; if they do, suction is not continuously applied)
		  Continuous ECG reading or apical/radical pulse for arrhythmias and irregular rhythm; note concurrent signs of decreased cardiac output
		  For signs/symptoms of heart failure, right ventricular strain and hypertrophy

Potential problems	Expected outcomes	Nursing activities

■ Respiratory insufficiency related to improper positioning in the *lobectomy and segmental resection patients;* if the operated side is down, full expansion of the remaining lobe(s) is impaired	■ Respiratory function sufficient to maintain Pa_{O_2} and Pa_{CO_2} within normal limits
	Respiratory rate and depth within normal limits
	Auscultation and chest radiograph reveal full expansion of remaining lung tissue, such that operative area is filled with the remaining lung tissue
		■ Assess patient's respirations, q½-1 hr until stable for rate and quality
		Observe for dyspnea
		Prevent by
		  Providing for maximum diaphragmatic excursion
		    Semi-Fowler's position
		    Frequent (q1-2 hr) repositioning
		    Support for chest around chest tube insertion site (if present) to prevent tension on tube and surrounding tissues and to give support for deep breathing and coughing
		  Positioning
		    Lobectomy and segmental resection patients—in the early postoperative period many physicians preferentially position patient so that operated side is up to facilitate expansion of the lobes adjacent to the resected lobe; after the first 1 to 2 days, the patient is usually permitted to turn to either side
		    Bullectomy patients—can be turned to either side

■ Respiratory insufficiency in the *pneumonectomy patient* related to compression of the remaining lung by accumulation of drainage on the operated side as revealed by a mediastinal shift
Cardiac output may be compromised and contribute to respiratory insufficiency and hypoxia
	■ Mediastinum in midline position as revealed by observation, chest radiograph, and auscultation
	Full expansion of remaining lung tissue
		■ Prevent by positioning *pneumonectomy patient* on back or slightly turned to operative side; this position is usually preferred for the first 1 to 2 days after surgery
		Monitor
		  Tracheal position q½-1 hr until stable; note if not in midline position, indicating a mediastinal shift
		  Breath sounds q1-2 hr in the remaining lung tissue
		  For arterial blood gas results indicating hypoxemia, hypercapnia
		  Results of chest radiograph, indicating mediastinal shift
		If mediastinal shift present, note concurrent signs of compromised cardiac output, hemodynamic instability
		Notify physician for abnormalities in these parameters
		If problem occurs and the mediastinal shift is toward the operated side, assist physician with injection of air into the operated side to move the mediastinium back into midline position
		If problem occurs and the mediastinal shift occurs away from the operated side
		  Assist physician with removal of drainage from the operated side or if a chest tube is in place and clamped, release clamp as ordered to allow some drainage to flow out the chest tube
		  Assist with insertion of chest tube if procedure required

■ Respiratory insufficiency related to
  Inadequate chest drainage
  Hemothorax
	■ Absence or resolution of inadequate drainage and hemothorax
	Full expansion of remaining lung tissue
		■ Maintain a patent draining chest tube system; "milk" or "strip" (i.e., squeeze) chest tubes as needed to move thick drainage, clots down the tube
		Monitor
		  For effective suction in the chest tube system
		  For thick drainage, clots that need to be mobilized
		  For fluctuation of drainage in the chest tube ("tidaling"); this fluctuation will decrease gradually as the space being drained decreases in size and the amount of drainage subsides
		  Chest radiograph results for any collection compatible with a hemothorax

Potential problems	Expected outcomes	Nursing activities

		Notify physician for abnormalities in any of the aforementioned
		If hemothorax occurs
		    Assist with chest tube insertion if needed; monitor subsequent chest tube drainage
		    Monitor for resolution of hemothorax by auscultation and according to chest radiograph results and improved respiratory function

■ Respiratory insufficiency related to
  Atelectasis
  Hypoventilation
  Airway obstruction associated with secretions, tracheal edema (e.g., tracheal resection)
	■ Absence of signs and symptoms of respiratory distress, atelectasis
	Adequate oxygenation and ventilation with Pa_{O_2} and Pa_{CO_2} levels within patient's normal limits
		■ Prevent by
		    Providing for pain relief sufficient to allow for optimal pulmonary toilet while avoiding respiratory depression
		    Encouraging deep breathing and coughing q½-1 hr in the early postoperative period
		    Supporting patient's chest
		    Administering gentle chest physiotherapy q2-4 hr and prn as ordered
		    Administering humidified O_2 as ordered to enhance oxygenation and to liquefy secretions (adequate systemic hydration also assists in liquefying secretions)
		  Monitor
		    Respirations q½-1 hr and prn until stable; note presence of dyspnea, tachypnea, stridorous breathing
		    Breath sounds q1 hr until stable; note presence of abnormal or adventitious breath sounds in the remaining lung tissue
		    Arterial blood gas results; note hypoxemia, hypercapnia, or acidemia
		    For signs/symptoms of hypoxia (tachypnea, tachycardia, restlessness)
		    Results of sputum C and S; if sputum changes in character, send additional specimens as ordered
		    Results of serial inspiratory pressures if determined
		    Results of chest radiographs for presence of atelectasis and absence of full lung expansion
		    BP, P q½-1 hr until stable; note presence of hypotension, tachycardia
		Notify physician for the presence of any of these abnormalities
		If atelectasis occurs
		    Augment chest physiotherapy to affected areas
		    Assist patient with coughing and deep breathing; suction secretions if patient unable to cough
		    Administer bronchodilators, mucolytic agents if ordered
		    Monitor patient's response to these interventions
		If airway obstruction occurs
		    Position head to open airway
		    Augment chest physiotherapy to affected areas
		    Aspirate secretions with suctioning as necessary
		    Administer bronchodilators, mucolytic agents as ordered
		    Assist with bronchoscopy if procedure required for diagnosis and for aspiration of a mucous plug
		    Monitor patient's response to these measures

■ Respiratory insufficiency related to air leak, particularly in patients with the following
  Lobectomy
  Segmental resection
  Bullectomy
	■ No inspired air leaks out through incision or out chest tube
	While chest tube(s) is in situ, drainage bottle indicates no air with inspiration (ventilated patient) or with expiration (extubated patient)
		■ Monitor
		    For air bubbling down the chest tube into the underwater seal bottle/chamber
		    The amount of air lost in the artificially ventilated patient by measuring the difference between the preset volume to be delivered and the expired volume
		If an air leak is present, monitor progression/resolution of by observing changes in amount of air lost
		The tidal volume (V_T) to be delivered by the ventilator may be

Potential problems	Expected outcomes	Nursing activities
	While patient is intubated, the amount of air expired approximates the amount of air inspired	increased as ordered so that the expired volume, or the volume that does not leak out the chest tube, is equal to the desired V_T Monitor for inadequate drainage of air leak (signs/symptoms of pneumothorax); notify physician if this occurs Assist with chest tube insertion if necessary
■ Respiratory insufficiency related to pulmonary interstitial edema resulting from an acute increase in blood flow to the remaining lung tissue in the initial postoperative period (the *pneumonectomy patient* is particularly susceptible to this complication)	■ Clear lungs Arterial blood gas levels within normal limits Weight remains the same or decreases postoperatively (if weight gain occurred intraoperatively)	■ Prevent by administering fluids and blood products as ordered to maintain intravascular volume and hemodynamic stability, taking care to avoid administration of nonessential fluids that can contribute to pulmonary interstitial edema, ventricular strain, and/or heart failure Monitor Intake and output q1 hr Daily weights Hemodynamic parameters every hour, particularly closely in the pneumonectomy patient; correlate abnormalities with the presence of abnormal or adventitious breath sounds Arterial blood gas levels for hypoxemia Notify physician of significant imbalance in the fluid intake and output flow sheet and in the daily weight pattern If pulmonary interstitial edema and associated hypoxemia occur, artificial ventilation with the use of small amounts PEEP may be ordered and instituted to achieve adequate oxygenation; see Standards: *Mechanical ventilation; Positive end expiratory pressure* Administer diuretics as ordered, and closely monitor response in terms of Urine output BP, P, CVP, and PAP measurements Weight loss or gain Arterial blood gas results Improved oxygenation
■ Respiratory insufficiency related to bronchial stump leakage due to extra tension on stump in a *pneumonectomy patient*	■ Bronchial stump intact	■ Prevention When inserting suction catheter to aspirate secretions, stop before the point of resistance (which may be the bronchial stump suture line) V_Ts are reduced according to the amount of lung tissue resected; the pneumonectomy patient receives a little more than one half of the predicted V_T for his/her weight (approximately 10 cc/kg) Monitor for Expectoration of old, partially clotted blood Sudden respiratory distress, including shortness of breath, with restlessness, tachycardia, hypotension If signs of bronchial stump leakage occur Notify physician at once Monitor arterial blood gas results Monitor results of emergency chest radiograph if done Prepare patient for emergency surgery to oversew the bronchial stump if procedure is planned

Potential problems	Expected outcomes	Nursing activities

■ Respiratory insufficiency related to breakdown of the anastomosis from infection, poor healing, and bronchopleural fistula in patients with *tracheal resection*	■ Tracheal anastomosis intact	■ Prevent anastomotic breakdown in tracheal resection patient by
		  Avoiding tension, torsion of fresh suture line by keeping patient's head flexed
		  Avoiding rotation of patient's head by placement of a suture from chin to chest or some other stabilizing measure
		  Avoiding endotracheal intubation, which puts undue pressure against suture line
		  Administering vigorous pulmonary toilet with modified chest physiotherapy, deep breathing and coughing as needed q2-4 hr and prn
		  Humidified O_2 supplements as ordered
		Monitor
		  For acute respiratory distress
		  For pneumothorax, subcutaneous emphysema
		  Chest radiograph results
		If problem occurs
		  Assist physician with insertion of chest tube
		  Prepare patient for surgery if planned
		  Administer antibiotics as ordered

■ Pneumothorax	■ Full lung expansion with adequate oxygenation and ventilation	■ Monitor for signs and symptoms of pneumothorax, including
		  Respiratory distress—shortness of breath, dyspnea, tachypnea
		  Anxiety, diaphoresis, pallor, vertigo
		  Asymmetrical chest movements, distant or absent breath sounds on affected side
		  Pleural pain
		  Tachycardia with weak pulse
		  Cyanosis and hypotension if severe
		Notify physician if these abnormalities occur
		If pneumothorax occurs, administer therapy as ordered, which may include
		  Staying with patient
		  Placing patient in semi- to high Fowler's position
		  Administering O_2 therapy as ordered
		  Assisting with insertion of chest tube; if done, note loss of air from patient's lung into chest tube and signs of resolution of pneumothorax with reexpansion of lung
		  Monitoring q1-2 hr for continued lung expansion
		  Auscultation of breath sounds q1-2 hr

■ Subcutaneous emphysema associated with collection of air and/or blood in the operative area	■ Absence of an air or blood collection in the operative area
	  Absence of subcutaneous emphysema
	  Full expansion of remaining lung tissue
		■ Monitor for
		  Subcutaneous emphysema over chest wall, which may indicate presence of additional air or blood in the operative area
		  Chest radiograph results, indicating air or blood in operative area
		  Breath sounds consistent with air or blood in operative area (distant, dull)
		If subcutaneous emphysema occurs associated with air in operative area, see Problem, Pneumothorax, for nursing activities
		If subcutaneous emphysema occurs in association with a collection of blood in the operative area
		  Place patient in semi- to high Fowler's position
		  Assist physician with insertion of chest tube
		  Monitor patient's response, including
		    BP, P q1-2 hr
		    Nature and amount of blood lost through chest tube; notify physician of blood loss greater than 200 ml/hour in adults
		    Hct levels q1-3 hr, depending on presence of active bleeding

Potential problems	Expected outcomes	Nursing activities
		Milk chest tube q1-2 hr Assist patient to cough and deep breathe q1-2 hr and prn, splinting patient's chest when patient coughs Auscultate breath sounds q1-2 hr for degree of lung expansion Monitor chest radiograph results for lung expansion

■ Muscle spasm of neck associated with neck flexion and shoulder immobility
The tracheal resection patient is particularly prone to this complication
	■ Absence of muscle spasm and discomfort of neck/shoulder muscles	■ Prevent muscle spasm by
		  Supporting patient's head and neck while maintaining them in a flexed position, usually with the aid of a suture line from chin to chest
		  Massaging back and shoulder muscles frequently
		Monitor for tight neck and shoulder muscles, including patient complaints of discomfort in some muscles
		Notify physician if spasm occurs
		If neck spasm occurs
		  Continue massaging muscles and providing support of neck and shoulder
		  Administer a muscle relaxant if needed, as ordered

■ Infection, pneumonia	■ Infection free
	Afebrile
	Arterial blood gas levels within patient's normal limits
	Chest radiograph clear with full lung expansion
		■ Prevention
		  Administer pain medication if needed, as ordered, to avoid patient splinting and reduced respiratory excursion
		  Administer maximal chest physiotherapy, including
		    Turning q1-2 hr
		    Chest physiotherapy q2 hr with turning
		    Auscultation of breath sounds q1 hr with suctioning as needed
		    Using pillows for support and comfort, particularly around chest tubes
		    In addition, after extubation
		      1. Incentive spirometry q1-2 hr
		      2. Deep breathing and coughing q1-2 hr
		      3. Assisting and supporting patient as needed
		      4. Promoting optimal chest expansion by positioning patient in semi-Fowler's position
		      5. Ambulation as soon as possible
		  Monitor
		    Respirations q½-1 hr for rate and quality; note tachypnea, dyspnea
		    Secretions for color, amount, consistency; particularly note copious, tenacious, and/or abnormally colored sputum
		    Temperature q1-2 hr; note fever
		    For pleuritic chest pain
		    For unequal chest movements
		    Breath sounds q1 hr; note presence and nature of—particularly the presence of rales, rhonchi, and other adventitious breath sounds—or the absence of breath sounds altogether
		    Color for cyanosis
		    Arterial blood gas levels; note presence of hypoxemia, hypercapnia
		    Chest radiograph results revealing infiltrates, atelectasis
		    Sputum C and S results
		    Pulse q½-1 hr for tachycardia
		  Notify physician for abnormalities in these parameters
		  If pneumonia occurs
		    Administer antibiotics as ordered
		    Administer analgesics, antipyretics, and/or expectorant, if needed, as ordered
		    Liquefy tenacious secretions by administering additional systemic fluid or instilling of small amounts of saline solution into endotracheal tube, followed by manual inflations

Potential problems	**Expected outcomes**	**Nursing activities**

■ Infection, empyema, which may be related to bacteria introduced during surgery	■ Infection free
	Afebrile
	Absence of abnormal collection in operative area as revealed by chest radiograph, auscultation
		■ Prevent by
		  Avoiding opening closed chest drainage system (except if necessary to change the system)
		  Evacuating drainage from chest; keep drainage flowing down chest tubes by frequently "milking" (squeezing) the chest tubes
		Monitor
		  Temperature q1-2 hr; note fever
		  Results of chest radiograph for results compatible with empyema
		  CBC results for leukocytosis
		  Erythrocyte sedimentation rate for elevation
		If problem occurs
		  Send cultures of drainage, sputum as ordered
		  Administer antibiotics as ordered
		  Prepare patient for surgery if necessary

■ Hoarseness related to tumor compression of laryngeal nerve or surgical damage of laryngeal nerve in the *esophagogastrectomy patient*	■ Patient's speaking voice is unchanged from preoperative level
	Absence of hoarseness
		■ Monitor
		  For hoarseness
		  Patient's voice if hoarseness develops
		  For difficulty in coughing
		Notify physician of any of these abnormalities
		If problem occurs, administer therapy as ordered to facilitate patient's ability to phonate

■ Limited ROM on operated side of thoracic surgery patients related to position used during surgery; arm is usually in a very extended position taped over head or to table, occasionally causing nerve damage and brachial plexus palsy and limited ROM related to shoulder pain, particularly for people who have had a significant amount of muscle cut	■ Patient adequately performs breathing and body exercises
	Patient has full ROM of extremity on operated side
		■ Prevent by
		  Reviewing breathing, shoulder/arm and leg exercises preoperatively
		  Instructing patient in and encouraging skeletal exercises to promote abduction and mobilization of shoulder and arm
		  Administering pain medication, if needed, as ordered
		  Encouraging ambulation as soon as possible as ordered, particularly after the chest tubes are removed; pneumonectomy patients are mobilized more slowly because of the greater cardiopulmonary adjustments that occur
		Monitor for
		  Limited ROM of upper extremity
		  Shoulder pain with associated decrease in movement of upper extremity
		Notify physician if these occur
		If problem occurs
		  Administer pain medication if needed, and institute an aggressive exercise program as ordered
		  Arrange for physical therapy consultation as ordered

■ Thrombophlebitis, pulmonary embolism, other types of emboli	■ Coagulation studies within normal limits
	No signs/symptoms of thrombophlebitis, pulmonary embolism, or other types of emboli
		■ Prevent by
		  Encouraging early postoperative mobilization as ordered
		  Monitoring for signs and symptoms of thrombophlebitis and pulmonary embolism; if either problem occurs, see Standard: *Embolic phenomena*

Potential problems	Expected outcomes	Nursing activities
■ Insufficient knowledge to comply with discharge regimen*	■ Patient/family has sufficient information to comply with discharge regimen Patient/family accurately describes dietary and medication regimen and particular precautions for activities Patient/family accurately describes plan for follow-up care	■ Assess patient/family's level of understanding regarding the postdischarge regimen Describe the follow-up plan of care, including medications and their purpose, identification, route, dosage, frequency and timing, and potential adverse effects Instruct patient in activity progression, cautioning the sternotomy or thoracotomy patient not to progress to activities faster than physician recommends; resumption of such activities as driving, vacuuming, lifting objects of a prescribed weight range, or sports should be discussed with physician If appropriate, explain that some intercostal discomfort may normally continue for a few weeks and that it can be relieved by heat and, if necessary, a mild analgesic Instruct patient/family in suture line care if appropriate; provide opportunity for practice and return demonstration Instruct the esophagogastrectomy patient not to bend over at waist but rather to bend at knees and squat to pick up items, tie shoes, and so on Identify signs/symptoms that require medical attention, depending on the outcome of surgery and residual pulmonary dysfunction; instruct patient to seek medical attention for any untoward signs and symptoms Provide opportunity for and encourage patient/family questions and verbalization of anxiety regarding discharge regimen Describe the plan for follow-up visits, including the purpose of visits, when and where to go, who to see, and what specimens to bring Assess patient/family's potential compliance with discharge regimen

*If responsibility of critical care nurse includes this type of follow-up care.

4 □ Near drowning

Drowning is the third most common cause of accidental death in the United States and one of the most common causes of death in children over 1 year of age.

Approximately 10% of all near-drowning victims do not aspirate water because of laryngospasm or forced breath holding. These individuals respond best to immediate mouth-to-mouth resuscitation and often recover spontaneous respirations within minutes. Once the patient aspirates water, however, hypoxemia, acidosis, pulmonary edema, red cell lysis, and death can result if adequate ventilation is not quickly established and skillfully maintained.

There are theoretical differences between fresh and salt water aspiration. When the patient aspirates *fresh* water, alveolar surfactants are displaced or removed, alveolar surface tensions become high, and atelectasis can occur. Aspirated fresh water tends to be absorbed quickly into the vascular space; consequently, with greater amounts of fresh water aspiration, a mild, transient hemodilution and increase in blood volume may occur. In addition, if the fresh water was from a chlorinated swimming pool, the chlorine can destroy alveolar membranes and cause a chemical pneumonitis. *Salt* water aspiration may also interfere with alveolar surfactants; however, the predominant effect is pulmonary edema because the hypertonic salt water draws more fluid from the vascular space into the alveoli. With this fluid shift, hemoconcentration and severe hypovolemia may occur.

The end result of any significant aspiration is decreased alveolar ventilation. Aspiration causes inflammation, obstruction, and collapse of smaller airways and destruction of alveolar and capillary membranes. This produces pulmonary edema, a severe decrease in lung compliance, and alveolar hypoventilation. Arterial oxygen desaturation occurs, due to the ventilation/perfusion abnormalities (perfusion of nonventilated alveoli). Healing of injured membranes can result in fibrosis and loss of intrapulmonary diffusion surface. Corticosteroid administration is thought to reduce the severity of this membrane destruction and fibrosis.

The most serious complication of near drowning is hypoxia. The patient with severe pulmonary involvement will require mechanical ventilation with high inspiratory pressures and high (up to 30 cm H_2O) PEEP to maintain adequate ventilation despite low lung compliance and pulmonary edema. Such high ventilatory pressures make the patient extremely susceptible to the development of pneumothoraces and other air leaks (pneumomediastinum, subcutaneous emphysema). Acidosis may be severe and must be managed aggressively. End stage hypoxemia produces depression of cardiac, cerebral, renal, hepatic, and metabolic functions.

Beyond the second day of care, pulmonary infections can become problematic. If the patient aspirated contaminated water, severe infections can result. Many victims vomit and aspirate gastric contents during the near-drowning episode; initially, this can cause airway obstruction and later can result in severe chemical pneumonitis and pneumonia. Antibiotics will be required if evidence of pulmonary infection or lung abscess occurs.

The severity of neurological sequelae following near drowning depends on the severity and duration of hypoxemia and on the temperature of the immersion water. Cold water submersion produces hypothermia prior to the hypoxic insult; this hypothermia may reduce tissue oxygen requirements and may result in increased patient tolerance of brief respiratory arrest. Because reports of neurological sequelae following near drowning vary considerably, aggressive management of the near-drowning victim is recommended. In the absence of as-

sociated neurological injury, if spontaneous respirations and cranial nerve reflexes do not return within hours of resuscitation (and rewarming of the patient if necessary), the prognosis for the patient is grave.

Companions or family members of the near-drowning victim may feel frustrated and guilty. Parents often will need special support as they feel responsible for their child's condition.

ASSESSMENT

1. Circumstances of near drowning
   a. Duration of submersion
   b. Water temperature
   c. Type of water—fresh, salt, or contaminated
   d. Condition of patient when rescued
      (1) Presence/absence of spontaneous respirations and heart rate
      (2) Level of consciousness
      (3) Patient temperature
   e. Evidence of associated neurological injury (concussion, skull fracture)
2. Resuscitation attempts and patient's response
   a. At scene of near drowning
   b. During transportation to the hospital
   c. On arrival in the hospital
3. Respiratory status
   a. Presence of pulmonary congestion or airway obstruction
   b. Evidence of bronchospasm, aspiration, or pulmonary edema with clinical examination or on chest radiograph
   c. Presence and efficiency of independent respiratory effort (lung aeration, use of accessory muscles)
   d. Arterial blood gas levels and acid-base balance
   e. Mechanical ventilatory assistance required (and inspiratory pressures and PEEP necessary)
   f. Chest radiograph
   g. Quantity and characteristics of respiratory secretions or sputum
4. Cardiovascular status
   a. Indirect evidence of circulating blood volume
      (1) CVP and/or left atrial pressure
      (2) PCWP
      (3) Urine output (and specific gravity)
      (4) Hct and Hgb
   b. Evidence of cardiac output
      (1) BP
      (2) Tissue perfusion
      (3) Urine output

c. Consequences of severe hypoxemia
   (1) Progressive acidosis
   (2) Decreased myocardial function and increased irritability (and arrhythmias)
   (3) Red cell lysis and increase in serum potassium level
   (4) Decreased BP
5. Neurological status
   a. Level of consciousness
   b. Presence of cranial nerve or brain stem reflexes (gag, corneal reflex, withdrawal from pain)
   c. Seizure activity
   d. Evidence of increased intracranial pressure (due to traumatic or hypoxic cerebral edema)
   e. Pathological posturing (decorticate or decerebrate)
   f. Pupil response to light and pupil size
6. Fluid and electrolyte balance
   a. Fluid balance (level of hydration, hypervolemia, hypovolemia)
   b. Electrolyte concentrations
      (1) Increased concentration indicative of hemoconcentration and hypovolemia
      (2) Decreased concentration indicative of hemodilution and hypervolemia
      (3) Increased serum potassium concentration with red cell lysis
      (4) Serum potassium concentration changes with acid-base imbalance
   c. Serum glucose level (especially important in infants, who have little glucose storage)

d. Renal function (especially consequences of hypoxia and acute tubular necrosis)
7. Recent history of illness
   a. Respiratory (pneumonia, emphysema, asthma)
   b. Cardiovascular (myocardial infarction, coronary arteriosclerosis, congenital heart disease, arrhythmias, hypertension)
8. Current medications and allergies
9. Family members and their locations
10. Level of patient/family's anxiety

GOALS

1. Patent airway
2. Adequate ventilation
3. Adequate cardiac output
   a. Appropriate intravascular volume
   b. Effective cardiac rhythm
   c. Adequate tissue perfusion and BP
   d. Adequate Hct and Hgb
4. Normal electrolyte and acid-base balance
5. Optimal CNS function
6. Absence or resolution of pulmonary infection
7. Adequate renal function
8. Absence of nosocomial or opportunistic infection
9. Patient/family's comprehension of patient's health status with realistic discussion of patient's prognosis
10. Patient/family's participation in hospital plan of care as appropriate
11. Patient/family's demonstration of ability to provide appropriate home health care

Potential problems	Expected outcomes	Nursing activities
■ Airway obstruction related to fluid aspiration, bronchospasm, pulmonary edema	■ Patent airway	■ Monitor for evidence of obstruction of airway Stridor Coughing Retractions (and other evidence of use of accessory muscles of respiration) Nasal flaring Cyanosis (or pallor if patient is anemic or an infant) Excessive respiratory secretions Decreased lung aeration and chest expansion If the aforementioned occur, suction the patient's airway immediately, request that a physician be called, and begin emergency resuscitation measures if patient does not respond If endotracheal tube is in place, maintain tube patency with sterile suction technique, and secure tube to prevent accidental dislodgement Keep suction, resuscitator bag, O_2, and appropriate sizes of prepared endotracheal tubes at bedside (tube will need to be cut to appropriate size for children) Keep patient's head turned to the side with neck slightly extended to keep upper airway as straight as possible

Potential problems	Expected outcomes	Nursing activities

If patient is mechanically ventilated, see Standard: *Mechanical ventilation;* keep in mind that these patients require higher ventilatory and PEEP pressures

See also Standard: *Positive end expiratory pressure*

NOTE: If the patient requires high inspiratory and end expiratory pressures, sedation will be required to ensure ventilatory control of patient (sedatives, muscle relaxants, or paralyzing agents may be used); once patient is sedated, the nurse must be sure to carefully maintain adequate ventilation because patient is totally ventilator-dependent

If the patient requires long-term ventilation, a tracheostomy may be indicated; see Standard: *The patient with a tracheostomy*

■ Hypoxemia and respiratory distress related to pulmonary edema, bronchospasm, surfactant elimination, chemical pneumonitis, destruction or fibrosis of alveolar membrane, pneumonia, pneumothorax, and possible CNS depression

■ Adequate ventilation as measured by
Satisfactory arterial blood gas levels
Equal and adequate lung aeration
Pink color
Minimal use of accessory muscles of respiration
Absence of pulmonary congestion on radiograph and with clinical examination

■ Monitor for evidence of hypoxemia
Altered patient level of consciousness (patient may become more agitated or more lethargic)
Increased heart rate (consider patient's normal range)
Increased respiratory rate (consider patient's normal range)
Increased respiratory effort; increased use of accessory muscles of respiration and "fighting" of ventilator will occur if patient is not sedated
Decreased arterial PO_2 and decreased pH (with hypoxia, the respiratory rate is stimulated, so initial *hypocapnia* may occur)
Peripheral vasoconstriction
Cyanosis or pallor (cyanosis will appear only if sufficient hemoglobin is present)
If the aforementioned occur, notify physician and increase patient ventilation through resuscitator bagging (once patent airway is assured as in Problem, Airway obstruction)
Monitor for evidence of increased respiratory distress
Symptoms noted above
Decreased lung aeration
Increased pulmonary congestion
Decreased chest excursion during inspiration
Arterial O_2 desaturation and/or hypercapnia
If the aforementioned occur, ensure patent airway (as in Problem, Airway obstruction), bag patient with resuscitator bag and mask (or bag and adaptor if patient is intubated), request that physician be called, and begin emergency resuscitation measures as needed (be prepared for emergency intubation or reintubation of patient)
If a mechanically ventilated patient demonstrates the aforementioned evidence of increased distress, the following problems should be considered
Tube may be blocked; if you are unable to produce adequate ventilation by hand bagging and much resistance to ventilation is felt, the tube is probably blocked; suction patient immediately; if tube remains blocked, it should be removed to allow the patient to be ventilated by mask until reintubation can be accomplished
If the tube is patent and patient remains severely distressed, a *pneumothorax* is the next consideration; the physician should be notified while hand bagging is attempted and a chest radiograph is obtained; the nurse should have equipment in the room for emergency insertion of chest tubes
NOTE: In small infants, breath sounds are easily transmitted through the thin chest wall, so adequate breath sounds may

Potential problems	Expected outcomes	Nursing activities

appear to be present despite a pneumothorax because of transmission of breath sounds from other areas; *since a pneumothorax can appear suddenly and cause rapid, severe compromise of cardiorespiratory function, the health care team must be prepared to act quickly*

Maintain mechanical ventilation as ordered; see Standards: *Mechanical ventilation* and *Positive end expiratory pressure* but note that these patients will require higher ventilatory pressures

Monitor blood gas levels and make ventilatory changes as ordered; hypercapnia, hypoxemia, and acidosis indicate increased respiratory failure

Check ventilator settings at least q1 hr if patient is mechanically ventilated

Monitor for evidence of increased pulmonary edema

  Increased pulmonary congestion (by radiograph or clinical examination)

  Decreased lung aeration at same ventilator inspiratory pressures, or increased ventilator inspiratory pressures at same set V_T (if patient is mechanically ventilated)

  Increased respiratory effort (if patient is breathing spontaneously)

  Increased respiratory secretions or sputum production

  Increased PCWP

  Tachycardia (increased from patient's normal range)

  Tachypnea (increased from patient's previous rate, if patient is not mechanically ventilated)

  Falling arterial Po_2 and pH and rising arterial Pco_2 with increasing alveolar-arterial O_2 difference

If the aforementioned occur, notify physician, restrict fluid intake, and administer diuretic therapy as ordered

Plasma oncotic agents may be prescribed with diuretics to help reduce pulmonary edema; if ordered, be sure to include them as part of patient fluid intake and monitor patient response

Weaning of the patient from mechanical ventilation must be performed in a structured, meticulous fashion

  Initially, inspiratory or PEEP pressures will be decreased; *this must be done very slowly in patients who have aspirated fresh water to make sure that they have had adequate regeneration of surfactant*

  If patient tolerance permits, rate or V_T is then decreased

  Only one ventilator variable should be changed at any given time, and a thorough evaluation of patient response should be made before any other change is introduced

  During weaning, monitor the patient closely for clinical evidence of hypoxia

  If possible, monitor patient's end-tidal CO_2 (it should be representative of the arterial Pco_2 unless severe pulmonary disease is present) with arterial blood gas results

  Arterial *hypocapnia* (and falling end-tidal CO_2) during weaning may indicate patient hyperventilation in response to hypoxia

  Arterial *hypercapnia* (and rising end-tidal CO_2) or falling arterial Pa_{O_2} reflects respiratory insufficiency and intolerance of weaning

  Monitor alveolar-arterial O_2 difference; increased gradient suggests increased intrapulmonary shunting and decreased alveolar ventilation

Potential problems	Expected outcomes	Nursing activities

■ Possible inadequate cardiac output related to inadequate circulating blood volume, peripheral and pulmonary vasoconstriction, arrhythmias, hypoxemia, acidosis, and possible pneumomediastinum	■ Stable cardiac output as measured by
	Effective cardiac rhythm
	Adequate BP
	Warm, pink extremities
	Adequate urine output (1 to 2 ml/kg/hour) in children; 25 to 30 ml/hour in adults)
	Adequate cerebral perfusion
		■ Monitor for evidence of decreased cardiac output
		  Adults—systolic BP less than 100 mm Hg (consider patient's normal range)
		  Children—systolic BP less than 85 mm Hg (consider patient's normal range)
		  Infants—systolic BP less than 70 mm Hg (consider patient's normal range)
		  Tachycardia
		  Poor peripheral perfusion (cold, clammy extremities, decreased urine output with high—greater than 1.015—specific gravity, decreased peripheral pulses)
		  Pallor or cyanosis
		  Increased central or pulmonary venous pressures may indicate hypervolemia, cardiac failure, or pneumomediastinum
		  Decreased central or pulmonary venous pressures may indicate hypovolemia
		  Arrhythmias (monitor and document any arrhythmias with rhythm strip—note BP during arrhythmias—and notify physician); be aware of electrolyte imbalance, which may precipitate arrhythmias; see Standard: *Arrhythmias*
		If symptomatic pnemomediastinum is present, it should be aspirated immediately
		Assess circulating blood volume
		  Monitor Hct—notify physician and prepare to administer packed red blood cells (RBC) or whole blood if Hct is less than 30% (40% in infants) or falling rapidly
		  Increased Hct and serum electrolyte concentrations may indicate hemoconcentration and decreased blood volume, requiring increased fluid intake
		  Decreased serum Hct and serum electrolyte concentrations may indicate hemodilution and increased blood volume, requiring diuresis
		Monitor urine output—decreased urine output (less than 1 to 2 ml/kg/hour despite adequate intake) with increased specific gravity may indicate cardiac failure
		Administer vasopressors as ordered—note their effect on heart rate, central and pulmonary venous pressures, arterial pressure, and urine output and titrate accordingly
		See Standard: *Shock*
		With CNS injury, *inappropriate antidiuretic hormone (ADH) secretion* may occur; this causes increased loss of sodium (Na^+) in the urine and decreased serum Na^+ concentration (H_2O intoxication); urine volume may be increased, decreased, or unchanged, but will be more concentrated (specific gravity greater than 1.015); the treatment of choice is fluid restriction
		With CNS injury (especially following hypoxic insult), *diabetes insipidus* may occur; the patient loses enormous amounts of dilute urine (less than 1.010 specific gravity), and hypovolemia will result if fluid replacement is not rapid; the treatment is fluid replacement and administration of vasopressin (pituitary hormone)

■ Possible cerebral edema related to hypoxemia, acidosis, fluid shifts, electrolyte imbalance, traumatic cranial injury, and extremely high ventilatory PEEP	■ Optimal CNS function as measured by
	Absence of seizures
	Absence of signs of increased intracranial pressure
		■ Monitor for evidence of increased intracranial pressure
		  Increased systolic BP
		  Decreased heart rate (although initially it may increase)
		  Depressed respirations
		  Altered level of consciousness (increased irritability or lethargy)
		  Decreased pupil response to light

Potential problems	Expected outcomes	Nursing activities
		If the aforementioned symptoms occur, notify physician at once and be prepared to begin emergency resuscitative measures should further deterioration and respiratory arrest occur; see also Standard: *Increased intracranial pressure*
		Perform neurological assessment q1 hr (or as indicated by patient's condition)
		Monitor pupil response to light and notify physician of any change in response or new pupil inequality (these findings may indicate severe cerebral edema and increased intracranial pressure)
		Monitor intracranial pressure if intracranial pressure monitoring line is in place; see Standard: *Increased intracranial pressure*
		Note any pathological posturing by the patient; notify physician immediately if deterioration occurs
		Monitor for seizure activity
		Ensure safety of patient environment (pad side rails, remove sharp objects, tape all tubes securely)
		If seizures occur, note duration, extent, and muscle involvement and notify physician
		Notify physician immediately if seizure activity increases in frequency or duration (additional anticonvulsants may be required)
		See Standard: *Seizures*
		Administer anticonvulsants as ordered (check patient's dosage and monitor patient's response)
		Intravenous fluids with low salt content may be ordered to decrease the posttraumatic or posthypoxic tendency to fluid retention and cerebral edema
		Diabetes insipidus or inappropriate ADH secretion may occur; see Nursing activities, Possible inadequate cardiac output
■ Nutritional compromise related to prolonged nasotracheal intubation, bed rest, and stress	■ Adequate nutritional status as measured by Appropriate weight gain Adequate subcutaneous tissue Moist mucous membranes Good skin turgor Adequate wound healing Normal Hgb	■ Calculate patient's daily caloric requirements; ensure adequate caloric intake via parenteral alimentation or gavage feedings if oral intake is impossible
		Monitor infant's serum glucose or Dextrostix* as needed; notify physician of any evidence of hypoglycemia (glucose storage in infants is minimal)
		NOTE: Dextrose solutions of 5% provide only 200 kcal/liter and thus are inadequate for long-term nutrition
		If patient is placed on parenteral alimentation, see Standard: *Total parenteral nutrition through central venous catheter*
		Turn patient frequently, and keep skin warm and dry to prevent skin breakdown; massage any bony prominences to improve skin circulation
		Monitor patient's Hct and Hgb, and notify physician of any significant changes
		Weigh patient daily (or twice daily if indicated), and notify physician of any significant weight gain or loss (greater than 1 kg/24 hours in adults, greater than 200 g/24 hours in children, and greater than 50 g/24 hours in infants)
		Monitor patient's fluid intake and output; calculate patient's daily fluid requirements, and notify physician if patient is not receiving them
		Monitor for evidence of dehydration; notify physician if present

*Dextrostix, Ames Co., Elkhart, Ind.

Potential problems	Expected outcomes	Nursing activities

■ Possible infection related to aspiration of contaminated H_2O, pulmonary compromise, and multiple invasive procedures	■ Absence of local signs of infection
	  Fever (or hypothermia in infant)
	  Possible leukocytosis
	  Redness, heat, or discharge at wound site
		■ If patient aspirated contaminated water obtain daily sputum cultures and notify physician of any abnormalities
		Monitor
		  For evidence of systemic infection
		    Fever or temperature instability in the infant
		    Possible leukocytosis
		    With severe systemic infection, a fall in BP and cardiac output can occur; see Standard: *Shock*
		  For evidence of respiratory infection
		    Increased pulmonary congestion by radiograph or physical examination
		    Increased respiratory distress (increased respiratory rate and effort, decreased lung aeration, and cyanosis or pallor)
		    Increased color, thickness, and odor of secretions (obtain specimen for C and S and gram stain)
		  For evidence of urinary tract infection
		    Fever
		    Cloudy, malodorous urine (obtain clean catch specimen for C and S and gram stain)
		    Pain with urination
		    In children, frequent voiding in small amounts is seen
		  For evidence of wound infection
		    Erythema at wound edges
		    Fluctuation of wound margins
		    Wound drainage (obtain C and S and gram stain)
		    Heat around area of wound
		Administer antibiotics as ordered

■ Possible electrolyte imbalance related to acidosis, hemodilution, hemoconcentration, red cell lysis, or fluid shifts	■ Normal serum electrolytes	■ Monitor serum electrolyte levels; notify physician if abnormal
		  Potassium (K^+) shifts will occur with changes in pH; therefore, before initiating any K^+ replacement, consider acid-base balance
		  With acidosis, serum K^+ rises (K^+ shifts out of the cells and into the serum); conversely, with correction of acidosis, the serum K^+ concentration falls
		  With alkalosis, serum K^+ falls (K^+ shifts into the cells and out of the serum); conversely, with correction of alkalosis, serum K^+ concentration rises
		  With hemodilution, serum electrolyte concentrations fall; will return to normal when diuresis occurs
		  With hemoconcentration, serum electrolyte concentrations rise; will fall again with hydration
		  Infants who are severely ill are particularly prone to development of hypoglycemia (they have little glucose storage); monitor their glucose level carefully and ensure adequate source of caloric intake (5% dextrose IV solutions provide only 200 kcal/liter)
		  With red cell lysis, serum K^+ will rise and hemoglobinuria will be seen; notify physician and monitor renal function

■ Possible hypothermia or hyperthermia related to patient submersion in cold water, CNS damage, or infection	■ Normal rectal temperature	■ Monitor patient's rectal temperature; if fever (greater than 38° C) is present, notify physician; note blood culture results If hyperthermia is present, this will increase patient's O_2 requirements; therefore, once the source of fever is established, application of hypothermia blanket may be indicated to control patient temperature; if such a blanket is used, it should never be set below 72° F (22° C) and should not cool patient enough to cause shivering (or frostbite)

Potential problems	Expected outcomes	Nursing activities
		If hypothermia is present, rewarming of patient should be accomplished gradually; rewarming should never be accomplished by application of a warm object to the patient's skin, as severe burns can result, particularly if cardiac output (and skin perfusion) is decreased; overbed warmers are preferred
■ Patient/family's anxiety related to near drowning, critical patient status, and intensive care environment and equipment (in children, separation from parents will also add to the child's fear)	■ Patient/family's comprehension of diagnosis and therapeutic regimen as demonstrated by their discussions and questions Patient/family's support of one another with demonstration of appropriate behavior	■ Determine concerns of patient/family Prepare family members for the sight of the patient with multiple IVs and many pieces of monitoring equipment Assess patient/family's understanding of condition and prognosis; elicit their opinions and comments, and attempt to clarify any misconceptions Attempt to elicit patient/family's response to the patient's near drowning; provide support and reassurance to family's discussion of anger or guilt Be present when patient prognosis is discussed by physician, and encourage patient/family's questions, as needed Involve family in patient care as appropriate; note that family members may not have enough emotional energy to provide physical care for the patient Make appropriate referrals to the chaplain and to social services Assist family in anticipatory mourning and/or realistic appraisal of patient's prognosis, as appropriate

■ Patient/family may have inadequate information to provide appropriate home care for the patient after discharge	■ Patient/family will possess sufficient information to enable them to demonstrate and discuss home care techniques	■ Include patient/family in discharge planning as they demonstrate readiness
		 Keep family informed of plans for patient discharge
		 Allow sufficient time to permit teaching at a relaxed pace, with adequate time for patient/family to perform return demonstration
		 Provide encouragement and support as needed
		 By the time of patient discharge, family should be able to discuss
		     Amount, schedule, and route of administration of any medications
		     Side effects of medications (if appropriate)
		     What to do if medication dose is forgotten (i.e., should it be given late or omitted)
		     Indications for contacting physician or primary nurse
		     Follow-up appointments and telephone numbers of health care personnel
		 Provide family and patient with written information as needed
		 By the time of patient discharge, patient/family should be able to demonstrate
		     Wound care techniques, including appropriate dressing changes
		     Any required airway care (if appropriate, see Standard: *The patient with a tracheostomy*)
		 Make appropriate referrals to community health services (public health nursing, visiting nurse, community groups)
		 Assist family in obtaining needed home health care equipment
		 If patient will be institutionalized following discharge, involve physician and social services or chaplain in the family's decision as appropriate; support the patient/family in their decision, once it has been made

5 □ The patient with a tracheostomy

A tracheostomy is a procedure in which an artificial opening is created between the second and fourth tracheal rings to provide an airway that bypasses upper airway structures and facilitates tracheobronchial toilet. The most common indication for a tracheostomy is upper airway obstruction (due to congenital stricture, trauma, carcinoma, infection, hemangioma, or long-term mechanical ventilation). A tracheostomy may also be performed to enable management of respiratory secretions that cannot be removed effectively by patient cough or nasopharyngeal suction. The tracheostomy may be temporary or permanent. Generally, uncuffed tubes are used in children to avoid later tracheal stenosis. Silastic tubes are popular for this age-group because they conform easily to the shape of the child's trachea; since they have no inner cannula, however, such tubes are unsuitable for home-going tracheostomy intubation. Metal or cuffed tubes are more commonly used in the adult patient or the patient requiring high ventilatory pressures (cuffs prevent air leaks). The type of tube and specific methods of stomal care will depend on the experience and the preference of the physician.

Since the tracheostomy allows air to bypass the upper airway, the functions of these structures—humidification, filtration, and warming of the air—must be artificially provided until cells in the trachea can compensate. Aseptic technique is essential in all phases of tracheostomy care during hospitalization, especially since multiple caretakers will be involved in the patient's care. When the patient returns home and the caretakers are limited, a clean technique will usually be satisfactory.

Complications of the actual tracheostomy include infection, airway obstruction, hemorrhage, tracheal ulceration or stenosis, subcutaneous emphysema, tube dislodgement or displacement, increased viscosity of respiratory secretions, peristomal skin breakdown, and laryngeal injury.

ASSESSMENT

1. Purpose of tracheostomy and intended duration
2. Evidence of respiratory distress—tachypnea, increased use of accessory muscles of respiration, nasal flaring, head bobbing (in infant less than 4 months old), jaw tugging, cyanosis or pallor, copious tracheal secretions, pulmonary congestion (by radiograph or clinical examination), decreased breath sounds, decreased feeding tolerance, diaphoresis, grunting
3. Level of hydration—skin turgor, mucous membranes, fontanelle (in infants less than 18 months old), tearing (in patient more than 3 months old), urine output and specific gravity (should be 1 to 2 ml/kg/hour with specific gravity less than 1.020 if fluid is adequate), consistency of tracheal secretions
4. Presence of stomal or pulmonary infection—pulmonary congestion, fever (or hypothermia in infants), purulent or malodorous secretions, leukocytosis, redness or fluctuance of edges of stoma
5. Appearance of stoma—retraction sutures, inflammation, size of orifice, evidence of bleeding
6. Nutritional status—weight, wound healing, amount of subcutaneous fat, serum glucose (in infants)
7. Current medications and allergies
8. Patient/family's response to tracheostomy (and comprehension of reasons for and consequences of the tracheostomy)
9. Patient/family's concerns and fears

GOALS

1. Patent airway and adequate ventilation
2. Absence of stomal or pulmonary infection
3. Absence of tracheal stenosis or damage
4. Adequate patient hydration and nutrition
5. Patient/family's comprehension of tracheostomy procedure and necessary postoperative and home care
6. Appropriate and constructive patient/family verbalization of concerns regarding patient alterations in body image and change in life-style.
7. Patient/family's ability to provide home care of patient's tracheostomy as appropriate
8. Effective patient communication with health team members and family

Potential problems	Expected outcomes	Nursing activities
■ Possible airway obstruction related to copious or dried tracheal secretions, pneumonia, atelectasis, hemorrhage, aspiration, or tracheostomy tube dislodgement	■ Patent airway	■ Tape spare tracheostomy tube of same size (and one a size larger and one a size smaller) to head of bed, and document size of tracheostomy tube in place

Keep tracheal dilator with extra tube for older children and adults at bedside

Keep suction equipment and resuscitator bag *with appropriate adaptor* at bedside

Tape retraction sutures securely to neck or to chest wall so that they are readily accessible

Provide humidity to inspired air as ordered; increase if secretions appear tenacious or dried

Initially suction tracheostomy frequently, then less often as amount of mucus decreases

Use O_2 as needed

Irrigate tube with sterile saline solution (0.5 to 1 ml) if secretions are thick

Once stoma is healing (after the first postoperative days) and as the patient's level of consciousness permits, encourage patient to cough out secretions to stomal orifice so that they may be removed without suctioning

Insert catheter *much less deeply* for tracheostomy suctioning than for endotracheal tube suctioning; irritation of the carina with the catheter will cause severe coughing spasm, pain, and possibly mucosal damage

Warm inspired air for infants and young children to prevent heat loss through respiratory tract

Restrain patient as needed to prevent removal of tube (mittens may be useful for children)

Tie tracheostomy tube in place securely with twill or umbilical tape

Use square knots, and allow only one small finger-breadth of room between tape and patient's neck (tie tapes in back of child's neck to prevent loosening or dislodgement by child)

Remember that cotton tape stretches when wet so it may have to be changed frequently to prevent loosening

When changing the tape, do not remove old ties until new ties are securely in place—generally two people are necessary to anchor tube and to secure new ties (especially with an anxious child or a combative adult)

Remove and clean inner cannula (if present)* q2-4 hr and prn; use sterile technique and hydrogen peroxide or boiling as indicated by hospital policies

Change tube weekly or according to hospital policies, using sterile technique (the tubes are generally changed for the first time 5 to 7 days following the tracheotomy)

After tracheostomy is created (especially in small children), the physician may gradually increase the size of the tube in place to provide a larger patent airway; have a larger tube ready as requested

When tracheostomy is to be closed, often the size of the tube will be reduced slowly to allow assessment of patient tolerance and gradual reduction in size of stoma; have smaller tube ready at physician's request, but monitor patient tolerance and keep larger tubes ready to insert if patient demonstrates intolerance of smaller tube

---

*Silastic tubes do not have an inner cannula.

Potential problems	Expected outcomes	Nursing activities

		Monitor for signs of respiratory distress—cyanosis, agitation, tachypnea, retractions, nasal flaring, use of accessory muscles for respiration
		   Normal adult respiratory rate: 10 to 15/minute (consider patient's normal range)
		   Normal pediatric respiratory rate: 18 to 30/minute (consider patient's normal range)
		   Normal infant respiratory rate: 20 to 30/minute (consider patient's normal range)
		   Normal newborn respiratory rate: 30 to 50/minute
		If patient demonstrates the aforementioned symptoms of increased respiratory distress, request that physician be notified immediately and prepare to institute emergency measures
		   Suction tracheostomy and oropharynx with O_2 support; remove inner cannula if present
		   Check position of tube and lung aeration; replace tube if needed
		   Change tube if unable to suction; use caution and retraction sutures in first 5 to 7 days (as stomal tract is not yet healed)
		   Prepare for intubation of patient if these efforts are unsuccessful
		NOTE: If you are unable to replace tracheostomy tube, an endotracheal tube may even be used *only in an emergency* (and can only be inserted a *short* distance into the tracheostomy) to provide an airway until proper reintubation can be accomplished
		   Ventilate patient with resuscitator bag and mask *only if upper airway is intact and relatively unobstructed*
		   Provide O_2 support as needed

■ Respiratory distress related to hypoventilation, pneumonia, pneumothorax, tracheostomy leakage, or perioperative sedation	■ Adequate ventilation as measured by equal and adequate lung aeration bilaterally, pink color, absence of pulmonary congestion, and absence of increased respiratory effort	■ Maintain patent airway as in Problem, Possible airway obstruction
		Monitor patient for lower airway problems
		   Pneumonia
		      Decreased breath sounds (indicating atelectasis)
		      Increased breath sounds (indicating consolidation)
		      Increase in thickness, quantity, and odor of secretions
		      Fever (or thermolability in the infant)
		      Increased respiratory effort (retractions or use of other accessory muscles of respiration)
		      Pulmonary congestion (by radiograph or physical examination)
		   Pneumothorax
		      Decreased or absent breath sounds
		      Cyanosis or pallor
		      Increased respiratory effort
		      Agitation
		      Increased respiratory rate (compare to previous rate)
		      Increased heart rate (compare to previous rate)
		      Possible shift in mediastinum
		      Hyperresonance to percussion
		      If the aforementioned are present, notify physician immediately, obtain chest radiograph, and prepare to assist with tapping of pneumothorax or insertion of chest tubes if necessary
		   Subcutaneous emphysema
		      Swelling of neck, face, and/or trunk (results from subcutaneous air leak and is usually self-limiting, but may result in airway compression)

Potential problems	Expected outcomes	Nursing activities
		Crackling with palpation
		Appearance of subcutaneous air on radiograph
		Administer chest physiotherapy including percussion, vibration, postural drainage (as tolerated), rib springing in infants and children, and suctioning as needed
		Provide humidity with or without O_2 continuously or during sleep
		Keep resuscitator bag *with appropriate adaptor* at bedside
■ Possible pneumonia related to contamination and aspiration (aspiration is much more likely if the patient is neurologically impaired or if fenestrated tube is used)	■ Absence of radiographic or clinical evidence of pulmonary infection	■ Monitor for signs of pulmonary infection (congestion, fever, leukocytosis, increased respiratory distress)
		Use sterile suctioning technique
		Change humidification equipment daily; use only sterile distilled water to fill nebulizers
		Send tracheal aspirates for C and S and gram stain if infection is suspected (pulmonary tree is generally thought to be colonized with gram-negative bacteria within 48 hours of intubation)
		Administer antibiotics as ordered (double check patient dosage and allergies prior to administration)
		Prevent aspiration with careful attention during feedings
		If cuffed tube is in place, keep cuff inflated when patient is eating, drinking, or receiving gastrostomy feedings
		Administer chest physiotherapy before feedings, but no sooner than 1 hour prior to feeding (so patient is not coughing during feeding) or 1 hour after feeding
		If NG or gastrostomy feeding is required, check gastric tube position prior to each feeding, and leave gastric tube unclamped for 30 to 45 minutes following each feeding
		Have suction equipment at hand
		Keep patient in high Fowler's position or on right side during feedings and for 1 hour following feedings; do not allow patient to recline on back (flat) for 1 hour following feeding
		Avoid disturbing patient for 1 hour after feeding (no blood tests, chest physiotherapy, injections)
		Monitor for signs of aspiration
		Coughing
		Increased respiratory distress
		Cyanosis
		Vomiting
		Agitation
		If the aforementioned occur, discontinue feedings immediately, suction oropharynx (but try not to cause gag reflex, which may result in further vomiting and aspiration), lower feeding tube orifice (to allow reflux), turn patient prone and slap the back sharply, request that physician be notified, obtain chest radiograph (will not be positive for at least 6 to 12 hours), and prepare to institute emergency measures
		If patient has history of aspiration during feeding, add food coloring to feeding and notify physician if this coloring appears in tracheal secretions
■ Stomal infection or peristomal skin breakdown	■ Absence of stomal infection (no signs of inflammation of stoma, no discharge)	■ Observe stoma for erythema, exudates, odor, and crusting lesions
		Notify physician and culture stoma if inflammation appears (yeast infections are most commonly detected around stoma)
		Cleanse stoma q8 hr and as needed with hydrogen peroxide and rinse with sterile water
		Apply dressing to protect stoma during feeding and if patient has constant drooling

Potential problems	Expected outcomes	Nursing activities
		Change tapes daily and as needed; use two people for the procedure with children and uncooperative adults
		Do not allow secretions to pool around stoma; suction or wipe them to keep stoma as dry as possible
		Apply topical antifungal or antibiotic agent only if ordered; prophylactic administration may encourage growth of resistant strains of bacteria or fungi
		Change all humidification equipment daily and as needed
		Use sterile technique to suction and care for stoma
		Keep skin under tracheal ties as clean and dry as possible, as skin is prone to breakdown due to abrasion and secretions
■ Stomal bleeding related to erosion of tube through blood vessel wall or incomplete cautery of skin vessel during tracheostomy procedure	■ No excessive stomal bleeding	■ Monitor site for bleeding; notify physician if bleeding is occurring
		If bleeding is profuse, apply pressure to site to control bleeding; suction as needed to keep airway patent
		Change dressings as needed and weigh dressings before and after use to document amount of bleeding
■ Possible tracheal erosion related to tube movement or high-pressure cuff	■ Absence of tracheal damage and ability to resume upper airway ventilation following closure of tracheostomy	■ Keep cuff deflated whenever possible
		Maintain small air leak around tracheostomy tube to prevent excessive pressure on trachea by cuff or tube
		Avoid movement of tube or torsion of the tracheal collar when suctioning, changing tapes, and cleansing site
		Prevent tube dislodgement (especially in first week), as frequent tube replacement causes tracheal irritation
		Monitor tube shape and position; discuss with physician if tube does not conform to angle of patient's airway—a different brand of tube may be required; Silastic tubes tend to become more flexible when warmed and moistened in the patient's airway, so these tubes conform most easily to the angle of the pediatric airway; however, these tubes are expensive and can only be used for one 2-month period (approximately); for home tracheostomy care, metal tubes with inner cannulas are more advisable
		Tracheostomy tube *must* be changed frequently enough to ensure its cleanliness; a dirty tube will cause chronic tracheal inflammation, resulting in tracheal scarring and granulomatous tissue formation
■ Possible dehydration related to inadequate humidification of inspired air or inadequate fluid intake	■ Patent airway and adequate hydration as measured by Moist, easily suctioned secretions Moist mucous membranes Good skin turgor	■ Assess level of patient hydration—mucous membranes should be moist; fontanelle in infant under 18 months should be flat but not sunken; adequate eye tearing should be present in patient over 3 months of age; skin should not "tent" when pinched; urine output should be adequate
		Increase humidification of inspired air as needed
		Calculate patient's maintenance fluid requirements and ensure that patient receives them (through oral, IV, or gavage route); discuss requirements and route of administration with physician
		If secretions are dry, provide humidification via tracheal cuff
■ Poor nutritional status related to prolonged hospitalization, dysphagia, anorexia, or CNS disease	■ Adequate nutritional status as measured by Appropriate weight gain Adequate subcutaneous fat	■ Calculate patient's daily caloric requirements and ensure that patient receives them (discuss with physician)
		Monitor infant's serum glucose, and notify physician of hypoglycemia (infant glucose stores are low)
		If patient is placed on parenteral alimentation, see Standard: *Total parenteral nutrition through central venous catheter*

Potential problems	Expected outcomes	Nursing activities
	Moist mucous membranes Good skin turgor Adequate wound healing Normal Hgb	Monitor patient's Hct and Hgb, and notify physician of abnormalities Weigh patient daily and notify physician of any significant weight loss (greater than 1.0 kg/24 hours in adults, greater than 200 g/24 hours in children, and greater than 50 g/24 hours in infants) Make food and mealtimes as appetizing for the patient as possible; provide small, tasty, frequent feedings rather than large "hospital tray" ones
■ Inability of patient to communicate verbally	■ Patient can communicate his/her needs to caregivers in manners appropriate to patient's level of consciousness and conceptual development	■ Assess patient's level of consciousness If patient is alert Provide a call bell within easy reach at all times Provide for easy observation of patient by nursing staff (and of nursing staff by patient) Provide "magic slate" or pad and pencil if patient is able to write (or communications board if unable to write) Provide communications board with illustrations if patient is preverbal or aphasic In children, assess growth and developmental level and utilize aforementioned strategies as appropriate Provide patient with reassurance and patience; tell the patient which nurses are nearby so that patient will not feel alone As appropriate teach patient to briefly occlude airway to speak
■ Patient/family's anxiety related to patient's inability to speak, patient care required, and alterations in patient's appearance	■ Patient/family able to discuss concerns and to support one another and function appropriately	■ Explain all activities and procedures as appropriate (utilize play for teaching of children) Initiate appropriate referrals to social services, chaplain, and clinical specialist as needed Provide patient/family with daily reports of patient's progress (it is important to provide them with concrete daily goals and positive reinforcement) Be present when physicians discuss patient's progress with patient/family; clarify information as needed Begin to involve patient/family in decision making and patient care as appropriate Assist patient/family in development of realistic plan for patient home health care or postdischarge care
■ Patient/family may have insufficient information to provide adequate patient home health care	■ Patient/family will be able to realistically assess their abilities to provide adequate patient home health care If patient will be discharged to the home, patient/family will demonstrate adequate skills in patient health care If patient will be discharged to an institution for health care, patient/family will demonstrate acceptance of this solution, while maintaining support for one another	■ Critically assess patient/family's ability to provide adequate home health care of patient's tracheostomy and to respond to any emergency situations that may arise; most families will be able to assume appropriate care; however, if both parents of an infant are blind, for example, some alternative method of care for the patient may need to be explored If patient cannot be discharged to the home, assist patient/family in exploring alternative forms of patient care Make appropriate referrals to community health and social service agencies If patient will be discharged to the home or if patient or family will be involved in posthospital care of the patient's tracheostomy, assess their readiness to learn, and begin teaching skills for home health care slowly Assessment of patient's respiratory status Maintenance of patient's airway Clean suction technique (if patient is at special risk for development of respiratory infection, sterile technique may be required—check with patient's physician) NOTE: A double lumen metal tube is generally safest for home care

Potential problems	Expected outcomes	Nursing activities
		Stomal care
		Changing of tracheal tapes
		Changing or replacement of tracheostomy tube
		Emergency resuscitation measures
		Medications
		Physician and nursing follow-up appointments
		Where, when, and why to contact physician, emergency personnel, nurse
		If family does not speak English, arrangements must be made to have interpreter readily available (relative, hospital personnel, etc.)
		Provide frequent and consistant reinforcement throughout teaching
		Document teaching plan and patient/family's progress
		Assist patient/family in obtaining needed home care equipment
		Ensure effective follow-up of patient following discharge; check frequently with patient/family in person and by telephone following patient's discharge

6 □ Mechanical ventilation

Mechanical ventilation is the process in which a positive force is generated (in the airway) to inflate the lungs with humidified, oxygenated air to achieve adequate oxygenation and ventilation. It is necessary for patients who are unable to provide enough force for their own respirations, such as patients with compromised lungs or chest wall and apneic or nearly apneic patients.

Mechanical ventilation is employed to provide adequate exchange of blood gases in patients with a variety of abnormalities. Indications for mechanical ventilation include

Apnea or depressed respirations with respiratory acidosis

Hypoxemia due to excessive work of breathing, ineffective breathing patterns, and decreased functional residual capacity, or hypoxemia due to pulmonary interstitial abnormalities

Abnormalities in respiratory function that may require ventilatory assistance include severe pulmonary disease, massive aspiration of gastric contents, smoke inhalation, flail chest, after major thoracic surgery, and patients in coma, to name a few.

Mechanical ventilation is accomplished with the use of ventilators that inflate the lungs with a predetermined volume or preset pressure. There is a large variety of ventilators available. The volume-cycled ventilators are preferred by most clinicians because of their ability to ventilate the alveoli readily.

Guidelines for effectively administering mechanical ventilation include

Appropriate choice of ventilator, based on thorough assessment of the patient's needs

Serial monitoring of arterial blood gas levels

Adjustment of ventilator settings according to patient's response

Continuous assessment and evaluation of the patient's vital signs, color, general appearance, and other responses

Constant supervision of proper functioning of the ventilator

ASSESSMENT

1. History that notes presence of underlying conditions, including
   a. Respiratory failure
   b. Renal insufficiency

c. Cardiac disease

d. Neurological abnormalities

2. Problem necessitating mechanical ventilation

   a. Cardiac and/or respiratory arrest

   b. Presence of apnea

   c. Acute ventilatory failure

   d. Impending acute ventilatory failure

   e. Inadequate oxygenation

   f. Severe trauma

3. Current active medical and/or respiratory problems

4. Presence, nature, severity of abnormalities in the following systems

   a. Pulmonary

      (1) Degree of respiratory distress

      (2) Respiratory rate, quality; note tachypnea, dyspnea

      (3) Rales, wheezes, and other adventitious sounds

      (4) Ability to expectorate secretions

      (5) Amount, color, and consistency of sputum

      (6) Bedside pulmonary function; note those not within normal limits, including V_T, VC, minute volume, and inspiratory force

   b. Cardiovascular

      (1) BP, heart rate, CVP, PAP, PCWP, and cardiac output for any abnormalities

      (2) ECG for arrhythmias

   c. Neurological

      (1) Level of consciousness; note signs of hypoxia (e. g., restlessness, disorientation) or signs of hypercapnia (e.g., drowsiness)

      (2) Changes in pupillary size and light reflex

      (3) Abnormal motor and sensory function

   d. Renal

      (1) Increase or decrease in urine output; specific gravity, pH

      (2) Presence of any drainage, for example, ostomies

5. Patient's perception of and reaction to mechanical ventilation and intubation procedure

6. Temperature

7. Weight

8. Results of lab and diagnostic tests

   a. Arterial blood gas values

   b. Electrolyte levels

   c. C and S of blood, tracheobronchial secretions

   d. CBC and differential

e. Hgb and Hct

f. Serum creatinine, BUN, total protein

g. Chest radiograph

h. ECG

i. Bronchoscopy

9. Ventilation system

   a. Position of endotracheal tube

   b. Type of ventilator

   c. Settings

      (1) Oxygen percentage

      (2) V_T

      (3) Inspiratory-expiratory ratio

      (4) Sensitivity

      (5) PEEP

      (6) Airway pressure

      (7) Sigh

      (8) Mechanical dead space

      (9) Flow rate

      (10) Humidity and temperature

      (11) Expiratory retard (if used)

      (12) Rate

10. Patient/family's level of anxiety and understanding of mechanical ventilation and disease process necessitating ventilation

GOALS

1. Reduction of patient/family's anxiety with provision of information, explanations, and encouragement

2. Adequate oxygenation and ventilation with Pa_{O_2} and Pa_{CO_2} levels within patient's normal limits

3. Adequate oxygenation and perfusion of organs and tissues for maximum function

4. Hemodynamic stability

   a. Adequate cardiac output

   b. Normovolemia

   c. Absence of arrhythmias

5. Infection free; absence of pneumonia

6. Electrolytes and blood count results within normal limits

7. Resolution of underlying disease condition necessitating mechanical ventilation

8. Absence of complications associated with mechanical ventilation

9. Ventilator system functioning properly

10. Synchronization of patient's breathing with ventilator

Potential problems	Expected outcomes	Nursing activities

■ Patient/family's anxiety related to
Disease process, diagnostic tests and procedures, therapy
Mechanical ventilation
	■ Reduction of anxiety with provision of sufficient information, explanations, and encouragement	■ Ongoing assessment of level of anxiety, knowledge base, and understanding
		Collaborate with physician in providing
		  Realistic information for patient/family
		  Information relevant to level of understanding
		  Explanation of disease process, diagnostic tests and procedures, therapy
		  Explanation of the need for mechanical ventilation
		Encourage verbalization of questions, fears, and anxieties
		Provide for
		  Patient decisions and participation in care
		  Periods of uninterrupted sleep
		  As much sleep as possible
		  Minimal overstimulation with meaningless noise

Inability to talk	Patient effectively communicates with alternate means	Set up alternate means of communication Relay the alternate means of communication to staff, family; assist in effective use of means Reassure patient that after tube is removed, he/she will be able to talk Encourage patient to speak once tube is removed If appropriate, reassure patient that hoarseness and raspy voice will gradually subside Anticipate patient's needs Reassure and support patient/family Encourage staff/family to communicate with patient Evaluate effectiveness of alternate means of communication Provide ongoing explanation of care

■ Ventilator malfunction	■ Ventilator functioning properly
	Ventilator delivers requisite volume of humified O_2
		■ Ensure that respiratory therapist changes ventilator tubing and evaluates functioning daily
		Monitor for (q2-4 hr)
		  Correct ventilator settings (i.e., V_T, rate, O_2 percentage, sigh)
		  Delivery of correct concentration of O_2
		  Presence of any leaks (humidifier, tubing, endotracheal or tracheal cuff, nebulizer connection)
		  Patency of tubings; note condensation of H_2O in tubing or kinked, compressed, or stretched tubing
		  Functioning and setting of alarm systems (i.e., spirometer, pressure, ratio)
		  Correct temperature of H_2O vapor—95° to 100° F
		  Proper needle movement on pressure gauge
		  Sufficient H_2O content in cascade
		  Secure attachment of O_2 tubing to ventilator
		  Functioning panel light indicators
		If ventilator malfunction occurs and patient is not receiving adequate V_T and/or O_2 concentrations, hand ventilate patient and ask someone to assess the problem; call physical therapist if unable to resolve problem

■ Airway obstruction related to
Thick secretions
 	
Improper positioning of endotracheal tube
Bronchospasm
	■ Airway patency
	
	Effective mobilization of secretions
	Proper positioning of endotracheal tube
	Absence or resolution of bronchospasm
		■ Prevention
		  Administer chest physiotherapy q2 hr unless contraindicated
		  Suction endotracheal/tracheal tube and mouth q1-2 hr for secretions; if secretions are thick, it may be necessary to instill normal saline solution into endotracheal/tracheal tube and infuse more parenteral fluids, as ordered
		  Auscultate lungs to ascertain bilateral expansion q2-4 hr; note decreased or absent sounds or the presence of rales, rhonchi, or wheezing
		  Ensure proper positioning of endotracheal tube; monitor radiograph results for proper tube position

Potential problems	Expected outcomes	Nursing activities
		Monitor for bilateral, full expansion of lungs (by auscultation, observation, and chest radiograph)
		Provide for patency of ventilator tubings, i.e., H_2O accumulation, kinking, compression
		Monitor arterial blood gas levels q3-6 hr and prn until stable
		Place airway or orotracheal tube if patient is biting or gumming on the tube; remind patient not to bite or gum on the tube; reassure and sedate patient if necessary
		If bronchospasm occurs, hand ventilate, relax patient by reassuring and/or administering sedative; administer aminophylline, if needed, as ordered
		If bronchoscopy is necessary, assist with the procedure
■ Excessive accumulation of secretions above endotracheal/tracheal cuff	■ Minimal secretion accumulation above endotracheal/tracheal cuff Absence of tracheal wall irritation	■ Prevent by employing constant oral suction, using oral aspirator or intermittent oropharyngeal suctioning
		For secretions not aspirated by the aforementioned methods, deflate the endotracheal cuff q4-8 hr (more frequently if high-pressure, hard cuffs are used); simultaneously administer vigorous manual ventilations with a breathing bag, and suction oropharynx
		NOTE: This procedure may stimulate the gag reflex in alert patients; in these patients, deflate the cuff and as soon as the secretions reach the trachea, suction them out
■ Accidental extubation	■ Intubation maintained	■ Reassure patient; sedate and/or restrain if necessary
		Position intubation tray and breathing bag nearby
		Keep a spare tracheal tube of the same size and type at the bedside
		If extubation occurs, hand ventilate patient with a mask, and call physician immediately
■ Infection related to Bypass of the normal filtering system (the nose) Breach of aseptic technique for suctioning through tracheal tube Repeated, traumatic intrusive suctioning procedures	■ Infection free Afebrile	■ Prevention Employ sterile technique in suctioning Ensure that ventilator tubing is changed daily Ensure that tracheostomy tube is changed every week Change manual breathing bag at least every 3 days; keep inside plastic container Change position of patient q1-2 hr; administer chest physiotherapy when turning patient to mobilize secretions Frequent oral hygiene
		Monitor TPR, BP q2-4 hr For change in secretions—color, amount, consistency, and odor Results of C and S tests of secretions every 3 days or whenever changes in color and consistency occur
		Notify physician of any abnormality
		If infection occurs Send specimen (e.g., blood, tracheal aspirate, urine) for C and S Administer fluid, antibiotic, and/or antipyretic as ordered Monitor for patient response to therapy
■ Tension pneumothorax	■ Absence or resolution of pneumothorax Full expansion of lungs	■ Monitor Arterial blood gas results For signs and symptoms of tension pneumothorax, including respiratory distress, unequal breath sounds, decreased or distant breath sounds, crepitant rales during inspiration and/or expiration, subcutaneous emphysema, unilateral chest expansion, tracheal deviation, decreased cardiac output and BP, tachycardia, increased CVP, and distended neck veins Chest radiograph results for pneumothorax

Potential problems	Expected outcomes	Nursing activities
		Notify physician of any abnormality
		If tension pneumothorax occurs
		Disconnect patient from ventilator and hand ventilate with self-inflating bag
		Reassure and stay with patient
		Have someone else notify physician immediately; obtain chest tube and chest bottle/chamber setup
		Increase FI_{O_2} to 1.00
		Ensure that chest radiograph is done to confirm diagnosis and after insertion of the chest tube; note radiographic evidence of resolution
		Monitor arterial blood gas results q1-2 hr until stable

■ Fluid overload, weight gain from retention of inspired water vapor
 	
Pulmonary interstitial edema related to fluid overload
	■ Optimum fluid balance Weight remains stable
	
	Absence of pulmonary interstitial edema; Pa_{O_2} level within patient's normal limits
		■ Prevent by
		   Administering fluids as ordered to keep fluid balance parameters within normal limits
		   Ensuring inspired air temperature controlled to 95° to 100° F
		Monitor
		   Daily weights
		   Intake and output q1-2 hr
		Monitor for pulmonary interstitial edema
		   Breath sounds for rales, wheezing
		   Signs/symptoms of hypoxia
		   Chest radiograph for diffuse haziness
		Notify physician for any of these abnormalities
		Administer therapy as ordered, which may include
		   Diuretics, fluid restriction
		   CPAP or PEEP
		   Increased inspired O_2 concentrations

■ Atelectasis	■ Full lung expansion without atelectasis	■ Prevention
		   Ensure that sigh mode is on 4 to 10/hour, if ordered
		   Administer vigorous chest physiotherapy q2-4 hr
		   Turn patient q1-2 hr
		Monitor
		   Arterial blood gas results q3-6 hr for any abnormality until stable
		   TPR and BP q2-4 hr
		   For presence of any abnormal and/or adventitious breath sounds q2-3 hr
		   For altered level of consciousness
		If atelectasis occurs, notify physician and administer therapy as ordered

■ O_2 toxicity related to high inspired O_2 concentrations	■ Absence and/or resolution of O_2 toxicity	■ Progressively decrease FI_{O_2} to below 0.5 within 24 to 48 hours of initiation of mechanical ventilation or institute other remedial measures (i.e., PEEP) to achieve adequate oxygenation, as ordered
		Keep Pa_{O_2} level within patient's normal limits
		Monitor
		   Arterial blood gas results q2-3 hr for any abnormality until stable
		   Results of alveolar-arterial gradient determinations
		   Actual inspired O_2 content
		   Level of consciousness
		Notify physician of any abnormality and institute therapy as ordered

Potential problems	Expected outcomes	Nursing activities

■ Hyperventilation (low Pa_{CO_2} levels)	■ Normal ventilatory rate with values for Pa_{CO_2} within patient's normal limits	■ Prevent by
		  Providing frequent reassurance and explanations
		  Administering medications for pain and/or sedation if needed, as ordered
		Monitor
		  Respiratory rate, quality for tachypnea, dyspnea
		  Arterial blood gas results q2-3 hr until stable
		If hyperventilation occurs, notify physician; therapy is symptomatic
		  Administer sedation if needed, as ordered
		  Add dead space if patient is not breathing spontaneously
		  Decrease V_T and rate if ordered
		  Administer medication to paralyze patient if needed, as ordered

■ Hypoventilation (high Pa_{CO_2} levels)	■ Ventilatory rate and Pa_{CO_2} levels within patient's normal limits
	Full lung expansion by auscultation, observation, and chest radiograph
		■ Monitor
		  Respiratory rate q½-1 hr
		  Arterial blood gas results for hypercapnia
		  Breath sounds for decreased or absent sounds; presence of rales, rhonchi, or wheezes
		If hypoventilation occurs, notify physician; therapy is symptomatic
		  Increase V_T and rate as ordered
		  Augment chest physiotherapy as needed

■ Transient hypotension related to
  Increased intrathoracic pressures associated with mechanical ventilation (and PEEP if used)
  Hypovolemia
	■ Hemodynamic stability
	BP within patient's normal limits
		■ Monitor
		  BP, CVP, and urine volume q2 hr and prn
		  Arterial blood gas results for any abnormality q2-3 hr until stable
		If transient hypotension occurs, notify physician
		  Administer fluids and/or inotropic agents, i.e., digoxin and/or dopamine as ordered; closely monitor patient's response
		  Reassure patient

■ GI malfunction related to stress ulcers and bleeding	■ Absence of GI distress, malfunction	■ Prevent by administering antacid and/or milk as ordered, particularly to patients with NG tubes and those prone to increased anxiety
		Encourage and support patient; sedate if needed, as ordered
		Administer tube feeding if ordered
		Monitor for
		  Decreased Hgb and Hct daily
		  Positive Hematest results from NG aspirate and stool
		If GI malfunction occurs, notify physician of any abnormality and administer therapy as ordered

■ Hypoxia—inadequate oxygenation	■ Adequate oxygenation	■ Monitor
		  For signs and symptoms of hypoxia, including change in personality, decreased judgment, headache, restlessness, lack of concentration, paranoia, tachycardia, tachypnea, sudden increase in BP, cardiac arrhythmias, and cyanosis
		  For signs of respiratory distress
		  For adequate oxygenation; monitor Pa_{O_2} levels
		  Arterial blood gas results 15 to 20 minutes after any change in ventilator settings; note concurrent signs of adequate oxygenation
		If hypoxia occurs, notify physician and administer therapy as ordered

Potential problems	Expected outcomes	Nursing activities
■ Renal failure related to Decreased cardiac output associated with use of positive pressures Increased production of antidiuretic hormone	■ Absence and/or resolution of renal failure	■ Ensure adequate hydration as ordered Monitor Vital signs and temperature q2 hr CVP, PAP q1-2 hr and prn; cardiac output measurements, if available Urine output q1-2 hr; note oliguria Daily weights for weight gain Electrolyte levels q6-12 hr until stable Notify physician of any abnormality If renal failure occurs, administer therapy as ordered; see Standard: *Acute renal failure*
■ Pressure sores on side of mouth, nose, and tracheotomy site Hyperplasia and inflammation, scarring and stenosis of trachea due to trauma of endotracheal/tracheal tube	■ Minimal trauma caused by endotracheal/tracheal tube	■ Prevention Change tape that secures tube daily and as necessary Support tubing and maintain tracheal tube in proper alignment Reposition endotracheal tube from side to side of mouth daily Assist with change of tracheal tube every 7 days Change tracheotomy dressings q2-4 hr and as necessary; clean skin around tube Monitor for presence of sores on mouth and around tracheotomy site If trauma occurs, reevaluate preventive measures employed and alter regimen if needed, as ordered Administer supportive care as ordered
■ Tracheal esophageal fistula (TE fistula) and tracheal stenosis (ischemia, inflammation, and eventual narrowing of the orifice) related to Use of high-pressure cuffs Inadequate cuff care Concurrent presence of NG tube, resulting in pressure on the tracheoesophageal membrane from both sides	■ Adequate cuff care Absence of TE fistula and tracheal stenosis	■ Ensure use of low-pressure cuff on endotracheal/tracheal tube Inflate cuff so as to permit an air leak around cuff during sigh inspirations Monitor cuff pressure q4-8 hr; cuff pressure should not exceed 30 mm Hg Maintain cuff pressure at less than 30 mm Hg, lower if possible, with a minimal leak; remove NG tube as soon as feasible, as ordered Monitor contrast chest radiograph results for presence of TE fistula and tracheal stenosis Notify physician for presence of any of the aforementioned, and implement therapy as ordered

7 □ Positive end expiratory pressure

Positive end expiratory pressure (PEEP) therapy is designed as an adjunct to mechanical ventilation to maintain a prescribed amount of pressure in the patient-ventilator system at the end of each expiration. It is used to achieve adequate alveolar expansion in patients with ate-lectasis or pulmonary interstitial edema. Maintaining alveolar expansion helps to prevent shunting of blood through unventilated areas of lungs, thus providing an optimal ventilation/perfusion ratio for gas exchange in an already compromised environment. The increased volume of interstitial fluid is shifted to the intravascular space, thus reducing the diffusion distance between the alveolar membrane and the pulmonary capillary. Oxygenation is therefore enhanced.

PEEP levels are titrated to achieve adequate oxygenation without a diminution of venous return and subsequent decrease in cardiac output. As the physiologic problems requiring PEEP therapy subside, progressively lower levels of PEEP are required for adequate oxygenation.

Low levels of PEEP (3 to 5 cm water pressure) can be used prophylactically to promote alveolar patency in patients with borderline pulmonary status.

During PEEP therapy the patient's arterial blood gas levels are monitored for adequate oxygenation. Circulatory parameters are simultaneously monitored for signs of reduced cardiac output.

ASSESSMENT

1. History to include
   a. Presence of physiologic problems frequently associated with respiratory compromise
      (1) Surgery
      (2) Heart failure
      (3) Shock
      (4) Sepsis
      (5) Pulmonary trauma
      (6) Acute pancreatitis
   b. Relative contraindications to PEEP therapy, for example
      (1) Chronic lung disease
      (2) Bullous lung disease
         (3) Hypotension
         (4) Pneumothorax
2. Respiratory function
   a. Respirations—rate, depth, quality
   b. Secretions—amount, color, consistency
   c. Breath sounds
   d. Signs of adequate oxygenation, particularly color
   e. Inspection of thorax for abnormalities
   f. Blood gas values
   g. Chest radiograph results
   h. Inflation pressures
   i. Lung compliance
   j. Alveolar-arterial oxygen gradient
3. Circulatory parameters
   a. BP, P
   b. CVP and PAP, if available
   c. Urine output
   d. Peripheral circulation
   e. Weight
4. Level of patient/family's anxiety regarding PEEP therapy and aspects of mechanical ventilation, including inability to talk

GOALS

1. Adequate oxygenation, with arterial oxygen levels within patient's normal limits
2. Delivery of prescribed levels of PEEP
3. Absence or resolution of potential complications associated with use of PEEP
4. Reduction in patient/family's anxiety with provision of information and encouragement

Potential problems	Expected outcomes	Nursing activities
■ Patient/family's anxiety related to Hospitalization Disease process Intubation and consequent inability to talk Prolonged immobilization	■ Reduction in level of anxiety with provision of information, explanations, and encouragement	■ Ongoing assessment of level of anxiety Stay with the patient or reassure patient that nurse will be close at hand Provide for alternate means of communication Explain disease process and need for intubation and use of PEEP Encourage patient/family's questions and communication of anxiety or fears related to inability to talk, course of therapy, and so on Encourage participation in care as tolerated Perform treatments in an unhurried manner, allowing rest periods between treatments Provide comfort measures
■ Inadequate oxygenation	■ Adequate oxygenation Pa_{O_2} 80 to 100 mm Hg Clear sensorium Good color Good peripheral circulation	■ Monitor Serial blood gas results for hypoxemia Color, sensorium, peripheral circulation for signs of hypoxia For signs and symptoms of hypoxia—restlessness, headache, change in personality, loss of judgment-making ability, lack of concentration, tachycardia, cardiac arrhythmias, tachypnea, and sudden elevation in BP; late signs include cyanosis, bradycardia, hypotension, and unconsciousness

Potential problems	Expected outcomes	Nursing activities
		Select correct level of PEEP by Serial measurement of arterial O_2 levels (Pa_{O_2}) Volume of shunted blood in lungs (Qs/Qt) Capillary O_2 levels (Ca_{O_2}) Mixed venous blood O_2 levels Adequacy of cardiac output (by direct measurements and by BP, P, peripheral circulation, sensorium, urine output)
■ Inadequate oxygenation related to inadequate levels of PEEP	■ Adequate levels of PEEP	■ Monitor for Intact ventilatory-PEEP system; correct leaks if they occur Expiratory pressures on ventilator for maintenance of prescribed PEEP; adjust PEEP dial as needed Patient resistance to PEEP and patient anxiety; explain procedure and reassure patient as needed Administer light sedation if necessary, as ordered
■ Inadequate oxygenation related to worsening pulmonary interstitial edema	■ Resolution of pulmonary interstitial edema Fl_{O_2} progressively decreased to 0.4 PEEP no longer needed Extubation Clear chest radiograph *Secondary:* diminution of total body water	■ Monitor For maintenance of prescribed PEEP levels Daily weights for gain or loss For adventitious breath sounds Results of serial chest radiographs Arterial blood gas results for low Pa_{O_2} levels Progression of inspiratory pressures (become higher as interstitial edema worsens) If problem occurs Provide for maintenance of prescribed PEEP levels; increase if needed, as ordered Administer diuretics as ordered to decrease total body H_2O
■ Patient incoordination with ventilator Positive pressure maintained throughout expiration is not natural so the patient may resist it (often called ''bucking'' the ventilator) With higher levels of PEEP, pain is often felt in the intercostal region; pain and fear cause sympathetic stimulation, which increases O_2 requirements in an already hypoxic patient	■ Patient breathes in coordination with the ventilator Patient relaxed, calm	■ Prevent by Explaining procedure, what patient will experience Talking with and reassuring patient during PEEP therapy Sedating patient only if necessary, as ordered Changing sensitivity or flow rate on ventilator if indicated Monitor For patient incoordination with ventilator system; patient breathing out of sequence with ventilator breaths For low and varying V_T (in the absence of an intermittent mandatory ventilation system) Apparent patient resistance to ventilator breaths For factors contributing to patient restlessness, such as Hypoxia (monitor for signs and symptoms of; arterial blood gas results indicating hypoxemia) Acid-base imbalance (monitor serum electrolyte levels, arterial blood gas results for acidosis or alkalosis) Fears and anxieties (see Problem, Patient/family's anxiety) Pain Frustration because of inability to talk during intubation Notify physician of these abnormalities If patient incoordination with ventilator occurs Talk with patient; reassure and comfort him/her Reevaluate sensitivity settings and flow rates; make appropriate alterations Employ a system for intermittent mandatory ventilation to allow patient to breath spontaneously from a reservoir of humidified, oxygenated air with the addition of a predetermined number of mandatory breaths per minute, if ordered Administer sedation if needed, as ordered

Potential problems	Expected outcomes	Nursing activities
■ Decreased cardiac output with hypotension Hypotension may occur with initiation of or an increase in the level of PEEP; it reflects decreased venous return caused by the additional positive intrathoracic pressure; the sympathetic nervous system is stimulated, causing vasoconstriction and an elevation of BP; if the patient is hypovolemic, the sympathetic stimulation may be insufficient to elevate the BP to a physiological range	■ Adequate cardiac output Hemodynamic stability Adequate venous return Adequate pulmonary blood flow Adequate blood flow to kidneys	■ Prevent by instituting PEEP in gradual increments Monitor for signs of reduced cardiac output (hypotension, tachycardia, elevated CVP, oliguria, signs of reduced peripheral circulation) when PEEP initiated or when increments in PEEP levels are made Notify physician if any of the aforementioned occur If decreased cardiac output with hypotension occurs Increase levels of PEEP in smaller increments and over longer intervals of time Administer fluid and/or a cardiotonic/inotropic agent if ordered, and closely monitor patient's response
■ Hyperventilation, indicated by hypocapnia (low Pa_{CO_2}); occurs as a result of high inspired minute ventilation	■ Optimal Pa_{CO_2} and minute ventilation	■ Prevent by Explaining procedure to patient Calming and reassuring patient Monitor R q15-30 min for tachypnea Arterial blood gas levels for hypocapnia For patient resistance to ventilatory pressures being maintained If problem occurs Reassure and calm patient Administer light sedation if necessary Add "dead space" tubing to ventilatory system to elevate Pa_{CO_2} levels if necessary, as ordered
■ Atelectasis related to Immobility Primarily constant volume ventilation Secretions that tend to remain in periphery of lung because of high mean airway pressures	■ No atelectasis by auscultation or radiograph Full lung expansion as measured by pulmonary function tests	■ Prevent by administering vigorous pulmonary toilet, including Turn patient q1-2hr Chest physiotherapy q2-4 hr Monitor R for tachypnea, dyspnea Breath sounds for localized decrease, dullness, and adventitious sounds Chest radiograph results for signs indicating atelectasis Arterial blood gas results for hypoxemia If atelectasis occurs Increase chest physiotherapy to affected areas Assist patient with coughing and deep breathing Administer humidified O_2 to liquefy secretions and to achieve adequate oxygenation
■ Pneumothorax related to high alveolar pressures When the walls of the alveoli cannot withstand the positive pressure, perforation may occur; air leaks into the pleural space causing a pneumothorax, into the mediastinum, and/or into the subcutaneous spaces	■ Absence of pneumothorax Full lung expansion by auscultation, chest radiograph, and clinical examination	■ Prevent by Maintaining the minimum PEEP levels necessary for adequate oxygenation Employing an intermittent mandatory ventilation system to reduce mean intrathoracic pressures as ordered Monitor for signs and symptoms of pneumothorax Sudden sharp chest pain; pleuritic pain Anxiety, diaphoresis Dyspnea Asymmetrical chest movements Diminished or absent breath sounds on affected side Tachycardia with weak pulse

Potential problems	Expected outcomes	Nursing activities
		Vertigo, pallor
		Cyanosis, hypotension
		Chest radiograph results indicating a pneumothorax
		Notify physician if any of the aforementioned occur
		If a pneumothorax occurs
		Monitor for resolution of a small pneumothorax
		Assist with insertion of chest tube and monitor for air bubbling in the drainage chamber/bottle as it is drawn from the chest; monitor for resolution of pneumothorax by noting alleviation of respiratory distress and less asymmetrical-chest movement on the affected side; breath sounds become less resonant and distant, and chest radiograph shows resolution
■ Mediastinal emphysema	■ Absence of mediastinal emphysema or widened mediastinum on chest radiograph	■ Monitor
		Chest radiograph results revealing widened mediastinum
		Breath sounds for decreased lung expansion
	Full lung expansion by auscultation and chest radiograph	For signs and symptoms of respiratory distress associated with a decrease in lung volume
		For signs of reduced cardiac output and impaired venous return that may result from mediastinal emphysema
		Notify physician for any of these abnormalities
■ Subcutaneous emphysema	■ Absence of subcutaneous emphysema	■ Monitor for air accumulation under skin, elevation of skin, "cracking" sound when skin is pressed
	Full lung expansion by auscultation and chest radiograph	Notify physician if any of the aforementioned occur
		If subcutaneous emphysema occurs, the air usually resorbs without treatment; if emphysema is marked, subcutaneous needles may be inserted to release some of the air

8 □ Chest physiotherapy

Chest physiotherapy is a coordinated series of actions consisting of manipulations designed to prevent and/or reduce respiratory complications. Chest physiotherapy also improves pulmonary function in patients with acute and chronic respiratory diseases.

This coordinated series of manipulative actions (percussion and vibration) instituted to each lung segment with the aid of gravity and coughing can mobilize secretions from a peripheral portion of the lungs into the large bronchi where they can be coughed out or removed by suctioning.

In *percussion*, cupped hands lightly strike the chest wall in a rhythmical fashion with wrists alternately flexed and extended. A linen or towel is placed over the segment of the chest that is being cupped to prevent discomfort. The sudden compression of air between the hand and the chest wall during percussion produces an energy wave that is transmitted through the chest wall tissues to the lung tissue. This energy wave helps to dislodge adherent mucous plugs and moves them toward the main bronchus or trachea where they can be easily coughed out or suctioned.

Vibration is accomplished by placing hands on the chest wall and producing a rapid vibratory motion in the arms while gently compressing the chest wall. This aids in mobilizing secretions to the main bronchus or trachea. It is performed on exhalation after a deep inhalation.

Coughing is a pulmonary defense mechanism that aids in effective mobilization of retained secretions. Cough is utilized after percussion and/or vibration. Instructions on effective coughing begin with proper breathing exercises followed by the mechanical components of coughing. The sequence starts with a deep breath, an inspiratory pause, and glottic closure. These actions result in increased intrathoracic pressure and expectoration of secretions when the glottis opens. Sterile suctioning is utilized if the patient is unable to cough.

Postural drainage is accomplished with the aid of gravity by different body positions. Because of the variability and complexity of the tracheobronchial branching, practical postural drainage positions are best limited to areas of the lungs that commonly retain secretions. Precautions are to be considered when applying postural drainage to patients with recent myocardial infarction, postoperative neurosurgical patients, and in patients with known intracranial disease, recent spinal fusion, and/or skin graft. Techniques of postural drainage will depend on the physician's/therapist's clinical evaluation.

SEQUENCE OF THERAPY
For intubated patient

1. Auscultate to assess affected areas requiring therapy
2. Administer pain medication if needed, as ordered
3. Suction endotracheal tube and mouth
4. Position according to location of involved area and condition of patient
5. Percuss involved area for 2 minutes
6. Sigh patient two to three times
7. Vibrate on exhalation; do vibrations five times after each exhalation
8. Suction endotracheal tube
9. Auscultate lungs for evaluation of therapy

For nonintubated patient

1. Give instructions to patient on effective deep breathing and coughing exercises
2. Auscultate to assess affected areas requiring therapy
3. Administer pain medication if needed, as ordered
4. Position according to location of involved area and condition of patient
5. Percuss involved area for approximately 2 minutes
6. Instruct patient to inhale deeply, and as he/she exhales, vibrate the chest wall; do vibrations five times after each exhalation
7. Instruct patient to cough
8. If patient is unable to cough effectively, do nasotracheal suctioning
9. Auscultate lungs for evaluation of therapy

ASSESSMENT

1. Pulmonary status—quality of breath sounds, existence of full lung expansion, significance of abnormal breath sounds, and areas of pulmonary tree with abnormal or absent breath sounds
2. Presence of disease or conditions
   a. That indicate the need for chest physiotherapy, that is, COPD, pneumonia, acute atelectasis, lung abscess, bronchiectasis, cystic fibrosis, and ventilator care; postoperative patients and patients who have been on prolonged bed rest
   b. That necessitate caution in administering chest physiotherapy, that is, recent myocardial infarction, increased tendency to bronchospasm, neurological conditions, spinal fusion, and/or a skin graft
   c. That contraindicate physiotherapy, that is, hypotension, unstable vital signs, dialysis, severe bleeding from esophageal varices, medical and surgical catastrophies
3. Results of lab and diagnostic tests, including
   a. Arterial blood gas levels
   b. Prothrombin time
   c. Chest radiograph
   d. ECG
4. Ability of patient to tolerate modified chest physiotherapy positions

GOALS

1. Optimal efficiency and distribution of ventilation/perfusion
2. Effective mobilization of secretions
3. Arterial blood gas and chest radiograph results within patient's normal limits
4. Hemodynamic stability; absence of arrhythmias
5. Infection free; absence of pneumonia

Potential problems	Expected outcomes	Nursing activities
■ Anxiety related to limited understanding of therapy	■ Patient verbalizes understanding of therapy Patient's behavior indicates reduction in anxiety with provision of information, explanations, and encouragement	■ Ongoing assessment of level of anxiety and understanding Explain procedure and reassure patient Provide time for and encourage questions Administer pain medication 30 minutes before therapy if needed, as ordered Position for therapy, ensuring minimal discomfort If patient is unable to tolerate percussion, do vibration only

■ Retention of secretions	■ Effective mobilization of secretions
	Absence of atelectasis
		■ Auscultate affected areas
		Percuss affected area effectively
		  Maintain straight alignment of patient's body; support with pillows prn
		  Stand so that patient is facing you
		  Use muscle of shoulder and with cupped hands strike chest wall lightly in a rhythmical fashion, flexing wrists
		  Minimize tension of muscles in forearms
		  Produce a hollow sound without causing pain to the patient
		Vibrate effectively
		  Place hand flat over segments that have just been percussed
		  Rhythmically tense and relax muscles of wrist and forearm (isometric movement) during exhalation
		  Instruct patient to take two to three deep breaths and cough; deliver a sigh ventilation to intubated patients
		Instruct patient to cough out secretions; if patient is unable to do this, suction patient nasotracheally; suction intubated patients

■ Arrhythmias	■ Absence of arrhythmias Regular pulse rate	■ Avoid head-down position If ECG monitor is being used, increase audibility of QRS beeps and observe for arrhythmias Monitor BP and P intermittently during procedure until patient toleration is established If arterial line is in situ, set alarm limits closely and monitor BP during therapy Notify physician for significant incidence of arrhythmias Avoid percussion and emphasize vibration If problem occurs, see Standard: *Arrhythmias* Obtain ECG monitor if one is not already in use

CARDIOVASCULAR

9 □ Angina pectoris

Angina is chest pain or discomfort that results from an imbalance of myocardial oxygen supply and demand. The myocardial need for oxygen may increase, as with exercise, excitement, ingestion of a heavy meal, or exposure to cold; or the supply may decrease, as with progressive atherosclerotic coronary heart disease. Angina is often the first clinical manifestation of coronary heart disease. However the term *angina* should not imply etiology, for it may also be the result of severe ventricular hypertrophy due to aortic stenosis or regurgitation, coronary arteritis, coronary ostial stenosis, and anemia. Angina can appear abruptly or gradually. It can precede or follow an acute myocardial infarction (AMI). It does not always progress to myocardial infarction (MI), although specific patterns may be a warning and preinfarction angina may or may not continue following infarction.

Since myocardial metabolism is primarily aerobic and 70% to 80% of oxygen is extracted by the myocardium, increased blood flow is necessary to increase oxygen supply. Blood flow to the myocardium occurs predominantly in diastole and is determined by cardiac output, diastolic arterial pressure, coronary artery resistance, and intramyocardial pressure. The major determinants of myocardial oxygen consumption (MVO_2) are heart rate, systolic blood pressure, ventricular volume (myocardial tension), and the contractile state.

Angina that occurs with a changing pattern in terms of frequency, severity, precipitating factors, and response to rest and nitroglycerin has been given different names including *unstable angina, crescendo angina, preinfarction angina* and the *intermediate syndrome. Decubitus angina pectoris* is that which occurs at rest without any identifiable precipitating cause, and *nocturnal angina* is that which awakens a patient from sleep. *Prinzmetal's angina,* or *atypical angina,* is a variant form, which may occur in the absence of exertion and may not respond promptly to rest and nitroglycerin. ECG changes also differ from "typical" angina.

Causes of chest discomfort from which angina needs to be differentiated include anxiety; disorders involving the bony skeleton, joints, and skeletal muscle; pulmonary problems; esophageal disorders; pericarditis; Dressler's syndrome; and AMI.

Management of angina is directed toward minimizing the imbalance between oxygen supply and demand. When the patient's condition is stable, this includes use of medications such as nitroglycerin, long-acting nitrites, and propranolol; vagal stimulation; and avoidance of provoking situations and/or use of prophylactic medication. Also to be included are correction of factors known to aggravate or accelerate angina such as smoking, obesity, hypertension, and anemia.

Management of unstable angina is more aggressive, since the course is unpredictable. This includes hospitalization, often in a coronary care unit, ECG monitoring, drug therapy, diagnostic tests such as coronary arteriography and, more and more frequently, coronary artery bypass grafting (CABG). Indications for surgery are still evolving, but usually if coronary arteriography verifies occlusion greater than 75% of one (particularly a left main stem artery lesion) or more arteries coupled with failure of aggressive medical treatment to control pain or if the angina is significantly altering the patient's lifestyle, bypass surgery is recommended.

Usually angina is seen in critical care units when it has progressed to an unstable state, if arrhythmias develop, or when it is associated with another disease requiring critical care.

ASSESSMENT

1. History of angina, hypertension, MI, left ventricular failure, aortic valve disease, or anemia
2. Patient profile, including risk factors and information regarding life-style, habits, and emotions
3. Patient's perception of and reaction to diagnosis, progression of disease, and assessment and treatment modalities
4. Precise history and description of chest pain or discomfort
   a. Location, radiation, quality

b. Duration

c. Frequency

d. Precipitating factors and any recent changes

e. Relief mechanisms and any recent changes

f. Indicators of progression

5. Presence of other symptoms with episodes of pain

6. Evaluation of hemodynamic status

7. Monitor ECG for
   a. Changes characteristic of angina or Prinzmetal's angina
   b. Arrhythmias

8. Lab data results if indicated
   a. Chest radiograph
   b. Coronary arteriography
   c. Left ventriculography
   d. Exercise ECG test

9. Signs and symptoms of complications
   a. AMI
   b. Left heart failure
   c. Arrhythmias

10. Ongoing and final evaluation of effectiveness of teaching program

11. Determinants of patient compliance

GOALS

1. Absence and/or control of pain or discomfort and any associated symptoms

2. Hemodynamic stability

3. Maintenance of optimal activity level

4. Patient's behavior demonstrates reduction of anxiety with provision of information

5. Before discharge the patient/family
   a. Demonstrates comprehension of the knowledge components of the teaching program when evaluated by testing or questioning
   b. Identifies own risk factors and of those agreed on by health care team and patient, describes methods of modification
   c. Identifies own precipitating factors and/or those that frequently precipitate angina and describes appropriate action to take to avoid or treat prophylactically
   d. Lists methods for monitoring activity—demonstrates accurately skill of counting pulse, identifying own maximal heart rate
   e. Describes symptoms requiring immediate medical attention and those suggesting disease progression that should be reported to the physician within 48 to 72 hours
   f. States necessary information for compliance with discharge regimen
      (1) Medications
      (2) Follow-up

Potential problems	Expected outcomes	Nursing activities
■ Chest pain or discomfort related to ischemic myocardium	■ Verbalizes relief and/or absence of pain Absence of associated symptoms	■ Minimize discrepancy between O_2 supply and demand Provide periods of rest Regulate activities of patient and health care team as condition allows Determine visitor preferences with patient if unit policy allows Maintain comfortable, quiet environment Avoid heavy meals Prophylactic use of medication as ordered Assist patient in recognition of precipitating events and control if possible by avoidance or prophylactic use of medication; lower doses are usually required for prevention than for treatment Assess for verbal and nonverbal cues indicating presence of chest pain or discomfort; patient may refer to vague sensations or aches; instruct patient to inform nurse immediately when pain occurs Maintain patent IV line Administer O_2 as ordered If patient is admitted with unstable angina, generally treat as an AMI until ruled out; see Standard: *Acute myocardial infarction* If problem occurs Obtain clear description of chest pain, including Location, radiation: most often located in retrosternal region; may radiate to neck, jaw, clavicles, shoulders,

Potential problems	Expected outcomes	Nursing activities

		arms, and/or epigastrium; may be located only in areas of radiation without affecting retrosternal region
		Quality: may be described as pressure, heaviness, squeezing, smothering, burning, or indigestion; varying intensity from mild to severe
		Duration: usually lasts only 3 to 5 minutes; check carefully for change
		Precipitating factors: identify and compare to prior history; note particularly if these occur at rest or at a lower oxygen-expending activity
		Response to relief mechanism: usually relieved by rest and/or nitrites within 15 minutes
		Check heart rate and BP during episode of pain; there may be an initial rise in systolic BP in an attempt to compensate
		Assess for presence of associated symptoms
		  Dyspnea
		  Weakness, fatigue
		  Palpitations
		  Dizziness or near syncope
		Monitor ECG for
		  Characteristic S-T segment depression and inversion of T waves (not always seen)
		  Prinzmetal's angina: S-T segments may be elevated indicative of epicardial "injury current"
		  Arrhythmias
		Administer medications as ordered
		  Vasodilators and/or analgesics
		  1. Drug doses should be increased in increments as long as patient continues to have pain; response to therapy, type and dose, should be communicated to physician and recorded
		  2. Have patient in supine or semi-Fowler's position
		  3. Check BP at 1, 5, and 10 minutes after administration of medication for hypotension
		  4. Observe for and/or elicit from patient presence of headache, nausea, and vomiting, vertigo, and/or flushing of the skin; if necessary, give aspirin to increase headache threshold
		Maintain bed rest until pain pattern resolves
		If angina persists with minimal activity or after AMI, special studies may be ordered to assess potential candidacy for CABG; see Standards: *Cardiac catheterization; Cardiac surgery*

■ Anxiety related to
  Diagnosis and awareness of being "victim of heart disease" or that disease is progressing
  Pain and limited activity tolerance
  Uncertainties about future
  Diagnostic tests
  Pending surgery
  Other
	■ Verbalizes anxiety and/or fears
	Asks questions
	Behavior demonstrates decreased anxiety with provision of information and opportunities to ventilate feelings
		■ Continuous assessment of verbal and nonverbal clues of anxiety; attempt to identify source
		Assess relationship of anxiety to pain; role of anxiety as precipitating factor
		Provide information to patient/family regarding diagnosis, pain, and diagnostic procedures
		Encourage questions from patient/family
		Provide opportunities for patient to ventilate fears and discuss future management
		Explain purpose of and expectations from invasive studies if indicated; remember that patients generally want to know if it will hurt, how long it will take, what to expect
		If surgery is indicated, see Standard: *Cardiac surgery*
		Sedate if necessary and as ordered

Potential problems	Expected outcomes	Nursing activities
■ Hemodynamic instability related to left heart failure—some abnormalities of left heart function may occur transiently with ischemic episodes	■ Hemodynamic stability Absence of left heart failure	■ Check BP, P, and R q2 hr and with episodes of pain Observe for signs and symptoms of heart failure 　Dyspnea 　Fatigue 　Rales 　S_3 gallop 　Sinus tachycardia; if present differentiate from relationship to pain or anxiety 　Presence of interstitial edema on chest radiograph Inform physician of abnormalities If propranolol is being administered for angina, reevaluate its use with physician if indications of heart failure develop; may be contraindicated because of negative inotropic effect If problem occurs, see Standard: *Heart failure*
■ Arrhythmias	■ Absence of arrhythmias	■ Continuous monitoring of ECG for presence of arrhythmias; serious ventricular arrhythmias and AV block are common complications of Prinzmetal's angina Relate occurrence to pain Assess for presence of associated symptoms such as palpitations If problem occurs, see Standard: *Arrhythmias*
■ AMI	■ Absence of AMI	■ Differentiate pain of angina from that of AMI 　May or may not be more severe 　Duration longer than 20 minutes, although difficult to evaluate since pain is to be treated promptly 　Does not respond to nitroglycerin; requires analgesic 　Often accompanied by sense of impending doom or acute anxiety 　Associated symptoms often present Monitor daily 12 lead ECG for changes suggestive of myocardial infarction (MI) If AMI is suspected, serum enzymes should be evaluated for characteristic changes If problem occurs, see Standard: *Acute myocardial infarction*
■ Decreased activity tolerance	■ Maintenance of optimal activity level	■ Assess for indications of decreasing activity tolerance 　Lower levels of activity provoke onset of angina, increased pulse rate, and/or decrease in systolic BP 　3 to 5 minutes before, during, and immediately after (within 1 minute) activity, check P, BP, ECG for arrhythmias and for presence of symptoms indicative of intolerance; if changes occur, have patient cease activity and immediately provide rest and/or nitroglycerin 　Compare pulse in early evening to that on awakening for indications of cumulative stress; increased at rest Alternate periods of rest and activity 　Avoid activity for 1 hour after meals; remember that activities done to patient, e.g., bathing, often result in increased activity by patient 　Maintain level below anginal threshold; use nitroglycerin prophylactically if indicated, as ordered 　Administer long-acting nitrites as ordered When patient's condition is stabilized, gradually increase activity and record and report indices of tolerance

Potential problems	Expected outcomes	Nursing activities
		If prolonged bed rest is required, use preventive measures to avoid complications of increased immobility Passive/active range of motion (ROM) exercises Ensure that patient deep breathes q1 hr Ensure that patient changes position at least q2 hr Apply elastic or support stockings
■ Insufficient knowledge and skill to comply with discharge regimen	■ Evaluation by testing or questioning demonstrates patient/family's understanding of the knowledge components of the teaching program Asks pertinent questions regarding self-care	■ Institute teaching program for patient/family, including Nature and significance of angina
	Identifies own risk factors and of those agreed on by health care team and patient, describes methods of modification	Discussion of risk factors Meaning of risk factors Identification of patient's own risk factors Cost-benefit ratio of modification Methods of modification and sources of support
	Identifies own precipitating factors and/or those which frequently precipitate angina; describes appropriate action to take to avoid or treat prophylactically	Common precipitating factors of angina with emphasis on patient's own precipitating factors Activity Emotional stress Ingestion of a heavy meal Extremes of temperature Sexual activity Discussion of activities or situations to avoid and/or prophylactic use of nitroglycerin
	Lists methods for monitoring activity; demonstrates accurately skill of counting pulse, identifying own maximal heart rate	Importance of regulating activity to keep below threshold of angina Method of counting own pulse Identification of maximal heart rate Work simplification techniques
	Describes symptoms requiring immediate medical attention and those suggesting disease progression that should be reported to the physician within 48 to 72 hours	Symptoms requiring immediate medical attention Symptoms suggesting progression of disease to be reported to physician within 48 to 72 hours
	States necessary information for compliance with discharge regimen Medications Follow-up	Information regarding discharge medications Name and purpose Dosage Frequency Prophylactic use Storage Side effects Prophylactic use of aspirin to control headaches Follow-up information Provide opportunities for patient/family to ask questions and practice palpating pulse Assess patient/family's potential compliance

10 □ Acute myocardial infarction

Myocardial infarction (MI) is death of myocardial cells resulting from impaired coronary blood flow. The impairment is most frequently the result of atherosclerosis. The area of necrosis or infarction may be small and focal or large and diffuse. Generally the infarct does not involve the cells uniformly. It is thought that there is a central area of necrosis (nonviable tissue) surrounded by injured tissue that is viable if adequate circulation is reestablished but which will otherwise become necrotic. Current therapeutic research is directed toward salvaging this tissue, thereby limiting the size of infarcts. Surrounding this injured tissue is ischemic tissue, which is viable (assuming no further infarction) but "irritable" and may be the source of some of the arrhythmias that follow the acute event.

The hemodynamic consequences of infarction range from minimal changes in left ventricular function reflected by minimal changes in the left ventricular end diastolic filling pressure and cardiac output to major elevations of left ventricular end diastolic filling pressures with low cardiac output and blood pressure. In addition, any challenge to a compromised myocardium such as arrhythmias, hypertension, pain, and anxiety may tip the balance and result in rapid deterioration.

Healing begins immediately as the body's defense mechanisms mobilize to remove the "debris." In general necrotic tissue is replaced with young granulation tissue between the first and second weeks postinfarction; then this is replaced by fibrous tissue during the next few weeks and finally becomes a scar within 2 to 3 months.

Most key areas of the heart receive blood either from a dual arterial supply or from a coronary artery with important secondary sources. The site of infarction depends on which coronary artery is obstructed. Generally, obstruction of the left anterior descending coronary artery results in an anterior or anteroseptal MI affecting the apical portion of the anterior wall of the left ventricle and/or the contiguous portion of the ventricular septum. Obstruction of the left circumflex coronary artery produces a lateral MI affecting the lateral wall of the left ventricle, and obstruction of the right coronary artery produces an inferior MI that involves the inferior wall and contiguous septum. Infarctions of the atria and right ventricle are uncommon; therefore site classification refers to the left ventricle.

The terms *subendocardial* and *transmural* describe the amount of muscle wall involved at the site. A subendocardial infarction is one that is confined to a restricted segment of the myocardium, usually muscle in the endocardial half of the left ventricular wall. A transmural infarction is one that involves the entire (or almost entire) thickness of the muscle in the involved segment, that is, goes through the wall.

The diagnosis of MI is based on a characteristic clinical history, ECG changes, and enzyme elevations. If any one of these is positive, it warrants the patient being treated for a MI unless or until it is ruled out.

The characteristic clinical history is that of pain lasting longer than 20 to 30 minutes unrelieved by rest or nitroglycerin. Associated symptoms of dyspnea, nausea and vomiting, weakness, diaphoresis, and palpitations may or may not be present. Often the patient describes a sense of impending doom, and some degree of anxiety is present. In some cases pain is slight or absent altogether.

There are three types of characteristic ECG changes which may be seen: alterations of the QRS complexes, elevations of S-T segments, and serial T wave changes. S-T segment and T wave changes are thought to be related to the areas of injury and ischemia surrounding necrotic tissue. Alterations of the QRS complex include developing significant Q waves in leads facing the area of infarction or diminishing or disappearing R waves in one or more of the precordial leads. The exception is a true posterior infarction that usually produces broad R waves in the right precordial leads, V_1 and V_2. S-T segment elevation is temporary, occurring acutely in leads facing the area of infarction, usually with reciprocal S-T segment depression in the opposite leads. S-T segment depression that occurs for several days in all leads except aV_R suggests a subendocardial infarction. The serial T wave changes occur over several days. Initially they may be positive or biphasic, becoming negative in leads facing the infarction. The changes may not appear immediately but usually exist in some form by the fifth to seventh day. It is important to compare the ECG with a prior one if available to rule out nonspecific S-T and T wave changes.

Estimation of the site of infarction can be determined by the leads in which the ECG changes are seen. An inferior MI would be visible in leads II, III, and aV_F; an anteroseptal infarction in leads V_1, V_2, and V_3; an anterior infarction in leads V_2, V_3, and V_4; and an anterolateral MI in V_4, V_5, V_6 and leads I and aV_L. If the entire anterior wall is involved, all six V leads will reflect the changes. These are the most common sites of infarction.

Enzymes reflecting myocardial damage include CPK, LDH, and SGOT. These are not specific to cardiac muscle, so isoenzymes of CPK (MB band) and LDH (LDH_1 greater than LDH_2) that are more specific are more heavily relied on. Some or all of these may increase within 24 hours postinfarction and resolve within days or weeks at varying times.

Management decisions are based on maintaining optimal cardiac function by maintaining adequate coronary perfusion and decreasing myocardial oxygen demands. Electrophysiological stability is critical to both.

ASSESSMENT

1. History of angina pectoris, coronary insufficiency, MI, cardiac failure, hypertension, diabetes, arrhythmias, medications, and cardiac surgery
2. Results of special cardiac studies—past and current
   a. Coronary arteriography
   b. Left ventricular cineangiograms
   c. Exercise ECG studies; may be combined with cardiac catheterization or myocardial imaging
   d. Echocardiography
   e. Myocardial imaging with radioactive isotopes
3. Level of anxiety, depression, and denial
4. Chest pain
   a. Location, radiation, quality
   b. Duration
   c. Precipitating factors
   d. Relief mechanisms
   e. Relation to exertion, respiration, and movement
   f. Presence of associated symptoms
5. Hemodynamic status
   a. BP
   b. P
   c. Heart sounds
   d. Respiratory effort
      (1) Breath sounds
      (2) Adventitious sounds
   e. Fluid balance
   f. Venous pressure
   g. Mental status
   h. General appearance
   i. Invasive monitoring if appropriate
      (1) Intra-arterial pressure
      (2) PAP and PCWP
      (3) Cardiac output
      (4) CVP
6. Continuous monitoring and daily and prn 12 lead ECG for
   a. Arrhythmias
   b. Changes characteristic of evolving MI
   c. Changes characteristic of electrolyte imbalance
   d. Changes characteristic of drugs and their toxic effects
7. Lab data results of
   a. Serial cardiac enzymes and isoenzymes
   b. Blood gases
   c. Erythrocyte sedimentation rate
   d. White blood cell (WBC) count
   e. BUN and/or creatinine clearance
   f. Electrolyte values
   g. Drug levels
   h. Chest radiographs
   i. Cultures
8. Temperature
9. Signs and symptoms of complications
   a. Arrhythmias
   b. Heart failure; pulmonary edema
   c. Cardiogenic shock
   d. Angina
   e. Extension of MI
   f. Pericarditis
   g. Infections
   h. Pulmonary/systemic emboli
   i. Rupture
      (1) Cardiac
      (2) Ventricular septum
      (3) Papillary muscle
   j. Papillary muscle dysfunction
   k. Chordae tendineae tears
   l. Ventricular aneurysm
   m. Dressler's syndrome (post MI syndrome)
10. Information regarding patient's
    a. Risk factor profile
       (1) Family history of premature coronary heart disease
       (2) Cigarette smoking
       (3) Hypertension
       (4) Elevated serum lipids
       (5) Carbohydrate intolerance, diabetes
       (6) Obesity—greater likelihood of hyperten-

sion, elevated blood cholesterol, or diabetes
  (7) Sedentary life-style
  (8) Psychosocial factors
      (a) Type A personality
      (b) Recognition and management of stress
  b. Social support systems
  c. Health beliefs and perceptions
  d. Perception of impact of illness; cost-benefit ratio of therapy
  e. Life-style if anticipated adjustments required
11. Ongoing and final evaluation of effectiveness of teaching program

GOALS

1. Absence of chest pain—patient verbalizes comfort
2. Hemodynamic stability—absence of complications
3. Electrophysiological stability
4. Control of anxiety, denial, and/or depression
   a. Verbal and nonverbal behavior demonstrates decreased anxiety with provision of information
   b. Verbalizes understanding of disease process and purpose and expectations of equipment, procedures, and routines
   c. Asks pertinent questions regarding future; verbalizes fears and identifies sources of anxiety
   d. Utilizes support systems if available
5. Normal temperature after 72 hours
6. Maintains prescribed activity level
7. Performs exercises, including those to avoid deleterious effects of bed rest
8. Patient verbalizes acceptance of diagnosis and asks pertinent questions regarding future management
9. Before discharge the patient/family
   a. Demonstrates comprehension of the knowledge components of the teaching program when evaluated by testing or questioning
   b. Identifies own risk factors and of those agreed on by health care team and patient, describes methods of modification
   c. Describes home exercise program and work simplification techniques
   d. Describes parameters for monitoring own activity—symptoms and pulse; demonstrates accurately skill of counting pulse, identifying own maximal heart rate
   e. Describes symptoms requiring immediate medical attention, listing what steps to take to obtain it
   f. States necessary information for compliance with medication regimen and follow-up

Potential problems	Expected outcomes	Nursing activities

■ Chest pain related to MI	■ Absence of chest pain and associated symptoms
	
	If pain occurs, patient immediately notifies staff
		■ Patient should be admitted immediately to CCU
		   Attach patient to cardiac monitor using lead that gives clearest tracing; note lead used and settings of rate meters
		   Ensure that patent stable intravenous route is obtained using indwelling venous catheter
		   Administer O_2 as ordered
		If pain is present and severe, immediately inform physician and make medication available, and/or follow standing orders for treatment
		   Check BP, P, and R before and after medication administration, at 1, 5, and 10 minutes for hypotension, tachycardia, and respiratory depression; assess response to medication
		   Obtain a full description of pain including location, radiation, patient's description of quality, duration, precipitating factors, and relief mechanisms; determine if influenced by respiration or movement
		   Assess for presence of shortness of breath, sweating, weakness or fainting, nausea and vomiting, degree of anxiety or sense of impending doom; record and report information with the above data
		When patient's condition is stabilized, perform full admission assessment for baseline information
		   Check BP in both arms for equality and level
		   Check all pulses—carotid, brachial, radial, femoral, popliteal, dorsalis pedis, posterior tibial, and apical—for rate, rhythm, quality, and equality

Potential problems	Expected outcomes	Nursing activities

Respiratory rate and effort
Neck veins for jugular venous distention
Weight and presence of edema
Mental status
Temperature
General appearance
Auscultate precordium for
  Quality of heart sounds
  Rate and rhythm
  Murmurs*
  Rubs*
  Gallops*
    S_4 is usually present, reflecting an increased ventricular filling pressure resulting from temporary impairment of left ventricular function
Auscultate lungs for aeration and presence of rales
Palpate precordium for point of maximal impulse and abnormal precordial movements, e.g., lifts or heaves
Assess patient/family's level of anxiety
Obtain a 12 lead ECG and a rhythm strip from monitor noting rate, rhythm, P-R interval, QRS duration, and Q-T interval for baseline data
Ensure that blood samples are obtained and sent to lab for cardiac enzymes and isoenzymes, blood gases, and CBC
Obtain chest radiograph
Interview patient for information regarding past medical and surgical history and medications
Ongoing assessment and care
  Ensure that emergency equipment is functioning and readily accessible; check every shift
  Check q2 hr for 48 hours and then q4 hr, increasing the frequency as needed
    BP, P (apical and radial), and R
    Auscultate precordium for normal and abnormal sounds
    Auscultate lungs for aeration and rales
    Examine neck veins
    Mental status
    General appearance
    Be alert to development of pulsus alternans and pulsus paradoxus
  Check temperature q4 hr
  Check intake and output q8 hr
  Ongoing assessment of level of anxiety, depression, denial, and readiness to learn
  Monitor lab data for results of
    Enzymes and isoenzymes
    Blood gas levels
    WBC
    Sedimentation rate
    Chest radiograph
Instruct patient to inform team immediately of presence of chest pain or discomfort, emphasizing reasons why
  Relief of pain
  Importance of data collection during episode
  To prevent further muscle damage and side effects of nausea and vomiting, hypotension or hypertension

---

*If not nursing responsibility, review physician's notes to determine presence.

Potential problems	Expected outcomes	Nursing activities
		Daily 12-lead ECG for
		Changes characteristic of evolving MI
		Changes characteristic of electrolyte imbalance
		Changes characteristic of drugs and their toxicity
		Arrhythmias
		When patient is stable and rested, continue admission interview to obtain items listed in 10 in assessment; use information to determine compliance probability and tailor discharge plan
		Initiate measures to decrease O_2 consumption during acute phase
		Activity regulation
		Maintain bed rest for 24 hours
		Patient may feed self, wash face, and brush teeth if elbows are supported on table
		Place patient in semi-Fowler's position, which is generally most comfortable for patients and also physiologically preferable because it decreases venous return and increases lung expansion
		If condition is stable after 24 hours, the patient may be assisted to bedside commode after dangling, and men may stand to void after obtaining physician's order
		Check BP, P, R, and ECG before activity and within 1 minute after returning to bed; always be alert to symptoms of nontolerance
		Obtain physician's order to place patient on a graded exercise program to reduce complications of physical deconditioning; refer to hospital program or literature
		Emphasize to patient/family that activity will be progressively increased
		Give stool softeners and laxative if necessary and ordered
		Diet will vary according to patient's condition and danger of vomiting; for reinforcement purposes of discharge planning it is helpful to begin on low cholesterol, low fat diet
		Control calories if patient is overweight and salt if patient is hypertensive
		Avoid large meals
		If patient is retaining fluid, limit intake of fluids
		Maintain quiet, controlled environment; approach patient with calm, confident, reassuring manner
		Administer medications as ordered; prophylactic anticoagulation against venous thromboembolus and mural thrombi may be ordered

■ Chest pain related to angina
Preexisting angina may or may not continue after MI; new onset of angina may develop
	■ Absence and/or control of angina sufficient for maintenance of hemodynamic stability	■ Assess hemodynamic effect of pain; check P and BP
		With physician determine etiology of pain
		  Previous history of angina
		  Description of pain; may or may not be similar to that of MI in severity, location, and radiation; duration difficult to evaluate since chest pain should be treated promptly
		  Relief of pain by nitroglycerin suggests angina; however, failure of nitroglycerin to relieve pain does not confirm an MI
		  Appearance of chest pain in the absence of new or changing ECG, or enzyme evidence of MI suggests angina
		Treat pain as ordered, recording and reporting response; check P and BP
		Assess effect of reappearance of chest pain on patient's level of anxiety; often frightening

Potential problems	**Expected outcomes**	**Nursing activities**
■ Chest pain related to extension of infarction	■ Absence and/or control of extension sufficient for maintenance of hemodynamic stability	■ Assess hemodynamic effect of pain; check P and BP Determine etiology of pain with physician; continuation of pain beyond 24 hours requiring narcotic for relief and ECG or enzyme evidence of new evolution suggest extension Treat pain as ordered, recording and reporting response; check BP and P Increase frequency of observations reflecting hemodynamic instability because increased necrosis further reduces functional ventricular muscle Assess level of anxiety related to continued or reappearance of chest pain
■ Chest pain related to pericarditis More common with anterior or transmural infarctions	■ Absence and/or control of pericarditis sufficient for maintenance of hemodynamic stability	■ Assess hemodynamic effect of pain; check P and BP Assess for following characteristics of pain and associated symptoms useful for differentiating source Chest pain appearing 2 days to 1 week postinfarction that is influenced by deep inspiration or a change in position (may be relieved by leaning forward); note response to narcotics; lack of response may serve as clue Presence of pericardial friction rub; may not appear for 4 to 48 hours following onset of pain Presence of characteristic ECG changes of pericarditis; appearance of atrial arrhythmias Temperature elevation greater than 101° F for more than 72 hours post MI or new appearance of fever Treat pain as ordered; anti-inflammatory agents most commonly effective If patient is being treated with anticoagulants, check with physician regarding continuation; usually contraindicated because of risk of cardiac tamponade but this remains controversial Assess for complications of arrhythmias, heart failure, and cardiac tamponade; see Standard: *Pericarditis*
■ Chest pain related to Dressler's syndrome (post MI syndrome) Related to hypersensitivity reaction in which antigen is necrotic cardiac muscle	■ Absence of pain and associated complications	■ Patients occasionally admitted to critical care units for diagnostic differentiation Determine if recent history of MI; syndrome usually develops within few weeks to months post MI Assess for presence of pericardial-type pain, friction rub, and prolonged fever Assess for signs and symptoms of pleuritis or pneumonitis, which are sometimes present Assess for signs and symptoms of pericardial effusion or tamponade; anticoagulation usually contraindicated because of potential risk of tamponade; see Standard: *Pericarditis* If pain occurs, administer aspirin, indomethacin, or corticosteroids as ordered
■ Anxiety, depression, and denial related to Fear and concomitant symptoms Lack of information regarding condition, procedures and equipment, future impact of heart disease on life-style Matters left pending at work or home		■ Provide a comfortable, quiet environment; avoid use of audio alarms if not necessary for safety Limit nursing personnel caring for patient to allow for the benefit of continuity Orient patient/family to unit, equipment, daily routines, and expected progression of activities Stress that frequent assessments are part of the preventive purpose of the unit and do not necessarily imply a deteriorating condition Explain each new procedure as it is done Inform patient/family of 'team qualifications'—specially trained personnel

Potential problems	Expected outcomes	Nursing activities
Effect of illness on others		Maintain a confident manner Repeat information as needed because of reduced attention span associated with anxiety
	Patient/family verbalizes fears, concerns, and questions	Encourage patient/family to verbalize fears, concerns, and questions Provide private opportunities for both patient and family Answer questions when possible; do not avoid questions Remember that anxious families create anxious patients Allow patient as much control over environment, daily hygiene, and visitors as possible; observe effect of visitors on patient Sedate patient only if necessary and as ordered; heavy sedation makes it difficult to integrate realities of illness necessary for successful rehabilitation If pain occurs, treat promptly and stay with patient until resolved; narcotics also help reduce anxiety; explain source of pain
	Control or resolution of anxiety, depression, and denial with time and provision of information	Continually assess verbal and nonverbal clues of levels of anxiety, depression, and denial Differentiate from environmental and physiological factors, e.g., cerebral hypoxia Clues to *anxiety* include restlessness, sleeplessness, hostility, nonresponsiveness, incessant talking, difficulty concentrating, muscular tenseness or rigidity, and a watchful or frightened appearance Clues to *depression* include insomnia, constipation, anorexia, decreased energy drive, underresponsiveness, irritability, weeping or crying, verbalization of feelings of hopelessness about future, despondency, helplessness, depersonalization, decreased self-esteem, guilt, and a general lack of interest in everything Clues to *denial* include explicit verbal denial, stoic or inappropriately cheerful, unrealistic statements in the face of reality and outright refusal to comply with medical regimen Determine degree of denial and if it interferes with care; denial may be beneficial if it helps to reduce anxiety during acute state Search for sources of anxiety; may be related to matters left pending at home or work which can be resolved Assess hemodynamic consequences of anxiety

	Coping mechanisms adequate to help control anxiety while not interfering with care	Participate in management of coping mechanisms
		Denial
		  Accept patient's denial when it serves beneficial purpose of reducing acute anxiety, but do not reinforce it; may be inadvertently reinforced by delay of definite diagnosis pending ECG and enzyme results
		  Be specific when patient generalizes about, avoids, or attempts to change the subject
		  Identify and discuss ambiguities
		Hostility and/or sexual aggression
		  Maintain calm, matter-of-fact attitude
		  Avoid confrontation
		  Explore causes of feelings with patient and be supportive
		  Do not ignore overt behavior or overcompensate with kindness

	Acceptance of diagnosis	Begin teaching plan when patient indicates readiness
		  Priority of time in unit should be to move patient toward acceptance of diagnosis
		  Explain what a heart attack is and the healing process
		  Personalize teaching to patient
		Participate in ongoing preparation of patient/family for transfer from unit

Potential problems	Expected outcomes	Nursing activities
■ Arrhythmias related to Myocardial ischemia Increased sympathetic tone Abnormalities associated with reduced left ventricular function Treatment modalities	■ Electrophysiological stability Optimum cardiac rhythm	■ Continuous observation of ECG is essential

■ Continuous observation of ECG is essential
  Select best leads
    Clear QRS complexes and P waves
    Clear pacemaker artifact if present
    "Special" leads such as MCL$_1$ (modified V$_1$)
      1. Bundle branch blocks
      2. Differentiating aberrancy from intraventricular conduction problems
    Leads I and II—axis shifts
  Set rate alarms if necessary; if rate alarms are used, check rate limit indicators and alarm system regularly for accuracy and operation
Premature beats are often a warning sign of more serious arrhythmias
  Note site of origin, frequency, presence of patterns, coupling interval (relationship to preceding normal beat), and configuration (multiformed or uniformed)
  Check pulse to see if perfused
  Participate in management as ordered to avoid more lethal arrhythmias and negative hemodynamic consequences
Tachyarrhythmias
  Assess effect on cardiac output resulting from decreased coronary perfusion and increased myocardial O$_2$ demand; significance primarily dependent on ventricular rate
  A ventricular rate of 100 to 150 is usually the result of arrhythmias secondary to heart failure—sinus tachycardia, atrial flutter, and atrial fibrillation; with atrial fibrillation, assess effect of loss of atrial contraction on hemodynamic status in patients with left heart failure or mitral stenosis
  If the ventricular rate is greater than 150
    Institute treatment promptly as ordered to avoid potential circulatory collapse
    If countershock is required and time allows, assess for presence of acidosis, hypoxia, and digoxin toxicity
    If any of these are present, participate with physician in their correction, if possible, prior to countershock
Bradyarrhythmias
  Assess effect on cardiac output
    May be beneficial because of increased time for diastolic coronary artery filling and decreased O$_2$ consumption
    Ventricular rates below 50 more likely to decrease cardiac output because of inability of left ventricle to compensate with increased stroke volume
  Observe for and treat as ordered the occurrence of premature beats
For all arrhythmias, assess effect on cardiac output; check BP, P, and observe for changes that reflect increasing left ventricular dysfunction (see Problem, Ventricular dysfunction)
Check emergency equipment at every shift to ensure functioning and ready availability
Participate with physician in the identification and treatment of predisposing clinical conditions or factors
Administer antiarrhythmics as ordered; regulate IV infusions to avoid overdosing and serious side effects
Assist with pacemaker insertion if necessary
  Relate conduction problem to site of infarction

Potential problems	Expected outcomes	Nursing activities
		Anterior or anteroseptal MI—prophylactic insertion more common because there is a statistically higher probability of progression to complete heart block and less reliability of an escape ventricular pacemaker; the block is generally the result of extensive septal damage Inferior MI—AV block generally occurs in the AV node; should complete heart block develop, the escape pacemaker is usually junctional (more reliable than ventricular), and the block is more often transient, resolving within 14 days See Standard: *Pacemaker* For more detailed information, see Standard: *Arrhythmias*

■ Hypotension related to reflex mechanisms, probably vagal
Peripheral vascular resistance remains normal or decreases in response to hypotension resulting from decreased left ventricular function rather than increasing in normal manner to maintain BP and cardiac output
More commonly seen in patients with inferior or posterior MI
	■ Normal peripheral vascular response to compensate for hypotension, thereby maintaining BP and cardiac output	■ Assess for other indications of excessive vagal stimulation to differentiate from hypotension related to uncompensated left ventricular dysfunction
		Sinus bradycardia
		First degree or Wenckebach heart block
		Nausea
		Bronchospasm
		Tracheal burning
		Assess for consequences of decreased cardiac output and increased peripheral vascular resistance resulting in decreased peripheral vascular perfusion
		Monitor BP; frequency dependent on level and hemodynamic consequences
		Administer medications as ordered
		    Parasympatholytics, e.g., atropine; often abolishes symptoms and may be given in low doses to help with differentiation
		    Vasopressors; monitor closely to avoid hypertension, tachycardia, and ventricular arrhythmias

■ Ventricular dysfunction related to heart failure, pulmonary edema
Occurs in most patients following MI to some degree during first 4 days; on continuum from asymptomatic (with minimal compensatory rise in left ventricular filling pressure) to cardiogenic shock
	■ Hemodynamic stability	■ Observe for problems known to aggravate heart failure—arrhythmias, hypotension or hypertension, acidosis, hypoxemia, pain
		Report presence to physician
		Treat immediately according to physician's orders
		Assess for signs and symptoms of heart failure
		    Sinus tachycardia
		    Dyspnea
		    Tachypnea
		    Orthopnea
		    Pulmonary rales
		    S_3 gallop
		    Pulsus alternans
		    Elevation of jugular venous pressure, neck vein distention
		    Hepatic enlargement
		    Positive hepatojugular reflux
		    Peripheral or sacral edema
		    Persistent hypotension continuing after relief of pain
		    Displaced or diffuse apical impulse
		Review chest radiograph for signs of pulmonary congestion or enlargement; change may follow occurrence of symptoms by as much as 24 hours
		Therapy dependent on extent of failure and response to treatment; promptly inform physician of changes
		Administer O_2 as ordered, usually through nasal cannula 2 to 6 liters/minute; review results of blood gases for hypoxemia

Potential problems	Expected outcomes	Nursing activities

		Administer diuretics as ordered
		  Monitor intake and output, urine specific gravity and lab results for electrolytes and BUN or creatinine clearance
		Ensure sodium restricted diet adhered to if ordered; explain purpose to patient/family, particularly when latter bring ''treats'' from home
		Heart failure not responding to aforementioned will be more aggressively managed; invasive hemodynamic monitoring is recommended
		  Intra-arterial lines
		  PCWP (reflecting left ventricular end diastolic filling pressure)
		  Cardiac output
		  Foley catheter
		  See Standard: *Hemodynamic monitoring*

■ Ventricular dysfunction related to cardiogenic shock
Related to extensive myocardial necrosis resulting in impaired perfusion of body tissues and organs
Patients remaining in shock for over 1 hour have a significantly higher mortality rate
	■ Absence of cardiogenic shock	■ Assess for signs and symptoms of cardiogenic shock
		  Hypotension: systolic BP less than 90 mm Hg
		  Tachycardia with poor pulse contour
		  Urine output less than 20 ml/hour
		  Mental confusion
		  Decreased peripheral perfusion
		If cardiogenic shock develops
		  Report to physician immediately
		  Participate in aggressive management to interrupt shock cycle
		In the absence of cardiogenic shock, initiate with physician invasive hemodynamic monitoring essential for determining response to therapy, thereby guiding therapy
		  Intra-arterial pressures
		  PCWP
		  Cardiac output measurements
		  Foley catheter for hourly urine measurements
		Identify and treat as ordered abnormalities such as hypoxemia, acidosis, arrhythmias, pain
		Institute therapy as ordered; this may include vasopressors, vasodilators, inotropic agents, fluid challenge, O_2 administration, counterpulsation and/or surgical intervention
		Continuous assessment required to monitor rapidly changing hemodynamic status characteristic of cardiogenic shock
		SEE STANDARDS: *Cardiogenic shock*
		                Hemodynamic monitoring
		                Intra-aortic balloon pumping

■ Ventricular dysfunction related to papillary muscle dysfunction/rupture
Related to papillary muscle infarction
More commonly seen with inferior, lateral, and subendocardial infarctions
	■ Absence of or resolution of papillary muscle dysfunction/rupture	■ Assess for signs and symptoms of papillary muscle dysfunction, particularly during first few days after AMI
		  Transient systolic murmur at apex indicative of mitral insufficiency
		  Left heart failure
		If failure is hemodynamically significant, administer vasodilators as ordered, monitoring intraarterial pressure and PAP, urine output, etc.
		If mitral valve replacement is necessary due to continued heart failure, maintenance therapy with po or IV vasodilators may be required to delay surgery for at least 6 to 10 weeks post MI to allow time for healing
		Onset of sudden pulmonary edema resistant to drug therapy suggests papillary muscle rupture
		  Determine presence of
		    Sudden onset of loud holosystolic murmur best appreciated

Potential problems	Expected outcomes	Nursing activities
		at the apex with patient lying on left side; may radiate to left axilla or back Hypotension Barely palpable pulses Signs and symptoms of severe left heart failure Electromechanical dissociation Prepare patient for cardiac catheterization and coronary arteriography to determine feasibility of surgical correction Administer vasodilators as ordered, monitoring intra-arterial pressure and PAP If indicated, prepare patient for cardiac surgery; counterpulsation may be required SEE STANDARDS: *Pulmonary edema* *Hemodynamic monitoring* *Cardiac catheterization* *Cardiac surgery* *Intra-aortic balloon pumping*
■ Ventricular dysfunction related to rupture of the ventricular septum Rare complication usually occurring within 2 to 10 days after infarction Seen with anterior and inferior MI	■ Absence of ventricular septal rupture	■ Determine presence of Loud holosystolic murmur near lower left sternal border with palpable thrill; may be louder at apex, which makes differentiation from papillary muscle rupture more difficult Left to right shunting Heart failure of varying degrees dependent on amount of shunting Pulmonary congestion; pulmonary edema Hypotension Prepare patient for cardiac catheterization if necessary Administer afterload reducing agents to decrease shunting as ordered, monitoring intra-arterial pressure and PCWP Assist with insertion of intra-aortic balloon if ordered; maintain according to protocol and physician's orders Attempts will be made to delay surgery as long as possible after MI to allow infarcted tissue to heal; development of cardiogenic shock or drug-resistant heart failure mandates earlier repair SEE STANDARDS: *Heart failure* *Pulmonary edema* *Cardiac catheterization* *Intra-aortic balloon pumping* *Hemodynamic monitoring* *Cardiac surgery*
■ Ventricular dysfunction related to external cardiac rupture Usually results in sudden death	■ Absence of cardiac rupture	■ Has been noted in relation to coughing and straining to have a bowel movement; more common in absence of congestive heart failure Assess for signs and symptoms of cardiac tamponade and electromechanical dissociation Assist with emergency intervention Pericardiocentesis Constant drainage by intrapericardial catheter Rapid administration of dextran and norepinephrine Counterpulsation Surgery to close defect SEE STANDARDS: *Pericarditis* *Intra-aortic balloon pumping* *Cardiac surgery*

Potential problems	Expected outcomes	Nursing activities

■ Ventricular dysfunction related to left ventricular aneurysm
 	
Occurs more commonly with transmural infarction from few days to 6 weeks post MI
	■ Hemodynamic stability	■ Determine presence of the following indications suggestive of aneurysm
		  Palpable prolonged outward systolic impulse medial and/or superior to point of maximal impulse
		  Persistent S-T segment elevation in precordial leads; occasionally can be produced by exercise
		  Abnormal contour of left cardiac border on posterior-anterior chest radiograph
		  Paradoxical movement of left ventricle during fluoroscopy
		  Drug-resistant ventricular arrhythmias, particularly ventricular tachycardia
		  Refractory congestive heart failure
		Prepare patient for radioisotope scanning studies and/or left ventricular angiography, which may be ordered to confirm impression
		If surgery is indicated (cardiac failure and ventricular arrhythmias persist threatening hemodynamic stability; surface area involved less than 50%), it will be delayed at least 4 to 10 weeks following MI if possible
		Administer treatments directed toward controlling heart failure and arrhythmias as ordered
		Observe for signs and symptoms of systemic arterial embolization resulting from intra-aneurysmal thrombosis
		SEE STANDARDS: *Heart failure*
		                  Cardiac catheterization
		                  Cardiac surgery
		                  Embolic phenomena
		                  Arrhythmias

■ Thromboembolism related to deep vein thrombosis or mural thrombi from the infarcted endocardium	■ Absence or resolution of thromboembolism	■ Institute preventive measures particularly for patients with severe or chronic congestive heart failure, shock, preexisting thromboembolic disease, and obesity and older (over 70) or inactive patients
		  Anticoagulate as ordered; observe for signs of bleeding
		  Assist patient with passive exercises while in bed; place footboard on bed for patient to press toes against 10 times every hour
		  Instruct patient not to cross legs or ankles
		  Use elastic stockings and measure calf for correct size
		    Remove twice a day
		    Make certain that stockings do not roll down, creating a "tourniquet"
		  Have patient ambulate as early as possible
		Observe for signs of venous thrombosis
		  Positive Homans' sign
		  Change in color, temperature, or girth of extremity
		  Presence of tenderness and/or cords
		Assess for signs and symptoms of pulmonary embolus—sudden unexplained dyspnea, tachypnea, anxiety, hypotension, tachycardia, atrial arrhythmias, elevation of jugular venous pressure, elevation of PAP (if line is in place), and expiratory or fixed splitting of S_2
		Assess for signs and symptoms of pulmonary infarction—hemoptysis, pleural friction rub, dyspnea, or signs of pulmonary consolidation
		Prepare patient for lung scan if ordered
		If problem occurs
		  Inform physician

Potential problems	Expected outcomes	Nursing activities

		Administer anticoagulants as ordered
		Observe for appearance of heart failure or pulmonary edema, which may be aggravated or precipitated by pulmonary emboli
		Assess for signs and symptoms of systemic emboli; often not recognized unless of large size or cerebral
		If systemic emboli occur
		  Inform physician
		  Administer anticoagulants as ordered
		  Treat complications
		SEE STANDARD: *Embolic phenomena*

▪ Temperature elevation related to
  Myocardial tissue necrosis
  Pericarditis
  Infection
	▪ Normal temperature after 72 hours	▪ Encourage patient to cough and deep breathe every hour while on bed rest and awake
		Foley catheters should not remain in place over 2 weeks and depending on appearance may need to be changed more frequently
		IV lines should be changed q48 hr
		Monitoring lines should be changed as indicated in the following unless detrimental to patient; employ strict aseptic technique for tubing and transducer changes
		  Pulmonary artery lines: at least every 72 hours
		  Arterial lines: at least every 7 days
		  CVP lines: at least every 7 days
		Check temperature q4 hr while patient is awake, increasing frequency as needed
		If temperature is elevated
		  Observe for associated chills and diaphoresis
		  Keep patient warm and dry
		  Administer antipyretics as ordered
		  Review lab results of WBC and sedimentation rate
		  Inform patient that temperature elevation is expected during first 48 to 72 hours
		If temperature is elevated beyond 101° F or persists beyond 48 to 72 hours, observe for other sources of infection
		  Assess for signs and symptoms of pericarditis (see Problem, Chest pain related to pericarditis)
		  Assess for other sources of infection—lungs, urine, monitoring lines
		  Obtain cultures if necessary
		  Culture tips of monitoring lines when removed if serum culture positive
		  Administer antibiotics or other medications as ordered

▪ Insufficient knowledge to comply with discharge regimen	▪ Evaluation by testing or questioning demonstrates patient/family's understanding of the knowledge components of the teaching program
	Asks pertinent questions about self-care
	Identifies own risk factors and of those agreed on by health care team and patient, describes plans for modification
		▪ Institute teaching program for patient/family, including
		  Normal heart function
		  Explanation of what a heart attack is and process of healing; relate to symptoms
		
		  Discussion of risk factors
		    Meaning and significance of
		    Identification of patient's own
		    Cost-benefit ratio of modification
		    Methods of modification and sources of support
		      Tailor to patient
		        1. Smoking

Potential problems	**Expected outcomes**	**Nursing activities**
		2. Diet
		3. Recognition and management of stress
		Control of coexisting disease if present
		Hypertension
		Diabetes
		Arrhythmias
		Heart failure
		Angina
	Describes home exercise program and work simplification techniques; demonstrates exercises	Activity regulation
		Significance of activity regulation related to healing process
		Purpose of home exercise program, providing opportunity for practice
	Describes how own symptoms and pulse will be used to monitor activity; demonstrates accurately how to count own pulse and state maximal heart rate	Work simplification techniques
		Importance of avoiding or modifying activity following meals, stress, or in extremes of temperature
		Prophylactic measures if appropriate
		Method of counting pulse; meaning and significance of maximal heart rate
		Symptoms suggesting lack of tolerance and what to do if these occur
		Sexual activity: include both partners
	Describes those symptoms requiring immediate medical attention and what steps should be taken to obtain it	Symptoms requiring immediate medical attention; sources of help available to patient and how to obtain; be as specific as possible after discussion with physician
	States necessary information for compliance with medication regimen and follow-up	Information regarding discharge medications
		Name and purpose
		Dosage
		Frequency: tailor to patient's routine schedule
		Prophylactic use of and storage of nitroglycerin
		Side effects
		Group timing of medications if possible to decrease complexity of scheduling
		Follow-up information
		Include discussion of future tests if ordered
		1. Exercise ECG
		2. Cardiac catheterization
		Helpful for patient/family to be aware that periods of depression and fatigue are not uncommon, particularly during first few weeks at home
	Patient/family discusses future realistically	Provide frequent opportunities for patient/family to ask questions and express concerns or fears
		Provide opportunities for skills practice
		Assess patient's potential compliance with discharge regimen

11 □ Heart failure (low cardiac output)

Heart failure occurs when the heart is unable to perform normally as a pump, which may render it unable to maintain a cardiac output sufficient to meet the body's needs at rest and/or during normal activity.

The multiple etiologies of heart failure can be organized into three major groups, depending on the way they interfere with ventricular function. These are as follows:

1. Conditions resulting in direct myocardial damage such as occurs with MI, myocarditis, myocardial fibrosis, or ventricular aneurysm.
2. Conditions resulting in ventricular overload either by increasing the pressure against which the ventricle must work (afterload) or increasing the volume with which it must deal (preload). Increased afterload may be created by systemic or pulmonic hypertension, aortic or pulmonic stenosis, and coarctation of the aorta. Increased preload may occur with rapid infusion of intravenous solutions, mitral or aortic regurgitation, atrial or ventricular septal defects, and patent ductus arteriosus.
3. Conditions resulting in restriction to ventricular diastolic filling created by cardiac tamponade, constrictive pericarditis, or restrictive cardiomyopathies.

The ventricles may fail independently, but the most common cause of right heart failure is left heart failure. Right heart failure may result from pulmonary hypertension independent of left heart failure.

Failure of the ventricle results in an increase in the ventricular end diastolic filling pressure. The heart will attempt to compensate and maintain cardiac output through several mechanisms. These include increasing sympathetic nervous system activity, which results in an increase in heart rate, vascular resistance, and myocardial contractility; increasing contractility as a result of increased fiber length according to the Frank-Starling principle; and, chronically, increasing ventricular mass, resulting in ventricular hypertrophy. Hypertrophy is usually not evidenced in heart failure resulting from acute causes in intensive care units unless there is preexisting heart disease.

Compensated heart failure occurs when these mechanisms are able to prevent an abnormal elevation of left ventricular end diastolic pressure and a fall in cardiac output below resting systemic requirements. Decompensation occurs as the left ventricular end diastolic filling pressure increases. If cardiac output declines with decompensation, then in addition to the pulmonary vascular congestion due to the elevated left ventricular end diastolic pressure, there will also be a fall in renal perfusion pressure and a fall in glomerular filtration rate that initiate renal compensatory mechanisms. The result is salt and water retention in an attempt to increase the effective intravascular volume to maintain normal renal perfusion pressure.

The early signs of cardiac failure, sinus tachycardia, S_3 gallop, dyspnea, and bibasilar rales are related to compensatory mechanisms as are many of the later complications. Recognition at this early stage with appropriate intervention may prevent complications such as arrhythmias, pulmonary edema, cardiogenic shock, and those occurring as a result of congestion and ultimate dysfunction of organs other than the heart.

There are many degrees of heart failure, and the stage the patient is in will primarily determine the selection and aggressiveness of hemodynamic assessment and therapeutic intervention. Therapy is directed toward identifying and treating or removing precipitating or aggravating factors, reducing the work load on the heart, improving the force and efficiency of contraction, and treating the symptoms and complications resulting from congestion.

ASSESSMENT

1. History of rheumatic fever, congenital heart disease, valvular heart disease, coronary heart disease, systemic or pulmonic hypertension, myocardial disease, heart failure, endocarditis, constrictive pericarditis, infiltrative diseases, and pulmonary disease
2. Presence of factors that may precipitate or aggravate heart failure
   a. Acute MI
   b. Recent open heart surgery
   c. Arrhythmias
   d. Hemorrhage
   e. Anemia
   f. Respiratory infections

g. Pulmonary embolism
h. Thyrotoxicosis
i. Fever
j. Hypoxia
k. Excessive salt intake
l. Excessive or rapid administration of parenteral fluids
m. Emotional stress
n. Activity
o. Corticosteroid administration
p. Administration of drugs that may cause cardiac depression such as propranolol or quinidine
3. Patient's perception of and reaction to diagnosis, progression of disease, assessment, and treatment modalities
4. Level of anxiety
5. Level of activity tolerance
6. Signs and symptoms of decreasing cardiac function
7. Signs and symptoms of pulmonary venous congestion
8. Signs and symptoms of systemic venous congestion
9. Monitor ECG for
   a. Arrhythmias
   b. P wave changes, indicating acute elevations in left atrial pressure
   c. Changes indicative of ventricular hypertrophy
   d. Changes indicative of myocardial damage, e.g., AMI or ischemia
   e. Drug effects
10. Lab data results of
    a. Electrolytes, particularly potassium
    b. BUN/creatinine clearance
    c. Blood gases
    d. Chest radiograph for cardiac dimensions and pulmonary congestion
    e. Cardiac catheterization
    f. Echocardiography
    g. Drug levels, particularly digitalis
    h. Cultures
    i. Any other tests performed to evaluate precipitating or aggravating factors, e.g., cardiac enzymes or isoenzymes, thyroid or lung scans
11. Signs and symptoms of complications
    a. Infection
    b. Thromboembolism
    c. Pulmonary edema
    d. Cardiogenic shock
12. Ongoing and final evaluation of teaching program
13. Determinants of patient compliance with discharge regimen

GOALS

1. Hemodynamic stability
2. Absence of complications of congestion
   a. Pulmonary
   b. Systemic
   c. Renal
   d. Hepatic
   e. Intestinal
   f. Peripheral
3. Electrophysiological stability
4. Absence or resolution of complications of
   a. Infection
   b. Thromboembolic disease
   c. Pulmonary edema
   d. Cardiogenic shock
5. Patient's verbal and nonverbal behavior demonstrates reduction of anxiety with provision of information
6. Before discharge the patient/family*
   a. Demonstrates comprehension of the knowledge components of the teaching program when evaluated by testing or questioning
   b. Identifies own risk factors and/or precipitating factors, describing methods of modification or avoidance
   c. States information necessary for compliance with discharge regimen related to
      (1) Activity management
      (2) Diet
      (3) Medications
      (4) Follow-up care
   d. Accurately demonstrates skill of counting pulse, stating acceptable ranges of rate and rhythm; identifies when it is appropriate to check with physician or nurse before taking digoxin
   e. Lists symptoms requiring medical attention and appropriate actions to take to obtain it
   f. Asks pertinent questions regarding self-care

---

*Applies when chronic management is required.

Potential problems	Expected outcomes	Nursing activities
■ Cardiac decompensation related to increased ventricular volume and filling pressure	■ Hemodynamic stability	■ Monitor closely for early signs and symptoms of heart failure in patient with predisposing history; early intervention and removal of aggravating factors may prevent further problems; symptom onset varies depending on ventricle involved, acute versus chronic nature, and the cause

Check BP for hypotension, pulsus alternans, and changes in pulse pressure

Check P for compensatory tachycardia, rate and regularity, and pulsus alternans; check apical and radial P for deficit

Observe for signs and symptoms of decreased perfusion
    Diaphoresis, cool skin
    Restlessness, confusion
    Cheyne-Stokes respirations

Monitor intake and output and presence of nocturia for indication of decreased renal perfusion
    Check urine specific gravity
    Estimate diaphoretic fluid loss
    Report to physician if output is less than 30 ml/hour

Obtain history of and observe for indications of decreasing activity tolerance and presence of fatigue (particularly significant if felt on awakening)

Auscultate precordium or review chart for presence of S_3 and/or S_4 gallop; S_3 gallop can be normal in children and young adults

Palpate apical impulse, noting position and quality; with ventricular hypertrophy, it becomes large and displaced to left

Review 12-lead ECG for changes associated with ventricular hypertrophy and increased atrial filling pressure (prominent negative P waves in V_1 and V_2)

Review chest radiograph results for evidence of ventricular hypertrophy and/or pulmonary congestion

Observe for the signs and symptoms of pulmonary and systemic venous congestion listed in Problems, Pulmonary venous congestion and systemic venous congestion

Frequency of these observations dependent on degree of stability

Treatment plan dependent on severity of failure
    Participate in identification and correction of aggravating factors
        AMI
        Pain
        Arrhythmias
        Hemorrhage
        Anemia
        Respiratory infections
        Pulmonary embolism
        Thyrotoxicosis
        Fever
        Hypoxia
        Excessive salt intake
        Excessive or rapid administration of parenteral fluids
        Emotional stress
        Activity
        Corticosteroid administration
        Administration of drugs that may cause cardiac depression such as propranolol or quinidine

If patient is receiving medications with negative inotropic effect, check with physician regarding discontinuing

Ensure that emergency equipment is functioning and available at every shift

Potential problems	Expected outcomes	Nursing activities

If IV fluids or medications are ordered, use microdrip or infusion pump; avoid rapid or excessive hydration

Institute measures to reduce work load of heart

    Maintain bed rest; semi-Fowler's or high Fowler's position generally most comfortable and physiologically preferable because venous return is decreased and lung expansion is increased

    Organize care to allow frequent rest periods

    Maintain quiet, controlled environment and approach patient with calm, confident, reassuring manner

Administer medications as ordered

    Agents to increase contractility and/or to decrease afterload or preload generally given

    Monitor closely the effect of medication and for hypotension and arrhythmias

    Invasive hemodynamic monitoring is essential for safe administration and therapeutic regulation with medications such as sodium nitroprusside, hydralazine, phentolamine, isoproterenol (Isuprel), or dopamine

    Monitor pulmonary artery diastolic pressure or mean PCWP, reflecting left atrial and left ventricular diastolic filling pressures; filling pressures between 15 to 20 mm Hg are good for maintaining stroke volume; if the filling pressures are above 20 mm Hg, myocardial O_2 demand probably exceeds benefit of improved stroke volume

    Intra-arterial pressure monitoring and cardiac output measurements may also be indicated

Participate with insertion and monitoring of left ventricular assist devices, which may be indicated to prevent further deterioration until patient's condition is stabilized and/or surgical correction is undertaken

Prepare patient for and monitor results of special studies to assess ventricular function if ordered

SEE STANDARDS: *Hemodynamic monitoring*
                     Intra-aortic balloon pumping
                     Cardiac catheterization

■ Pulmonary venous congestion related to increased left ventricular filling pressure

■ Absence or resolution of pulmonary venous congestion and associated symptoms

■ Observe for signs and symptoms indicating pulmonary venous congestion

Dyspnea

    Relate to level of activity and changing pattern; usually begins with exertion progressing to dyspnea at rest

    Cough with dyspnea on exertion

    Orthopnea—dyspnea occurring when patient is recumbent and relieved by patient sitting up

    Paroxysmal nocturnal dyspnea—may or may not be associated with cough; extreme form of orthopnea; patient awakens breathless, which may be relieved in minutes by sitting or standing or may progress to pulmonary edema

Tachypnea

Auscultate lungs for presence of adventitious sounds q1-2 hr

Monitor results of chest radiograph for indications of pulmonary venous congestion; radiographic changes can be delayed up to 24 hours after onset of symptoms of pulmonary congestion

Monitor PCWP to determine left ventricular filling pressure

Administer O_2 as ordered

Continue measures to reduce left ventricular filling pressure identified in Problem, Cardiac decompensation

Potential problems	Expected outcomes	Nursing activities

■ Systemic venous congestion related to increased right ventricular filling pressure and/ or decreased renal perfusion pressure	■ Absence or resolution of systemic venous congestion and associated symptoms	■ Observe for signs and symptoms indicative of systemic venous congestion
		   Distention of neck veins
		   Peripheral or sacral edema
		   Ascites (more common with tamponade, constrictive pericarditis, or tricuspid stenosis)
		   Hepatic congestion
		     Right upper quadrant pain or tenderness
		     Hepatomegaly
		     Hepatic pulsation
		     Jaundice
		     Serum enzymes reflecting hepatic dysfunction
		   Visceral congestion
		     Anorexia
		     Nausea
		     Constipation
		     Bloating
		   Decreased urine output
		     Increased BUN
		     Proteinuria
		     High urine specific gravity
		   Pleural effusion (more common in right pleural space)
		 Assess effect of systemic congestion on drug metabolism and excretion; adjust medication dosages as ordered
		   Medications given po may not be absorbed in presence of intestinal congestion
		   Renal and hepatic congestion will interfere with metabolism and excretion
		   Circulatory congestion reduces volume of distribution for medications, resulting in higher concentrations
		 Administer diuretics to decrease intravascular volume as ordered
		   Measure intake and output q2 hr; Foley catheter may be needed; check specific gravity
		   Daily weights; notify physician if greater than 500 g/day
		   Monitor lab results for BUN and electrolytes, particularly potassium and sodium
		     Administer potassium supplements if ordered
		     If patient is receiving digoxin, observe closely for toxicity, particularly in presence of hypokalemia
		   Observe for side effects of diuretic therapy; these vary with the type used; loop diuretic is most potent
		     Hypokalemia and hyponatremia
		     Hypovolemia
		     Lethargic
		     Postural hypotension
		     Muscle cramps
		     Metabolic alkalosis
		 Maintain fluid restriction if ordered (more likely if patient is hyponatremic)
		 Ensure adherence to low sodium diet if ordered
		 Encourage foods high in potassium
		 If anorexic, do not force patient to eat but allow food preferences if compatible with diet; provide smaller more frequent meals and frequent oral hygiene
		 Maintain bed rest if necessary to promote diuresis
		 Elevate feet when patient is up in chair
		 Continue measures to improve pump efficiency indicated in Problem, Cardiac decompensation

Potential problems	Expected outcomes	Nursing activities

Potential problems

- Arrhythmias related to
  Cardiac compensatory
    response to de-
    creased stroke vol-
    ume
  Hypoxia
  Electrolyte distur-
    bances
  Etiological condition
    precipitating heart
    failure
  Digitalis toxicity

Expected outcomes

- Electrophysiological sta-
    bility
  Optimum cardiac rhythm

Nursing activities

- Maintain continuous ECG monitoring
    Select lead best exhibiting atrial and ventricular complexes
    Set rate alarms
  Participate with physician in identifying etiology of arrhythmia
    and treat as ordered
    Assess ECG changes indicating developing or progressing
      cardiac failure
      Sinus tachycardia as compensatory mechanism
      Atrial arrhythmias related to increased atrial pressures
    Monitor lab results for
      Hypoxia
      Electrolyte disturbances, particularly potassium
      Acidosis/alkalosis
      Serum digitalis levels
  Assess effect of arrhythmia on cardiac output and heart failure
    Check BP and P and observe for changes reflecting increasing
      left ventricular dysfunction; see Problem, Cardiac decom-
      pensation
    Bradycardias may decrease cardiac output when ventricle is
      not able to increase stroke volume
    Persistent tachycardias reduce ventricular filling time, in-
      crease myocardial O_2 consumption, and can contribute to
      disordered synchrony of ventricular contraction
    Loss of effective atrial contraction with atrial fibrillation, atri-
      al flutter, and AV dissociation in presence of elevated left
      ventricular diastolic pressure can markedly reduce ventricu-
      lar filling
  Check emergency equipment every shift, ensuring proper func-
    tioning and availability
  If it is necessary to treat arrhythmia, e.g., adversely compromis-
    ing cardiac output and/or treatment of underlying problem not
    sufficient, proceed as ordered; therapy may include antiar-
    rhythmics, cardioversion, or pacing; if cardioversion is rec-
    ommended, assess for presence of digoxin toxicity; if digoxin
    toxicity is a possibility, inform the physician; cardioversion
    then is contraindicated; patients with long-standing atrial fi-
    brillation may be anticoagulated prophylactically
  SEE STANDARD: *Arrhythmias*

- Decreased activity toler-
    ance related to de-
    creased cardiac output
    and/or dyspnea

- Activity level below fail-
    ure threshold
  Absence of complications
    related to bed rest
  Patient verbalizes com-
    fort

- Assess level of activity tolerance; relate to fatigue or dyspnea;
    New York Heart Association classification helpful and may be
    appropriately used
    Class I: patients with heart disease who are asymptomatic
    Class II: slight limitation of physical activity; symptoms pro-
      duced only with more than ordinary physical activity
    Class III: marked limitation; symptoms produced with ordi-
      nary physical activity
    Class IV: symptoms while patient is resting
  Maintain ordered activity level
    Higher degrees of failure require bed rest during acute man-
      agement; semi-Fowler's position usually most comfortable
      for patient and physiologically preferable because venous
      return is decreased and lung expansion is increased
    Change position q2 hr and administer skin care, particularly if
      edematous; observe for early indications of breakdown of
      skin—reddened or marked areas
    Increase activity as ordered and as tolerated by patient; check
      BP, P, R, and ECG before each level increase and after
      activity (within 1 minute); observe for symptoms indicating
      poor tolerance

Potential problems	Expected outcomes	Nursing activities
		Provide opportunities for patient to verbalize feelings regarding activity limitations Institute preventive measures to reduce thromboembolic complications of bed rest; see Problem, Thromboembolism
■ Anxiety and frustration related to 　Awareness that heart is not functioning properly, that "heart is failing" 　Resultant symptoms, particularly difficulty with breathing 　Lack of information regarding condition, equipment, procedures, and treatment modalities 　Decreased activity tolerance 　If heart failure is a transient problem secondary to an acute noncardiac problem, the patient may be less aware of diagnosis	■ Verbalizes anxiety and fears Asks questions Reduction of anxiety with sufficient information, resolution of symptoms, and future planning	■ Ongoing assessment and recording of level of anxiety Encourage patient/family to verbalize concerns and to ask questions Explain nature of heart failure relating to etiology if known and to symptoms experienced 　If probability exists that this will be a chronic problem, more information will be necessary as condition stabilizes and anxiety decreases 　If problem is transient and not related to cardiac disease, clarify for patient 　If problem is recurrent, it is particularly important to identify precipitating factors with patient, allowing time for verbalization of fears and frustrations and discussion of past and future impact on life-style Explain purpose and expectations of monitoring equipment, frequency of assessments, and treatment modalities utilized Maintain as quiet and relaxed an environment as possible Assess hemodynamic consequences of anxiety Administer sedatives as ordered when necessary
■ Infection related to 　Pulmonary congestion 　Systemic lines 　Foley catheter	■ Absence or resolution of infection	■ Initiate preventive measures or precautions as appropriate 　Prevent atelectasis by 　　Instituting measures or drugs as ordered to reduce pulmonary congestion 　　Administering pain medication promptly 　　Encouraging patient to cough and deep breathe every hour while on bed rest and awake 　　Providing chest physiotherapy q2 hr if necessary 　　Turning patient at least q2 hr if immobile 　　Sterile suctioning as needed 　Increase level of activity as soon as possible and as ordered 　Maintain strict aseptic technique during insertion of hemodynamic monitoring lines and during any change of tubing or transducers 　　Record date of insertion of each line 　　Monitoring lines should be changed as follows unless detrimental to patient 　　　Pulmonary artery lines: at least q72 hr 　　　Arterial lines: at least every 7 days 　　　CVP lines: at least every 7 days 　　IV lines for fluid administration should be changed q48 hr or earlier if site becomes inflamed 　　Maintain sterile technique when inserting Foley catheter and apply antibiotic ointment to meatus; maintain closed system; should be removed as soon as possible and never left in place more than 14 days; bladder irrigations with antibiotic solution may be ordered; provide perineal care q8 hr; change drainage system q24 hr Check temperature q4 hr while patient is awake; increase frequency as needed; report elevation to physician If temperature is elevated, observe for associated chills or diaphoresis; keep patient warm and dry

Potential problems	Expected outcomes	Nursing activities

		Collect data to determine source of infection
		   Increased atelectasis on chest radiograph
		   Increased pulmonary secretions, which may be purulent
		   Localized signs of inflammation at IV or line insertion sites
		   Changes in character of urine—cloudy, foul smelling, persistent hematuria, flank pain
		   Obtain cultures and send to lab as ordered
		   Culture tips of lines or catheters when removed if indicated
		Administer antipyretics and antibiotics as ordered

■ Thromboembolism
   Pulmonary embolus related to
      Systemic venous congestion
      Prolonged bed rest
	■ Absence or resolution of pulmonary embolus	■ Initiate preventive measures for patients assessed to be high risk candidates for embolization
		   Severe or chronic congestive heart failure with long-standing lower extremity edema or atrial fibrillation
		   History of preexisting thromboembolic disease
		   Obese
		   Over 70 years old
		   Prolonged bed rest anticipated
		Administer prophylactic anticoagulation as ordered
		   Observe for signs of bleeding
		   Hematest all stools, urine, and secretions
		Assist patient with passive/active exercises while on bed rest
		   Place footboard on bed for patient to press toes against 10 times q1 hr
		   Instruct patient not to cross legs or ankles
		   Avoid use of knee gatch on bed
		   Use elastic stockings, measuring calf for correct size
		      Remove twice a day
		      Make certain stockings do not roll down, creating a tourniquet
		   Have patient ambulate as early as possible
		Observe for signs of venous thrombosis
		   Positive Homans' sign
		   Change in color, temperature, or girth of extremity
		   Presence of cords or tenderness
		Assess for signs and symptoms of pulmonary embolus—sudden unexplained dyspnea, tachypnea, anxiety, hypotension, tachycardia, atrial arrhythmias, elevation of jugular venous pressure, elevation of PAP (if line in place), and expiratory or fixed splitting of S_2
		Assess for signs and symptoms of pulmonary infarction—hemoptysis, pleural friction rub, dyspnea, or signs of pulmonary consolidation
		Prepare patient for lung scan if ordered
		If problem occurs
		   Inform physician
		   Administer anticoagulants as ordered
		   Assess for signs and symptoms suggesting further cardiac decompensation including pulmonary edema, which may be result of pulmonary emboli
		SEE STANDARDS: *Embolic phenomena*
		                           Pulmonary edema

■ Pulmonary edema related to pulmonary capillary pressures that exceed oncotic pressure of lungs and result in the transudation of fluid into the alveoli	■ Absence of pulmonary edema	■ Assess for signs and symptoms of pulmonary edema
		   Respiratory distress
		   Increased distribution of rales
		   Cough and increased secretions with severe pulmonary congestion; may have blood-tinged frothy sputum
		   Bulging neck veins
		   Pallor; cyanosis

Potential problems	Expected outcomes	Nursing activities

		Diaphoresis
		Apprehension
		Restlessness
		Tachycardia
		PCWP above 25 to 30 mm Hg
		If problem occurs
		  Elevate head of bed
		  Inform physician immediately—cardiac emergency
		  Administer medications and O_2 as ordered
		  Apply rotating tourniquets if ordered
		  Have someone remain with patient if at all possible
		SEE STANDARD: *Pulmonary edema*

■ Cardiogenic shock related to left ventricular dysfunction, resulting in inadequate tissue perfusion	■ Absence of cardiogenic shock	■ Assess for signs and symptoms of cardiogenic shock
		  Hypotension: systolic BP less than 90 mm Hg
		  Tachycardia with poor pulse contour
		  Urine output less than 20 ml/hour
		  Mental confusion
		  Decreased peripheral perfusion
		If problem develops, inform physician immediately
		  Aggressive management and invasive hemodynamic monitoring must be initiated immediately to interrupt shock cycle
		  Identify and treat, as ordered, abnormalities resulting from and promoting decompensation including hypoxemia, acidosis, arrhythmias, and pain
		SEE STANDARD: *Cardiogenic shock*

■ Insufficient knowledge to comply with discharge regimen*	■ Evaluation by testing or questioning demonstrates patient/family's understanding of the knowledge components of the teaching program
	Identifies own risk factors and/or precipitating factors with methods for modification or avoidance
	States information necessary for compliance with discharge regimen
	  Activity
	  Diet
	  Medications
	  Follow-up care
	Accurately demonstrates skill of counting pulse
	Lists symptoms requiring medical attention
	Asks pertinent questions regarding self-care
	Patient/family discusses future realistically
		■ If heart failure requires chronic management, institute a teaching program for patient/family, including
		  Explanation of normal heart function
		  Explanation of heart failure and related signs and symptoms
		  Discussion of risk factors for atherosclerotic heart disease including purpose and meaning; identification of patient's own and cost-benefit ratio of modification; if risk factor modification is indicated, discuss methods of modification and sources of support
		  Control of precipitating or aggravating factors of heart failure including diseases, e.g., hypertension or valvular heart disease
		  Activity regulation
		    Work simplification techniques
		    Importance of avoiding or modifying activity following meals, with stress, or in extremes of temperature
		    Symptoms suggesting intolerance and actions to take
		  Need for avoiding activities or clothing that promote circulatory stasis
		  Diet instruction if a special diet has been ordered; give patient list of foods and beverages high in potassium if diuretic therapy is indicated, unless potassium-sparing diuretic has been ordered
		  Information regarding discharge medications
		    Name and purpose
		    Dosage
		    Frequency—tailor timing to patient's routine schedule
		    Side effects

*If patient follow-up is the responsibility of the critical care unit nurse.

Potential problems	Expected outcomes	Nursing activities
		1. Signs and symptoms of digoxin toxicity
		2. Signs and symptoms of hypokalemia unless potassium-sparing diuretic has been ordered
		Method and significance of counting pulse if patient receiving digoxin when discharged
		Signs and symptoms of recurring heart failure and appropriate action to take; importance of daily weights
		Information regarding follow-up
		Provide frequent opportunities for patient/family to ask questions and express concerns
		Provide opportunities for skills practice
		Assess patient's potential compliance and make referrals for home follow-up if necessary

12 □ Cardiogenic shock

Cardiogenic shock is a syndrome that results from inadequate tissue perfusion secondary to heart disease. It is most often the result of an AMI or cumulative infarctions in which 40% or more of the left ventricle is destroyed. It can also occur as a result of decompensating left heart failure or following cardiac surgery. In the presence of impaired left ventricular function, other factors may promote the shock syndrome including arrhythmias, drugs depressing myocardial contractility, hypoxia, acidosis, hypovolemia, and abnormalities in peripheral vascular regulation.

Cardiogenic shock consists of sustained systemic arterial hypotension with evidence of inadequate tissue perfusion of the kidneys, brain, and skin. Indications of inadequate tissue perfusion include decreased urine output (less than 20 ml/hour); changes in sensorium (restlessness, apprehension, confusion); cool, clammy skin; thready, weak brachial and radial pulses; sinus tachycardia; and hyperventilation as a compensatory mechanism for rising blood lactate levels. Most of these symptoms are due to the redistribution of blood volume as the body attempts to maintain blood pressure in the presence of decreasing cardiac output.

Hypotension has been defined in this context by the Myocardial Infarction Research Unit Program as an arterial pressure less than 90 mm Hg for a previously normotensive person or a fall of greater than 80 mm Hg for a previously hypertensive person. Once hypotension occurs, rapid deterioration usually evolves as the "cycle" of shock begins. Coronary blood flow decreases as the blood pressure decreases, resulting in further deterioration of left ventricular function and elevation of left ventricular filling pressures. As the gradient (aortic diastolic pressure minus left ventricular diastolic pressure) diminishes, decreasing the effective coronary perfusion pressure, further impairment to coronary blood flow occurs resulting in progressive subendocardial ischemia, progressive left ventricular dysfunction, and peripheral flow deficiencies. Hypoxemia and acidosis are established as a result and contribute to further deterioration.

Cardiogenic shock lasting more than 1 hour associated with a prior MI has a mortality rate greater than 80%. It is the most frequent cause of in-hospital death following AMI. Therefore early recognition, ideally before the cycle is established, and aggressive intervention are imperative. Invasive monitoring is essential for assessing the rapid and generally unpredictable changes in status and response to the therapeutic modalities used. Minimally this includes accurate determinations of intra-arterial blood pressure, left ventricular filling pressures

(PCWP), hourly urine output, and arterial blood gas levels.

The problems and therapies employed for cardiogenic shock are interrelated and cannot be considered in isolation.

ASSESSMENT

1. Historical and current data necessary for assessing concomitant disease states and medications that contribute to or cause shock syndrome
2. Intake and output (urine via Foley catheter); urine specific gravities
3. Level of consciousness—neurological status
4. Color, temperature, and moisture of skin
5. Pulses: rate, rhythm, quality, and equality
6. Respiration: rate, pattern, depth, and sound
7. BP and MAP with intra-arterial line
8. Measurement of pressures
   a. Pulmonary artery diastolic pressure
   b. PCWP
   c. CVP
   d. Mean aortic pressure
9. Cardiac output measurements
   a. Ejection fraction
   b. Cardiac index
10. Signs and symptoms of elevated right ventricular filling pressure
    a. Neck vein distention
    b. Positive hepatojugular reflux
    c. Increased CVP
11. Signs and symptoms of pulmonary congestion
12. Pain
13. Temperature
14. Intensity of heart sounds, presence of S_3 or S_4 gallops and murmurs
15. Lab data results for
    a. Blood gas levels
    b. Electrolytes
    c. BUN/creatinine clearance
    d. Hct
    e. Serial cardiac enzymes and isoenzymes
    f. Chest radiographs
    g. Drug levels
16. Monitor ECG for
    a. Arrhythmias

b. Changes characteristic of myocardial ischemia and necrosis
c. Changes characteristic of electrolyte imbalance
d. Changes characteristic of drugs and their toxic effects
17. Results of special studies employed to determine cardiac status
    a. Radioisotope scanning
    b. Coronary arteriography
    c. Left ventricular cineangiography
    d. Two-dimensional echocardiogram

GOALS

1. Hemodynamic stability
   a. Systolic BP: 90 to 110 mm Hg
   b. Diastolic BP: 60 to 90 mm Hg
   c. Pulse pressure within normal limits
   d. Left ventricular filling pressure: 15 to 20 mm Hg
   e. Cardiac output sufficient to maintain adequate tissue perfusion
2. Adequate tissue perfusion and tissue integrity
   a. Urine output minimally 20 to 30 ml/hour; BUN/creatinine clearance and urine specific gravity within normal limits
   b. Skin warm and dry with no pallor or cyanosis
   c. Patient is oriented and able to communicate—neurological system intact
   d. Adequate coronary perfusion pressure
   e. Peripheral resistance sufficient to maintain BP without deleterious effects or decreased tissue perfusion
3. pH, Pa_{O_2}, and Pa_{CO_2} within normal limits
4. Serum electrolytes within normal limits
5. Electrophysiological stability
6. Normal temperature
7. Absence of signs and symptoms of pulmonary congestion
8. Absence or control of pain
9. Patient/family verbalizes fears and concerns
   a. Reduction of patient/family's level of anxiety with provision of information and emotional support
   b. Family calmly visits with patient
   c. Clergyman of choice available if desired by patient/family

Potential problems	Expected outcomes	Nursing activities
■ Inadequate tissue perfusion related to Depressed ventricular function Body's compensatory redistribution of blood volume Hypoxia Acidosis	■ Adequate tissue perfusion and tissue integrity Urine output minimally 20 to 30 ml/hour BUN/creatinine clearance and specific gravity within normal limits	■ Assess for signs and symptoms indicating degree of tissue perfusion and peripheral resistance Renal perfusion 　Measure intake and output; include sources other than urine 　Measure urine output q1 hr; Foley catheter required for accuracy 　　1. Report output less than 30 ml/hour 　　2. Output less than 20 ml/hour is indicative of shock; intervention is required to prevent ischemia and renal failure 　Assess for indications of renal failure 　　1. Lack of response to sufficient dosages of diuretics 　　2. Anuria and azotemia 　　3. Elevated BUN or creatinine clearance 　　4. Decreased specific gravity 　　5. See Standard: *Acute renal failure*
	Skin warm and dry with no pallor or cyanosis	Cutaneous perfusion: check color, temperature, and hydration of skin for changes consistent with decreased perfusion—cool, pale, cyanotic, moist, or clammy
	pH within normal limits	Skeletal muscle and splanchnic perfusion: check blood gas levels for evidence of metabolic acidosis resulting from rise in blood lactate levels; may be initial isolated reduction in Pa_{CO_2} in response to compensatory hyperventilation; subsequently the pH falls
	Absence of abdominal or cardiac pain	Gastrointestinal perfusion: check for presence of recurring abdominal pain and rigidity associated with ischemia of the bowel, which may lead to necrosis and bleeding
	Patient oriented and able to communicate; neurological system intact	Cerebral and coronary perfusion are affected more by aortic perfusion pressure than by sympathetic nervous system compensatory activity; therefore signs and symptoms of inadequate perfusion more often occur with imminently pending or concurrent hypotension Cerebral perfusion Observe for changes indicating altered sensorium 　　1. Restlessness 　　2. Confusion 　　3. Somnolence 　　4. Psychosis Assess neurological status 　　1. Level of consciousness 　　2. Pupils and extraocular movements 　　3. Presence of spontaneous movement of extremities 　　4. Response to stimuli—verbal, tactile, pain 　　5. Presence of gag reflex 　　6. Respiratory rate and pattern; absence of spontaneous respiration
	Absence or stabilization of arrhythmias and congestive heart failure Adequate coronary perfusion pressure 60 to 80 mm Hg Pa_{O_2} and Pa_{CO_2} within normal limits	Coronary perfusion: observe for arrhythmias, signs and symptoms of congestive heart failure, and extension of MI Check pulses; poorly palpable brachial and radial pulses with bounding central pulsations may indicate intense upper extremity vasoconstriction, which may precipitate hypotension Check R for indications of hypoventilation or hyperventilation Check blood gas results for acidosis, decreased Pa_{O_2}, or increased Pa_{CO_2}; acidosis further promotes inadequate tissue perfusion
	Peripheral resistance sufficient to maintain BP without deleterious effects of decreased tis-	Monitor pressures for indication of increased peripheral resistance; intra-arterial line is required for accuracy Decreased pulse pressure; more significant finding with concurrent increased venous pressure, which helps to differen-

Potential problems	Expected outcomes	Nursing activities
	sue perfusion Pulse pressure within normal limits Diastolic pressure maintained at 60 to 90 mm Hg Systolic pressure maintained at 90 to 110 mm Hg	tiate etiology of change from depressed myocardial function or hypovolemia Increased diastolic pressure (also influenced by heart rate, which determines duration of diastole) Increased MAP If measurements are available, total peripheral vascular resistance can be calculated with the following formula:

$$\frac{\text{Mean aortic pressure} - \text{Mean right atrial pressure (mm Hg)}}{\text{Cardiac output (liters/minute)}}$$

Keep physician informed of patient's status and changes indicating deterioration

Participate in management directed toward improving tissue perfusion before hypotension, acidosis, and hypoxemia become established, and toward treating complications of inadequate perfusion

Maintain patent intra-arterial line; maintain patent intravenous line for administration of drugs; use soluset or infusion pump for control

Administer medications as ordered

Vasodilators may be ordered when blood flow is reduced and when patient is still normotensive to decrease afterload and O_2 consumption

Sodium nitroprusside most commonly used

Nitroglycerin and long-acting nitrates more difficult to titrate

High doses of corticosteroids may be ordered in an attempt to produce same effects

Monitor effectiveness of medication according to the improvement in patient's perfusion and left ventricular performance reflected by a decrease in left ventricular filling pressures and an increase in cardiac output without hypotension being produced

Titrate medication as ordered to maintain systolic BP 90 to 110 mm Hg

Inotropic agents with vasodilator effects such as isoproterenol (Isuprel); dobutamine, and dopamine (dosage dependent); observe for side effects resulting from increased myocardial O_2 consumption

Initiate measures to prevent renal failure as ordered by maintaining urine output greater than 20 ml/hour

Administer diuretics ordered by physician such as furosemide

Administer if ordered an osmotic diuretic such as mannitol to increase renal blood flow if output is less than 30 ml/hour in an attempt to prevent renal ischemia; inform physician if this fails to induce diuresis; an osmotic diuretic does not enter cells and metabolize so if it is not excreted, it may cause blood volume to overexpand and result in pulmonary edema

Dopamine or dobutamine may be ordered specifically because of the ability of these drugs to increase renal blood flow

If acute renal failure develops, hemodialysis or peritoneal dialysis may be indicated

See Standard: *Acute renal failure*

The smallest amount of any medication that will produce the desired effect should be used; inadequate renal or hepatic perfusion may interfere with metabolism and excretion of drugs and result in accumulation and toxicity

Monitor ECG for arrhythmias, a frequent complication of medications

Potential problems	Expected outcomes	Nursing activities
		Monitor PCWP to determine left ventricular filling pressure; see Problem, Depressed myocardial function
		Monitor cardiac output; see Problem, Depressed myocardial function
		If cerebral hypoxia results in inadequate spontaneous respiration or its absence, patient will require intubation and mechanical ventilation
		If pharmacological management is not effective, counterpulsation may be instituted to decrease afterload during systole, to increase aortic pressure during diastole resulting in increased coronary perfusion, and to increase peripheral arterial blood flow

SEE STANDARDS: *Hemodynamic monitoring*
Mechanical ventilation
Intra-aortic balloon pumping

■ Hypotension resulting in inadequate venous return related to Depressed myocardial function
Hypovolemia
Vasodilator therapy
Inadequate vasoconstriction—inability to compensate for decreasing cardiac output most common with elderly or diabetic patients

■ Systolic pressure 90 to 110 mm Hg
Adequate circulating blood volume
Peripheral resistance sufficient to maintain BP without deleterious effects of decreased tissue perfusion
Left ventricular filling pressure 15 to 20 mm Hg
Absence of signs and symptoms of pulmonary edema

■ Monitor arterial BP and MAP with intra-arterial pressure lines; MAP can also be calculated using the following formula:

$$\frac{\text{Diastolic pressure} \times 2 + \text{Systolic pressure}}{3}$$

Monitor CVP to determine blood volume and adequacy of central venous return
Check P for compensatory sinus tachycardia
Check for signs and symptoms of reduced cerebral or coronary blood flow, both of which are directly affected by mean aortic pressure; see Problem, Inadequate tissue perfusion
Check urine output and specific gravity q1 hr; follow lab data noted in Problem, Inadequate tissue perfusion; if tubular necrosis develops secondary to hypotension (lack of response to diuretics), urine output is a less specific indicator of renal blood flow because of nephron abnormalities
Assess for presence of hypovolemia
    Review intake and output records and acute weight changes; with AMI, fluid loss can occur as a result of reduced intake related to pain, nausea and vomiting, and analgesic therapy or secondary to diaphoresis, diuretic therapy, and diarrhea resulting from medications
Check for signs and symptoms indicating elevated right ventricular filling pressures
    Elevated CVP
    Neck vein distention
    Positive hepatojugular reflux
    Hepatomegaly
    Ascites
    Peripheral or sacral edema
Participate in fluid challenge as ordered to help distinguish hypovolemic shock from that due to left ventricular dysfunction
    Contraindicated if PCWP is greater than 18 to 22 mm Hg or CVP is greater than 12 cm H_2O
    Administer colloidal solution (dextran or albumin) or normal saline solution in 50 to 100 ml boluses at 5- to 10-minute intervals; the challenge must be carried out rapidly to ensure vascular compartment expansion
    Check PCWP and CVP after each bolus; a rise in PCWP to 20 to 22 mm Hg or an increase in CVP by 2 cm H_2O is considered a reasonable challenge
    Continue challenge until these pressures are reached or until the flow deficiency is corrected, whichever comes first; earlier cessation is an inadequate challenge
    Hypovolemia is indicated if a favorable response is achieved without much increase in PCWP

Potential problems	Expected outcomes	Nursing activities
		Cardiac dysfunction is indicated if PCWP increases without clinical improvement
		Participate as ordered in management directed toward maintaining an adequate circulating volume either by supplementing fluid or altering redistribution
		Maintain systolic arterial BP at 90 to 110 mm Hg
		If a problem related to hypovolemia occurs, continue fluid challenge, using guidelines described before
		Monitor
		PCWP
		CVP
		Intra-arterial pressure
		Indices of perfusion noted in Problem, Inadequate tissue perfusion
		Signs and symptoms of pulmonary edema
		Administer vasoconstrictors if ordered; the only indication for these drugs in patients with depressed myocardial function following AMI is hypotension; norepinephrine is the usual drug of choice because it also has inotropic properties; metaraminol may also be ordered
		Monitor BP at least q15 min
		Monitor PCWP: with left ventricular dysfunction, left ventricular filling pressures at 15 to 20 mm Hg are desired to enhance contractility according to Starling's law
		Monitor ECG for arrhythmias continuously
		Monitor signs and symptoms of inadequate perfusion (see Problem, Inadequate tissue perfusion)
		Titrate to smallest dosage that raises BP and increases urine output; attempt to titrate off medication as soon as possible; if medication is necessary for a prolonged period, dextran or plasma expanders may be ordered to maintain adequate left ventricular filling pressures
		Check blood gas levels for acidosis, which decreases the effect of vasoconstrictor agents; adjust dosages as ordered
■ Depressed myocardial function related to Loss of functional cardiac muscle Adverse effect of medications Acidosis Hypoxemia Hyperkalemia Arrhythmias	■ Left ventricular filling pressure 15 to 20 mm Hg Cardiac output sufficient to maintain adequate tissue perfusion Cardiac index 2.5 to 4.0 liters/minute/m² Ejection fraction 60% to 75% of end diastolic volume Electrophysiological stability Normal temperature pH, Pa_{O_2}, and Pa_{CO_2} within normal limits Serum K^+ within normal limits	■ Determine if the patient is receiving any medications that may depress myocardial function such as propranolol, quinidine, or procainamide (Pronestyl)
		Participate with physician in monitoring hemodynamic measurements essential for evaluating serial changes in left ventricular function and response to therapy
		PCWP reflecting left ventricular filling pressure; ideally maintained at 15 to 20 mm Hg
		Cardiac output measurements—several methods for determining cardiac output are available, including thermodilution, Fick principle that measures arterial-venous O_2 difference, the indicator dilution method, and radioisotope scanning method if equipment is available
		Cardiac index is a more specific determinant of the adequacy of cardiac output because body size is considered; it may be calculated using the DuBois body surface chart after measuring cardiac output, height, and weight; a normal cardiac index is 2.5 to 4.0 liters/minute/m²
		Ejection fraction may be calculated by the following formula:

$$\frac{\text{Stroke volume}}{\text{End diastolic volume}} \times 100\%$$

The normal range is 60% to 75% of the end diastolic volume; a decreased ejection fraction reveals inability of left ventricle to empty adequately

Potential problems	Expected outcomes	Nursing activities

Intra-arterial measurements of BP and mean aortic pressure; decrease in mean aortic pressure and increase in left ventricular filling pressure result in decreased coronary artery perfusion, promoting further myocardial ischemia and necrosis

Assess for indices of inadequate perfusion noted in Problem, Inadequate tissue perfusion

Assess for signs and symptoms indicative of myocardial ischemia or extension of infarction

Auscultate precordium for
  Intensity of heart sounds
  Presence of S_3 or S_4 gallops
  Murmurs

Continuously monitor ECG for
  Arrhythmias
  Changes consistent with myocardial ischemia or extension of infarction
  Drug effects

Check temperature q4 hr or as indicated; if temperature is elevated, observe for indications of increased cardiac work and myocardial O_2 demands and a potential decrease in peripheral vascular resistance

Monitor blood gas levels and electrolytes for acidosis, hypoxemia, and hyperkalemia

Keep physician informed of patient's status, reporting any changes in data

Participate with physician in measures to improve myocardial function, and correct aggravating factors as ordered

Eliminate myocardial depressant drugs

Place patient in supine position; avoid Trendelenburg position

Maintain patent IV line for drug and fluid infusions

Maintain patent hemodynamic monitoring lines
  Observe for signs and symptoms of complications resulting from lines; see Standard: *Hemodynamic monitoring;* interpret results relating to therapeutic interventions

Administer antipyretics as ordered if temperature is elevated; keep patient warm and dry

Continue activities to correct perfusion abnormalities, acidosis, and hyperkalemia (noted in Problems, Inadequate tissue perfusion, Hypoxia-hypoxemia, and Acidosis) if present

Treat arrhythmias as ordered

Administer medications to improve myocardial function; inotropic agents with either vasoconstricting (only in presence of hypotension) or vasodilating actions will be ordered
  Monitor hemodynamic parameters indicated previously to determine response to therapy
  Be alert to development of arrhythmias, particularly ventricular arrhythmias, which are a frequent side effect of medications

Observe for toxic effects of all medications that patient is receiving if reduced circulation and redistribution of blood flow are present; the result is a decreased volume of distribution whereby smaller concentrations may be required to avoid toxicity

If patient does not respond to therapy, aortic balloon counterpulsation in conjunction with medications may be employed to stabilize patient for cardiac catheterization and

Potential problems	Expected outcomes	Nursing activities
		possible emergency surgery if correctable lesions are found; see Standards: *Intra-aortic balloon pumping; Cardiac catheterization; Cardiac surgery*
■ Hypoxia-hypoxemia related to Pulmonary congestion Hypoventilation Decreased cardiac output Altered cerebral function	■ pH, Pa_{O_2}, and Pa_{CO_2} within normal limits Absence of signs and symptoms of pulmonary congestion Adequate circulating blood volume to maintain cardiac output Absence of pain Serum K^+ within normal limits	■ Frequently monitor blood gas levels via intra-arterial line; ensure that factors which alter blood gas results are stabilized at least 20 minutes before sampling Patient's comfort if the patient is conscious Endotracheal suctioning Changes in O_2 concentration Adjustments to mechanical ventilator Administer O_2 as ordered If pulmonary congestion is present, use a high flow rate and rebreathing mask If Pa_{O_2} does not respond and remains less than 70 to 75 mm Hg, probably intubation and mechanical ventilation will be required Observe for signs and symptoms of pulmonary congestion; if present, institute measures as ordered to decrease congestion to improve oxygenation Administer diuretics as ordered following precautions noted in Problem, Inadequate tissue perfusion; hypovolemia and electrolyte imbalance augment shock state Deliver positive pressure if ordered, monitoring closely for indications of decreasing venous return which may augment shock state Monitor respiratory effort noting rate, pattern, depth, and sound If tachypnea is present, it may indicate atelectasis, bronchospasm, pulmonary edema, or compensatory response to acidosis; if patient is being mechanically ventilated, check for increased secretions, cuff integrity, placement of tube, adequacy of ventilator settings, and patient's response Changes in patterns of respiration generally reflect cerebral perfusion problems If pain is present, treat immediately; if opiates are ordered, administer with great caution because of their respiratory depressant and hypotensive effects Review results of arterial and venous blood sampling for arterial-venous O_2 difference if performed; an increase or widening of the difference indicates that more O_2 is being extracted by tissues during circulation as an autoregulatory response to decreased cardiac output Continue measures for improving cardiac output and perfusion noted in Problems, Inadequate tissue perfusion and Depressed myocardial function Observe for complications of hypoxia, which will promote shock cycle if they occur and are not corrected immediately Hypercapnia—always occurs with hypoventilation; results in respiratory acidosis and a compensatory increase in respiration; administration of O_2 will not remove excess CO_2 so measures noted before to improve ventilation must be continued Hypotension—see Problem, Hypotension resulting in inadequate venous return Tachycardia and arrhythmias—see Problem, Arrhythmias Metabolic acidosis/hyperkalemia—see Problem, Acidosis SEE STANDARD: *Mechanical ventilation*

Potential problems	Expected outcomes	Nursing activities
■ Acidosis related to Hypercapnia Increased lactate acid production resulting from anaerobic metabolism of glucose	■ pH, Pa_{O_2}, and Pa_{CO_2} within normal limits Left ventricular filling pressure 15 to 20 mm Hg Absence of signs and symptoms of pulmonary congestion Electrophysiological stability Serum K^+ within normal limits	■ Frequent monitoring of blood gas levels via intra-arterial line; initially a decrease in arterial Pa_{CO_2} may be seen in response to compensatory hyperventilation; if ventilation is not improved and the Pa_{CO_2} lowered sufficiently, the pH will fall, indicating acidosis If problem occurs, inform physician immediately and make available sodium bicarbonate IV for administration to maintain normal pH; participate with physician in correction of factors producing acidosis; check blood gas levels and pH frequently for resolution of acidosis and/or for development of metabolic alkalosis resulting from too vigorous therapy Monitor PCWP for increased left ventricular filling pressure and for signs of pulmonary congestion Observe for complications produced or aggravated by acidosis Decreased cardiac contractility Arrhythmias Hyperkalemia, which further impairs cardiac contractility and promotes arrhythmias Adjust dosages of vasoconstrictor drugs as ordered, the effect of which is lessened by acidosis Continue therapeutic modalities as ordered for improving myocardial function and tissue perfusion
■ Arrhythmias related to Inadequate tissue perfusion, particularly cardiac Hypotension Diminished myocardial function Hypoxia Acidosis Hyperkalemia Pain	■ Electrophysiological stability	■ Continuous ECG monitoring is essential Select lead best demonstrating atrial and ventricular activity Set rate alarms If arrhythmia occurs, assess effect on cardiac output; bradyarrhythmias, tachyarrhythmias, ventricular premature beats, and those resulting in loss of sequential atrial ventricular contraction may seriously alter an already compromised status and promote progressive deterioration If problem occurs, inform physician immediately; continue measures to correct precipitating factor Administer antiarrhythmics as ordered through soluset or infusion pump for exact dosage control and prevention of fluid overload; remember that many antiarrhythmics further depress myocardial contractility, particularly procainamide, quinidine, and propranolol; in addition, in a patient with diminished circulating volume and diminished renal or hepatic function, lower than usual doses may produce toxicity Ensure that emergency equipment is available and functioning for immediate correction of ventricular tachycardia or ventricular fibrillation SEE STANDARD: *Arrhythmias*
■ Pain related to decreased tissue perfusion	■ Absence or control of pain	■ Assess for verbal and nonverbal cues of pain If patient is able to communicate and is coherent, instruct patient to inform nurse immediately of the presence of pain If patient is not able to communicate but is coherent, develop signals indicating presence of pain If pain is present Inform physician Determine location Cardiac Abdominal Peripheral Administer medication as ordered using as small a dose as possible

Potential problems	Expected outcomes	Nursing activities
		If morphine is administered, monitor closely for depressive effect on cardiac and respiratory functions; it is safer to use if the patient is being mechanically ventilated
■ Patient/family's anxiety related to severity of condition	■ Patient/family verbalizes fears and concerns Reduction of patient/family's level of anxiety with provision of information and emotional support Family calmly visits with patient	■ Continuous assessment of level of anxiety made difficult by altered levels of consciousness of patient and inability to speak if intubation is required Maintain a quiet, controlled environment as much as possible If patient is able to speak, provide opportunities and encourage verbalization of fears, concerns, and confrontation with death but do not force communication Provide frequent explanations of who the team members are and their qualifications, the purpose of multiple monitoring systems and treatment modalities, and what to expect before intervention or procedure is initiated; comment on condition and presence or communications from family members Provide family with frequent information about patient; provide opportunities for family to be with patient; if desired and possible without compromising safety, provide time alone for patient and family; if possible, provide someone to whom family can talk, if not a health professional, then perhaps clergy or a trained volunteer; often the threat of death is sudden and unexpected, and the patient/family has not been allowed time for any emotional preparation
	Clergyman of choice available if desired by patient/family	Determine if patient/family desires a religious representative, e.g., priest, rabbi, minister

13 □ Shock

Shock is a clinical syndrome characterized by a reduction in the effective circulating blood volume, leading to a generalized inadequacy of perfusion to the vital body organs. An acceleration of circulatory impairment and progressive organ dysfunction may result in irreversible damage and death.

The common findings in all forms of shock include hypovolemia (absolute or relative) and significantly altered peripheral resistance.

Generally the patient is acutely ill and confused, restless, or stuporous, with cool extremities. The blood pressure is low (less than 90 mm Hg) with a narrow pulse pressure. Tachycardia is often present, with weak and thready pulses. Only the larger, more central vessel pulses may be palpable. Signs of peripheral hypoperfusion and vasoconstriction may be present, including cool and clammy skin. On the other hand, septic shock may be associated with capillary dilatation and warm skin. Urine output is diminished or absent as a result of decreased renal perfusion. Metabolic acidosis is usually present. Temperature may be below normal, normal, or slightly elevated. Dyspnea may be present, with rapid and shallow respirations.

The major types of shock include
1. Hypovolemic or oligemic shock with a blood volume relative to vascular space deficit; etiological factors include
   a. External fluid losses
      (1) Severe vomiting
      (2) Diarrhea
      (3) Gastrointestinal bleeding
   b. Internal losses; largely losses of intravascular

fluid volume to the interstitial and intracellular spaces
   (1) Ileus
   (2) Intestinal obstruction
   (3) Burns
   (4) Peritonitis
2. Cardiogenic shock or inadequate cardiac output
   a. MI
   b. Acute arrhythmias
   c. Acute pericardial tamponade
   d. Severe heart valve malfunction
   e. Massive pulmonary embolus
   f. Tension pneumothorax
3. Bacteremic shock or sepsis, especially gram-negative sepsis
   a. Pyelonephritis
   b. Acute cholecystitis
   c. Pneumonia in the alcoholic patient and in the patient with COPD
   d. Burn sepsis
   e. Bacterial endocarditis
   f. Nosocomial sepsis
4. Neurogenic or vasogenic shock involves the loss of neurogenic tone to vessels
   a. Spinal cord injury
   b. Anesthetic paralysis (vasodilation)
   c. Reflex vasodilation
5. Anaphylactic shock, which results from an antigen-antibody reaction that damages capillaries and results in histamine release and associated vasodilation
   a. Drugs
   b. Pollen
   c. Insect sting
   d. Foreign proteins in serum
6. Endocrine abnormalities inducing shock
   a. Diabetic ketoacidosis
   b. Adrenal crisis

Therapy for shock of any cause is directed toward improvement of arterial pressure to 90 mm Hg to restore blood flow to vital organs and management of accompanying hypoxemia, azotemia, acidosis, and other complications.

ASSESSMENT

1. History and nature of
   a. Gastrointestinal problem, that is, ulcers, varices, and gastritis
   b. Severe infection with either gram-positive or gram-negative organisms, including severe respiratory infections, peritonitis, meningitis, etc.
   c. MI, cardiac failure, valvular disease, hypertension, arrhythmias, and cardiac surgery
   d. Diabetes mellitus, hypoglycemia, renal insufficiency, coagulation disorders
   e. Recent spinal cord injury
   f. Severe reactions to anesthetics, drugs, diagnostic agents, vaccine, insect bites, etc.
   g. Endocrine disorders
   h. Nutritional status
2. Presence of signs and symptoms, including
   a. Severe hypotension
   b. Abnormally low or high CVP and PAP, if measurements are available
   c. Weak and thready or bounding pulse
   d. Cool, clammy skin
   e. Pallor, cyanosis
   f. Oliguria
   g. Acidosis and/or azotemia
   h. Restlessness, confusion
   i. Decreased or absent reflexes
   j. Labored, shallow respirations
   k. Chest pain
   l. Jugular venous distention
   m. Hemorrhage
   n. Severe burn injury
   o. Open wound
   p. Embolic episodes
   q. Rashes or erythema
   r. Abdominal pain and/or tenderness
3. Results of lab and diagnostic tests, including
   a. Hct level
   b. WBC count
   c. Erythrocyte sedimentation rate (ESR)
   d. BUN and/or creatinine clearance
   e. Electrolyte values
   f. Drug levels
   g. Arterial blood gas levels
   h. Cultures: sputum, blood, wound, and urine
   i. Cardiac enzymes
   j. Clotting profile
   k. Lactic acid levels
   l. Urinary electrolytes
   m. Chest and abdominal radiographs
   n. Lumbar puncture
   o. Arterial BP, CVP, PCWP
   p. Cardiac output
   q. ECG
   r. Gastroscopy or endoscopy
   s. Arteriogram
4. Patient/family's anxiety related to perception of and reaction to disease process, signs and symptoms,

diagnostic procedures, therapy employed, and prognosis

GOALS

1. Patient/family's behavior indicates reduction in anxiety with provision of information and explanations
2. Hemodynamic stability; adequate cardiac output
   a. Adequate tissue perfusion of vital organs
   b. Normovolemia
3. Respiratory function sufficient to maintain
   a. Adequate oxygenation and ventilation
   b. Acid-base balance within normal limits
   c. Absence of respiratory distress syndrome
4. Serum electrolyte levels and blood count within normal limits
5. Gastrointestinal, neuromuscular, and integumentary function within normal limits

6. Infection free; absence of septicemia
7. Resolution and/or control of etiological factors
8. Prevention and/or resolution of accompanying complications, that is, disseminated intravascular coagulation (DIC), acute respiratory distress syndrome, etc.
9. Patient/family supplied with sufficient information for compliance with discharge regimen; before discharge the patient/family will be able to
   a. Identify factors specific to the patient that might precipitate a recurrence of shock and ways to prevent or avoid these precipitating factors
   b. Describe medications, dietary and activity regimen
   c. State signs and symptoms requiring medical intervention
   d. Describe plan for follow-up care

Potential problems	Expected outcomes	Nursing activities
■ Anxiety related to Insufficient knowledge Monitoring equipment Diagnostic procedures	■ Reduction in level of anxiety with provision of information, explanations	■ Ongoing assessment of level of anxiety Describe nature of disease process, signs and symptoms, and therapy employed Explain anticipated diagnostic procedures, monitoring equipment, and plan of care Encourage questions and verbalization of anxieties, fears, and concerns Involve patient/family in plan of care Demonstrate concern and warmth in providing care to the patient Keep patient warm and comfortable Anticipate needs to minimize patient efforts and energy expenditure Position and turn patient q2 hr Encourage coughing and deep breathing Allow uninterrupted rest periods between procedures Evaluate for decrease in level of anxiety with provision of information and explanations
■ Hypovolemia related to External blood volume losses Wound GI bleeding Hemorrhage Internal losses with "third spacing" Peritonitis Burns Intestinal obstruction	■ Normovolemia—adequate volume expansion Hemodynamic parameters within normal limits	■ Monitor for Severe hypotension; note vital signs q1 hr and prn Low CVP and PAP (note q½-1 hr until stable) and low cardiac output measurements if available Oliguria; note urine output with specific gravity q1 hr Signs of inadequate peripheral perfusion Poor skin turgor, dry mucous membranes Signs and symptoms of GI hemorrhage; see Standard: *Acute upper gastrointestinal bleeding* Signs and symptoms of peritonitis and intestinal obstruction; see Standard: *Peritonitis; Gastrointestinal surgery* Signs and symptoms of excessive fluid loss from burns; see Standard: *Burns* Lab data results q6 hr Electrolyte levels, particularly Na^+, and Hct levels BUN level and creatinine clearance Notify physician for any abnormality If hypovolemia occurs

Potential problems	Expected outcomes	Nursing activities
		Administer volume expanders as ordered, i.e., blood, plasma, saline solution, and dextran; high caloric solution, proteins and fats Administer vasopressors as ordered Place patient in a position to maximize blood flow to central organs; keep patient supine until signs of hypovolemia resolve Administer corticosteroids to increase tissue perfusion if ordered

■ Infection
  Systemic sepsis or bacteremia
  Local infection
	■ Absence of or early resolution of sepsis
	  Absence of clinical manifestations of infection
		■ Observe and monitor q½-1 hr for
		  Hyperthermia/hypothermia
		  Skin—warm and dry or cool and clammy
		  Tachycardia
		  Sudden, unexplained hypotension
		  Decreased, normal, or increased peripheral resistance, CVP, and cardiac output
		  Tachypnea, hyperventilation
		  Gastrointestinal symptoms, including vomiting, abdominal cramps, distention
		  Altered mental status—check level of consciousness
		  Any swelling, redness, abnormal secretions from wounds or any part of the body
		  Abnormal bleeding indicative of DIC; see Standard: *Disseminated intravascular coagulation*
		  Monitor lab data daily for results of
		  C and S of organism growing in sputum, urine, blood, and/or wound
		  WBC count
		  ESR
		  Chest and abdominal radiographs
		  Clotting profile, Hct
		  Notify physician for any abnormalities
		  Maintain a patent airway for efficient ventilation
		  Administer antibiotic and corticosteroid therapy as ordered
		  Administer vasoactive amine if shock persists, if ordered
		  Administer volume replacement if ordered
		  Prepare patient for surgery as ordered, if needed

■ Neurogenic or vasogenic shock related to spinal cord injury and/or spinal anesthesia, leading to vasodilation and hypotension	■ Absence of or resolution of vasogenic shock
	  Adequate cardiac output
	  Hemodynamic stability
	  BP and peripheral perfusion within normal limits
		■ Observe for
		  Sudden hypotension associated with precipitating event (q½-1 hr until stable)
		  Syncopal episode(s)
		  Altered mental status; monitor ongoing level of consciousness
		  Notify physician for any abnormality
		  Administer volume expanders if ordered
		  Administer vasopressors if ordered (e.g., phenylephrine [Neo-Synephrine] or methamphetamine [Methedrine] to reverse the reflex and depressive, vasodilating effect of anesthetic drugs)

■ Anaphylactic shock related to a severe drug reaction—vaccine, serum, insect bite, etc.	■ Absence of or resolution of anaphylactic shock
	  Hemodynamic stability
		■ Delay absorption of antigen with forced emesis when appropriate or by applying a tourniquet above the injection site
		  Observe for
		  Severe hypotension; check vital signs, including temperature, q30 min if reaction is suspected
		  Signs and symptoms of respiratory distress including choking, wheezing, and coughing
		  Apprehension and restlessness
		  Generalized urticaria and pruritus

Potential problems	Expected outcomes	Nursing activities
		Edema and cyanosis Paresthesia and altered level of consciousness Notify physician for any abnormality Maintain an adequate airway—assist with intubation if needed; see Standard: *Mechanical ventilation* Administer epinephrine (0.5 ml—1:1000 in 10 ml saline solution as ordered, usually q5-15 min) until adequate response is elicited Administer bronchodilator as ordered to relieve bronchospasm Administer antihistamines if ordered to shorten the duration of drug reaction and prevent relapses Administer hydrocortisone for prolonged reactions as ordered Administer a volume expander rapidly, using saline, albumin, and/or dextran solution Treat acidosis with bicarbonate as ordered Alert health team to adverse reaction of patient to offending agent If appropriate, advise patient to avoid offending agent in the future and inform future health care providers of his/her adverse reaction/allergy
■ Cardiogenic shock	■ Adequate cardiac contractility and output	■ Observe for Signs of decreased cardiac output (e.g., hypotension, oliguria) Signs of increased peripheral resistance with high CVP Atrial and ventricular arrhythmias Severe crushing pain radiating to arms and back Notify physician for any of these abnormalities If cardiogenic shock occurs, see Standard: *Cardiogenic shock*
■ Acute respiratory failure leading to acidosis	■ Absence of respiratory distress Respiratory function sufficient for adequate oxygenation and ventilation Arterial blood gas levels within normal limits	■ Monitor Arterial blood gas results q1-2 hr and prn until stable; note hypoxemia, hypercapnia, and acidemia Respirations q½-1 hr; note tachypnea, dyspnea Ongoing level of consciousness Notify physician for any of these abnormalities Maintain a patent airway Administer O_2 as ordered to maintain the arterial Pa_{O_2} at 90 to 100 mm Hg; desirable safe Pa_{O_2} levels are lower in patients with chronic lung disease Suction secretions as needed Administer bicarbonate as ordered Prepare for mechanical ventilation as ordered, if needed; see Standard: *Mechanical ventilation; Acute respiratory failure*
■ Renal failure related to inadequate perfusion	■ Adequate renal perfusion Indices of renal function and electrolyte levels within normal limits	■ Observe for signs and symptoms of acute renal failure Note urine output q1 hr If urine output is less than ½ ml/kg/hour in adults or 1 to 2 ml/kg/hour in children and infants, respectively, notify physician Fixed specific gravity at or about 1.010 Daily weights revealing steady weight gain Notify physician for any of these abnormalities Monitor lab data for Elevated BUN and creatinine levels Acid-base imbalance Electrolyte balance, particularly sodium (Na^+) and potassium (K^+) Administer fluids as ordered If problem occurs, see Standard: *Acute renal failure*

Potential problems	Expected outcomes	Nursing activities

■ Insufficient knowledge to comply with discharge regimen*	■ Sufficient information to comply with discharge regimen
	
	Patient/family correctly verbalizes postdischarge regimen regarding medications, diet, and activity progression
	
	If appropriate, patient/family identifies etiological factors for shock, accompanying signs and symptoms, and ways to avoid or prevent a recurrence
	
	Patient/family correctly describes plan for follow-up care
		■ Assess patient/family's level of understanding regarding discharge regimen
		Explain the discharge regimen, including
		  Medications—identify each medication, actions, side effects, routes, dose, schedule, and any precautionary or safety measures necessary
		  Dietary therapy
		  Activity progression—avoid overfatigue; allow for rest and relaxation
		Describe etiological factors for patient's shock episode, if appropriate, and ways to prevent or avoid a recurrence
		Explain need for medical alert identification bracelet indicating allergy
		Review plan for follow-up care, including purpose of the visits, when to come, where to go, who to see, and what specimens to bring
		Evaluate the potential compliance of the patient/family with the discharge regimen

*If this type of follow-up care is the responsibility of the critical care unit nurse.

14 □ **Pericarditis**

The heart is enclosed by a pericardial sac, which is composed of two surfaces. The inner surface encasing the heart is called the *visceral pericardium,* or *epicardium.* The outer surface, which is attached to different structures in the chest including the manubrium, ziphoid process, vertebral column, and diaphragm, is called the *parietal pericardium.* Normally there is 10 to 20 ml of thin, clear pericardial fluid between the contacting surfaces of the visceral and parietal pericardium. This fluid serves as a lubricant, allowing the heart to move freely within the pericardial sac.

Pericarditis refers to an alteration of the pericardium regardless of etiology. Known etiologies of acute pericarditis include infection (viral, bacterial, tuberculosis, fungal), AMI, postmyocardial thoracotomy syndrome, trauma, connective tissue diseases, neoplastic disease, systemic disease such as uremia, and drugs such as procainamide, hydralazine, and phenytoin (Dilantin). Frequently the etiology is not known, and the disease is labeled *idiopathic* or *nonspecific* pericarditis. Since few

diseases affect the pericardium alone, the etiology or associated disease must be sought.

The onset of pericarditis may be insidious or abrupt. Signs and symptoms frequently present include fever, pericardial pain, pericardial friction rub, and a typical ECG picture that will be described later. The pain must be differentiated from that of AMI, dissecting aortic aneurysm, and pulmonary embolism. Pericardial pain is classicially described as sharp or knifelike; of moderate to severe intensity; precordial, often referred to the back and shoulders; and aggravated by deep inspiration or movement.

Inflammation of the pericardium may result in localized or generalized deposition of fibrin. This can produce constrictive pericarditis whereby the pericardium becomes rigid and unable to stretch. More commonly, the pericardial sac, normally a potential space with only a few drops of fluid, may fill with sufficient fluid to produce pericardial restriction (effusion or tamponade). Compression of the heart either by fibrosis or pericardial fluid results in the heart not being able to fill completely. Consequently, the systemic and pulmonary venous pressures increase and systemic blood pressure decreases, producing a compensatory sinus tachycardia. Eventually cardiac output will decrease.

The hemodynamic consequence of fluid accumulation in the pericardial sac is a result of the amount and speed of accumulation. The faster the accumulation, the less the volume necessary to produce hemodynamic instability and changes in intrapericardial pressure. Therefore, severe tamponade can occur when a small volume of fluid rapidly enters the pericardial sac or when large volumes accumulate over time. Early identification and treatment of effusions may prevent tamponade.

Management of pericarditis is usually achieved by appropriate analgesics for pain and/or anti-inflammatory agents. Some patients require steroid therapy. Treatment of the causative disease may be sufficient. Patients with frequent relapses may be considered for elective pericardiectomy. Generally, anticoagulants are contraindicated in the presence of pericarditis because they may precipitate bleeding into the pericardial sac and tamponade if the fluid is sanguineous.

If constrictive pericarditis occurs, a pericardial resection is usually recommended. The earlier this is done, the lower the mortality and the better the prognosis.

The prognosis of pericarditis is dependent on the causative disease and/or the complications of tamponade or constriction if present.

ASSESSMENT

1. Recent history of upper respiratory tract infection
2. Presence, nature, and extent of characteristic signs and symptoms of pericarditis
   a. Temperature—diaphoresis and chills
   b. Chest pain
   c. Pericardial friction rub
   d. Respiratory status
      (1) Breath sounds
      (2) Dyspnea
      (3) Orthopnea on leaning forward
   e. Fatigue
3. Monitor ECG for
   a. Changes specific for pericarditis
   b. Tachycardia
4. Patient's perception of and reaction to the diagnosis and/or required therapy
5. Signs and symptoms and lab data changes consistent with complications
   a. Pericardial effusion
   b. Pericardial tamponade
   c. Constrictive pericarditis

GOALS

1. Absence of pain
2. Afebrile
3. Hemodynamic stability
4. Patient asks questions and verbalizes understanding of disease process and required therapy
5. Patient's behavior demonstrates decreased anxiety with provision of information
6. Absence of or resolution of complications
7. Before discharge, the patient/family
   a. Lists symptoms suggestive of recurrence to be reported to physician
   b. Asks pertinent questions regarding self-care
   c. Identifies reasons why and methods for avoiding fatigue
   d. States the information necessary for compliance with medication regimen
   e. States necessary information regarding follow-up visits to physician and/or clinic
   f. States why he/she should avoid unnecessary exposure to those with upper respiratory infections and report symptoms of colds or cough to physician

Potential problems	Expected outcomes	Nursing activities

■ Alterations of the pericardium related to inflammation	■ Absence of pain	■ Assess for presence of pain
		  Observe patient for nonverbal cues
		  Instruct patient to inform health care team if pain is present
		If pain occurs
		  Obtain a clear description to assist in differentiation from AMI, dissecting aortic aneurysm, and/or pulmonary embolus; the description should include
		  Onset
		  Quality
		  Severity
		  Site

Potential problems	Expected outcomes	Nursing activities
		Radiation
		Influence of movement or deep inspiration
		Administer analgesics as ordered
		Administer anti-inflammatory agents or steroid therapy, which may be selectively used as ordered
		Participate in the treatment of underlying disease, e.g., uremia, which may be sufficient
		Position patient in high Fowler's or leaning forward on a padded overbed table for comfort
		Record and report occurrence, description of pain, and response to interventions

	Normal temperature
	Absence of diaphoresis and/or chills
	Absence of signs or symptoms of hidden infection
		Check temperature q4 hr or as indicated
		Observe for any signs or symptoms of hidden infection
		If problem occurs
		  Keep patient warm and dry
		  Observe for diaphoresis and/or chills
		  Administer antipyretics if indicated, and institute cooling measures if needed
		Maintain bed rest while chest pain, fever, and friction rub are present
		Assist patient to increase activity gradually after symptoms disappear while monitoring level of fatigue

■ Alterations of the pericardium related to parietal and visceral surfaces of the inflamed pericardium rubbing against each other	■ Absence of a pericardial friction rub	■ Auscultate the precordium q2-4 hr for presence of a friction rub; the sound is similar to that produced by rubbing pieces of hair together over your ear and is described as grating or scratchy
		Press diaphragm of the stethoscope firmly against the chest
		Determine location of rub; usually is best appreciated along the lower left sternal border to the apex but may be more diffuse
		Determine if rub is intermittent or continuous
		Determine number of components; it usually has three components related to the movement of the heart during atrial systole, ventricular systole and diastole
		If a rub is present
		  Report to physician
		  Record full description, including
		    Location
		    Number of components
		    Whether intermittent or continuous
		    Whether changing patient's position alters it

■ Alterations of the pericardium related to alterations in cardiac electrophysiology	■ Resolution of ECG changes characteristic of pericarditis	■ Monitor 12-lead ECGs serially for characteristic changes of pericarditis if suspicious of presence and/or documented by diagnosis
		  S-T segment elevation in two or three of the standard leads and in some or all of the V leads; this occurs early in the course followed by S-T segments returning to baseline and T waves becoming flattened and then inverted in all leads except aVr
		  The *absence* of abnormal Q waves, the loss of R wave voltage in V leads, and the presence of a general distribution of S-T segment changes helps differentiate pericarditis from an MI; in addition, the S-T segment elevation of pericarditis has a concave curvature as opposed to the convex curvature typical of an MI
		If changes occur, save recorded strip and report to physician

Potential problems	Expected outcomes	Nursing activities
■ Anxiety related to Limited understanding of the disease and its effect on the body Nature and degree of pain	■ Patient verbalizes anxiety and asks questions Reduction of anxiety with sufficient information Patient notifies health care team of pain when present	■ Ongoing assessment of level of anxiety Explain simply the nature of the disease and subsequent pain and fatigue, stressing that the resolution of one will resolve the other; also stress improvement in measurable parameters, indicating progress Explain reasons for monitoring and/or examination procedures used Encourage questions from patient/family
■ Collection of fluid in the pericardial sac related to pericardial effusion Gradual accumulation of fluid in the pericardium; may be small or large in volume	■ Absence or resolution of effusion or tamponade	■ Monitor carefully for changes in hemodynamic status; speed and amount of fluid accumulation determines onset of symptoms and frequency of observations Observe for the following indices of pericardial restrictions Increased venous pressure* Jugular vein distention Elevated CVP NOTE: If patient is receiving diuretic therapy, the venous pressure elevation may be less obvious Patient complaints of dyspnea or fullness in the chest Decreased BP* Narrowing pulse pressure Sinus tachycardia resulting from decreased stroke volume Weakening and/or absent peripheral pulse (decreased circulating blood volume) Pulsus paradoxus: decrease in pulse volume and systolic BP (greater than 10 mm Hg) during normal inspiration related to changes in left ventricular filling; produced by pericardial restriction and accentuated by inspiration* Palpate pulse for decrease in pulse amplitude with inspiration; check BP to confirm presence and to determine degree of pulsus paradoxus present Have patient breathe normally; inflate cuff Deflate cuff slowly and evenly, relating systolic reading to phase of inspiration Identify and record point at which first systolic sounds are heard regardless of phase of respiration; the mm Hg difference represents the millimeters of paradoxus Increasing restlessness or anxiety Signs of decreasing cerebral perfusion Record serial 12-lead ECG to detect decreases in QRS voltages and/or the development of electrical alternans (every other complex varies between two configurations) Report and record occurrence of any of the aforementioned, and change timing of observations appropriately Prepare patient for special tests used to determine the presence and amount of pericardial fluid, and monitor results if ordered Echocardiography Chest radiograph (enlarged heart with clear lung fields) Radioisotope angiography Contrast studies Ensure that equipment for a pericardiocentesis is readily available if an effusion is present and there is indication of increasing hemodynamic instability, or if the presence of pus in the pericardial sac is suspected Maintain patent IV line Administer steroids to treat recurrent effusions accompanied by fever and pain as ordered

*Indicates classic triad of tamponade.

Potential problems	Expected outcomes	Nursing activities
		If tamponade develops
		Place patient in low Fowler's position; administer O₂ as ordered
		Have CPR equipment and medications available for immediate use
		Monitor venous pressure, BP, and P q15-30 min
		Check peripheral pulses for perfusion q30 min
		Check for changes in degree of pulsus paradoxus, q15 min
		Monitor rhythm strips particularly for signs of tachycardia; take 12-lead ECG q30 min or as indicated
		Observe for and record changes in mental status
		Check for presence of Kussmaul's sign resulting from restriction to diastolic filling (absence of normal fall in pressure during inspiration)
		Assist with pericardiocentesis (removal of 100 to 200 ml usually results in dramatic improvement)
		Administer medications and IVs as ordered for
		Pain
		Arrhythmias
		Remain with patient as much as possible and provide emotional support
		Prepare for potential surgery, which may be indicated particularly if tamponade recurs after successful pericardiocentesis
■ Constrictive pericarditis related to fibrosis of the pericardium Usually develops slowly as a chronic disease but also may be subacute occurring in days or weeks even while effusion and/or tamponade is still present	■ Absence or resolution of constriction	■ Determine if patient has past history of constrictive pericarditis
		Observe for
		Fluid retention related to elevated systemic venous pressure
		Ascites
		Peripheral edema—may be pitting
		Patient complaints of abdominal swelling, lassitude, and exertional dyspnea
		Elevated jugular venous pressure
		Decreased pulse pressure
		Jaundice secondary to liver congestion and/or cardiac cirrhosis
		Pulsus paradoxus (less common than in tamponade)
		Auscultate precordium for "the precordial knock," a loud third heart sound
		Chronic, severe cachexia
		Kussmaul's sign (more common in patients with chronic pericarditis)
		Monitor ECG for
		Atrial fibrillation—common in patients with chronic pericarditis
		Low QRS voltage and flattened or inverted T waves
		Conduction disturbances and pathological Q waves related to involvement of myocardium, conduction system, and/or coronary arteries
		Notched P waves in lead II
		Prepare patient for and review results of the following, if ordered
		Chest radiograph—useful only when pericardium is heavily calcified
		Liver function studies—presence of hepatic insufficiency
		Cardiac catheterization—to confirm absence of myocardial and/or valvular disease in presence of restricted ventricular filling
		If diagnosis is made, assist in preparation of patient for a pericardial resection if indicated

Potential problems	Expected outcomes	Nursing activities
■ Insufficient knowledge to comply with discharge regimen*	■ Evaluation by testing or questioning demonstrates patient/family's understanding of the knowledge components of the teaching program Patient asks pertinent questions regarding self-care	■ Institute teaching program for patient/family, including Nature of disease and effect on body; relate explanation to the symptoms that patient experienced Signs and symptoms suggestive of recurrence to be reported to physician Increased fatigue without cause Elevated temperature and how to take it Chest pain Dyspnea Reasons for avoiding unnecessary exposure to people with upper respiratory infections and the necessity of reporting to physician cold or flu symptoms Importance of avoiding fatigue and suggestions for doing so related to patient's pattern of activity Information regarding discharge medications, if any Follow-up information including why important; what visits involve; where to go; whom to see and when Provide opportunities for patient/family to ask questions Assess patient/family's potential compliance

*If this type of follow-up care is the responsibility of the critical care unit nurse.

15 □ Endocarditis

Endocarditis is an infection of the endothelium and/or valves of the heart. It occurs most often in persons with structural abnormalities of the heart or great vessels but can occur in persons with normal hearts. The infection may occur on the valves or on the endocardium near congenital anatomical defects such as a ventricular septal defect. Since organisms other than bacteria, that is, fungi, viruses, and *Rickettsia,* may be responsible, it is most descriptive to use the term *endocarditis* preceded by the name of the appropriate microorganism.

The term *acute endocarditis* traditionally has been used to designate the time of fulminating onset or rapid progression of the disease. However, since even persons with subacute cases may suddenly develop serious complications, once the diagnosis is made appropriate therapy should be instituted and the differentiation loses significance.

Bacteria and other organisms can gain access to the circulation and hence the endothelium by many routes. The reason why the reticuloendothelial system, which normally handles transient bacteremia, is not successful in some people is not completely clear. People with a known predisposition to development of the disease are those with rheumatic valvular, congenital, or syphilitic cardiovascular disease. There is also a higher incidence in persons who have prosthetic valves or patches and in those who self-inject narcotics or diabetic medications. These people are particularly susceptible to bacteremia secondary to dental work, genitourinary manipulation (including catheterization), obstetrical and gynecological procedures, upper respiratory tract infections, pyoderma, and open heart surgery. Prophylactic treatment with an antibiotic should be considered. The selection of the drug is dependent on the kind of microorganisms likely to enter the bloodstream from the given site.

Endothelial vegetations develop as the bacteria multiply, initiating fibrin and platelet thrombi aggregation and deposition. If the process continues, the result can lead to valvular injury or deformity. The mitral valve is most frequently involved followed by the aortic, tricuspid, and pulmonic valves. Cardiac failure can develop or be aggravated by the resultant valvular damage or associated myocarditis. Peripheral complications may arise from endogenous immunological reactions to the chronic infection or from emboli released from the vegetations to various organs and tissues.

The diagnosis of endocarditis is often difficult. The disease may present itself acutely and dramatically or more commonly as an insidious but progressive process. The subacute form in particular may mimic almost any systemic disease, depending on the nature of the infecting organism, site of the vegetation, and the complications that have developed. Patients are often admitted to a critical care unit as a result of the complications with the diagnosis of endocarditis not yet established.

Fever, often low grade, is found in almost all cases, and cardiac murmurs are heard in the majority of patients. Once suspicion is aroused, blood cultures are drawn to confirm the diagnosis (they are not always positive) and to select the appropriate antibiotic. An echocardiogram may reveal vegetations on infected valves.

Endocarditis is managed by the selection of an appropriate antibiotic for the involved microorganism, given in sufficient doses over a period of time to eradicate the infecting organism.

Relapses may occur in a small percent of patients following treatment; therefore follow-up cultures are obtained every 1 to 2 weeks up to 6 weeks and the patient's temperature is monitored. The prognosis after successful treatment generally depends on the residual valvular damage.

ASSESSMENT

1. History of rheumatic, congenital, syphilitic heart disease, prosthetic cardiac valves or patches, frequent self-injections (narcotics or diabetics medication), and/or previously diagnosed endocarditis
2. Recent history of dental treatment and/or surgical procedures or instrumentation involving the upper respiratory tract, genitourinary tract, or lower gastrointestinal tract
3. Signs and symptoms of infection
   a. Temperature above normal
   b. Diaphoresis and/or chills (most common at night)
   c. Anorexia; weight loss
   d. Malaise
   e. Arthralgias
4. New murmurs, particularly those characteristic of mitral, aortic, or tricuspid regurgitation
5. Petechiae in mucous membranes of mouth, conjunctiva, necklace area, or about wrists and ankles

6. Lab data results, including
   a. Blood culture reports
   b. Antibiotic sensitivity reports
   c. Hgb and Hct values for anemia
   d. Positive rheumatoid factor (latex agglutination titer)
   e. Echocardiograph report
7. Signs and symptoms of complications
   a. Cardiac decompensation
   b. Embolization to
      (1) Spleen
      (2) Kidneys
      (3) Brain
      (4) Coronary arteries
      (5) Peripheral arterial circulation
      (6) Lungs (right-sided endocarditis)
   c. Splenomegaly
   d. Pericarditis
8. Patient's perception of and reaction to the diagnosis and requirements of therapy

GOALS

1. Absence of infecting organism
2. Hemodynamic stability
3. Absence of or resolution of embolic complications
4. Patient asks questions and verbalizes understanding of disease, need for frequent blood samples, and therapy
5. Patient's behavior demonstrates decreased anxiety with provision of information
6. Before discharge, the patient/family
   a. Lists symptoms requiring physician notification with reasons why
   b. Asks pertinent questions regarding self-care
   c. Describes the activity regimen given him/her by the health care team
   d. Identifies methods for maintaining oral hygiene
   e. States the information necessary for compliance with the antibiotic regimen
   f. States necessary information regarding follow-up visits to physician and/or clinic
   g. Identifies situations or procedures for which prophylactic antibiotics may be indicated and whom to inform

Potential problems	Expected outcomes	Nursing activities

■ Infection	■ Normal temperature
	Absence of diaphoresis and/or chills
	Absence of arthralgias related to bacteremia
	Normal appetite
	Negative blood cultures
		■ Check temperature q4 hr or as indicated
		Administer antipyretics/analgesics as ordered for elevated temperature or arthralgias; if there is little or no response, inform physician
		Institute cooling measures if needed
		Encourage fluid intake when temperature is elevated if there is no evidence of heart failure
		Avoid chills
		  Keep patient warm and dry
		  Avoid exposing body to differences in temperature
		  Change clothes and linen frequently while patient is diaphoretic
		Administer bactericidal antibiotic as ordered after checking patient's history for allergies; large doses may be required over 4 to 8 weeks
		  Maintain IV route or heparin lock; protect with armboard if necessary; check site and change dressing daily; change IV site q48 hr
		  Check for drug reaction—toxicity, rash, fever
		  Give drug on time; if patient is to be off the floor unavoidably, give it early; if dose is delayed due to IV infiltration, give it promptly, inform physician, and change schedule only if necessary

■ Discomfort from IV related to phlebitis or immobilization of extremity	■ Absence of phlebitis
	Patient verbalizes comfort
		■ Observe regularly for phlebitis; if problem occurs
		  Remove IV promptly
		  Apply warm soaks
		  Culture if area is suppurating
		  Ensure that new IV is started before time of next antibiotic dose
		Alternate arms if possible when changing IV
		Provide active/passive ROM exercises
		Explore possibility of heparin lock

■ Malaise related to
Cardiac infection
Anemia
Prolonged bed rest (if necessary)
	■ Continuous increase in activity tolerance without fatigue	■ Evaluate extent of malaise related to immobility versus chronic infection versus anemia
		Maintain level of physical activity ordered during treatment as determined by the patient's situation/status
		  If bed rest is necessary during the acute phase or when evidence of heart failure is present
		    Assist patient to turn, cough, and deep breathe q2-4 hr
		    Assist with active or passive ROM exercises
		    Apply elastic stockings
		  Gradually increase activity level, monitoring cardiac tolerance
		  Plan for rest periods between activities
		  Avoid fatigue
		  Provide for a mobile IV stand or heparin lock, allowing greater freedom for ambulating patients
		Caution patient to avoid strenuous exercise (be specific) for several weeks following treatment

■ Anemia related to depressed bone marrow from chronic infection	■ Normal Hgb and Hct	■ Monitor serial Hgb and Hct values Administer blood products if ordered
■ Splenomegaly related to increased reticuloendothelial function resulting from duration of infection	■ Absence of or resolution of splenomegaly	■ Observe for indications of abdominal discomfort . Spleen may be palpable 4 to 6 weeks into course of disease

Potential problems	Expected outcomes	Nursing activities
■ Anxiety related to Limited understanding of disease and its effect on body Need for frequent blood samples and/or loss of blood	■ Patient verbalizes anxiety and asks questions Reduction of anxiety with sufficient information	■ Ongoing assessment of level of anxiety Encourage questions from patient/family Explain in simple terms the nature of the infection, relating explanation to patient's symptoms Explain purpose of frequent blood cultures and how often they will be drawn to determine the organism and check response to antibiotics; note that amount drawn each time is equal to only 1 tablespoon (blood C and S tube holds 10 to 15 ml blood)
■ Valvular insufficiency related to complications of valve infection Perforation of cusp from infection eroding through leaflet Scarring may occur causing retraction/stenosis of valve Enlargement of vegetations can lead to poor closure of valve leaflets Necrosis and rupture of chordae tendineae or papillary muscles secondary to spread of infection	■ Absence of or correction of valvular insufficiency	■ Monitor for signs and symptoms suggestive of mitral, aortic, or tricuspid regurgitation; rarely are two or more valves infected simultaneously Mitral regurgitation Review chart and/or auscultate precordium for a high-pitched, blowing holosystolic murmur best appreciated at the apex or along the lower left sternal border and which may radiate to the axilla or back; turn patient to left lateral decubitus position to accentuate intensity; note also presence of S_3 and/or diminished S_1 Palpate precordium for apical impulse, which may be large, sustained, and displaced laterally Monitor for indications of left ventricular dilatation, hypertrophy, or failure, noting in particular rapid development of pulmonary congestion Aortic regurgitation Review chart and/or auscultate precordium for a blowing, decrescendo diastolic murmur best appreciated in the third and fourth intercostal spaces along the left sternal border with the patient leaning forward and the breath expelled and which may radiate to the cardiac apex Palpate precordium for apical impulse, which may be large, forceful, sustained, and displaced downward and laterally Monitor for 1. Wide pulse pressure 2. Water-hammer pulse (bounding pulse with rapid rise and fall) 3. Signs and symptoms of left ventricular failure Tricuspid regurgitation Review chart and/or auscultate precordium for an atrial gallop (S_4) and/or a medium-pitched, blowing, holosystolic murmur best appreciated in the fourth or fifth intercostal space close to or over the sternum, accentuated by inspiration Monitor for indications of right atrial enlargement and systemic venous congestion If problem occurs Notify physician if physician is unaware of findings Continue or initiate treatment as ordered for endocarditis and/or heart failure Prepare patient/family for surgical replacement of artificial valve when applicable SEE STANDARDS: *Heart failure* *Cardiac surgery*
■ Cardiac decompensation related to altered hemodynamics from poorly functioning valves or myocarditis	■ Absence of or controlled left heart disease	■ Check BP, P, and R q4 hr or as indicated Auscultate chest for breath sounds at every shift Observe for early signs and symptoms of left heart failure Sinus tachycardia S_3 gallop

Potential problems	Expected outcomes	Nursing activities
		Bibasilar rales
		Dyspnea
		If problem develops, see Standard: *Heart failure*
■ Embolic episodes	■ Absence of or resolution of embolic problem	■ Check report of echocardiogram if ordered; if vegetations are seen on valves, there is a higher risk for embolization
		Observe for signs of embolization described in the following section at every shift and prn; report positive signs to physician immediately
		If embolic episode occurs; see Standard: *Embolic phenomena*
		Further diagnostic evaluation and antiembolic thrombolytic therapy may be instituted
Spleen		Observe for
		Pain in left upper quadrant (LUQ) with radiation to left shoulder
		Local tenderness, abdominal rigidity, and friction rub
Kidney		Observe for
		Persistent hematuria
		Oliguria
		Costovertebral angle pain (lower back discomfort or flank pain
Brain		Observe for
		Altered level of consciousness
		Paralysis; hemiplegia
		Aphasia
		Ptosis of eyelids, mouth droop
		Incontinence
		Seizures
		Nausea and vomiting
		Elevated BP
		Abnormalities in respiratory pattern
Coronary arteries		Observe for signs/symptoms of MI, abscess, or pericarditis
		If problem occurs, see Standards: *Acute myocardial infarction; Pericarditis*
Peripheral arterial circulation		Observe extremities at every shift or prn for
		Positive Homans' sign
		Tenderness; pain
		Swelling
		Erythema
		Signs of acute arterial insufficiency to an extremity
		Decreased or absent pulse
		Coolness
		Blanching
		Decrease in capillary refilling time
		Observe acral portions of body (tip of nose, pinna of ear, fingers, and toes) for gangrenous infarctions
Lungs related to right-sided endocarditis		Observe for signs and symptoms related to hypoxia and pain
		Dyspnea
		Tachypnea
		Sudden pleuritic chest pain
		Tachycardia
		Pallor, cyanosis
		If symptoms occur
		Notify physician
		Assist with or draw arterial blood gas sample (look specifically for sudden drop in Po_2)

Potential problems	Expected outcomes	Nursing activities
■ Insufficient knowledge to comply with discharge regimen*	■ Evaluation by testing or questioning demonstrates patient/family's understanding of the knowledge components of the teaching program Patient lists symptoms requiring physician notification Patient asks pertinent questions regarding self-care	■ Institute teaching program for patient/family, including 　Nature of infection and effect on heart 　Relationship of predisposing factors to future susceptibility 　Signs and symptoms of the disease with specific indications regarding notification of health team 　Self-care instructions 　　Activity instructions 　　Oral hygiene 　　Suggestions for avoiding upper respiratory tract infections 　　Notification of other physicians and dentists of history 　　Situations that may require prophylactic antibiotic therapy 　Antibiotic regimen 　　Purpose of drug 　　Dosage 　　Timing and importance of 　　Discuss importance of completing even though patient feels better 　　Side effects 　Follow-up 　　Necessity of and timing 　　What is involved 　　Where to go and whom to see Provide opportunities for patient/family to ask questions Assess patient/family's potential compliance

*If this type of follow-up care is the responsibility of the critical care unit nurse.

16 □ **Arrhythmias**

Arrhythmias are disturbances of impulse formation and/or conduction within the electrical system of the heart. To understand the pathogenesis of arrhythmias, it is necessary to review the electrophysiology of the heart.

Automaticity (diastolic depolarization) refers to the ability of cardiac cells to discharge spontaneously, not requiring an external or propagated impulse to fire. Certain specialized cells such as those in the sinus node, the conductive pathways of the atria, the AV junctional tissue, and the His-Purkinje system have this capability. This creates the potential for these cells to act as the dominant pacemaker, depolarizing the rest of the heart. Normally, the sinus node acts as the dominant pacemaker, since it spontaneously discharges faster than the other specialized cells, often called *latent* or *secondary* pacemakers. Should one of the other areas discharge more rapidly than the sinus node, it may depolarize the atria, ventricles, or both. This may occur in two ways. If the sinus node discharges at a slower rate than a latent pacemaker or if the sinus impulse is blocked before reaching the latent pacemaker site, the latent pacemaker may *passively* escape sinus domination and discharge automatically at its own intrinsic rate. These escape beats or escape rhythms will be slower than normal sinus rhythm because the intrinsic rate of the junctional tissue is 40 to 55 times/minute and that of the His-Purkinje system is 20 to 40 times/minute. The other mechanism by which a latent pacemaker may take control is if it abnormally accelerates its discharge rate (increased automaticity) and *actively* usurps control from the sinus node. This results in a premature beat and may occur in the specialized cells of the atria, junctional tissue, or ventricles. A series of three premature beats in a row is considered a tachycardia.

For a pacemaker to depolarize the myocardium, it must be conducted from its site of origin through the heart. Excitability is property of the cell receiving a stimulus which determines whether the cell will be discharged by that impulse. Many factors may influence excitability but the most important is at what point during the recovery period following depolarization the heart is restimulated. Stages of the recovery period are related to the refractoriness of heart muscle. Immediately following depolarization is the *absolute refractory period,* during which excitability is zero and the tissue will not respond to a stimulus regardless of how intense it is. This is followed by the *relative refractory period* in which excitability is improving and a strong stimulus can evoke a response. Following this period, the heart will be fully excitable, and a relatively weak stimulus could evoke a response.

The speed at which the impulse spreads through the heart is the *conduction velocity,* which varies considerably depending on the inherent properties of different portions of the specialized conduction system and the myocardium. Velocity is most rapid in Purkinje fibers and slowest in the midportion of the AV node. If conduction becomes uneven due to a difference in refractoriness, block may occur in some areas and not in others, or block may occur in a tissue but only in one direction (unidirectional). When the block is unidirectional, this uneven conduction may allow the initial impulse to reenter areas previously unexcitable that are now recovered. Should the reentering impulse then be able to depolarize the entire atria and/or ventricles, a corresponding extra systole (an ectopic beat, dependent on and coupled to the preceding beat) results. Maintenance of the reentrant excitation establishes a tachycardia.

Changes in automaticity and/or conduction can conceivably occur as a result of almost any disease state or system imbalance, making them a common problem in critically ill patients, even those with normal hearts. Any form of cardiac disease may be complicated or compensated by arrhythmias, the latter often resulting in response to decreased stroke volume or hypotension. Other conditions often implicated include alterations in body temperature; hypoxia; hypercapnia; hypovolemia; abnormal potassium and calcium concentrations; drugs, particularly digitalis; stress; and during or following surgery, particularly cardiac.

The clinical or hemodynamic significance of an arrhythmia is ultimately dependent on its effect on the cardiac output. This is primarily determined by the patient's cardiovascular status, the duration of the arrhythmia, and the site of origin and its effect on the ventricular rate. Arrhythmias resulting in rapid ventricular rates in-

crease myocardial oxygen consumption while decreasing the availability of oxygen to the myocardium by shortening diastole (ventricular filling time) and thereby reducing stroke volume. Those resulting in slow ventricular rates if not compensated for by increased stroke volume also result in decreased cardiac output and the consequent problems of underperfusion of vital organs and the peripheral vessels. The loss of the sequential atrial-ventricular contraction sequence can be particularly detrimental to patients with left heart failure and/or mitral valve disease who are dependent on atrial contraction for adequate ventricular filling. Finally, the electrical stability of an arrhythmia is also an important factor in determining significance, particularly in patients with AMI in whom experience has documented the incidence of one arrhythmia creating opportunities for, or resulting in, the development of other more threatening arrhythmias.

The management of an arrhythmia is dependent on its effect on the patient; accurate interpretation of the rhythm; its etiology; its natural history and stability, e.g., transient or degenerative; the presence and nature of myocardial disease; the patient's electrolyte status; concomitant drug therapy; and the status of organ systems influencing drug metabolism. Based on these considerations, a number of treatment modalities may be employed. If the arrhythmia is not life-threatening, and particularly in the absence of heart disease, treatment of the underlying problem may be sufficient, such as correction of hypoxia or electrolyte imbalance. Treatment modalities include pharmacological agents; electrical intervention including pacing, cardioversion, or defibrillation; vagal maneuvers such as Valsalva or carotid sinus massage; and surgery. Combinations of modalities may be required.

Arrhythmias related to cardiac problems as opposed to those relating to acute imbalances and/or therapeutic modalities are more likely to require chronic management.

ASSESSMENT

1. History, including
   a. Preexisting arrhythmias
      (1) Precipitating factors if known
      (2) Associated symptoms
      (3) Onset, frequency, and duration
      (4) Therapeutic interventions, if any, and effectiveness
      (5) Relationship, if any, to current event
   b. Preexisting organic heart disease
   c. Medications
   d. Smoking and/or caffeine habits

2. Current medical and/or cardiovascular problems
3. Current forms of treatment, particularly pharmacological agents employed
4. Presence of factors that predispose to arrhythmias and/or influence therapy
   a. Electrolyte imbalance—potassium and calcium
   b. Hypoxia; hypercapnia
   c. Pain
   d. Anxiety
   e. Fever
   f. Infection
   g. Hypovolemia
   h. Anemia
   i. Endocrine disorders—hypoglycemia and diabetes
   j. Hypothyroidism or hyperthyroidism
   k. Impaired organ function—liver, renal
5. Continuous monitoring and/or full ECG for accurate interpretation of arrhythmia; old tracings may be helpful
6. Results of special procedures for interpretation if required
   a. Vagal maneuvers
   b. His bundle studies
   c. Pacing studies
7. Duration and frequency of arrhythmia
8. Patient's description of associated symptoms
9. Hemodynamic consequences of arrhythmia
   a. BP changes
   b. Apical and radial pulse deficit
   c. Fatigue
   d. Changes in heart sounds
10. Patient's perception of and reaction to the diagnosis and therapy

11. Signs and symptoms of complications
    a. Decreased cardiac output
    b. Inadequate perfusion of
       (1) Heart
       (2) Brain
       (3) Kidneys
       (4) Peripheral vascular system
    c. Electrical instability
    d. Embolic episodes

GOALS

1. Absence and/or stability of arrhythmias—optimum cardiac rhythm
2. Hemodynamic stability—adequate perfusion of brain, heart, kidneys, and peripheral system
3. Absence of or resolution of embolic complications
4. Absence of identified precipitating factors
5. Patient's behavior demonstrates reduction of anxiety with provision of information
6. Before discharge, the patient/family*
   a. Identifies factors that might precipitate arrhythmias and steps to follow to avoid
   b. Lists symptoms suggestive of recurrence and describes appropriate actions
   c. Accurately demonstrates skill of counting pulse, stating acceptable ranges of rate and rhythm
   d. States necessary information for compliance with discharge regimen
   e. Asks pertinent questions

---

*Applies when chronic management and/or prevention is required.

Potential problems	Expected outcomes	Nursing activities
■ Anxiety related to 　Awareness of heart 　　activity 　Insufficient knowledge 　Fear of consequences 　Monitoring equipment 　Special diagnostic 　　procedures	■ Patient verbalizes anxiety 　and asks questions 　Reduction of anxiety with 　sufficient information 　and control of ar- 　rhythmia 　Absence of nonverbal 　responses suggestive 　of anxiety	■ Ongoing assessment of level of anxiety 　Encourage patient to verbalize fears; search for sources of anxiety; encourage questions from patient/family 　Maintain as quiet and relaxed an environment as possible; regulate bedside audio alarms to reduce additional stimuli without compromising patient's safety 　Sedate patient if necessary and as ordered 　Explain nature of arrhythmia to patient, stressing effectiveness of pump, i.e., difference between electrical and mechanical activity 　Elicit from patient indices of awareness 　　Sensation of irregular beat 　　Palpitations 　　Dyspnea 　　Feeling of fullness or throbbing in chest, neck, or head—sometimes manifested as sensation of choking

Potential problems	Expected outcomes	Nursing activities
		Discomfort in chest because of greater than normal contractile force of postectopic beats or beats following delay
		Feeling that heart has stopped during long pauses
		Explain symptoms in relation to arrhythmia being experienced
		If natural history of arrhythmia suggests that it will be transient, state this to patient
		Explain purpose of monitoring equipment and alarm systems
		Explain purpose and procedure of special studies or maneuvers that may be required to identify and/or treat arrhythmia
		Assess effect of anxiety on patient's rhythm

■ Electrical instability related to
  Very rapid or very slow ventricular rates
  Initiation of tachycardia by premature beats
  Degeneration of rhythms—ventricular tachycardia to ventricular fibrillation
  Underlying cardiac disease
	■ Electrical stability	■ Determine type of arrhythmia
		  Select best leads
		    Clear QRS complexes, P waves
		    Clear pacemaker artifact if present
		    "Special" leads such as MCL (modified V_1)
		      1. Bundle branch blocks
		      2. Differentiation of aberrancy from ventricular conduction problems
		    Leads I and II—axis shifts
		  Systematic inspection of rhythm strip—save for record
		  Obtain a 12-lead ECG if necessary, e.g., accurate interpretation of bundle branch block requires precordial leads
		  Maintain continuous ECG monitoring for prompt recognition of changes in rhythm and for determining duration and/or frequency of arrhythmia
		    Identify and record lead selected for monitoring
		    Note if lead is changed
		    Set high and low rate alarms
		  Participate with physician and monitor results if special maneuvers or procedures are required for accurate interpretation
		    Response to selected drugs, e.g., atropine, edrophonium (Tensilon)
		    Response to carotid sinus massage or other vagal maneuvers
		    Bundle of His ECG recording
		    Atrial pacing
		  Determine etiology of arrhythmia with physician
		    Past and present history of medical problems and treatment modalities, particularly drugs and recent surgical intervention; instability is more common in presence of underlying heart disease
		    Monitor lab data, signs and symptoms of conditions (regardless of their etiology) that are frequently associated with the development and/or perpetuation of arrhythmias
		      1. Hypotension
		      2. Alterations in K^+ and Ca^{2+} concentrations
		      3. Alterations in body temperature
		      4. Hypoxia
		      5. Hypercapnia
		      6. Hypovolemia
		      7. Anemia
		      8. Pain
		      9. Anxiety
		      10. Endocrine disorders
		      11. Hyperthyroidism/hypothyroidism
		    Relate identified etiology to natural history of arrhythmia when possible

Potential problems	Expected outcomes	Nursing activities
		Initiate with physician progressive management to treat arrhythmia and to prevent evolution or development of new arrhythmia; selection of intervention dependent on
		Correct interpretation of arrhythmia
		Etiology
		Effect of arrhythmia on patient's clinical status
		Functional state of organs influencing drug metabolism and excretion
		Concomitant drug therapy
		Therapeutic benefit versus potential toxicity
		Methods of intervention include
		Drugs
		Pacemaker—temporary or permanent
		Cardioversion
		Vagal maneuvers
		Respiratory maneuvers
		Carotid sinus massage/electrical stimulator
		When administering medications intravenously
		Ensure that IV remains patent
		Use soluset with microdrip administration setup or an IV pump
		Check q15 min to ensure adequate dosage being delivered
		Be alert to signs and symptoms of toxicity regardless of route of administration, since antiarrhythmics are potentially lethal and dosages may need to be adjusted as patient's status changes
		When cardioversion is required
		Prepare patient for procedure
		If patient has been (within the last 24 to 48 hours) or is receiving digitalis, check carefully for indications of toxicity
		If indications of toxicity are present, inform physician; procedure should be postponed for 24 to 48 hours
		If patient's status permits, explain the purpose of the procedure and that he/she will be given medication so that he/she will be asleep during procedure
		Ensure that IV line is in place and patent
		Have emergency equipment and drugs immediately available
		If pacemaker is required, see Standard: *Pacemaker*
		Be prepared to treat lethal arrhythmia
		Arrest cart and defibrillator should be immediately accessible
		Confirm occurrence—check for presence of P, BP, and/or audible heart sounds
		Initiate CPR and/or defibrillate (if unit policy permits) immediately while calling for team
		Prepare IV medications (usually lidocaine) to maintain stable rhythm
■ Decreased cardiac output related to Persistent tachycardia and/or marked bradycardia Loss of sequential AV contraction Loss of hemodynamic benefit of atrial contraction is particularly significant in patients	■ Adequate cardiac output to maintain hemodynamic stability	■ Check BP q2 hr for
		Decrease in systolic pressure
		Narrowed pulse pressure reflecting reduction in effective volume
		If hypotension occurs, report to physician and increase frequency of observation; consider other causes such as medications patient may be taking, MI, hypovolemia
		Check P q2 hr for
		Rate
		Regularity
		Quality—hyperkinetic or hypokinetic

Potential problems	Expected outcomes	Nursing activities

with left heart failure or mitral stenosis		Pulse deficit—most common with atrial fibrillation and non-perfused premature beats
		Bigeminal pulse—most common with ventricular bigeminy
		Auscultate precordium for abnormal changes in intensity of S_1 and apical pulse
		Check intake and output q8 hr or more frequently if indicated
		Elicit description of symptoms from patient suggesting decreasing cardiac output
		  Fatigue
		  Dyspnea
		  Nervousness
		  Dizziness—relate to position
		Assess for early signs of left heart failure, which may be precipitated by persistent tachycardia and/or loss of atrial contribution to ventricular filling; see Standard: *Heart failure*
		If problem of diminishing output occurs
		  Inform physician
		  Continuous observation of ECG to determine response to therapy or effect of decreased cardiac output on electrical stability
		  Anticipate more aggressive management of arrhythmia
		  Increase frequency of observations noted before and in Problem, Inadequate tissue perfusion related to decreased cardiac output
		  Administer O_2 as ordered
		  Ensure patent IV, and administer parenteral fluids as ordered
		  Restrict patient's activity
		  Give medications as ordered; in addition to those being used to treat arrhythmias, these may include drugs used to improve cardiac contractility; monitor closely to determine effectiveness on improvement of cardiac output because the increased contractility will increase myocardial O_2 consumption and therefore demand
		  Inform patient/family of reasons for changes in observation, symptoms, and therapy

▪ Inadequate tissue perfusion related to decreased cardiac output: cerebral	▪ Adequate cerebral perfusion	▪ Observe for signs and symptoms suggesting inadequate cerebral perfusion
		  Yawning
		  Mental confusion
		  Dizziness
		  Syncopal episodes (Stokes-Adams)
		  Convulsions; seizures
		  Cheyne-Stokes respirations
		  Stroke related to transient cerebral ischemia
		Rule out other causes, particularly use of class II antiarrhythmics, lidocaine, and phenytoin (Dilantin) which first manifest toxicity via the CNS; sensory deprivation; and organic syndrome of the aged

▪ Inadequate tissue perfusion related to decreased cardiac output; myocardium	▪ Adequate myocardial perfusion	▪ Observe for signs and symptoms suggesting inadequate myocardial perfusion
		  Angina—see Standard: *Angina pectoris*
		  MI or extension of—see Standard: *Acute myocardial infarction*
		  Left heart failure—see Standard: *Heart failure*
		  Pulmonary edema—see Standard: *Pulmonary edema*
		  Cardiogenic shock—see Standard: *Cardiogenic shock*
		  Greater electrical instability—see Problem, Electrical instability

Potential problems	**Expected outcomes**	**Nursing activities**

■ Inadequate tissue perfusion related to decreased cardiac output: renal	■ Adequate renal perfusion	■ Observe for signs and symptoms of acute renal ischemia
		Check urine output q8 hr
		  If oliguria develops, check output q1-2 hr
		  If anuria develops, check output q1 hr
		  Catheterize patient if indicated and/or ordered
		  Measure specific gravity of urine
		Daily weight
		Monitor lab data for results
		  BUN
		  Creatinine clearance
		  Electrolyte balance, particularly K^+
		  Acid-base balance
		Changes in mental status, e.g., lethargy, confusion
		Anorexia, nausea and vomiting
		SEE STANDARD: *Acute renal failure*

■ Inadequate tissue perfusion related to decreased cardiac output: peripheral system	■ Adequate peripheral perfusion	■ Observe for signs and symptoms indicative of inadequate peripheral perfusion
		Check all pulses for presence, equality, and quality
		Pallor, cyanosis, or cooling of extremities
		Sweating related to peripheral arterial constriction
		If any of the aforementioned problems occur
		  Inform the physician immediately and record data
		  Increase frequency of observations and collection of aforementioned lab data
		  Prepare for specific measures to assess and improve perfusion
		    Assist with insertion of intra-arterial lines and/or pulmonary artery line
		    See Standard: *Hemodynamic monitoring*
		If the problem is arrhythmia, prepare for more aggressive antiarrhythmic intervention
		Administer medications to improve cardiac function and perfusion; many of the pharmacological agents used for this purpose, e.g., inotropic agents and sympathomimetics may provoke arrhythmias
		Ascertain mode of excretion of drugs, adjusting medication dosages as ordered when hepatic or renal function is altered; the same amount of medication may produce toxicity if it is not metabolized and excreted because of altered hepatic or renal function

■ Embolic episodes	■ Absence or resolution of embolic complications	■ Determine if positive history of rheumatic mitral valve disease or chronic atrial fibrillation
		Initiate preventive measures for these patients and for those with previous history of thromboembolic disease or for whom prolonged bed rest is anticipated
		  Antithromboembolic stockings
		  ROM exercises, passive or active to extremities
		  Ambulate as soon as possible
		  Patients with chronic atrial fibrillation may be anticoagulated before cardioversion
		Observe for signs of emboli routinely at every shift in high-risk patients
		  Sudden onset of chest pain
		  Signs and symptoms of respiratory distress
		  Altered mental status
		  Unexplained restlessness or anxiety
		  Decreased temperature, sensation, or pulses in extremities
		If problem occurs, see Standard: *Embolic phenomena*

Potential problems	**Expected outcomes**	**Nursing activities**
■ Insufficient knowledge to comply with discharge regimen*	■ Evaluation by testing or questioning demonstrates patient/family's understanding of the knowledge components of the teaching program Patient takes own pulse correctly and states acceptable ranges Patient lists symptoms requiring physician notification Patient asks pertinent questions regarding self-care	■ If arrhythmia requires chronic management or if there is a strong probability of recurrence, institute a teaching program for patient/family, including Normal heart function—electrical and mechanical Nature of arrhythmias and potential effect on cardiovascular system Factors or situations that might precipitate arrhythmias and suggestions for avoiding discussed with patient/family Symptoms indicating recurrence and appropriate actions to take Medication regimen Purpose Dosage Timing and importance of—adjust schedule to patient's life-style Side effects and what to do about them Follow-up information Provide opportunities for patient/family to ask questions Assess patient/family's potential compliance

*If this type of follow-up care is the responsibility of critical care unit nurse when patient is transferred from the intensive care unit.

17 □ Pacemakers: temporary and permanent

A pacemaker is an electronic device that delivers an electrical stimulus to the myocardium to control or maintain heart rate when the natural pacemakers of the heart are unable to do so. The system consists of a pulse generator (energy source) and a unipolar or bipolar electrode catheter, which may be sewn on the epicardium or placed in contact with the endocardium.

When the atrium is being stimulated (paced), the pacing artifact is followed by a P wave; and when the ventricle is being paced, the pacing artifact is followed by a QRS complex.

In addition to the function of stimulation, some units also have a sensing mechanism to eliminate the problem of competition between paced and spontaneous beats, which could result in serious ventricular arrhythmias, fusion beats, or an iatrogenic parasystolic ventricular rhythm. The information that is sensed is relayed to the energy source via the same electrode that stimulates or through a second sensing electrode. The location of the electrode with this sensing capacity determines whether atrial or ventricular activity is sensed.

There are several types of pacemakers available.

1. Asynchronous or fixed rate: models without a sensing mechanism
2. Demand: models with a sensing mechanism that allows the pacemaker to behave as an escape focus when the natural pacemaker does not fire during a preset escape interval and that inhibits the pacemaker when the natural pacemaker functions
3. Synchronous: models with a sensing mechanism whereby sensing in the atrium results in stimulation of the ventricle

The approach to pacemaker implantation depends in part on whether pacing is to be a temporary or permanent measure and the acuteness of the situation. Approaches include external pacing, transthoracic pacing, epicardial pacing, and transvenous endocardial pacing. For temporary pacing the energy source is external. For permanent pacing, the energy source is implanted in a pocket under the skin and connected to the heart by epicardial or endocardial electrodes. With both methods, once the catheter is thought to be in position the stimulation threshold, the minimal current necessary to achieve one-to-one capture, is found; the sensitivity threshold is measured if the unit has a sensing mechanism; and the rate is set.

Therapeutic indications for permanent or temporary pacing include arrhythmias refractory to medication, resulting in an inadequate heart rate for the maintenance of an effective cardiac output. The rate may be too fast or too slow. The patient may be symptomatic or asymptomatic with an arrhythmia whose natural history supports pacing. "Overdrive" pacing may be employed to suppress dangerous ventricular tachyarrhythmias when medication is ineffective or when ventricular arrhythmias are related to a slow ventricular rate. Temporary pacing may also be employed prophylactically following open heart surgery or prior to permanent pacemaker implantation.

Diagnostically, temporary pacing (usually atrial) may be used to evaluate the electrophysiological response (particularly on AV conduction and sinus node function) and the hemodynamic response to increased heart rate. It also may be employed to determine the mechanism for tachyarrhythmias. A paced atrial premature beat may induce and terminate reentrant tachyarrhythmias while not affecting those resulting from enhanced automaticity.

Patients being paced temporarily are considered subject to microshock hazards. The pacemaker catheter itself is insulated and electrically safe, but the exposed metal tips are not. Because the usual protective resistance provided by the skin and other body tissues is bypassed, a very minimal current can potentially produce ventricular fibrillation.

Temporary pacemaker
ASSESSMENT
1. Problem necessitating pacemaker insertion
   a. Disease process
   b. ECG illustrating arrhythmia
   c. Symptoms associated with the arrhythmia
   d. Prognosis—temporary versus permanent need
2. Baseline information included in chart
   a. Date and method of insertion
   b. Location—atrial or ventricular
   c. Type—asynchronous, demand, etc.
   d. Rate and threshold (MA) settings
   e. Turned on or off
   f. Frequency of use
3. Patient's perception of and reaction to pacemaker and procedure
4. Monitor rhythm strips for
   a. Frequency of need for pacing
   b. Maintenance of preset rate
   c. Paced P or QRS configuration
   d. Capture
   e. Sensing
5. Stimulation and sensing thresholds and presence of influencing factors
6. State of equipment
   a. Battery
   b. Connections
   c. Integrity and position of catheter
7. Evaluation of hemodynamic status
8. Pulse perfusion distal to cutdown
9. Site of insertion for signs of infection, cellulitis, or phlebitis
10. Safety of electrical environment
11. Signs and symptoms of complications
    a. Aberrant pacemaker stimulation
    b. Cardiac tamponade
    c. Pulmonary embolus
    d. Pain or discomfort related to restricted mobility of extremity
    e. Cardiac arrhythmias, particularly ventricular

GOALS
1. Pacemaker unit functioning properly
2. Hemodynamic stability
3. Infection-free insertion site
4. Patient verbalizes comfort
5. Microshock-safe environment
6. Patient asks questions and verbalizes understanding of insertion procedure, reason for and function of pacemaker, and prognosis
7. Patient's behavior demonstrates decreased anxiety with provision of information
8. Absence of threatening arrhythmias

Potential problems	Expected outcomes	Nursing activities
■ Anxiety related to Procedure Lack of physiological self-control Lack of understanding of function of pacemaker unit Unknown prognosis (permanent versus temporary need for)	■ Patient verbalizes reasonable understanding of insertion procedure, reason for and function of pacemaker, and prognosis Patient verbalizes anxiety and asks questions Reduction of anxiety with sufficient information	■ Ongoing assessment of level of anxiety Encourage questions from patient/family Explain pacemaker insertion Explain function of and need for pacing; differentiate between electrical and mechanical functions of the heart Discuss prognosis—permanent versus temporary need Ongoing explanation of care required

■ Pacemaker malfunction related to	■ Pacemaker unit functioning properly
	Fires at preset rate
	Each pacemaker stimulus produces myocardial response (capture)
	Senses patient's own beats (models with sensing mechanism)
	Hemodynamic stability
		■ Continuous monitoring of ECG for
		  Frequency of need for pacing
		  Maintenance of preset rate
		  Capture
		  Paced QRS or P configuration
		  Sensing
		Check initially and q8 hr
		  Security of connections
		  Battery
		  Consistency between settings on pacemaker and those recorded in chart—rate, stimulation and sensitivity thresholds, and whether on or off
		  Pulse distal to insertion site for perfusion
		Check threshold q24 hr or as indicated
		Check vital signs q4 hr or as indicated
		Check sense/pace needle q4 hr with vital signs

Improper care of equipment		Keep box and wires dry and a plastic cover over dials Clean box with water, alcohol or gas sterilize; do not autoclave Clean nondisposable catheters in bactericidal solution and gas sterilize Check to see if pacemaker must be disconnected before defibrillating

Battery failure		Check battery q8 hr
		Observe for signs of battery failure
		  Complete or intermittent loss of capture
		  Failure to sense
		  Loss of pacing; box not discharging
		  Needle on box not moving fully to sense/pace
		  Alterations in discharge rate
		Ensure that fresh batteries are readily available
		Replace battery when low

Catheter displacement
Loss of contact between heart and electrode
		Secure wire and equipment
		Minimize motion of extremity or torso at site of insertion
		  Arm: do not raise above shoulder level or lift patient under arm thereby raising shoulder
		  Leg: avoid outward rotation and marked hip flexion
		Observe for signs of catheter displacement
		  Change in QRS configuration
		  Complete or intermittent loss of capture
		  Loss of pacing artifact on ECG—box continues to discharge
		  Failure to sense
		  Aberrant pacemaker stimulation—spasm of chest muscle or hiccups
		If problem occurs
		  Reposition patient (roll side to side)
		  Increase stimulation threshold
		  Inform physician of need to reposition

Potential problems	Expected outcomes	Nursing activities
Improper terminal connections		Check connections q8 hr Observe for loss of pacing artifact on ECG—box continues to discharge Tighten connections if necessary
Changes in threshold		Check threshold q24 hr Be alert to factors that alter threshold 　Decrease threshold 　　MI or ischemia 　　Electrolyte abnormalities (decreased K^+) 　　Frequent premature ventricular contractions 　　Sympathomimetic drugs or increased catecholamine excretion 　　Hypoxic states 　Increased threshold may occur 3 to 4 days postinsertion due to local inflammation and fibrosis at electrode tip Observe for 　Complete or intermittent loss of capture 　Loss of pacing artifact on ECG—box continues to discharge 　Failure to sense If problem occurs 　Increase output 　Inform physician—may reposition catheter to new site
Electrode failure		Observe for complete and intermittent loss of capture If problem occurs, convert bipolar to unipolar
Fractured electrode—more common with epicardial electrode		Observe for complete or intermittent loss of capture If problem occurs, electrode will be replaced by physician
Failure to sense when catheter properly positioned and battery not failing		Observe for competition between paced and spontaneous beats If problem occurs 　Reposition ECG electrodes if sensing another wave as the QRS 　If patient's own rhythm is adequate, turn pacemaker off and inform physician 　If patient's own rhythm is inadequate 　　Inform physician 　　Increase pacer rate to overdrive 　　Lidocaine for ectopics 　　Increase sensitivity 　　Unipolarize a bipolar system 　If pacemaker is fixed rate, turn to demand
■ Arrhythmias	■ Absence of threatening arrhythmias	■ Observe ECG for arrhythmias, particularly ventricular If premature ventricular contractions are present 　Measure coupling interval 　Treat with lidocaine as ordered
■ Perforation of right ventricle or septum by electrode tip	■ Electrode properly positioned	■ Observe for 　Change in paced QRS configuration 　Aberrant pacemaker stimulation, including hiccups 　Complete or intermittent loss of capture 　Loss of pacing artifact on ECG—box continues to discharge 　Signs and symptoms of tamponade (rare) 　　Decreased BP 　　Narrow pulse pressure 　　Increased venous pressure 　　Tachycardia 　　Restlessness, cyanosis 　　Decreased output

Potential problems	Expected outcomes	Nursing activities

		If problem occurs
		  Inform physician
		  Assist physician who may withdraw catheter
		  Reposition patient

■ Embolization	■ Absence of emboli related to pacing	■ SEE STANDARD: *Embolic phenomena*

■ Infection at insertion site	■ Absence of infection at insertion site	■ Maintain sterile technique with insertion
		Ensure clean/sterile equipment
		Change dressing q24 hr
		  Cleanse skin with antiseptic solution
		  Apply antibiotic ointment and dry sterile dressing
		Provide padding beneath wires to prevent ulceration of underlying tissue in predisposed patients
		Respond to patient's complaints
		Inspect regularly for signs of inflammation or infection
		  Tenderness
		  Redness
		  Swelling
		  Discoloration
		Check site q4 hr or as indicated
		Culture tip of catheter on removal if
		  Signs of infection present
		  Catheter in place over 1 week
		  Traumatic insertion

■ Pain or discomfort of affected extremity	■ Patient verbalizes comfort	■ Check pulse perfusion distal to cutdown q8 hr Position extremity comfortably Assist with exercises to avoid stiffness of extremity with restricted movement Administer medication as needed for pain

■ Tamponade related to removal of epicardial electrodes	■ Absence of tamponade	■ Closely monitor for signs and symptoms of tamponade for 3 to 4 hours following removal; note changes in
		  BP
		  Pulse pressure
		  Venous pressure
		  Heart rate
		  Urine output
		  Mentation

■ Microshock hazard	■ Electrically safe equipment and environment	■ Insulate the external metallic portions of the pacing catheter
		  Safe if embedded in the insulated pacemaker terminals of newer models
		  Cover with clear Scotch tape or dry surgical rubber glove
		Be certain all equipment properly grounded with three-prong plugs only and no adaptors
		  Common ground for all equipment used on patient; avoid extension cords
		Equipment with frayed wires or other signs of disrepair *must* not be used
		If there is any question, consult hospital electrician
		Protect patient from contact with metal
		  Patient should not control line-powered equipment, e.g., television or radio
		  Staff should not simultaneously touch the patient or bed while touching electrical equipment
		  Avoid electrical beds not specifically approved
		  Unplug bed lamps attached to metal beds
		  Electrical equipment should not touch bed, e.g., respirator

Potential problems	Expected outcomes	Nursing activities
		Identify patient as "microshock precaution" by placing sign on bed; explain to patient/family
		Wear intact rubber or plastic gloves when handling the external metallic portions of the pacing catheter
		Keep energy source and dressing dry

Permanent pacemaker

ASSESSMENT

1. Problem necessitating pacemaker insertion
   a. Disease process
   b. ECG illustrating arrhythmia
   c. Symptoms associated with the arrhythmia
2. Baseline information included in chart
   a. Date and location of implant
   b. Manufacturer's model and serial numbers for the generator and leads
   c. Set rate, ECG tracing with and without magnet held over generator
   d. Amplitude of pacemaker artifact
   e. Threshold measurements at time of implant
3. Monitor rhythm strips for
   a. Maintenance of preset rate
   b. Capture
   c. Paced QRS configuration
   d. Amplitude of pacemaker artifact
   e. Sensing
   f. Competition
4. Level of anxiety
5. Patient's perception of and reaction to pacemaker
6. Evaluation of hemodynamic status—signs and symptoms suggestive of pacemaker failure
7. Signs and symptoms of complications
   a. Aberrant pacemaker stimulation
   b. Discomfort at implant site and/or of affected shoulder
   c. Cardiac arrhythmias, particularly ventricular
8. Site of implantation for signs of inflammation or infection, bleeding, hematomas, and skin breakdown
9. Factors influencing learning
   a. Preexisting knowledge
   b. Level of education (formal and informal)
   c. Age
   d. Motivation
   e. State of health
   f. Level of anxiety
   g. Patient's life-style
10. Ongoing and final evaluation of effectiveness of teaching program
11. Determinants of compliance

GOALS

1. Pacemaker unit functioning properly
2. Hemodynamic stability
3. Clean, healing wound
4. Patient performs ROM exercises to affected shoulder
5. Absence of threatening arrhythmias
6. Patient verbalizes understanding of procedure, reason for and function of pacemaker
7. Patient's behavior demonstrates decreased anxiety with provision of information
8. Before discharge the patient/family
   a. Demonstrates comprehension of the knowledge components of the teaching program when evaluated by testing or questioning
   b. Takes pulse correctly, stating acceptable ranges
   c. Lists those symptoms requiring physician notification
   d. Asks pertinent questions regarding self-care
   e. Discusses future realistically, noting adjustments required
   f. States necessary information regarding follow-up visits to physician and/or clinic

Potential problems	Expected outcomes	Nursing activities
■ Anxiety related to Procedure Lack of physiological self-control Lack of understanding of function of pace- maker unit	■ Patient verbalizes anx- iety and/or fears Patient asks questions Patient verbalizes rea- sonable understand- ing of procedure, rea- son for pacemaker, and function (progression toward acceptance)	■ Ongoing assessment of level of anxiety Encourage questions from patient/family Explain procedure, preoperative and postoperative course ex- pectations Explain normal conduction system and relate explanation to pa- tient's arrhythmia which necessitates a pacemaker Relate patient's symptoms to arrhythmia, stressing difference the pacemaker will make Explain function and type of pacemaker to be implanted
■ Pacemaker malfunction	■ Pacemaker unit func- tioning properly Fires at preset rate Each pacemaker stimu- lus produces myo- cardial response (capture) Senses patient's own beat (models with sensing mechanism) Absence of competi- tion Hemodynamic stability	■ Continuous monitoring of ECG for first 24 hours; then analysis of ECG strip q4 hr or as indicated for Maintenance of preset rate Capture Paced QRS configuration Amplitude of pacemaker artifact Sensing Competition Ventricular arrhythmias Compare for consistency with baseline values in chart Check BP, R, and temperature q4 hr or as indicated Check apical and radial pulse q2 hr, then q4 hr Count for *1 full minute* Report rate below pacing rate or apical-radial pulse deficit Observe for signs and symptoms suggestive of pacemaker fail- ure Decreased BP Decreased urinary output Stokes-Adams syndrome Palpitations Chest pains Shortness of breath and fatigue Lightheadedness
Related to malposition- ing of pacing cath- eter		Bed rest for 24 hours and reduced activity for an additional 48 hours; then increase activity as tolerated Arm should not be raised above the shoulder until ROM exer- cises ordered (usually around third postoperative day) Observe for Intermittent or complete failure to pace Aberrant pacemaker stimulation
Related to generator problems—battery depletion or mal- function within electrical circuitry Related to malfunc- tioning pacing cath- eter Breaks in lead wire Fibrosis around site of lead tip MI in electrode area		Observe for Decrease in amplitude of pacemaker artifact Decrease in pulse from 5 to 10 beats/minute (rule out nonper- fused premature ventricular contractions as cause) "Runaway" pacemaker Observe for failure to pace If pacemaker malfunction occurs or is suspected, notify physi- cian
■ Problems at implant site related to Incisional pain Infection Hematoma	■ Patient verbalizes sense of comfort (lack of pain) Clean, healing wound	■ Ask patient of need for pain medication; administer medica- tion as needed Inspect site regularly (and respond to patient's complaints) for any signs of inflammation or infection, skin breakdown, or hematomas

Potential problems	Expected outcomes	Nursing activities
Erosion or skin break-down due to pressure Sterile abscesses around generator		Check temperature q4 hr or as indicated If hemovac is present, empty q8 hr or prn; report excessive bleeding When pressure dressing is removed, sterile dressings may be applied; if so, change daily Administer antibiotics as ordered for 5 to 7 days after implant procedure
■ Frozen shoulder	■ Patient performs ROM exercises to affected shoulder	■ Begin ROM exercises to affected shoulder after checking with physician, usually around the third postoperative day
■ Arrhythmias	■ Absence of threatening arrhythmias	■ Observe for ventricular premature beats; note frequency, coupling interval, whether sensing or competition occurs, and whether or not they perfuse If problem occurs, notify physician and treat with lidocaine as ordered or follow standing orders
■ Insufficient knowledge and skill to comply with discharge regimen*	■ Evaluation by testing or questioning demonstrates patient/family's understanding of the knowledge components of the teaching program Patient takes own pulse correctly and states acceptable ranges Patient lists symptoms requiring notification of physician Patient asks pertinent questions regarding self-care Patient discusses future realistically, noting adjustments required	■ Institute teaching program for patient/family, including Normal heart function—electrical and mechanical Patient's disease process/arrhythmia, which necessitates a pacemaker Pacemaker function Method of counting pulse Patient's own normal range Acceptable variations of pulse, noting specifically when to call physician Signs and symptoms indicative of pacemaker failure; relate to those patient had prior to pacemaker and identify when to call physician Activity instructions including work, sports, sex, and travel Necessity of identification ID card Medical alert jewelry Informing physician or dentist Electrical interference; precautions and actions to take if occurs Clothing suggestions—comfort and cosmetic Follow-up Necessity of and timing What is involved Expected battery life and procedure for generator change Provide opportunities for patient/family to ask questions and practice palpating pulse Assess patient/family's potential compliance and make referrals for home follow-up if necessary

*If this type of follow-up care is the responsibility of the critical care unit nurse when patient is transferred from intensive care unit.

18 □ Intra-aortic balloon pumping (counterpulsation)

The intra-aortic balloon is used for patients with marginal cardiac function when augmentation of coronary blood flow and a decrease in *afterload,* or resistance to cardiac ejection, is desired. *Preload,* or the resting pressure and stretch in the left ventricle, is decreased also. These actions result in a decreased myocardial work load and oxygen consumption.

Blood supply is augmented while oxygen demand is diminished, resulting in improved myocardial efficiency and augmented stroke volume and cardiac output.

The intra-aortic balloon pump is used when medical therapy is inadequate to support patients in the following clinical situations:

1. For high-risk patients requiring cardiac catheterization, particularly in the presence of unstable angina
2. Preoperatively, for patients with a recent MI and associated cardiogenic shock; mechanical defects such as mitral insufficiency, ruptured papillary muscle, septal defect; intractable angina; and arrhythmias
3. For intractable, unstable angina
4. As an adjunct to preoperative and postoperative management of surgical cardiac patients
5. When weaning from the cardiopulmonary bypass (CPB) machine is not possible using medical therapy alone; this situation occurs in patients with left ventricular failure and a low cardiac output syndrome*

Intra-aortic balloon pumping is avoided in patients with severe aortic insufficiency, aortic dissection, coarctation of the aorta, high-output shock, terminal noncardiac diseases, and in the presence of irreversible brain damage. Severe aortoiliac disease is a relative contraindication, although femoral-to-femoral grafts can be placed to increase blood to the extremity fed by the artery into which the balloon will be placed.

The intra-aortic balloon consists of a catheter with a balloon at the tip. This device can be placed in the descending aorta via an arteriotomy in the right or left femoral artery and then threaded up the descending aorta to a point 1 cm distal to the subclavian artery.

The balloon is alternately inflated and deflated with gas, such that inflation occurs during ventricular diastole when the aortic valve is closed, displacing blood into the upper torso arteries (unidirectional balloon system) or into both upper and lower torso arteries (bidirectional balloon system).

Knobs on the intra-aortic balloon console are adjusted so that the balloon inflates just when the aortic valve closes. The timing is usually done using the R wave of the QRS complex as the reference point, although the arterial waveform may be used also.

An arterial line and pulmonary artery catheter should be in place before the balloon is inserted. Antibiotics and heparin are administered before the procedure as prophylaxis against infection and thromboembolism.

Hemodynamic and circulatory monitoring activities are essential in assessing the benefit of intra-aortic balloon pumping and related therapeutic interventions. Based on these observations, alterations in the therapeutic regimen may be made. Problems that arise may also require alterations in the therapeutic regimen, including hemorrhage during insertion, laceration of the aortic vessel lining, thromboemboli, and infection.

ASSESSMENT

1. Level of patient/family's anxiety
2. Patient/family's understanding of the disease process and anticipated intervention
3. Presence, nature, and severity of problem necessitating balloon insertion, including
   a. Disease process
   b. Hemodynamic parameters
   c. Medical management that has been employed
4. Lab and diagnostic tests, including
   a. ECG abnormalities
   b. Echocardiographic studies
   c. Radionuclide studies
   d. Electrolyte levels
   e. Cardiac enzymes

---

*Bailin, M. T.: Lectures on intra-aortic balloon pumping, 1976-1979, Cardiovascular Laboratory, College of Physicians and Surgeons, Columbia-Presbyterian Medical Center, New York; Bregman, D.: Mechanical support of the failing heart, Curr. Probl. Surg. **13**(12):1-84, 1976; Durie, M. E.: Use of an intra-aortic balloon pump following postoperative pump failure and cardiac arrest: case presentation and discussion, Heart Lung **3**:971-975, 1974.

f. Complete blood count (CBC)

g. Cardiac catheterization results

h. Chest radiograph results

5. Integrity and general function of balloon system

    a. Connections

    b. Lamps (lights)

    c. Position of balloon and catheter

        (1) External—observe for slack in balloon line and moderately tight insertion of catheter into safety chamber (using no tape)

        (2) Internal

            (a) Chest radiograph

            (b) Note adequacy of circulation to left arm

            (c) Note adequacy of diastolic augmentation

6. Waveform and hemodynamic/circulatory status for optimal balloon pumping

    a. Proper timing

        (1) Augmented wave begins at dichrotic notch

        (2) Augmented wave reaches 5 to 10 mm Hg below zero baseline just before next beat begins

    b. Hemodynamic parameters

        (1) Drop in height of patient's own systolic wave (indicating decreased afterload and left ventricular work)

        (2) Decrease in aortic end diastolic pressures ("presystolic dip") of 5 to 10 mm Hg

        (3) Presence of hypotension, tachycardia, and/or abnormal CVP and PAP

        (4) CVP, PAP, and PCWP in comparison with pre–balloon pumping pressures

        (5) Urine output, mental status, and adequacy of peripheral circulation in relation to pre–balloon pumping measures; note presence of oliguria, abnormal mental status, and signs of inadequate peripheral circulation

        (6) Adequacy of circulation to extremities, particularly the extremities distal to the catheter insertion site and the balloon; in the left arm and affected leg note presence of

            (a) Decreased/weak pulses

            (b) Coolness, blanching, poor capillary filling

        (7) Insertion site for hematoma, signs of infection, or phlebitis

        (8) Signs and symptoms of complications, including

            (a) Aortic laceration

            (b) Thrombi

            (c) Microemboli

            (d) Coagulation abnormalities

        (9) Respiratory insufficiency—rate, rhythm, quality of respirations—noting presence of rales, rhonchi, wheezing, shortness of breath, dyspnea, tachypnea

GOALS

1. Reduction of patient/family's anxiety with provision of information, explanations, and encouragement; patient/family asks questions and verbalizes understanding of insertion procedures and reason for and function of intra-aortic balloon pumping

2. Adequate blood flow to extremity distal to site of balloon insertion

3. Absence of hematoma at site of balloon catheter insertion

4. Absence of hemorrhage from insertion site during insertion procedure

5. Absence of aortic, femoral injury

6. Signs of adequate circulation to left upper extremity and brain

7. Hemodynamic stability

8. Adequate cardiac output

9. Hemodynamic parameters and clinical signs indicate adequate perfusion of central and peripheral organs

10. Optimal function of intra-aortic balloon pumping system

11. Absence or resolution of signs and symptoms of renal failure

12. Absence or resolution of a thrombus

13. Sufficient circulatory flows to affected leg, arm

14. Pulses full, extremity warm, and color good

15. Coagulation studies within desired limits

16. Infection free; absence of signs of infection at insertion site

17. Respiratory function sufficient to maintain adequate oxygenation and ventilation

18. Absence of pulmonary infection

19. Absence of signs and symptoms of a gas embolism

Potential problems	Expected outcomes	Nursing activities
■ Anxiety related to disease process and deteriorating condition leading to need for intra-aortic balloon pumping	■ Reduction in patient/family's anxiety with provision of information, explanations, and encouragement Patient/family asks questions and verbalizes understanding of disease process, purpose for hospitalization, and need for intra-aortic balloon pumping	■ Assess patient/family's anxiety and understanding regarding disease process, purpose of hospitalization, deteriorating condition, anticipated balloon insertion, and diagnostic procedures (such as cardiac catheterization) Explain, in simple terms, each of the aforementioned as needed Prepare patient for and provide for ongoing support and encouragement during insertion of catheter and institution of balloon pumping Prepare patient for diagnostic tests and explain them as needed Evaluate for reduction in patient/family's anxiety with provision of information, explanations, reassurance, and comfort
■ Ischemic leg, which may be related to Low blood volume Severe atherosclerosis and circulatory insufficiency Spasm of vessel at insertion site	■ Adequate blood flow to affected extremities—to leg distal to insertion site and to arm distal to balloon tip Pulses in extremities full, color good, and extremity warm	■ Prevent by Administering therapy to provide for adequate blood volume and blood flow around balloon In patient with history of severe atherosclerosis and circulatory insufficiency, prepare patient for a prophylactic femoral bypass graft to augment blood flow to the leg below the planned insertion site, if planned During balloon catheter insertion, vessel spasm may occur; as the overall hemodynamic picture improves with counterpulsation, the spasm may subside; if not, assist in removal of balloon if procedure becomes necessary Monitor for ischemic leg Pulses (femoral, posterior tibial, and dorsalis pedis) before insertion of balloon, then q15-30 min (four times) and then q1-2 hr Absent pulses, which may indicate transient arterial spasm, femoral artery occlusion by the catheter or a thrombus, or an arterial embolus to the extremity; employ further evaluation for circulatory defects Color and temperature of extremity q30 min (four times) and then q1-2 hr Toe sensitivity and patient's ability to move toes Presence of claudication Complaints of pain and/or extreme restlessness along with signs of circulatory insufficiency to leg Notify physician for any of the aforementioned abnormalities If signs and symptoms of circulatory insufficiency to the extremity are marked, balloon removal may be required; assist with procedure as necessary Closely observe for continued or progressive circulatory insufficiency if pulses are weak and limb is cool; in this case reconstructive surgery may be accomplished after balloon removal to improve circulation to the leg; prepare patient for surgery if planned
■ Hematoma at insertion site related to anticoagulation necessary for balloon insertion and, in some cases, operative technique	■ Absence or resolution of hematoma at site of balloon catheter insertion Coagulation profile within normal limits	■ Prevention Monitor platelet, Hct, and Hgb levels prior to insertion; if any or all are low, administer blood and blood products as ordered to correct the abnormalities Administer anticoagulation as ordered to achieve moderately prolonged prothrombin time (PT), activated partial thromboplastin time (APTT), and bleeding time as appropriate; be aware of pertinent baseline values Proper surgical technique As soon as catheter is in place and skin incision is sutured closed, assist physician with application of a pressure dressing

Potential problems	Expected outcomes	Nursing activities
		Monitor for
		Development of signs of hematoma at insertion site; note presence of subcutaneous swelling, bruised (black and blue) skin and subcutaneous tissue, decreased Hct, Hgb
		Abnormally prolonged PT, APTT, and bleeding time
		If hematoma occurs
		If large hematoma develops during balloon insertion, assist physician with removal if necessary
		If smaller hematoma develops during and/or after insertion, maintain a pressure dressing

■ Hemorrhage from insertion site
Blood loss of more than 200 ml related to insertion of a catheter into a large artery
	■ Blood loss less than 200 ml
	Restoration of normal blood volume
	Hemodynamic stability
		■ Efforts to prevent hemorrhage include careful surgical technique during insertion procedure to reduce blood loss
		Monitor
		   For large amount of blood loss during insertion procedure
		   Serial Hct levels before, during, and after insertion procedure
		If hemorrhage occurs, administer blood replacement as ordered

■ Aortic injury: aortic rupture	■ Absence of aortic rupture	■ Prevent by
		   Assisting physician during balloon insertion
		   Avoiding head gatch of more than 30 degrees and angulation at groin when patient is turned; patients must remain in bed when the balloon is in place
		Monitor
		   Vital signs throughout insertion procedure
		   For signs and symptoms of shock and cardiovascular collapse associated with aortic rupture
		If aortic rupture occurs
		   Prepare patient for emergency surgery
		   Administer blood and sympathomimetic medications if needed, as ordered

■ Aortic/femoral artery injury related to
Dissection
Intimal hematoma
	■ Absence of aortic/femoral artery injury	■ Prevent by
		   Assisting physicians as they employ careful technique during balloon insertion
		   Avoiding head gatch of more than 30 degrees
		   Instructing patient not to flex the involved leg (leg restraints are rarely necessary)
		Monitor for
		   Difficult insertion procedure
		   Onset of patient discomfort, pain in lower back
		   Hematoma formation at or near insertion site
		   Hypotension, tachycardia, and falling Hct, with or without external bleeding, which may indicate a hemorrhagic process
		Notify physician for significant abnormalities
		If aortic/femoral artery injury occurs, administer blood replacement as ordered, and carefully monitor patient's response

■ Aortic/femoral artery injury related to inadvertent partial or total removal of catheter out of the artery into which it is inserted	■ Balloon and catheter remain in situ in desired location	■ Prevent by
		   Providing for slack in catheter once balloon is in place
		   Avoiding extremely tight connection of catheter to safety chamber; no tape should be used
		   Employing comfort, support measures, and pain/sedative medication as needed to minimize patient's restlessness
		Monitor
		   Tension/slack in intra-aortic balloon catheter; safety chamber connection
		   For inadvertent partial or total balloon catheter removal

Potential problems	Expected outcomes	Nursing activities

		If balloon displacement is suspected, obtain radiograph
		Notify physician if displacement is noted or suspected
		If catheter removal occurs
		  Apply, maintain pressure dressing as ordered
		  Monitor for development of hematoma at or near insertion site
		  Monitor for hemodynamic stability, stable Hct (note presence of hypotension and a falling Hct; notify physician if either occurs)

■ Partial or total occlusion of subclavian and/or carotid artery; ischemic arm and/or cerebral tissue	■ Adequate circulation to left upper extremity, brain
	Upper extremity pulses full; extremities are pink in color and warm
	Patient is alert and oriented
		■ Efforts to prevent occlusion of the subclavian or carotid artery include insertion of the balloon catheter using fluoroscopy or chest radiograph to achieve correct position
		Monitor
		  Pulses, circulation to left arm—note weak pulses, discomfort, pallor, and coolness of arm
		  Level of consciousness, orientation; note restlessness, confusion, irritability and other abnormalities
		Notify physician of these abnormalities
		If balloon occludes the subclavian or carotid artery, assist physician to pull it out a small distance to permit better circulation to upper extremity and brain

■ Hemodynamic instability related to inadequate diastolic augmentation Timing of balloon inflation/deflation inappropriate for patient's needs Improper timing, with too short a time of inflation, allows an interval of balloon deflation before the next beat begins; this encourages retrograde flow of blood from arteries, including the coronary arteries	■ Diastolic augmentation properly timed such that balloon inflation begins at the dicrotic notch when the aortic valve closes and deflation occurs just before the next systole when the aortic valve opens A decrease of about 5 to 10 mm Hg in presystolic aortic pressure occurs	■ Prevention Note heart rate before intra-aortic balloon counterpulsation begins and set timing intervals accordingly; if heart rate changes later by more than 7 to 10 beats/minute, retiming will be necessary The objective in proper timing of balloon inflation and deflation is to time inflation to occur at the dicrotic notch (or when the aortic valve closes and ventricular diastole begins); try to time the balloon deflation to achieve a 5 to 10 mm Hg drop in aortic end diastolic pressure Initial settings may be made according to the following guidelines Set filling time at 50 milliseconds (msec) to provide a small augmented tracing while inflation and deflation interval settings are made; the time for systole and balloon deflation is approximately one third of the cardiac cycle + 50 msec or $$\frac{\text{R to R interval in msec}}{3} + 50*$$ The time for diastole and balloon inflation is approximately two thirds of the cardiac cycle or $$\text{R} - \text{R interval} - \frac{\text{R} - \text{R interval}*}{3}$$ Check calibration and timing of balloon inflation and deflation at least q1 hr and prn

*Pastellopoulos, A. E., and Cullum, J.: Intra-aortic balloon assist for cardiogenic shock, J. Cardiovasc. Technol. **16:**21-30, 1974.

Potential problems	Expected outcomes	Nursing activities

		Monitor
		  Appearance of augmented pressure wave for placement and timing of inflation and deflation
		    This is easily done by momentarily turning ratio of augmented beats to 1:2
		    Note whether the augmented wave begins at the dichrotic notch and ends just before the next beat, with a 5 to 10 mm Hg drop in presystolic pressure
		  For arrhythmias—a mistimed balloon may be the cause (balloon inflation/deflation is also slightly less accurate in the presence of irregular cardiac rhythms)
		  For heart rate changes of more than 7 to 10 beats/minute
		Notify physician for any of these abnormalities
		If inappropriate timing occurs
		  Readjust timing
		  If cause of inappropriate timing can be found, resolve the problem as ordered (e.g., arrhythmias)

■ Hemodynamic instability related to inadequate amount of gas (CO_2, helium) in balloon
Approximately 1 to 2 cc gas lost from balloon q1 hr
	■ Sufficient diastolic augmentation to achieve BP in specified range
	When external balloon is filled, it is taut and smooth appearing
	Height of augmented wave remains at maximum height achieved immediately after balloon refilling (or in systems not requiring manual inflation, augmentation wave remains at maximum height)
		■ Provide for adequate amount of gas in balloon by
		  Refilling q2-4 hr as needed (if manual refilling system)
		  After filling, note height of diastolic augmentation
		Monitor for need to refill
		  A decrease in the height of the diastolic augmented wave
		  "Slave" balloon in external safety chamber is not taut when filled
		If there is an inadequate amount of gas in balloon, refill if system requires manual refilling

■ Hemodynamic instability related to kinked catheter	■ Sufficient diastolic augmentation to maintain BP in desired range
	Catheter not kinked
	Balloon/catheter system patent
		■ Prevent kinked catheter by
		  Providing for some, but not too much, slack in balloon catheter
		  Keeping system visible at all times
		  Checking for unkinked line when patient is repositioned
		Monitor for catheter patency, presence of kinks
		If kinked catheter occurs, straighten catheter

■ Problems in achieving proper diastolic augmentation related to
Difficulty in balancing/calibration
BP monitoring system
Faulty transducer
"Fuzzy" or "choppy" arterial trace
Missing arterial trace
	■ Transducer properly balanced/calibrated to console
	Appearance of crisp, normal appearing arterial tracing
	Console arterial BP approximates BP taken by cuff or Doppler sensor (usually there is as much as 10 to 15 mm Hg difference)
		■ Prevent by
		  Recalibrating transducer to console q4 hr and prn
		  Avoiding trauma to transducer
		  Being careful with bed rail movement so that it does not cut or damage transducer cable
		An extra transducer should be available for immediate use
		Compare balloon console pressures with cuff BP q4-8 hr; the transducer pressure is normally 10 mm Hg (5 to 15 mm Hg) higher than a cuff BP
		If a problem in achieving proper diastolic augmentation occurs
		  Try rebalancing, calibrating transducer
		  Transducer may need to be replaced

Potential problems	Expected outcomes	Nursing activities

■ Loss of pumping capability associated with leak in intra-aortic balloon with rapid depletion of gas (rare)	■ Balloon intact Absence of leak in balloon If leak occurs, balloon replaced immediately	■ Prevent by ensuring that the balloon catheter is not placed among surgical instruments after package is opened
		Monitor for
		  Rapid depletion of gas in external (safety chamber) balloon
		  Wrinkled appearance of external balloon instead of smooth, taut appearance
		  Loss of maximal diastolic augmentation capability (in comparison with postinsertion baseline augmentation)
		If loss of pumping capability occurs
		  Notify physician
		  Assist with balloon and catheter removal and replacement, if procedure becomes necessary

■ Balloon catheter becomes disconnected from external balloon
This may happen if great tension is applied between the internal balloon and catheter
Separation of the balloon catheter from the external balloon/console when undue tension is applied is preferable to inadvertent removal of the internal balloon
	■ Balloon/catheter system intact	■ Prevent by ensuring some slack in catheter; keep machine close to bed and provide for appropriate patient/catheter positioning
		Monitor for
		  Tension on external balloon line
		  Visible catheter system (so any disconnenction is seen immediately)
		If balloon catheter becomes disconnected from external balloon
		  Turn pump off
		  Quickly reconnect system and refill balloon (if manual method is necessary)
		  Turn pump on

■ Suboptimal pumping capability associated with poor ECG tracing related to
Inadequate height of R wave
ECG monitoring system not intact
Electrode displacement
	■ Intact ECG monitoring system, with crisp QRS picture; R wave of sufficient height for consistent, proper triggering of balloon inflation/deflation	■ Prevent by
		  Providing for intact ECG monitoring system and crisp ECG picture
		  Replacing electrodes as needed
		  Placing electrodes to maximize R-wave height (0.5 to 1.5 millivolts) relative to other ECG waves
		Monitor for need to replace electrodes including wide, hazy ECG baseline that may move all over screen
		If problem occurs and the intra-aortic balloon pumping console receives no ECG trigger stimulus, some units will automatically produce balloon deflation
		  Turn pump off (until electrodes can be replaced, etc.)
		  Switch trigger knob from ''ECG'' trigger to ''pressure'' or ''pulse'' trigger; turn machine on
		  Retime inflation/deflation using this pressure/pulse mode, since the pressure spike comes later in the cycle than the R wave
		  Replace electrodes or determine any other cause for problem in ECG picture; turn pump back to ''ECG'' trigger; and retime intervals

■ Suboptimal pumping capability associated with poor arterial tracing, which may be related to occluded arterial catheter or air in the system	■ Crisp, arterial waveform BP via arterial catheter is within 10 to 15 mm Hg of BP by cuff or Doppler sensor	■ Provide for continuous infusion of heparin solution through arterial line to prevent occlusion Prevent/monitor for air in transducer system or kinked catheter, which can reduce accuracy of pressure readings and affect proper timing (if the arterial waveform is used to trigger balloon inflation/deflation) Prevent/eliminate kinks in transducer-flush system q4-8 hr Compare cuff/Doppler pressure against monitor pressure q4-8 hr Rebalance transducer system q8 hr and prn Eliminate air from system if this problem occurs Flush solution through arterial catheter periodically if necessary If clot in arterial catheter is suspected, try withdrawing the clot back through the arterial catheter

Potential problems	Expected outcomes	Nursing activities

■ Arrhythmias
Irregular cardiac rhythm
Most intra-aortic balloon pumping models automatically deflate when a short coupling interval occurs
If the premature beat is not very close to the preceding beat, the intra-aortic balloon pumping system may continue to augment but at a reduced efficiency on the irregular beats
	■ Absence or control of arrhythmias	■ Prevent by avoiding/correcting factors that precipitate arrhythmias, such as hypoxia, acid-base imbalance, electrolyte imbalance, and anxiety
		If a sympathomimetic drug is the suspected offender, administer an alternative medication as ordered
		Monitor
		  ECG for arrhythmias, particularly supraventricular tachycardia and ventricular arrhythmias
		  Hemodynamic response to arrhythmias if present
		Notify physician for abnormalities
		If arrhythmias occur
		  Administer antiarrhythmic therapy if ordered
		  Administer therapy to correct hypoxia, acid-base imbalance, and electrolyte imbalance if needed, as ordered
		In patient with a pacemaker, if pacing artifact is sensed as an R wave, the timing for balloon inflation/deflation should be appropriately altered (delay will be increased due to increased time interval between trigger [pacing spike] and dichrotic notch [aortic valve closing])
		Until a supraventricular tachycardia can be resolved, the frequency of augmentation may be decreased to every other beat and 3 cc of CO_2 may be added to the balloon volume as ordered
		If a tachycardia develops, the timing intervals will need to be decreased
		In the presence of a very irregular rhythm, exhaust-pressure logic may be used with arrhythmias, following the procedure appropriate for the console in use
		An extremely irregular rhythm may require pacing to achieve a regular rhythm for proper timing of balloon counterpulsation; assist with procedure

■ Cardiac arrest during counterpulsation	■ Absence or resolution of cardiac arrest	■ Prevent by administering therapy to prevent and treat arrhythmias, thus reducing the likelihood of cardiac arrest
		Monitor for
		  Arrhythmias
		  Inadequate cardiac output, hemodynamic instability
		Notify physician if these abnormalities occur
		If cardiac arrest occurs
		  Assist in institution of CPR
		  The intra-aortic balloon pumping console may continue to pump in alternation with chest compressions, that is, the chest is compressed as the internal balloon deflates (and the external ''slave'' balloon in the safety chamber inflates)
		Check to see if intra-aortic balloon pumping console is protected against the electrical current used in cardioversion
		If cardiac arrest occurs and patient has a pacemaker, the balloon will continue to be triggered and filled; compress chest when internal balloon is deflated
		The intra-aortic balloon pumping machine can be turned to the ''internal'' trigger mode to trigger balloon inflation and deflation; chest compressions can be similarly interposed with inflations of the internal balloon

■ Continued hypotension related to low cardiac output after balloon is in place	■ Hemodynamic parameters within normal limits
	Hemodynamic/circulatory parameters in-
		■ Prevention
		  Review chart and radiograph results to determine if balloon is placed in optimal aortic position with its tip just distal to the subclavian artery
		  Monitor P, circulation, and BP to left arm and to brain during and after catheter insertion

Potential problems	Expected outcomes	Nursing activities

	dicate adequate cardiac output and perfusion of central and peripheral organs	Ensure scrupulous timing of balloon inflation and deflation; avoid delayed deflation and an associated increased afterload and resistance to cardiac ejection
		Monitor
		  BP, P, CVP, and PAP if available; jugular venous distention, urine output, peripheral circulation, and mentation q15-30 min for signs and symptoms of low cardiac output and/or hypotension
		  Daily weights
		  Serial arterial blood gas results (note acidosis)
		Notify physician for abnormalities in these parameters
		If hypotension related to low cardiac output occurs
		  Administer fluids as ordered, monitoring the patient's response very closely
		  Administer inotropic agents or an inotropic/vasodilating agent combination to achieve adequate cardiac output with a peak pressure of 100 to 110 mm Hg (systolic or augmented diastolic pressure, whichever is greater) and/or a mean pressure of 80 to 90 mm Hg, or as ordered

■ Renal failure, related to
  Low cardiac output
  Renal thromboemboli
	■ Absence or resolution of of signs and symptoms of renal failure
	Urine output at least 0.5 ml/kg/hour for an adult
	Indices of renal function, particularly BUN/creatinine, within normal limits
		■ Prevent by maintaining adequate cardiac output and renal blood flow by administering digitalis, fluids, blood products, inotropic agents, and balloon pumping as ordered
		Monitor
		  Fluid intake and output measurements q1 hr
		  Hemodynamic measurements to determine adequacy of cardiac output q1 hr
		  Results of daily lab studies, including BUN/creatinine levels
		If problem occurs, see Standard: *Acute renal failure*

■ Clotting abnormalities, thrombus formation, and thromboemboli, which may be related to any of several factors, including
Dislodgement of atheromatous material during balloon insertion
Balloon left in deflated position for more than 30 to 60 minutes
Turbulence of blood flowing around balloon
Hemolysis of RBC with platelet-fibrin aggregation enhanced by the turbulent blood flow around the balloon and by the balloon acting as a surface on which RBC-platelet-fibrin aggregates can adhere
	■ Absence of/or resolution of thrombus or thromboembolus
	Adequate circulation to affected leg and arm
	Pulses full, extremities warm, and color good
	Coagulation studies within desired limits
		■ Prevent by
		  Administering prophylactic anticoagulation if ordered (usually 4000 to 6000 units heparin q6 hr in most adults, except during the first 120 hours or so after surgery when 600 mg rectal aspirin may be given q4-6 hr)
		  Administering dextran (10 to 20 ml/hour), if ordered, to decrease platelet aggregation
		  Avoiding leg bending at groin or knee; when patient is turned on side keep groin and knee straight with pillows
		  Avoiding balloon deflation for more than 2 to 3 minutes and never for more than 30 to 60 minutes (maximum time depends on institutional policy)
		Monitor
		  Circulation to affected leg, arm q½-1 hr, noting presence and quality of pulses, color, and warmth
		  For signs of peripheral thromboembolus; arterial embolus; and embolus to kidneys, intestine, or brain, which may be followed by infarction; see Standard: *Embolic phenomena*
		  Serial PT, APTT, and bleeding time, often done approximately 3 to 4 hours after the morning dose of heparin
		  Results of serial platelet counts done at least q24 hr
		  Hct and Hgb levels at least q24 hr
		  For signs and symptoms of bleeding—internal or external; employ other anticoagulation precautions such as avoidance of bruising and so on
		  Record all blood loss, including blood samples
		If there are signs and symptoms of an embolus to any end organ, notify physician immediately and administer therapy as or-

Potential problems	Expected outcomes	Nursing activities
		dered; monitor for reduced function, signs of progressive ischemia of the end organ Administer fresh blood, fresh frozen plasma, platelets as ordered Procure a Fogarty thromboembolectomy balloon catheter and assist physician with insertion distal to the balloon insertion site to remove any thromboemboli (usually done immediately after balloon removal)
■ Infection related to indwelling catheters and the high frequency of invasive procedures	■ Infection free Absence of signs of local infection at insertion site	■ Prevent by Employing strict aseptic technique during the insertion of all lines, including the balloon, and for subsequent dressing changes Administering antibiotics, which are instituted before balloon insertion and continued for at least 48 hours thereafter Employing vigorous chest physiotherapy q2 hr and prn, to include turning, chest percussion and vibration, and coughing and deep breathing (if patient is extubated); if patient is intubated, see Standard: *Mechanical ventilation* Monitor For signs and symptoms of systemic and local infection, particularly of wounds or at insertion sites of invasive lines Temperature q1-3 hr, as indicated by patient's status The results of serial WBC counts, with differential Culture results If infection occurs Continue monitoring as described before Administer antibiotics and local care as ordered
■ Respiratory insufficiency related to Supine position Left ventricular power failure of any etiology leading to elevated PCWP and pulmonary edema Cardiac surgery with prolonged immobilization, minimal inflation of lungs intraoperatively, and decreased interstitial fluid/lymphatic drainage during surgery	■ Respiratory function sufficient to maintain adequate ventilation and oxygenation Pa_{O_2} and Pa_{CO_2} within patient's normal limits Absence of pulmonary infection Chest radiograph clear, indicating full lung expansion and absence of vascular congestion Absence of infection	■ Prevention Reposition patient q1-2 hr to avoid hypostatic pneumonia Administer chest physiotherapy q2-4 hr Administer humidified O_2 to liquefy secretions and to provide for adequate oxygenation Monitor relationship of hemodynamic parameters with pulmonary function; particularly note PCWP, if available, in relation to signs of adequate cardiac output If PCWP increases concurrent with signs of a falling cardiac output, notify physician Institute remedial measures as ordered, which may include fluids, cardiotonic/vasopressor and vasodilator agents to improve cardiac output and decrease pulmonary vascular congestion Administer blood products as ordered to increase the Hct (usually to 30%) to achieve an adequate oxygen-carrying ability and a sufficient intravascular colloid level Monitor Respiratory rate, rhythm, quality Breath sounds; note presence of rales, rhonchi, wheezing Arterial blood gas levels, noting presence of abnormal pH levels, hypoxemia, and abnormal CO_2 levels For signs and symptoms of hypoxia, hypocapnia, or hypercapnia Chest radiograph results for evidence of interstitial edema, atelectasis, pleural effusion, and other abnormalities Hemodynamic parameters q½-1 hr for adequacy of left ventricular function and for progress/resolution of pulmonary congestion Fluid intake and output q1 hr scrupulously

Potential problems	**Expected outcomes**	**Nursing activities**
		Notify physician of any significant abnormalities in these parameters
		If respiratory insufficiency occurs
		Provide for respiratory support to achieve adequate oxygenation and ventilation, including repositioning q1-2 hr, chest physiotherapy, coughing, and deep breathing
		Administer humidified O_2 supplement as needed and ordered
		If these measures are insufficient, mechanical ventilation with PEEP may be instituted until the precipitating cause is ameliorated (e.g., compromised myocardial function and pulmonary congestion); see Standards: *Mechanical ventilation* and *Positive end expiratory pressure* as appropriate
		Administer diuretic, inotropic, and vasodilating agents as ordered to improve myocardial efficiency
■ Gas embolism related to balloon rupture	■ Absence of signs and symptoms of gas embolism	■ Prevent by
		Ensuring that the balloon stays out of the operative field during the insertion procedure, thus avoiding a tiny tear by surgical instruments
	Balloon intact with adequate diastolic augmentation	Avoiding reuse of aortic balloons; as a balloon is withdrawn through the Dacron graft, tiny tears may occur; autoclaving changes the consistency and the integrity of the balloon; moreover, reuse may transmit the hepatitis antigen
		Monitor for proper, complete reinflation of the external balloon in the safety chamber
		If a significant loss of gas is noted, monitor for signs and symptoms of emboli to any of the central organs and the peripheral arterial vasculature (see Standard: *Embolic phenomena*)
		If gas embolism occurs
		Notify physician
		Assist with balloon catheter removal if the procedure is necessary

19 □ **Hemodynamic monitoring**

Hemodynamic monitoring involves the measurement of pressures including arterial, venous, pulmonary artery, and intracranial pressures to assist in the management of the critically ill patient. This is accomplished by placing catheters in an artery, vein, heart chamber, or cerebrospinal fluid and connecting them to pressure extension lines attached to the transducer in an airtight solution-filled system. The transducer is electrically connected to a pressure monitor, scope, and recorder. Pressure transducers are electronic devices that convert mechanical pressure waves into electrical signals. The monitor/amplifier receives electrical signals through the transducer cable and processes these signals to a meaningful form, for example, a standard unit of pressure measurement, which is then displayed on the digital meters on the front panel of the amplifier.

The scope/recorder allows for continuous display and trace of waveforms processed by the monitor. An alarm system is located in the monitor, and when appropriate alarm limits are set, abnormal pressures are revealed in 3 to 4 seconds.

This direct pressure determination permits continuous patient hemodynamic monitoring, allowing for a more precise diagnosis of patient problems and a rapid assessment of the patient's response to therapy.

The intra-arterial monitoring permits continuous blood pressure measurements in hemodynamically unstable patients, including those receiving potent vasoactive/inotropic medications. This permits immediate detection of changes in the blood pressure, thus guiding therapeutic alterations aimed at bringing the blood pressure into a consistently normal range. The waveform and pressures provide information for assessment of cardiac contraction, aortic valve closure, and perfusion of ectopic beats. The arterial catheter allows for easy access to blood specimens needed for monitoring a critically ill patient. Arterial lines may be inserted into the femoral, axillary, brachial, or radial artery. Generally, the radial artery is the vessel of choice because it has been associated with fewer complications.

The CVP measures the pressure in the vena cava or right atrium. CVP/right atrial pressures reflect mean right atrial filling pressures and right ventricular diastolic pressures (pressures at the end of the filling cycle, just before contraction). Normal CVP pressures range from 1 to 6 mm Hg or 5 to 12 cm H_2O pressure. The CVP is determined/affected by the relationship of blood volume, vascular tone, and ventricular (particularly right) function. Therapy that results in alterations in any of these three factors will alter the CVP measurement, and, therefore, it is a most useful guide in regulating fluid replacement and administration of diuretics, as well as vasopressors and vasodilators. CVP measurement is not an accurate index of left ventricular function when the functional efficiency of the two ventricles differs. An elevated CVP may signal right ventricular failure and indirectly reflect left ventricular failure, volume overload, increased vascular tone, tricuspid valve stenosis or regurgitation, constrictive pericarditis, cardiac tamponade, or pulmonary hypertension (due to chronic lung disease, pulmonary embolism, etc.). Other patient parameters must be assessed before diagnosis of the presence of any of these complications is made. Factors that produce low CVP/right atrial pressure include reduced blood volume and decreased venous tone.

A pulmonary artery catheter, called a *Swan-Ganz*, can measure pulmonary artery diastolic pressure, pulmonary artery systolic pressure, PCWP, left atrial filling pressure, CVP, and cardiac output. It also provides information about the competency of left ventricular function, and the response of the marginal left ventricle to particular therapeutic interventions, particularly fluid administration, diuretics, inotropic agents, and vasodilators. The pulmonary artery catheter is a pliable balloon-tipped, flow-directed catheter that is passed through a large vein, usually in the antecubital or neck area, into the right side of the heart to the pulmonary artery. There are three kinds of pulmonary artery catheters:

Double lumen catheter: monitors pulmonary artery and wedge pressures; used for obtaining samples of mixed venous blood; used for infusion of solutions

Triple lumen catheter: same capabilities as double lumen catheter; also monitors right atrial pressure (CVP)

Flow-directed thermodilution catheter: same capabilities as double and triple lumen catheters; also monitors cardiac output via a fourth lumen connected to a cardiac output computer

Pulmonary artery systolic pressures reflect the pressures of blood flow from the right ventricle and usually approximate the right ventricular systolic pressure in the absence of pulmonary artery stenosis. Pulmonary artery pressures (PAP) are elevated in the presence of increased pulmonary blood flow (e.g., hypervolemia), elevated pulmonary resistance, and/or left ventricular failure.

Left ventricular end diastolic pressure is reflected by the pulmonary artery diastolic and capillary wedge pressures. Left ventricular end diastolic pressure occurs at the end of the diastole when the valves on the left side of the heart open and the left ventricle, left atrium, and the pulmonary beds momentarily become a single chamber. The PCWP is obtained by inflating the balloon near the end of the catheter until the small pulmonary vessel is occluded and the catheter is said to be ''wedged.'' The pressure reflected on the monitor is called *PCWP*. It reflects the resting baseline pressures in the lungs, left atrium, and left ventricle, which are nearly the same in the absence of mitral valve disease or severely increased pulmonary vascular resistance. If severe mitral valve stenosis is present, the left atrial pressures are higher and reflect a greater degree of left ventricular failure than is actually present. Serial wedge pressure measurements are useful in determining the response of the left ventricle to fluids, diuretics, and vasopressor and vasodilator drug therapy. Pulmonary wedge pressures indicating heart failure range from 18 to 20 mm Hg; for frank heart failure from 22 to 25 mm Hg; and for pulmonary edema over 30 mm Hg. For normal PAP values see Table 1.

Table 1. Normal PAP values

Pressure	Value (mm Hg)
Right atrial mean	−1 to +7
Right ventricular	
Systolic	15 to 25
End diastolic	0 to 8
Pulmonary artery	
Systolic	15 to 25
Diastolic	8 to 15
Mean	10 to 20
Pulmonary wedge mean	5 to 12

Elevated PAP may occur with pulmonary embolism, which is associated with increased pulmonary vascular resistance and increased PAP. It can also be elevated in the presence of pulmonary hypertension of chronic lung disease. Pulmonary artery pressures are useful in the diagnosis of these and in the differentiation of hypovolemic shock (low PAP), cardiogenic shock (high PAP), and spinal shock (normal PAP). They also provide accurate quantification of the degree of myocardial depression after an MI, thereby permitting more precise, individualized therapy. Heart failure can be quantitated for each ventricle, and the response to therapy can be followed. Pericardial disease can be confirmed as a result of characteristic pressure changes. The presence of ventricular septal rupture can be verified with the aid of oxygen content determinations, where a step up in oxygen content between the right atrium and the pulmonary artery can be seen.

Cardiac output is the amount of blood pumped by the ventricle in 1 minute. The cardiac output of the left and right ventricles is essentially the same, since each ventricle usually pumps equal amounts of blood/minute. The two determinants of cardiac output are stroke volume (amount of blood a ventricle pumps to the body during each contraction measured in milliliters of blood/contraction) and heart rate.

Stroke volume (milliliters/beat) ×
Heart rate(beats/minute) =
Cardiac output (milliliters/minute)

The normal cardiac output ranges from 4 to 7 liters/minute in the adult, depending on body size and the effect of variables that influence the demand for cardiac output.

The determination is accomplished with the use of a pulmonary artery flow-directed thermodilution catheter connected to a cardiac output computer. An exact amount of solution of known temperature is injected into the proximal catheter lumen, which empties into the right atrium or vena cava. The change in blood temperature is detected by the thermistor at the distal end of the catheter and then transmitted to the cardiac output computer for calculation and display of the cardiac output measurement.

A left atrial catheter is used to measure the pressure in the left atrium, which is a direct reflection of the left ventricular end diastolic pressure or filling pressure. It is usually placed in patients with very marginal heart function, actual or anticipated low cardiac output, rapid blood loss, or impaired cardiac contractility and in those for whom determination of fluid administration will be partly based on the direct response of the left atrial pressures. Like the PAP, the left atrial pressure is an index to the function of the left ventricle and a guide to fluid and blood replacement. It is critical that air not enter the atrium through this catheter because an air embolus can flow directly to the brain, heart, or other organs without being filtered by the lungs.

Intracranial pressure (ICP) monitoring is useful in patients who have signs/symptoms of increased intracranial pressure or who are likely to develop increased ICP to provide early detection of ICP elevation, which may not be obvious clinically until irreversible brain damage has occurred.

Normal ICP is less than 15 mm Hg. Cerebral perfusion pressure is determined by subtracting the mean intracranial pressure from the mean arterial blood pressure. The normal value is at least 50 mm Hg. The waveforms resemble an arterial waveform, with variations occurring with cardiac and respiratory movements/pressure changes.

ASSESSMENT

1. Level of patient/family's anxiety
2. Problem necessitating hemodynamic monitoring
   a. Disease process
   b. Hemodynamic parameters
   c. Medical management employed
3. Site of insertion for pain, ecchymosis, hematoma, infection, and phlebitis
4. Signs and symptoms of complications
   a. Arterial monitoring: dissection, external hemorrhage, sepsis, plaque dislodgement, false aneurysm, local obstruction with distal ischemia, cerebral infarction (carotid artery catheter), renal dysfunction (femoral artery catheter)
   b. CVP monitoring: infection, catheter breakage, thromboembolic phenomena, air embolism, perforation of right ventricle, arrhythmias if catheter in right atrium
   c. PCWP and cardiac output monitoring: infection, pulmonary artery perforation, thromboembolic complications, pulmonary ischemic lesions, pulmonary infarction, pneumothorax, arrhythmias, catheter kinking, and intracardiac knotting
   d. Left atrial pressure monitoring: air embolism
   e. Intracranial pressure monitoring: uncontrolled loss of CSF, infection, leakage of brain matter, brain trauma

5. Integrity and general function of hemodynamic monitoring system
   a. Patency of catheter
   b. Proper placement of catheter verified by chest radiograph results, fluoroscopy, waveforms, characteristics on the scope, pressures
   c. Accuracy of transducer
   d. Proper balancing and calibration of the system
   e. Airtight system of pressure tubings, stopcocks, adaptors or valves; absence of bubbles
   f. Proper function of amplifier/monitor
   g. Proper function of oscilloscope and/or recorder
   h. Measurement problems, including
      (1) Overdamping of waveforms
      (2) Influence of respiratory pressures
      (3) Migration of catheter tip
      (4) Drift of electronic zero or loss of calibration
      (5) Catheter whip artifact
      (6) Low pulmonary artery diastolic pressure
      (7) Faulty catheter system

6. Hemodynamic status in relation to patient's condition and therapy employed

GOALS

1. Reduction of patient/family's anxiety with provision of information and explanations
2. Hemodynamic stability—clinical signs and parameters indicate adequate central and peripheral perfusion
3. Infection free—absence of infection at insertion site or secondary sepsis
4. Absence and/or resolution of complications as stated in assessment for specific monitoring technique
5. Patient verbalizes comfort
6. Monitoring system functioning properly
7. Absence of measurement problems; waveforms correlate with patient's hemodynamic status

Potential problems	**Expected outcomes**	**Nursing activities**
■ Patient/family's anxiety related to disease process and procedures	■ Reduction in patient/family's anxiety with provision of information and explanations Patient/family asks questions and verbalizes understanding of disease process and need for hemodynamic monitoring	■ Assess patient/family's anxiety and understanding regarding disease process, hemodynamic monitoring, and diagnostic and lab studies Explain each of the aforementioned Prepare patient for and assist with diagnostic and lab studies as appropriate Prepare patient for hemodynamic monitoring and explain procedure Provide support, reassurance, and comfort for patient/family Evaluate reduction in patient/family's anxiety with provision of information and explanations
■ Problem during catheter insertion: arrhythmias, which usually result from catheter irritation of the right ventricular wall	■ Absence or minimal arrhythmia occurrence Absence of threatening arrhythmias	■ Prevention 　Monitor waveforms during insertion of catheter (or visually follow catheter under fluoroscopy) 　Physician will partially inflate balloon as catheter is advanced to the right ventricle to blunt catheter tip and prevent irritation of the endocardium 　Physician will advance catheter slowly and cautiously 　Administer therapy to resolve factors predisposing patient to arrhythmias including hypoxemia, acid-base imbalance, electrolyte imbalance, anxiety Monitor for any arrhythmia during insertion, particularly presence of premature ventricular contractions Have lidocaine and defibrillator available in case sudden hypotension or tachycardia develops If problem occurs 　Notify physician for significant incidence of ventricular arrhythmias 　Administer antiarrhythmic agent if needed, as ordered 　Physician may pull catheter back slightly and wait until arrhythmia subsides before attempting to advance the catheter

Potential problems	Expected outcomes	Nursing activities
■ Problem during catheter insertion: catheter curls, kinks, or knots in atrium, ventricle; more apt to occur in low-flow cardiac output states and with rapid insertion and manipulation	■ Absence/resolution of curling, kinking, or knotting of catheter Uneventful catheter insertion	■ Assist physician in partial inflation of the balloon once the catheter passes through the tricuspid valve so that flow of blood will carry the catheter into the pulmonary artery Catheter is advanced slowly; rapid advancement may cause curling or kinking of catheter so that further manipulation may result in knotting If knotting occurs in the atrium, the catheter can be carefully withdrawn by the physician to the insertion site, and knot can be removed through a small incision If knotting occurs in the ventricle, a thoracotomy may be required to remove the catheter
■ Problem during catheter insertion: perforation of the pulmonary artery; may be related to insufficient air in the catheter balloon such that catheter tip may injure the pulmonary artery	■ Absence or resolution of pulmonary artery perforation Pulmonary artery intact	■ Prevention Inflate balloon only with the specified amount of air or CO_2 Anchor the catheter firmly at insertion site Observe waveform before balloon inflation; do not inflate if waveform is flattened as this may indicate wedging If wedging occurs, turn patient to side and/or stimulate coughing in an attempt to dislodge the catheter from the wedged position Monitor For chest pain, hemoptysis, hypotension, cardiovascular collapse, and respiratory distress; notify physician immediately if any of these occur Chest radiograph results for catheter placement If problem occurs Administer medication and fluids as ordered Monitor BP and P continuously Prepare patient for emergency surgery if planned
■ Problem during catheter insertion: pneumothorax may be associated with subclavian insertion Where air inadvertently enters pleural space Inadvertent laceration of the apex of lung occurs	■ Pulmonary sufficiency Absence/resolution of pneumothorax Proper catheter placement	■ Prevention Place patient in supine or slightly Trendelenburg position for catheter insertion Keep patient still during insertion Physician employs careful technique so that the desired artery is entered, avoiding the pleural space and lung tissue Monitor For signs and symptoms of pneumothorax, including Anxiety and diaphoresis Sudden sharp chest pain, pleural pain Dyspnea and tachycardia Absent or distant breath sounds, asymmetrical chest movement, pallor, cyanosis Hypotension Vital signs q15-30 min and more often during acute episodes Notify physician for any of these abnormalities If problem occurs Stay with patient and have someone quickly procure equipment for chest tube insertion Check vital signs and respiratory status q15-30 min and prn Reassure and try to calm patient Assist with chest tube insertion Administer O_2 therapy as ordered Place patient in semi-to high Fowler's position Administer pain medication if needed, as ordered

Potential problems	Expected outcomes	Nursing activities
■ Pulmonary infarction related to occlusion of pulmonary artery by the catheter as a result of Balloon inadvertently left inflated with air Catheter drifts too far into the artery	■ Absence/resolution of pulmonary infarction Adequate pulmonary artery blood flow as indicated by waveform and pressure reading	■ Prevention Inflate balloon for a few seconds only Ensure that balloon is deflated after every wedging Observe waveform frequently to detect a damping (flattening) of the waveform, which may indicate a drift of the catheter farther into the artery Ensure that catheter is secured at desired length and that physician sutures catheter well on skin Limit frequency of wedging catheter to q2 hr if possible Avoid flushing catheter vigorously while it is being wedged Monitor for Chest pain with dyspnea, tachypnea, hemoptysis Chest pain with hypertension/hypotension and tachycardia If problem is suspected, monitor for Arterial blood gas results indicating hypoxemia (precipitous drop in Pa_{O_2}) Chest pain with dyspnea, tachypnea, hemoptysis If catheter drifts in too far Induce a quick increase, then decrease in intrathoracic pressure by turning patient; have patient cough If patient is intubated, manually inflate lungs vigorously a few times If pulmonary infarction occurs, administer supportive therapy as ordered, usually including humidified O_2
■ Pulmonary thromboembolism may be related to Clot formation around the catheter Patients with low cardiac output, hypercoagulability (e.g., with recent surgery) or other coagulation abnormalities are especially prone to this complication	■ Normal breath sounds Chest radiograph clear Infusion fluid system working properly	■ Prevention Avoid arterial blood sampling unless necessary Ensure a functioning, constant, slow infusion flush system with Tight connections Proper tubing (high-pressure tubing) and stopcocks Heparin is added to crystalloid solution, infused at 3 to 6 ml/hour, and regulated by a (Sorenson) flush System is pressurized—periodically check that pressure bag gauge is at 300 mm Hg Anticoagulation therapy may be employed for patients with a high risk for thrombus formation Monitor for Damping of waveforms Signs and symptoms of pulmonary thromboembolism, including severe substernal pain, dyspnea, tachypnea, diaphoresis, cyanosis, pallor, tachycardia, hypotension, hemoptysis, anxiety, diminished breath sounds, arrhythmias Notify physician for occurrence of the aforementioned If thrombus formation at catheter tip is suspected, an attempt should be made to withdraw blood and any clots through the catheter
■ Air or CO_2 embolism, which may be related to Balloon rupture: a high incidence after 72 or more inflations After catheter and balloon in situ for 3 or more days, lipids in the blood begin decomposing the balloon	■ Absence of air or CO_2 embolism	■ Prevention Prefill all lumens of catheter except balloon with fluid solution before insertion Ensure that balloon is inflated gradually with specified amount of air or CO_2 Immediate detection of balloon rupture; if no resistance is felt during balloon inflation and waveforms indicate that catheter has not wedged, balloon rupture may have occurred Use CO_2 for all patients with intracardiac shunt Remove catheter after 3 days in situ or with anything near 70 inflations If air or CO_2 embolism is suspected, notify physician and do not inject additional air or CO_2 into the balloon

Potential problems	Expected outcomes	Nursing activities
Lumens of catheter, except for balloon lumen, not prefilled with flush solution before insertion		
■ Infection Endocarditis, which may be related to catheter irritation of the endocardium and associated bacterial invasion Septicemia Infection at insertion site	■ Absence/resolution of infection Absence of any clinical manifestation of infection	■ Prevention Before insertion, assist physician in adequately cleaning skin for insertion Maintain aseptic technique during insertion Prepare and change flush solution system down to the catheter site q24 hr, using sterile technique Cleanse insertion site with antiseptic solution and change dressing daily, using sterile technique Secure catheter well in place If continuous flush system is not used, maintain sterile technique in intermittent flushing procedure Arterial and CVP lines should not remain in situ for more than 5 days; pulmonary, left atrial or ICP lines should not remain in situ for more than 3 days or longer than its use is justified Insertion of other lines into the involved extremity should be avoided Prophylactic antibiotics may be ordered in the presence of known valvular abnormality Monitor for Redness, inflammation, unusual warmth, pain, and purulent drainage at insertion site Any changes in temperature ECG changes consistent with endocarditis (see Standard: *Endocarditis*) Altered level of consciousness Notify physician for occurrence of any abnormalities If problem occurs Monitor C and S results of blood, sputum, and wound Remove catheter if infection at catheter insertion site Administer antibiotics as ordered
■ Ischemia distal to line insertion, particularly with radial lines, related to Insufficient ulnar artery blood flow Microemboli	■ Absence of ischemic episode distal to line insertion Absence of microemboli	■ Prevention Before cannulation of the radial artery, the Allen test should be done to assess adequacy of blood flow through ulnar artery Allen test 1. Occlude both radial and ulnar artery 2. Have patient close hand tightly several times until hand is blanched 3. Release ulnar artery 4. Note length of time for normal color on hand to return (should be approximately 5 seconds) Remove arterial line after 5 to 7 days or as soon as its use is not justified Monitor Circulation distal to arterial line insertion site for color, capillary filling, pulses, and sensation For any complaint of severe pain at and around the catheter site, with a blanched appearance of the limb distal to the catheter If ischemia occurs Apply warm compress to increase blood flow to the hand Increasing BP in hypotensive patient may help resolve ischemia to hand

Potential problems	Expected outcomes	Nursing activities
		If ischemia does not resolve, notify physician The catheter may be removed
■ Hematoma related to Trauma to vessel dur- ing insertion Patients with abnormal coagulation are at particularly high risk Insufficient external pressure after cathe- ter removal	■ Absence/resolution of hematoma Atraumatic catheter in- sertion procedure	■ Prevention Physician avoids traumatic injury to vessel during insertion Extra precaution used for patients with abnormal clotting abil- ity When catheter is removed, 10 to 15 minutes of direct pressure is applied to insertion site followed by placement of a pres- sure dressing Monitor for any Signs of hematoma near insertion site—note presence of sub- cutaneous swelling, bruised (black and blue) appearance Abnormally prolonged PT, APTT, and bleeding time; de- creased Hct and Hgb If hematoma occurs, catheter may be removed and compresses applied to assist in resolution
■ Arterial spasm—more common with arterial catheters that have been in place 3 or more days	■ Absence/resolution of spasm	■ Prevent by early removal of catheter or as soon as use is not justified Monitor for complaints of severe pain at or around catheter in- sertion site Observe circulation distal to catheter insertion site; blanching and decreased pulses may indicate spasm If problem occurs, apply heat locally; if not relieved, notify physican; the line may have to be removed
■ Hemorrhage, which may be related to Inadvertent system dis- connection Insertion technique	■ Absence/resolution of hemorrhage Flush system, including connections, tight and intact Hemodynamic stability	■ Prevention Careful technique is employed during insertion procedure to reduce blood loss Monitoring system alarms functioning properly with appro- priate alarm limits set Set limits on monitor closely (within 20 mm Hg of patient's BP) so that staff is quickly alerted of a BP drop associated with possible hemorrhage Insertion site and system should be visible at all times Ensure tight connections with no apparent leaks Tape catheter system securely All connections should be of the Luer-Lock or Linden type, which are not easily disconnected Monitor for Hemorrhage from disconnected system Alarm limits and their activation if pressure drops Blood backing up in system, caused by a leak in the system; tighten all connections and inspect for leaks If problem occurs If an arterial line comes out, apply pressure on insertion site immediately and maintain for 10 to 15 minutes If a connection comes apart, clamp the tubing going to the pa- tient, ask someone to procure another system or another part of the system, change the contaminated portion, and reinstitute an intact system
■ Abnormal intracranial pressure readings, which may be related to Loss of CSF Leakage of brain matter	■ Intracranial pressure readings are within normal limits Absence of CSF loss, leakage of brain mat- ter, and brain trauma	■ Prevention Careful and meticulous insertion technique employed by physician Keep patient quiet and cooperative during procedures Secure catheter/sensor/transducer in place to prevent any in- advertent removal Lumen of catheter is filled with solution before insertion

Potential problems	Expected outcomes	Nursing activities
Brain trauma Blockage of ICP monitoring catheter		Employ care in intermittent flushing of catheter Monitor for Any abnormal secretions from insertion site Abnormal changes in mental status Notify physician if changes occur If problem occurs, assist in removal of catheter/sensor/transducer
■ Monitoring problems: damped waveform resulting from Air in system Small thrombus at catheter tip Kinked catheter	■ Normal waveforms	■ Prevention Of air in system Ensure that all air is removed when system is assembled Ensure that all connections are tight Avoid vigorous flushing of the line; this tends to draw some of the air left in the drip chamber into the line Of clot in system Heparin is added to crystalloid solution, infused at 3 to 6 ml/hour, and regulated by a (Sorenson) flush System is pressurized; periodically check that pressure bag gauge is at 300 mm Hg Catheter is secured to skin at insertion site to prevent kinking Monitor for Decreased amplitude of the pressure waveform in which the systolic is usually decreased and the diastolic increased with each pressure reading and prn Any bleeding back to system from catheter If problem occurs Check system and transducer connection for air Check system for any kinks In the absence of the first two problems in the system, the catheter may have drifted further into the pulmonary artery; turn patient, have patient cough, or if he/she is intubated, manually inflate patient's lungs to encourage catheter to dislodge from small artery If aforementioned activities are unsuccessful, try to gently flush solution through catheter Aspirate catheter to remove any possibility of clot
■ Monitoring problems: inaccurate BP readings Arterial pressure is usually 5 to 15 mm Hg higher than a cuff BP reading Monitor "drift"; need for recalibration Inaccurate PCWP readings	■ BP readings accurately reflect patient's actual BP Accurate PCWP readings PCWP readings accurately reflect patient's actual PCWP	■ Prevention Balance and recalibrate transducer and monitor to air and to a known pressure (use of sphygmomanometer), with upper part of transducer dome placed at right atrial level q8 hr Check arterial monitor pressures with cuff or Doppler pressures q8 hr and prn Ensure absence of air in system Allow monitor-amplifier to warm up for 15 to 20 minutes before balancing/calibration and attachment to patient Monitor for Intra-arterial pressures that are more than 5 to 15 mm Hg higher or lower than cuff BP; take cuff BP in both arms, noting any differences Observe for entry of air into the system or for leaks If problem occurs, take action depending on the cause of the problem Flush air out of system Allow monitor, amplifier to warm up fully Recalibrate system

Potential problems	Expected outcomes	Nursing activities

■ Monitoring problems: pulmonary wedge tracing not obtainable
Balloon rupture
Catheter not in proper position; may flip back into ventricle
	■ PCWP readings obtainable and accurately reflect patient's PCWP	■ Prevention
		  Inflate balloon with the prescribed amount of air or CO_2 to avoid rupture
		  Leave catheter in place 3 days or less; since balloon deterioration is unavoidable, balloon rupture is likely to occur after 3 days or close to 70 inflations
		  Catheter must be placed into distal pulmonary artery during initial insertions
		Monitor for
		  Absence of resistance encountered on balloon inflation and wedge pressure tracing
		  Result of chest radiograph as to position of catheter
		If signs of balloon rupture occur, leave stopcock closed to balloon and notify physician

■ Monitoring problems: artifact or catheter whip
May be related to long connecting line between transducer and catheter
Related to motion of catheter caused by right ventricular contraction
	■ Pressure reading accurately reflects patient's pulmonary pressures	■ Monitor for fuzzy, unclear pressure readings on the oscilloscope
		If catheter whip artifact occurs
		  Use the pulmonary artery mean pressure reading
		  Obtain calibrated recording of the pressure tracing over a longer period of time to achieve the most representative pressures
		  Reduce length of connecting/extension line if possible

20 □ Cardiac catheterization

Cardiac catheterization is a procedure involving insertion under fluoroscopy of a radiopaque catheter through an artery or vein into the heart. Vessels in the antecubital fossa, axilla, or inguinal region are generally used, although the umbilical vessels may be utilized in the neonate. Pressure measurements are made and blood samples are drawn via the catheter to provide information regarding hemodynamics and oxygen saturations within the heart and great vessels. Pressure measurements can demonstrate the presence of resistance to blood flow (such as that caused by valvular stenosis), and abnormal oxygen saturations confirm intracardiac or intrapulmonary shunting. Specific structures (cardiac chambers, valves, great vessels, coronary arteries) can be visualized through injection of a radiopaque contrast agent; rapid, sequential radiographs, called angiograms, record the flow of the agent through these structures. Left heart and aortic catheterization can be performed through insertion of the catheter retrograde through an artery. In children and some adults, left heart catheterization may also be accomplished by passage of the catheter from the right atrium to the left atrium through the probe-patent foramen ovale. Right heart catheterization is accomplished through insertion of the catheter through a vein and into the right atrium. Percutaneous puncture or cutdown may be performed to gain access to the artery or vein.

Usually catheterization with blood gas and pressure measurements is performed first. If anomalies are detected or if further visualization of structures is needed, the angiogram is then performed. Angiograms are especially useful in the diagnosis of congenital heart defects, coronary artery disease, postinfarction ventricular septal defect, valvular insufficiency, and poor ventricular contractility.

Associated procedures may be accomplished during cardiac catheterization. His bundle mapping can be performed using an electrically sensitive catheter within the ventricles. Transvenous intracardiac pacing wires may also be inserted. Atrial septal defects may be created (through use of a balloon-tipped catheter) or closed (using an umbrella or plug-tipped catheter). Patients may be exercised during the catheterization to monitor effects of exercise on cardiac output and coronary artery circulation. Nitrogen inhalation may also be performed; timing of nitrogen circulation can provide information regarding the presence or absence of intracardiac shunts. Medication may be administered during the catheterization to allow detailed monitoring of the patient's hemodynamic response to specific drugs.

Cardiac catheterization may be performed on an elective or an emergency basis. The patient generally receives a sedative prior to the procedure and local anesthetic during the catheterization.

With the increased sophistication of catheterization equipment, mortality following elective catheterization is less than 1%; risk following emergency catheterization of the sick patient, however, is somewhat higher. Risk is also increased for patients with pulmonary hypertension, arrhythmias, hypoxia, or severe coronary arteriosclerosis and for children prone to periodic hypoxic episodes (severe tetralogy of Fallot).

Morbidity is caused by intracardiac catheter manipulation (causing arrhythmias, cardiac perforation, or increased myocardial ischemia), infection, contrast agent reactions, and impaired distal perfusion of the catheterized extremity.

ASSESSMENT

1. Patient/family's comprehension of patient's cardiovascular health problem
2. Patient/family's comprehension of catheterization procedure
3. Patient/family's anxiety and concerns
4. History of cardiovascular symptoms (including unstable angina, recent MI, cyanotic episodes, or pulmonary hypertension)
5. Previous illness or hospitalizations and patient/family's response to them
6. Current health status
   a. Current medications (especially cardiovascular medications and anticoagulants) and allergies
   b. Current diseases of other body systems: renal, pulmonary, gastrointestinal, neurological, musculoskeletal
7. Cardiovascular status
   a. Systemic perfusion: warmth of extremities, peripheral pulses and BP, urine output, color, level of consciousness, exercise tolerance, growth
   b. Heart rate and rhythm and presence of any heart murmurs or thrills
   c. Evidence of systemic venous engorgement: neck vein distention, periorbital edema, hepatomegaly, dependent edema (not often seen in children), or ascites
   d. Evidence of pulmonary venous engorgement: tachypnea, increased respiratory effort, rales on auscultation (not seen in children until late in the clinical course), cyanosis
   e. Presence and characteristics (precipitating or alleviating factors, severity, distribution) of angina or palpitations
   f. Presence or history of syncopal episodes, fatigue with minimal exercise
   g. Cardiac isoenzymes (if appropriate)
   h. If signs/symptoms of heart failure are present, see Standard: *Heart failure*
8. Fluid balance
   a. Presence of edema or recent large weight gain
   b. Level of hydration (mucous membranes, tearing in patients beyond 3 months, fontanelle in infants up to 18 months, skin turgor)
9. Nutritional status
   a. Growth
   b. Serum glucose level in infants
   c. Potassium balance (particularly if patient is receiving diuretics)
10. Respiratory status
    a. Evidence of pulmonary edema or pulmonary venous engorgement
    b. Evidence of concurrent respiratory infection (especially in children)
    c. Arterial blood gas results
11. Postcatheterization assessment
    a. Cardiovascular status: heart rate and rhythm, BP and peripheral perfusion, urine output, presence of any angina, signs of pulmonary or systemic venous engorgement, level of consciousness

b. Appearance of catheterization site: appearance of wound, presence of bleeding or hematoma, pain

c. Circulation of catheterized extremity: warmth, color, peripheral pulses, edema, pain, sensation

d. Evidence of any infection

GOALS

1. Patient/family demonstrates comprehension of patient's condition and catheterization procedure

2. Stable cardiovascular status

3. Absence of untoward response to contrast medium

4. Adequate circulation to catheterized extremity

5. Absence of infection

6. Patient/family demonstrates and comprehends patient's home health care routine (including wound care, medications, and health maintenance measures)

7. Appropriate fluid balance

Potential problems	Expected outcomes	Nursing activities
■ Decrease in cardiac output related to underlying cardiac disease, hemorrhage, cardiac perforation, reaction to sedation or contrast medium, or MI (for arrhythmias, see Problem, Cardiac arrhythmia)	■ Stable cardiac output as measured by Adequate BP Good peripheral perfusion Regular cardiac rate and rhythm Minimal bleeding from catheterization site Good urine output (25 ml/hour for adults; 1 to 2 ml/kg/hour for children) Absence of systemic or pulmonary venous engorgement Absence of incapacitating angina	■ Note occurrence of any arrhythmias during catheterization procedure Monitor vital signs, level of consciousness, and signs of peripheral perfusion frequently (q15 min initially, then q1-2 hr as appropriate) Heart rate ranges Newborn: 110 to 160/minute Toddler: 100 to 130/minute Preschooler: 90 to 120/minute School-age child: 80 to 110/minute Adolescent: 60 to 90/minute Adult: 50 to 95/minute Blood pressure ranges (systolic) Newborn: 60 to 100 mm Hg Toddler: 80 to 112 mm Hg Preschooler: 82 to 112 mm Hg School-age child: 84 to 130 mm Hg Adolescent: 100 to 142 mm Hg Adult: 105 to 145 mm Hg NOTE: Consider your patient's normal ranges when determining abnormalities If abnormalities are present, notify physician and be prepared to institute emergency measures as needed Notify physician of any arrhythmias (see problem, Cardiac arrhythmia) Monitor catheterization site and dressing for evidence of bleeding (dressing saturated with blood or developing hematoma); if bleeding is excessive and does not stop with application of pressure, notify physician immediately Obtain Hct as ordered Continue to apply pressure to site Closely monitor BP and peripheral perfusion Monitor for evidence of low cardiac output: cool, clammy extremities; decreased urine output; altered level of consciousness; cyanosis, mottling, or pallor; evidence of pulmonary or systemic venous engorgement; decreasing BP; notify physician immediately if these occur Monitor for signs of cardiac tamponade: pallor, tachycardia, jugular venous distention, decreased BP or decreased pulse pressure, decreased heart sounds, restlessness, cool extremities, tachypnea; notify physician immediately if they occur and be prepared for emergency measures if necessary SEE STANDARDS: *Pericarditis* *Arrhythmias* *Acute myocardial infarction* *Heart failure*

Potential problems	Expected outcomes	Nursing activities
		Infants must be kept warm during and following cardiac catheterization, especially if they have low cardiac output; their O_2 consumption increases dramatically if their rectal temperature is above or below 37° C; small infants with little subcutaneous fat are especially prone to heat loss
		Notify physician of any complaints of angina or palpitations; check cardiac isoenzymes and ECG if angina occurs, and monitor BP
■ Cardiac arrhythmia related to preexisting cardiac ischemia, intracardiac catheter manipulation, intramyocardial contrast medium injection, or further compromise of coronary circulation with contrast medium injection	■ Appropriate cardiac rate and rhythm	■ Record patient's rhythm prior to cardiac catheterization and use this strip for later comparison
		Check apical and peripheral pulses frequently following catheterization procedure; if any irregularities or pulse discrepancies exist, notify physician and obtain BP and rhythm strip
		If arrhythmia exists, note its effect on cardiac output (note if BP drops with aberrant beat), any precipitating or alleviating factors, and response to medications
		Monitor level of consciousness and be prepared to institute emergency measures as needed
		Assess heart rate—is it adequate for good cardiac output; see normal ranges given before; notify physician if heart rate is excessive or insufficient
		If arrhythmia occurs, see Standard: Arrhythmias
■ Compromise of circulation to catheterized extremity	■ Perfusion of catheterized extremity remains good as measured by Warmth Pink color Good pulses Adequate movement and sensation (use opposite limb for comparison)	■ If *arterial* catheterization was performed
		Monitor pulses of extremity distal to catheterization site; notify physician *immediately* of any decrease in pulses (if spasm or thrombus occurs in artery, the distal artery can rapidly become thrombosed and ischemia of extremity will result; this may ultimately require amputation of extremity if allowed to progress, so *prompt* attention must be given)
		Monitor color and warmth of extremity for reasons noted before
		NOTE: When arterial circulation is compromised, extremity usually will become *pale* or *mottled*—rather than cyanotic—and cool; notify physician immediately if either occurs; heat to *contralateral* extremity may help maintain circulation to catheterized extremity (by producing reflex vasodilation), but heat should *never* be applied to *involved* extremity as it merely increases O_2 consumption of already compromised tissue
		If thrombus is present, it may require surgical removal; a heparin drip may be ordered to prevent further thrombus (monitor for bleeding if heparin is ordered)
		Attempt to prevent flexion of catheterized extremity at catheterization site for 6 hours or as ordered
		Maintain bed rest for 6 to 12 hours following catheterization (or as ordered)
		Administer pain medication as ordered (and needed); monitor patient's response and cardiac output
		Monitor for evidence of excessive edema or hemorrhage at catheterization site; notify physician if hemorrhage is not stopped by application of pressure
		Apply ice to catheterization site as needed
		If *venous* catheterization was performed
		Monitor pulses of extremity distal to catheterization site
		NOTE: When a cutdown is performed, often the vein used for the catheterization is tied off at the end of the procedure, especially in small infants; in this case, the extremity distal

Potential problems	Expected outcomes	Nursing activities
		to the catheterization site would become edematous and slightly cyanotic as venous blood is trapped in the extremity; collateral veins will quickly provide venous drainage, but initial discomfort should be expected If edema is present, elevate extremity to facilitate venous return; *notify physician immediately if edema causes decrease in pulses* (this would indicate compromise of arterial circulation) Monitor for evidence of hemorrhage at catheterization site and notify physician if it is not relieved by pressure Maintain bed rest for 4 to 6 hours following catheterization (as ordered)
■ Possible infection of Catheterization site Intracardiac structures	■ Patient will remain free of symptoms of infection Fever Leukocytosis Erythema or drainage from catheterization site Evidence of endocarditis or pericarditis	■ Monitor catheterization site for edema, erythema, heat, or discharge; notify physician if present Monitor patient's temperature; blood cultures are usually recommended if fever higher than 38.5° C Monitor WBC count if infection is suspected Monitor for evidence of endocarditis (high fever, appearance of new heart murmur, hematuria) and pericarditis (cardiac friction rub, loss of heart tones, ECG changes); see Standards: *Pericarditis* and *Endocarditis*
■ Patient/family's anxiety related to patient's health status and anticipated catheterization	■ Patient/family demonstrates comprehension of preparation for procedure, catheterization itself, and postcatheterization care Patient/family's anxiety does not interfere with appropriate activity	■ Orient patient/family to nursing care unit, policies, personnel, catheterization lab (as appropriate) Orient patient/family to precatheterization preparation Chest radiograph Blood tests Appropriate medications (including withholding of anticoagulants prior to catheterization) Need for NPO precatheterization Premedication (include possible side effects such as dry mouth, blurred vision as appropriate) Instruct patient (as appropriate to age) and family regarding procedure itself (especially in those aspects that patient will see, hear, or feel), length of procedure, and postcatheterization appearance of catheterization site Discuss postcatheterization care with patient (if appropriate to age) and family Need for bed rest Post catheterization feeding orders Required care of catheterization site (include need for immobility, ice packs, etc.) Frequency of vital sign measurements If patient is a child over the age of 2, toys or puppets may be used to demonstrate the experiences the child will remember; in preparing any child for catheterization, the nurse must be sensitive to the cues of the child and prepare the child with only the information he/she can handle; if the child has little concept of time intervals, preparation just prior to injections and separation from parents may be most appropriate During and following the catheterization procedure, provide support and simple explanations of catheterization results; orient patient to time and place frequently while patient is recovering from sedation

Potential problems	Expected outcomes	Nursing activities
■ Possible compromise in renal function related to response to contrast medium (the very concentrated contrast medium can cause an oliguria, which should soon be followed by an osmotic diuresis; an anuria may occur rarely)	■ Patient will demonstrate adequate urine output (25 ml/hour minimum for adults and 1 to 2 ml/kg/hour for children)	■ Monitor urine output; notify physician if urine output is inadequate *despite* sufficient fluid intake NOTE: A small child may become rapidly dehydrated when kept NPO for hours while awaiting catheterization; the nurse must ensure that parenteral and/or oral fluid intake is adequate during the period preceding and following the catheterization If patient is anuric despite sufficient intake, fluid intake will then have to be restricted to prevent overload Monitor for evidence of dehydration (depressed fontanelle in infants, dry mucous membranes, decreased urine output with high specific gravity, poor skin turgor)
■ Possible respiratory depression related to sedation	■ Patient will demonstrate adequate respiratory function Appropriate rate Adequate and equal lung aeration bilaterally	■ Check precatheterization order against recommended dosage for patient's age and weight; notify physician if sedation order is excessive Monitor respiratory rate and effort and notify physician if either is insufficient or excessive Normal adult respiratory rate: 10 to 15 (note precatheterization range) Normal pediatric respiratory rate: 12 to 30 (note precatheterization range) Normal infant respiratory rate: 18 to 45 (note precatheterization range) Auscultate lungs and encourage patient to change position frequently, cough, and breathe deeply; rib-springing exercises or other forms of chest physiotherapy may be necessary if aeration is insufficient; notify physician immediately if respiratory effort is insufficient and begin emergency resuscitative measures if needed
■ Patient/family may have inadequate information to provide adequate home health care for patient	■ Patient/family possesses adequate information to comply with post-catheterization care regimen and general health maintenance	■ Provide patient/family with appropriate instruction regarding wound care, physician follow-up appointments, signs of infection, activity restrictions (if any), and medications Discuss implications of catheterization results with patient/family to obtain their perceptions of physician's recommendations and to clarify any misconceptions they may have Provide patient/family with appropriate telephone numbers and locations of health team members (primary nurse, cardiologist, cardiac surgeon, etc.) If patient is an infant, discuss immunization schedule with parents; often the cardiologist will request delay of immunizations (consult physician)

21 □ Cardiac surgery

Cardiac surgery may be required for patients with congenital heart disease, coronary atherosclerosis, valvular dysfunction, great vessel abnormalities, or other degenerative or inflammatory cardiac disease.

Coronary artery bypass grafting (CABG) is a surgical technique used to shunt blood around stenotic portions of major coronary arteries. A segment of saphenous vein is usually used; the proximal end is anastomosed to the root of the aorta and the distal end is sutured to a patent portion of coronary artery beyond the area of stenosis.

Patients who receive CABG often have documented partial occlusion of the left coronary artery in the presence of severe angina that has failed to respond to routine medical management.

The replacement or revision of heart valves is done for two major conditions: severe valvular stenosis and valvular insufficiency. In valvular stenosis the size of the valvular orifice is reduced, obstructing the forward flow of blood. In valvular insufficiency the valve cannot completely close, resulting in inappropriate regurgitation of blood.

In both valvular stenosis and valvular insufficiency cardiac output is reduced. Valvular repair or replacement can improve valvular function and dramatically improve cardiac output. Often the simple surgical division of two partially fused leaflets of the mitral valve (commissurotomy) can significantly improve valve function, but this may be only a temporary measure as the valve will gradually restenose. Valve replacement with one of a variety of prosthetic devices may then be necessary.

Cardiac surgery is also performed for acquired defects such as ventricular aneurysms, which occur as a complication of transmural MI. A ventricular aneurysm consists of dead muscle that balloons outward during cardiac contraction rather than moving inward. This paradoxical movement of the nonviable myocardium can significantly reduce cardiac output. Resection of the dead muscle results in more effective contraction and improved cardiac output.

Cardiac surgery can be done to repair an acquired ventricular septal defect, which often occurs as a complication of an anteroseptal infarction. The septal defect permits shunting of blood from the left to the right ventricle, resulting in reduced cardiac output and pulmonary vascular congestion.

Placement of a pericardial patch or a synthetic graft over the interventricular opening restores normal intracardiac blood flows. Unfortunately, the entire septum is frequently ischemic, requiring placement of suture material into friable tissue. These sutures frequently tear postoperatively, permitting redevelopment of a septal defect.

Surgical outcome depends on preoperative cardiac function, the success of surgery, and postoperative problems that arise.

The postoperative cardiac patient is particularly prone to developing hemodynamic and fluid balance abnormalities. Persistent monitoring of the patient's volume status, serum electrolyte composition, and cardiac function is of great importance in assuring an uncomplicated course. Fluids, diuretics, vasopressors, vasodilators, and inotropic medications are common modalities for correcting postoperative problems such as hypovolemia/hypervolemia, heart failure, angina, MI, and arrhythmias. Other conditions such as pericardial tamponade may require surgical intervention.

The postoperative cardiac patient remains on mechanical ventilation until it is clear that blood oxygenation and cardiac and volume status have stabilized. Pulmonary problems that must be dealt with relate to the continual production of secretions from the tracheobronchial tree. Turning the patient, chest physiotherapy, tracheal suctioning, and humidification of inspired air are all directed toward mobilizing copious secretions. After extubation, coughing and deep breathing are necessary elements in pulmonary care.

Postoperative renal problems usually arise as a result of hypoperfusion of the kidneys during or immediately after surgery. The extent of renal compromise is variable and most of the time reversible. Volume and electrolyte status must receive special attention during this period.

Psychological difficulties may be devastating in a patient who has just had cardiac surgery. Total dependency on life-support systems and the often radical change in the patient's role in his/her family often give rise to depression and a feeling of futility, which require frequent encouragement to counteract.

CONGENITAL HEART DEFECTS

The following table is designed as a quick reference guide to several forms of congenital heart defects. It includes symptoms of a particular defect, its repair, and postoperative complications *specific* to that defect. General principles of care of the cardiovascular patient and postoperative complications of cardiopulmonary bypass are not given here.

When *CHF* is a problem, in children the following symptoms may be noted:

Tachycardia

Tachypnea

Increased respiratory effort (retractions, jaw tugging, head bobbing, grunting)

Diaphoresis

Decreased urine volume

Peripheral vasoconstriction

Poor feeding, slow weight gain

Decreased exercise tolerance

Rales, ascites, and dependent edema may be only very *late* signs of CHF in children. If rales are present, a concurrent respiratory infection should be suspected. Rales will be present, however, if severe left heart obstruction (mitral or aortic stenosis) is present.

The child with *cyanotic heart disease* and compensatory polycythemia has possible systemic complications. He/she is at increased risk for thromboembolus formation, particularly when the hematocrit level is above 60%. Dehydration can cause hemoconcentration and increased blood viscosity, so care should be taken to prevent dehydration in these children. No air should be allowed in the intravenous line because it could be shunted right to left and into arterial circulation, causing a cerebral embolus. These children are also at increased risk for the development of brain abscesses (especially beyond the age of 2 years). Their platelets are often decreased in number and/or function, so these patients are prone to bleeding postoperatively.

Possible postoperative complications of open heart surgery (bleeding, arrhythmias, respiratory insufficiency, renal failure, metabolic derangements, etc.) should still be anticipated in these children; Table 2 lists the *most common* complications seen with each defect.

When hypothermia and circulatory arrest are utilized for repair of congenital heart disease in infants, the following complications are more likely to occur:

Cardiac irritability or heart block

Neurological impairment or seizure activity

Respiratory insufficiency

Wide serum glucose fluctuations

Hypocalcemia

Decreased plasma protein levels

Bleeding

Text continued on p. 156.

Table 2. Congenital heart defects

Lesion	Preoperative problems	Surgical repair	Postoperative problems
Patent ductus arteriosus (PDA)	Increased pulmonary blood flow (from aorta into pulmonary artery) CHF may result in infancy (particularly in premature infants) Older children may be asymptomatic except for murmur and waterhammer pulses Patent ductus may be *lifesaving* in infants with cyanotic heart disease and compromised pulmonary blood flow	Ligation and/or division of ductus may be performed using a left thoracotomy incision (closed heart procedure) Indomethacin (a prostaglandin inhibitor) may be administered to neonates to promote ductus closure without surgery	CHF may be present (if it was present preoperatively) Other complications are those associated with thoracotomy incision (possible chylothorax, phrenic nerve paralysis, bleeding, etc.)
Coarctation of the aorta (preductal or infantile type); this defect may be associated with other left heart anomalies	If aortic arch is small, symptoms of severe CHF may be apparent within hours or days of birth If hypoplastic left heart is present, child will deteriorate rapidly If coarctation is in arch of the aorta, difference of BP between right and left arms may be present Lower extremities may be cyanotic (they will receive blood flow from the ductus)	Narrowed aortic segment must be excised using thoracotomy incision with aortic crossclamping Aorta is then either reanastomosed directly or closed using a patch If aortic arch must be extensively reconstructed, hypothermia and circulatory arrest may be used	CHF may be severe in postoperative period Transient upper extremity hypertension may be present Mesenteric arteritis may occur following restoration of strong, pulsatile blood flow to distal aorta Renal failure and ventricular irritability may occur
Coarctation of the aorta (postductal or adult type) NOTE: A bicuspid aortic valve is present in the majority of these patients and may become calcified and/or stenotic	CHF may occur in infancy if coarctation is severe or associated with another defect (PDA, VSD, etc.) Decreased BP in lower extremities will cause decreased pulses and may cause claudication Increased BP (hypertension) in upper extremities will be present (bounding pulses) Large collateral circulation will cause ''rib notching'' on radiograph in older children	Narrowed segment of aorta must be excised and aorta reanastomosed using left thoracotomy incision and aortic crossclamping (closed heart surgery) Patch may be necessary to achieve reanastomosis of aorta without stenosis	CHF (if present preoperatively) Tachycardia and transient upper extremity hypertension may be present for days postoperatively Mesenteric arteritis may occur following restoration of strong, pulsatile blood flow to descending aorta (monitor for ileus and begin feedings slowly) Movement of or sensation in lower extremities may be impaired, if spinal cord circulation is decreased during aortic crossclamping

Continued.

Table 2. Congenital heart defects—cont'd

Lesion	Preoperative problems	Surgical repair	Postoperative problems
Atrial septal defect (ASD)	Usually children are asymptomatic, although CHF may occur if right ventricular dysfunction is present. Right to left shunt will cause increased pulmonary blood flow under low pressure. Atrial arrhythmias, CHF, and pulmonary hypertension may occur in middle adulthood	Stitch or patch closure of ASD using cardiopulmonary bypass	Conduction disturbances (especially heart block). Complications of cardiopulmonary bypass (postcardiotomy syndrome, bleeding, tamponade, etc.). CHF is a rare complication but is more likely if it was present preoperatively or if pulmonary hypertension or small left ventricular size is present
Ventricular septal defect (VSD)	If VSD is small, child may be asymptomatic (except for murmur) and defect may close spontaneously. If VSD is large, increased pulmonary blood flow under high pressure and CHF will result once pulmonary vascular resistance has fallen (at approximately 6 weeks of age); CHF may be present earlier if second defect (such as PDA) is present. Pulmonary hypertension may result from large defect	Pulmonary artery banding may be performed as a palliative procedure (closed heart) to reduce volume and pressure of pulmonary blood flow (and alleviate CHF); later debanding and closure of VSD are required. Open heart patch or suture closure of the VSD is the definitive open heart repair. An atrial or ventricular cardiac incision may be used for definitive repair	CHF is more likely if it was present preoperatively, if ventriculotomy cardiac incision was used for repair, or if pulmonary hypertension is present. Conduction disturbances, especially heart block, may occur; right bundle branch block will result if a right ventriculotomy incision was used. Respiratory insufficiency may be present, particularly if CHF or pulmonary hypertension was present preoperatively
Endocardial cushion defect (partial or complete AV canal may be present), consisting of: 1. Primum ASD (low in atrial septum) 2. Cleft in anterior leaflet of mitral valve	If simple primum ASD and small mitral valve cleft are present, the child may be asymptomatic. With larger left to right shunt and mitral insufficiency (from cleft in mitral valve), greater increase in pulmonary blood flow and CHF may result	Pulmonary artery banding may be performed as a palliative procedure if large VSD has caused CHF; banding will *not* be performed if left ventricle to right atrial shunt is present	CHF is frequent complication. NOTE: With closure of ASD, severe residual mitral regurgitation can cause pulmonary edema and left ventricular failure
3. Possible common AV valve 4. Possible membranous ventricular septal defect	With large VSD component, CHF can be severe. Right bundle branch block and left axis deviation are common ECG findings	Definitive repair is patch closure of ASD and VSD (if present), repair of mitral insufficiency (using suture closure of valve cleft), and division of common AV valves (if necessary), using cardiopul-	Heart block may occur, as the conduction system (including AV node and His bundles) runs along margin of defect. Respiratory insufficiency may complicate CHF and pulmonary edema

5. A left ventricle to right atrial shunt may be present in addition to ASD and VSD shunting	Children are generally small for age with frequent upper respiratory infections This defect is the most common cardiac defect associated with children with Down's syndrome	monary bypass (and possible hypothermia and circulatory arrest in infants, if necessary)	Preoperative pulmonary hypertension will make postoperative right ventricular failure and respiratory insufficiency more likely
Truncus arteriosus (types I, II, and III consist of direct branching of pulmonary artery[ies] and aorta from common trunk; VSD is present)	Increased pulmonary blood flow usually occurs under high pressure, and CHF results Cyanosis may be present (if so, compensatory polycythemia may make child more prone to embolic phenomena)	Pulmonary artery banding may be performed as palliative measure to reduce volume and pressure of pulmonary blood flow (later debanding and repair will be necessary) Open heart repair involves closure of VSD to allow left ventricular and aortic continuity; right ventricular to pulmonary artery continuity is established through insertion of a valved conduit; a ventriculotomy cardiac incision is used Deep hypothermia and circulatory arrest may be used in infants	CHF is present postoperatively Arrhythmias (especially heart block) may occur; right bundle branch block will be present due to ventriculotomy incision Respiratory insufficiency may be present (especially if severe CHF and pulmonary hypertension are present preoperatively) Preoperative cyanosis and compensatory polycythemia will make child more prone to bleeding and thromboembolus postoperatively
Truncus type IV or pseudotruncus (pulmonary atresia); only the aorta arises from the ventricles (any existing proximal main pulmonary artery is usually rudimentary) and distal pulmonary vessels are perfused only through collateral circulation	Pulmonary blood flow is accomplished only through PDA or collateral circulation, so pulmonary blood flow is *decreased* Cyanosis is present (may be mild until ductus begins to close)	Palliative procedure may be performed to increase pulmonary blood flow (Waterston or Blalock-Taussig shunt) Repair involves closure of any associated septal defects and/or PDA, and establishment of right ventricle to pulmonary artery blood flow through use of valved conduit or gusset patch in existing pulmonary artery	CHF will be present Arrhythmias may be present (particularly due to ventriculotomy cardiac incision and closure of septal defects) Cyanosis and compensatory polycythemia will make child prone to bleeding (decreased platelet function) and thrombus formation perioperatively Respiratory insufficiency may be increased by presence of severe cyanosis preoperatively (causing pulmonary microthrombi), by CHF postoperatively, and by adjustment of pulmonary vasculature to increased flow NOTE: Alveolar hypoxia may cause pulmonary arterial vasoconstriction and increased right ventricular afterload, so these children should be weaned from mechanical ventilation carefully

Continued.

Table 2. Congenital heart defects—cont'd

Lesion	Preoperative problems	Surgical repair	Postoperative problems
Pulmonary valvular stenosis or atresia without VSD	With pulmonary valvular atresia, there is no continuity between right ventricle and pulmonary artery, so blood must pass into left heart (via a patent, or "stretched," foramen ovale) and then back into the pulmonary artery via the ductus arteriosus; signs of systemic venous engorgement may be present; severe cyanosis and sudden deterioration may occur if ductus closes Right ventricular hypertrophy will be present With pulmonary stenosis, pulmonary blood flow may be normal or decreased	Emergency pulmonary valvulotomy in neonatal period is called the *Brock procedure*; no bypass is used, and a curved blade is inserted in the right ventricle (surrounded by pursestring sutures) to cut open the atretic pulmonary valve Hypothermia and circulatory arrest may be utilized to perform emergency valvulotomy under direct visualization Open heart surgery allows pulmonary valvulotomy in direct vision NOTE: If pulmonary atresia is present and a neonate is rapidly decompensating as the ductus is closing, prostaglandin E may be administered by continuous IV infusion to keep the ductus open until the neonate can be brought to surgery	CHF may be present due to reduction in right ventricular afterload If child has cyanosis and compensatory polycythemia preoperatively, bleeding and embolus formation are more likely postoperatively Respiratory insufficiency will be more likely if severe cyanosis was present preoperatively (pulmonary microthrombi may occur, and pulmonary vessels will react to increased flow) or if CHF is present postoperatively
Tetralogy of Fallot consists of four associated defects: 1. VSD 2. Pulmonary infundibular stenosis 3. Overriding aorta (overrides the VSD) 4. Right ventricular hypertrophy	Severity of cyanosis (and decrease in pulmonary blood flow) is related to severity of infundibular pulmonic stenosis Generally infants are mildly cyanotic at birth and become progressively more cyanotic during the first months of life as ductus closes and infundibular stenosis becomes relatively more severe Spasm of the infundibulum and the resultant severe decrease in pulmonary blood flow can cause severe cyanosis, hypoxia, and loss of consciousness; placing child in knee-chest position may promote increased pulmonary blood flow and alleviate the spell Compensatory polycythemia and right to left intracardiac shunting (allowing some venous blood to bypass the filtration of	Waterston shunt (ascending aorta to pulmonary artery shunt, as side to side anastomosis) or Blalock-Taussig shunt (subclavian artery to pulmonary artery shunt, as end to side anastomosis) may be created as palliative (closed heart) surgery to increase pulmonary blood flow Definitive (open heart) repair involves patch closure of the VSD, resection of the infundibular stenosis, and widening of the pulmonary outflow tract (a gusset or conduit may be required to produce a large enough pulmonary outflow tract); a right ventriculotomy incision is utilized for repair NOTE: If the neonate is rapidly deteriorating as the ductus closes, continuous IV infusion of prostaglandin E may be given to	CHF will occur postoperatively NOTE: If CHF is *severe* following surgery, a residual VSD should be suspected Arrhythmias, especially heart block, may be present Respiratory insufficiency may be present NOTE: Pulmonary vasoconstriction from alveolar hypoxia can produce increased right ventricular afterload (and increased right ventricular failure); pulmonary microthrombi can cause ventilation/perfusion abnormalities; CHF will increase work of breathing; thus, ventilatory support must be skilled Bleeding is more likely postoperatively as a result of preoperative cyanosis and compensatory polycythemia (these cause platelets to be decreased in number and

function)

Increased risk of postoperative thromboembolism is present

keep the ductus open until the neonate can be brought to surgery

CHF is likely; the right atrium will be acting as the right heart pumping chamber, so CVP will need to be high, but watched carefully; fluid management must be judicious

Preoperative cyanosis and compensatory polycythemia will make child more prone to development of postoperative bleeding and perioperative thromboembolism formation

Arrhythmias are likely, especially if VSD closure was performed

Atrial arrhythmias are common

Respiratory insufficiency can occur (related to CHF, pulmonary microthrombi, preoperative pulmonary hypertension, etc.)

pulmonary macrophages) makes these children more prone to thromboembolus formation and brain abscess

These children may instinctively squat during play to increase pulmonary blood flow

Clubbing of fingertips and toes will occur with severe cyanosis

Tricuspid atresia

NOTE: ASD and VSD will be present; other lesions (such as PDA, pulmonary stenosis, or transposition of the great vessels) may be present and complicate the clinical presentation and repair

Systemic venous return shunts from right atrium to left atrium; pulmonary blood flow depends on left to right shunt through VSD, PDA, or surgical shunt; thus, pulmonary blood flow is usually decreased (but *may* be increased if another large shunt is present)

Cyanosis is present to variable degree (depending on pulmonary blood flow); may be severe

Clubbing will be present in older cyanotic child

CHF may be present if large left to right shunt present through VSD

Compensatory polycythemia and right to left intracardiac shunt will make child more susceptible to spontaneous thromboembolus formation and (especially if child is over 2 years old) brain abscess

Signs of systemic venous engorgement will be present if ASD (patent foramen ovale) is restrictive

Palliative shunt may be performed to increase pulmonary blood flow—Waterston shunt is side to side anastomosis between aorta and pulmonary artery; Blalock-Taussig shunt is made by end to side anastomosis between subclavian and pulmonary artery; Glenn procedure is side to side anastomosis between superior vena cava and right pulmonary artery (formerly this was the shunt of choice for these patients but is done less frequently [is difficult to "take down" later])

If CHF due to large VSD is occurring, pulmonary artery banding may be performed as palliative procedure

If patent foramen ovale is too small to allow free right to left atrium shunting, a Rashkind balloon septostomy may be performed in the cardiac catheterization lab, or a Blalock-Hanlon septectomy may be performed (through a mediastinal incision but without use of cardiopulmonary bypass)

Corrective procedure is known as *Fontan procedure* and consists of valved conduit insertion between right atrium and main pulmonary artery; other existing shunts (ASD, VSD, Waterston, etc.) would be closed; surgical correction is ideally performed when child old enough (school age) to allow insertion of large conduit

Continued.

Table 2. Congenital heart defects—cont'd

Lesion	Preoperative problems	Surgical repair	Postoperative problems
Transposition of the great vessels (TGV) Other possible associated lesions (VSD, aortic or pulmonic stenosis, or coarctation of the aorta) will complicate the clinical picture and surgical repair	Since two "closed loops" (right heart with systemic circulation and left heart with pulmonary circulation) are present, communication must exist between two circuits to allow survival; often PDA provides the communication, and the child may decompensate rapidly once PDA closes Cyanosis is generally present within hours of birth and can be severe, depending on degree of mixing between arterial and venous blood Clubbing will be present in older children Compensatory polycythemia and intracardiac shunting will make child more susceptible to spontaneous thromboembolus formation and (especially beyond age 2) brain abscess formation	Rashkind balloon septostomy is usually performed in catheterization lab to facilitate intra-atrial mixing of arterial and venous blood Blalock-Hanlon septectomy may be performed as palliative surgery (via mediastinal incision but without use of cardiopulmonary bypass) to facilitate mixing between arterial and venous blood Corrective surgery will be the Mustard, Senning, or the great vessel switch operation 1. The Mustard procedure involves excision of atrial septum and use of a pericardial baffle to redirect venous return; the right ventricle remains the systemic ventricle and the left ventricle remains the pulmonary ventricle (the Senning is similar) 2. The great vessel switch operation involves closure of existing communication between the right ventricle and aorta; a conduit then connects the right ventricle to the distal pulmonary artery; the proximal pulmonary artery is anastomosed to the ascending aorta; so left ventricular output flows through this proximal portion of the pulmonary artery and into the aorta; the right ventricle is then the pulmonary ventricle and the left ventricle is the systemic ventricle If a VSD or pulmonary atresia is present, a Rastelli procedure may be employed for correction of the TGV; the VSD would be closed with a baffle, which allows left	CHF is likely, due to intra-atrial manipulation or ventriculotomy incision Arrhythmias are extremely common with any of the corrective procedures; atrial arrhythmias and heart block are particularly likely following the Mustard procedure; heart block and ventricular irritability are more common following the great vessel switch or Rastelli procedures; right bundle branch block will be present if ventriculotomy incision was made (in a great vessel switch or Rastelli) Preoperative compensatory polycythemia makes the child more prone to postoperative bleeding and perioperative thromboembolus formation If intra-atrial (Mustard) baffle is too restrictive, systemic venous engorgement and pulmonary venous engorgement will occur (will require reoperation) Respiratory insufficiency will be likely and will be worsened by pulmonary microthrombi and CHF; weaning from mechanical ventilation must be gradual (as pulmonary vasoconstriction due to hypoxia may increase right ventricular afterload)

Disorder	Assessment	Surgical intervention	Postoperative considerations
		ventricular output to flow through the VSD (under the baffle) and into the aorta; the pulmonary valve is sewn closed, and a conduit connects the right ventricle to the main pulmonary artery. Repair may be accomplished in infancy with the use of deep hypothermia and circulatory arrest	CHF will be present postoperatively; left atrium and ventricle generally are small and will need to adjust to normal pulmonary venous return; right ventricle has had change in Starling curve. Respiratory failure will be the most troublesome complication for infants who have had repair of TAPVR below the diaphragm; these infants should be monitored closely for pulmonary edema, atelectasis, and consolidation. Arrhythmias may occur (particularly atrial arrhythmias and evidence of ventricular irritability). Since the child has cyanosis and compensatory polycythemia preoperatively, he/she will have increased risk of postoperative bleeding and perioperative thromboembolus formation
Total anomalous pulmonary venous return (TAPVR) NOTE: TAPVR may be to vessel *above* the diaphragm or *below* the diaphragm; the infradiaphragmatic type is associated with much higher mortality	Since all venous return comes to right atrium and then passes into the left heart only through an ASD or VSD, right heart failure and evidence of systemic venous engorgement will usually be present. Cyanosis is present (as left heart blood is mixed with venous blood from right heart). If pulmonary veins drain *below* the diaphragm into portal venous system, severe pulmonary edema will result within weeks of birth	Rashkind balloon septostomy may be performed in catheterization lab to allow greater intra-atrial mixing (and more flow to left side of heart). Pulmonary veins must be anastomosed to left atrium (open heart). Repair is often accomplished through use of deep hypothermia and circulatory arrest in children	
Aortic stenosis/insufficiency	──── See adult open heart surgery ────		
Mitral stenosis/insufficiency	──── See adult open heart surgery ────		
Anomalous left coronary artery (left coronary artery arises from pulmonary artery, so venous blood is provided to left ventricle coronary artery supply)	Angina and infarction can occur in early childhood because of left ventricular ischemia. Ventricular arrhythmias or S-T segment changes also indicate ischemia	Coronary artery must be detached from pulmonary artery and reimplanted into aorta; a graft may be used. Cardiopulmonary bypass may be used if coronary artery is difficult to reanastomose to aorta	Myocardial ischemia and/or infarction. Left ventricular failure requiring vasopressor support. Arrhythmias (particularly those indicating ventricular irritability) may occur

ASSESSMENT

1. History, presence, and nature of
   a. Previous hospitalization and procedures, particularly
      (1) Cardiac catheterization
      (2) Cardiac surgery
   b. Related cardiac problems
      (1) Congenital heart disease; note presence of previous palliative or corrective surgery
      (2) Valvular disease; rheumatic fever
      (3) Coronary artery disease
      (4) Ventricular aneurysm
      (5) Septal defect
      (6) Risk factors for coronary heart disease
         (a) Hypertension
         (b) Glucose intolerance; diabetes
         (c) Hyperlipidemia
         (d) Cigarette smoking
         (e) Obesity, sedentary life-style, personality (type A), sex, age
      (7) Family history of any of the aforementioned risk factors
      (8) Past MI
      (9) Stroke, thrombophlebitis, pulmonary embolism
      (10) Angina, other signs of myocardial ischemia
      (11) Arrhythmias (palpitations)
   c. In children, note
      (1) Delayed motor milestones (in the presence of normal intellectual and social development)
      (2) Fainting spells, cyanotic episodes
      (3) Small stature, feeding difficulties (increased length of feeding, decreased volume of feeding, vomiting)
      (4) Decreased activity tolerance
      (5) Tachypnea, tachycardia
      (6) Frequent upper respiratory tract infections
      (7) Risk of or presence of endocarditis; known area of turbulent intracardiac blood flow
   d. Other organ dysfunction that may be related to cardiac compromise, particularly
      (1) Pulmonary
      (2) Renal
      (3) Neurological
2. Level of cardiac function/cardiac output
   a. Activity tolerance—note level of activity restriction; differentiate activity restrictions imposed by parents from those self-imposed by the child; presence of easy fatigability; in infants, slow feeding and tachypnea
   b. BP
   c. Pulse—note irregular rhythm, pulsus alternans, weak pulse
   d. Evaluate peripheral circulation, noting
      (1) Presence of pallor, duskiness, cyanosis
      (2) Temperature
      (3) Diaphoresis
      (4) Clubbing
   e. Heart sounds for murmurs, gallops
   f. ECG for hypertrophy, arrhythmias
   g. Level of consciousness, mentation for effects of inadequate cerebral perfusion
   h. Venous distention—sacral edema, dependent edema, distention of neck veins, ascites (unusual in children unless congestive heart failure [CHF] is severe), hepatomegaly (a particularly good indicator of CHF in children)
   i. Signs/symptoms of cardiomegaly, pulmonary vascular congestion
   j. Presence of a syndrome such as Down's or Marfan's, which is associated with certain types of congenital or acquired heart disease
   k. In children evaluate cognitive and social development to quantify a school-age child's illness; may ask parents about the number of school days the child has missed
3. Pulmonary status
   a. Rate, rhythm, quality of respirations; note presence of rales, rhonchi, wheezing, shortness of breath, tachypnea, dyspnea
   b. Inquire about presence of orthopnea (note that in children with CHF rales are a late sign of CHF or an upper respiratory infection)
4. Weight
5. Results of lab and diagnostic tests, including
   a. ECG evidence of
      (1) Myocardial ischemia
      (2) Ventricular aneurysm
      (3) Hypertrophy
      (4) Arrhythmias
      (5) Effects of inotropic/antiarrhythmic medications
      (6) Congenital heart disease; axis and ventricular/atrial hypertrophy consistent with defect
   b. Chest radiograph for
      (1) Cardiac hypertrophy, dilatation
      (2) Pulmonary vascular congestion
      (3) Location and configuration of great vessels
   c. Myocardial catheterization for objective evidence of
      (1) Coronary artery or valvular disease

(2) Cardiac hypertrophy; elevated intracardiac pressures

(3) Ventricular aneurysm

(4) Septal defect

(5) Congenital cardiac defect

d. Echocardiogram for evidence of

   (1) Valvular abnormalities

   (2) Hypertrophy of specific cardiac chambers

   (3) Contrast echo for intracardiac/great vessel shunts

e. Radionuclide studies

f. Cardiac enzymes (in adults)

g. Electrolyte levels

6. Patient/family's level of anxiety regarding disease process, medical therapy employed, purpose of hospitalization, need for surgery, postoperative management, and general follow-up plan of care

7. Patient/family's past alterations in roles, activities of daily living associated with patient's disease process

8. Parent's fears and concerns about their child's congenital heart disease

9. Patient/family's knowledge regarding operative therapy

a. What they have been told

b. Their expectations

c. Fears regarding surgery and the outcome

d. Previous experiences with surgery

e. Experience of other family members or friends with heart disease

10. Information and detail surgeon has provided patient/family about operative therapy, known pathology, and postoperative management

GOALS

1. a. Reduction in patient/family's anxiety with provision of information, explanations, and encouragement

b. Patient/family demonstrates understanding of disease process, purpose of hospitalization, surgery planned, preoperative and postoperative management, and expected outcomes

2. a. Adequate cardiac output

b. Hemodynamic stability

c. Absence of hypotension, hemorrhage, heart failure/low cardiac output syndrome, and cardiac tamponade

d. Absence of signs of hypervolemia, hypertension

e. Absence of MI

f. Absence of arrhythmias

3. a. Adequate perfusion to all vessels and end organs

b. Absence or resolution of emboli

4. a. Respiratory sufficiency with adequate alveolar ventilation and oxygenation; arterial pH, Pa_{O_2}, Pa_{CO_2} within normal limits

b. Absence of signs and symptoms of hypoxia, pain and splinting, atelectasis

c. Full lung expansion

d. Absence of pneumothorax, hemothorax, or pleural effusion

e. Absence of pulmonary edema, emboli

5. Acid-base status in balance and within normal limits

6. a. Absence of fluid imbalance

b. Serum electrolyte levels within normal limits

7. Indices of renal function within normal limits

8. a. Infection free

b. Absence or resolution of endocarditis

9. a. Absence or resolution of pericarditis

b. Absence or resolution of postcardiotomy syndrome

10. a. Patient alert and oriented to time, place, and person according to growth and development level

b. Patient returns to preoperative neurological status

11. Before discharge patient/family accurately describes

a. Dietary management

b. Plan for activity progression

c. Medications

   (1) Identification of

   (2) Dosage/number and schedule

   (3) Potential adverse effects and precautions

d. Care of and precautions for special devices such as the pacemaker

e. Plan for follow-up care

12. Before discharge patient/family safely performs special procedures such as suture line care

Potential problems	Expected outcomes	Nursing activities
Preoperative and postoperative periods		
■ Patient/family's anxiety related to Disease process Hospitalization	■ Reduction in patient/family's anxiety with provision of information, explanations, and encouragement	■ Ongoing assessment of level of anxiety Assess patient/family's understanding of disease process and need for surgery Describe nature of patient's cardiac problem and symptoms that patient is experiencing

Potential problems	Expected outcomes	Nursing activities

Medical therapy employed
Impending major surgery and associated risks
Diagnostic tests planned
Altered family roles
Separation from family members
Loss of job
	Anxiety does not interfere with patient/family's functioning
	Patient/family demonstrates understanding of disease process, purpose of hospitalization and surgery planned, preoperative and postoperative management, and expected outcomes
	Patient/family actively participates in planning and implementing care
		Provide opportunity for patient/family to discuss risks involved and the decision for open-heart surgery
		Collaborate with physician on patient teaching to be done
		Health team members should use the same terms when communicating with patient/family
		Explain the relationship of the disease process and the rationale for various therapeutic interventions
		Explain the anticipated procedures included in the diagnostic process and the plan of care, including what the patient will experience
		Assist in preparing patient for diagnostic procedures
		Encourage patient/family's questions, verbalization of fears and anxieties
		NOTE: More concrete feedback from the child may be obtained by asking him/her to name the one "scariest thing" about surgery
		Involve patient/family in planning for care
		For children
		  Ascertain what parents and others have told the child about the hospitalization and surgery
		  Determine how the parents think the child will best understand and accept the explanation about surgery
		  Consider the child's level of growth and development
		  Most children under 3 years of age do not benefit from understanding this explanation
		  For children over 3 years or so of age, use play and stories to prepare child and parents for postoperative period
		  For children under 3 years or so, direct most preparatory efforts to parents
		  NOTE: If child is fairly asymptomatic, health team should avoid telling the child that the surgery will "make him/her feel better," since the child will actually feel worse in the early postoperative period; the least threatening explanation may be to tell the child that the doctor will fix the "noise" in his/her heart rather than the "hole" in his/her heart, which may evoke thoughts of a "leaky" heart
		  Reassure parents, if appropriate, that they are not responsible for their child's congenital heart disease
		Provide comfort measures for parents and/or other family members
		Opportunity to visit recovery room/intensive care unit may be provided; patient/family should be acquainted with staff, visiting policies and, if possible, visit the critical care unit
		Describe the preoperative experience according to patient's need to know and readiness to learn
		NOTE: The timing of teaching is important; if a child's orientation to time is well-developed, prepare him/her gradually; if child does not have a well-defined sense of time, explanations may be limited to the evening prior to surgery
		Preoperative
		  Chest physiotherapy
		    1. Coughing and deep breathing
		    2. Incentive spirometry
		    3. Postural drainage
		  Shave
		  Have light dinner; then NPO after midnight

Potential problems	Expected outcomes	Nursing activities
		Medication for sleep if needed
		Morning bath/shower
		Preoperative medications
		Hospital gown
		Care of valuables
		Ride to operating room
		Scrub suits, masks, and hats worn by operating room staff
		Anesthesia
		Postoperative
		Waking up in the recovery room/intensive care unit
		1. Describe the general environment (size of unit, room, etc.)
		2. Nurse always nearby
		3. Dull, continuous noises
		4. Breathing tube temporarily in place to ease patient's work of breathing and the load on the heart; describe that speaking will not be possible while tube is in place but that other means of communication will be provided
		NPO until "breathing tube" removed
		Incision with bandage
		IV, arterial lines
		Chest tubes and bloody drainage expected
		ECG monitoring
		Medicine for discomfort, pain given as needed
		Policy on family visits
		As patient progresses
		Progression to the intermediate care unit, if appropriate (children—progression to the "getting better" room)
		Tubes out
		Eating again
		Chest physiotherapy, deep breathing, and coughing
		Getting stronger, ambulation
		Describe responsibility of patient for achieving a speedy recovery by taking an active role in coughing and deep breathing to keep lungs clear, and so on
		Home again
Postoperative period		
■ Anxiety in the postoperative period related to Pain Difficulty in communication during intubation Disorientation to time and place Feelings of helplessness	■ Reduction in anxiety	■ Postoperatively, continue the aforementioned measures as appropriate and, in addition Provide for pain relief, sedation if needed, as ordered Frequently orient patient to time and place Remind patient that operation is over Develop mode for patient communication during intubation period Encourage and provide for patient/family's participation in care
■ Hypovolemia related to Inadequate fluid replacement Use of deep hypothermia, which produces high peripheral resistance; with warming, peripheral vasodilatation occurs,	■ Hemodynamic stability, adequate cardiac output BP, P, CVP, and PAP within patient's normal limits Adequate peripheral perfusion Warm, dry skin	■ Prevent by Scrupulous monitoring of hemodynamic parameters (q5 min while patient is warming, then q15 min until stable, then q½-1 hr), including BP, P, PAP, and CVP Peripheral perfusion—skin temperature, color, peripheral pulses Urine output (q1 hr) Chest tube drainage (q½-1 hr)

Potential problems	Expected outcomes	Nursing activities

which may result in an inadequate circulating blood volume relative to vascular space	Full peripheral pulses
	Alert and oriented
	Urine output at least 0.5 ml/kg/hour for adults and 1 to 2 ml/kg/hour for children, infants
	
	Chest drainage less than 100 ml/hour for first few postoperative hours in adults, less than 2 ml/kg/hour in children
	Absence of bloody urine or secretions, or above-normal amounts of wound drainage
	Hct above 30% (above 35% to 40% in infants)
		Note above-normal amount of blood loss
		Notify physician for the following amounts of blood loss
		  Adults: more than 100 ml/hour in 2 or more consecutive hours or more than 150 ml in any 1 hour
		  Children: more than 2 ml/kg/hour in 2 or more hours or more than 5 ml/kg in any 1 hour
		    NOTE: Output of 3 ml/kg/hour in 3 hours constitutes greater than 10% blood loss
		Monitor for signs and symptoms of hypovolemia
		  Hypotension, tachycardia
		  Low CVP and PAP relative to patient's norm
		  Signs of peripheral hypoperfusion
		  Oliguria
		Notify physician for abnormalities
		If hypovolemia occurs
		  Administer fluids, blood, blood products as ordered, closely monitoring patient's response
		  If patient is hypovolemic in the presence of very marginal heart function, administer inotropic and/or vasodilator medications with concurrent fluid administration as ordered
		  Keep patient in supine position until hemodynamic parameters are within patient's normal limits

■ Hemorrhage/low Hct related to
  Inadequate blood replacement
  Platelet destruction in the CPB machine
  Blood replacement with old blood—deficient in platelet and clotting factors
  Inadequate reversal of heparin
  Liver congestion and deficient production of clotting factors in patient with right-sided congestion (heart failure)
  A missed bleeding artery and/or diffuse intrathoracic ooze, especially if chest has been entered before
NOTE: Children with cyanotic heart disease and compensatory polycythemia have an increased tendency to bleed postoperatively (related to inadequate platelet numbers and function); fresh whole blood and platelets may be required postoperatively
	■ Adequate cardiac output
	Hemodynamic parameters within patient's normal range
	Absence of inordinate blood loss, hemorrhage
	Chest drainage less than 100 ml/hour for first few postoperative hours in adults, less than 2 ml/kg/hour in children
	Absence of bloody urine or secretions, or above-normal amounts of wound drainage
	Hct above 30% (above 35% to 40% in infants)
		■ Monitor coagulation profile
		  Note dosage of protamine given to reverse heparin effects after CPB; administer additional protamine if needed, as ordered
		  Administer fresh blood, fresh frozen plasma, appropriate clotting factors if ordered
		Monitor for signs and symptoms of hemorrhage—
		  Brisk, large amounts of bright red drainage through chest tubes
		  Falling Hct (check q½-1 hr until stable)
		  Signs of hypovolemia
		Monitor for signs of coagulopathy, including
		  Blood oozing from incision site
		  Bloody secretions from endotracheal tube
		  Hematuria
		  Heme-positive NG aspirates and stool
		Notify physician for presence of these abnormalities
		Administer blood and blood products as ordered, closely monitoring patient's response

Potential problems	Expected outcomes	Nursing activities
■ Cardiac tamponade related to Inordinate blood loss Malposition of chest tube	■ Adequate cardiac output, peripheral perfusion Absence of cardiac tamponade	■ Monitor for signs and symptoms of cardiac tamponade, including Hypotension, tachycardia Venous congestion Increased CVP and left atrial pressure/PCWP Narrowing pulse pressure Distant heart sounds Decreased size of QRS complex Abrupt decrease in chest tube drainage (may occur if chest tubes are clotted) Chest radiograph—increased heart size, pulmonary vascular congestion If signs and symptoms of cardiac tamponade occur, notify physician immediately If chest tube losses abruptly decrease, milk tubes vigorously to remove clot Assist with pericardiocentesis if procedure is necessary Institute other remedial measures as ordered, including preparing patient for thoracotomy and return to operating room See Standard: *Pericarditis* (includes cardiac tamponade)
■ Myocardial failure, which may be associated with Ventriculotomy Cardiomyopathy (preexisting) Intraoperative myocardial ischemia Recent or perioperative infarction Tachyarrhythmias, bradyarrhythmias Hemopericardium with tamponade Residual cardiac depressant effects of anesthesia Metabolic abnormalities, including acid-base imbalance Thermolability in neonates and in infants who have an increased ratio of body surface area to body core, which tends to promote loss of heat and water to the environment Prematurity and malnutrition; these infants have reduced amounts of subcutaneous fat and thus have a reduced insulation and increased tendency to lose heat Pulmonary embolus	■ Adequate cardiac output	■ Reduce myocardial O_2 consumption by Bed rest in early postoperative period Providing for quiet, calm environment Comfort measures Administering pain medication Administering medications that directly reduce myocardial O_2 requirements (e.g., beta blockers) if ordered In infants—provide for consistently warm atmosphere, using Isolette, heat shield, or overbed warmer as appropriate In this thermoregulated environment, avoid covering infant Employ measures to avoid infection while using the open thermoregulating systems When using an Isolette, consolidate procedures to avoid repeatedly opening the enclosed system Monitor for signs/symptoms of heart failure, including Hypotension, tachycardia Elevated CVP and PCWP, venous congestion, pulmonary vascular congestion, pulmonary edema Peripheral hypoperfusion Lethargy, easy fatigability ECG changes associated with myocardial ischemia and/or infarction Signs of pulmonary congestion Rales in adults Tachypnea, increased respiratory effort in children Notify physician of significant abnormalities Administer therapy as ordered to achieve an adequate cardiac output Inotropic, vasopressor agents Vasodilator agents Diuretics Intra-aortic balloon pumping Monitor patient's response closely SEE STANDARD: *Heart failure*

Potential problems	Expected outcomes	Nursing activities

■ Hypertension, which may be related to
  Hypervolemia, fluid overload
  Delayed action of catecholamines stored in capillaries during deep hypothermia
  Continuing preoperative hypertension
	■ BP within patient's normal limits
	  Normovolemia
	  Blood volume within patient's normal limits
		■ Monitor hemodynamic parameters q5 min in early postoperative period (continuous monitoring via arterial, venous catheters whenever possible)
		Notify physician for presence of hypertension and administer therapy as ordered, including continuous intravenous infusion of antihypertensive agent
		Monitor for signs and symptoms of hypervolemia
		  Hypertension, tachycardia
		  Elevated CVP and PAP
		  Elevated urine output (if heart function is adequate)
		  Dramatic weight gain over preoperative weight (measure at least q24 hr)
		Notify physician for these abnormalities
		If hypertension occurs administer diuretic and/or vasodilator medication if needed, as ordered; institute fluid restriction if ordered

■ MI
  NOTE: MI is rare in children unless an anomalous coronary artery is present
	■ Absence of signs and symptoms of myocardial ischemia or infarction	■ Prevent by administering therapy as ordered to maintain adequate cardiac output/coronary artery blood flow and to maintain Hct at prescribed level (usually above 30%)
		Monitor for
		  ECG changes indicating myocardial ischemia/infarction
		  Restlessness, anxiety associated with signs/symptoms of low cardiac output, severe anginal pain, dyspnea, shortness of breath, wheezing, cough, rales
		  Results of serum cardiac enzyme levels
		    Presence of CPK (MB band)
		    Elevated lactate dehydrogenase (LD_1 and LD_2) isoenzyme levels
		If any of these abnormalities occur, notify physician
		If MI is suspected, see Standard: *Acute myocardial infarction*

■ Arrhythmias, which may be related to
  Cellular metabolic abnormalities
  Acid-base imbalance
  Hypoxia
  Intracellular shifts in K^+, Na^+, Ca^{2+}
  Circulating catecholamines and cardiotonic drugs
  Dilatation of cardiac chambers
  Surgical injury of conduction system
  Preoperative or postoperative atrial fibrillation, often associated with pericarditis, heart failure, and myocardial hypertrophy
  Sinus node injury, atrial ischemia, or infarction
  Pulmonary emboli
	■ Absence or resolution of arrhythmias, with adequate cardiac output	■ Prevent by monitoring for and administering therapy to correct factors that predispose patient to arrhythmias, including
		  Acid-base imbalance
		  Hypoxia
		  Electrolyte imbalance
		  Psychosocial stress
		Monitor
		  ECG continuously, with high and low rate alarms set at all times
		  Notify physician of any significant changes in rate and/or rhythm and of associated changes in cardiac output (BP, P, and/or peripheral perfusion)
		    NOTE: Patients with marginal heart function have limited cardiac reserve and are less able to maintain stroke volumes in the presence of bradyarrhythmias or tachyarrhythmias; thus heart rate must be kept within the patient's physiological range
		If arrhythmias occur
		  Document arrhythmias with rhythm strip in chart; compare ECG with baseline serial lab (12- or 15-lead) ECGs in chart
		  Administer therapy as ordered, which may include:
		    Antiarrhythmic agent
		    Correction of factors predisposing patient to arrhythmias
		  Document therapy given and patient's response
		  Make appropriate entries in nursing care plan
		  Assist with insertion of pacemaker, if necessary, for patients with complete heart block and/or unstable rhythms with

Potential problems	Expected outcomes	Nursing activities

poor cardiac output; for patients who have pacing wires in place for standby use, keep pacemaker at bedside
See Standard: *Pacemakers*
Administer humidified O_2 if needed, as ordered
Monitor Hct and Hgb for adequate oxygen-carrying capacity
Administer blood if needed, as ordered

■ Respiratory insufficiency related to hypoventilation and atelectasis, resulting from
Discomfort, pain, and splinting, with difficulty deep breathing and coughing
Thoracotomy with direct trauma to chest wall
Interstitial edema
Decreased compliance associated with interstitial edema and fibrosis

■ Adequate oxygenation and ventilation, with arterial pH, Pa_{O_2} and Pa_{CO_2} levels within normal limits
Absence of signs and symptoms of hypoxia, tachypnea, dyspnea, pain and splinting, and/or atelectasis
Lungs clear by auscultation and chest radiograph
Aeration equal and adequate bilaterally

■ Prevention
Administer pain medication, particularly in the first few postoperative days (administer sufficient medication to reduce pain, but not so much that respirations are depressed and shallow and the cough effort is weak)
Maintain patent airway by
Turning q1-2 hr
Chest physiotherapy q2 hr with turning
Auscultation of breath sounds q1 hr
Suctioning as needed
After extubation, also
Incentive spirometry q½ hr
Deep breathing and coughing q1-2 hr and prn
Promote optimal chest expansion by positioning patient in semi-Fowler's position
Maintain NG tube to prevent gastric distension with air and diaphragmatic elevation if needed, as ordered
Use pillows for support, comfort (considering placement of chest tubes)

■ Respiratory insufficiency related to *ventilation/perfusion abnormality*, which may result from
Postperfusion syndrome
Atelectasis
Microemboli
Residual intracardiac shunting
Respiratory insufficiency related to *impaired gas diffusion* in lung, resulting from pulmonary edema

■ Adequate oxygenation and ventilation, with Pa_{O_2} and Pa_{CO_2} within patient's normal limits

■ Monitor
Respiratory status q1 hr and prn, including
Presence of spontaneous respirations
Respiratory rate—note presence of tachypnea
Quality of respirations—note presence of dyspnea, shallow breathing
Respiratory effort (especially retractions in children)
Breath sounds—note presence of rales, rhonchi, wheezing
Color (note: cyanosis cannot be detected if patient is anemic)
Serial arterial blood gas levels q1-2 hr until stable and q15 min after any change in ventilator settings or O_2 concentration is made; note levels not within patient's normal limits and notify physician
For signs and symptoms of hypoxia, including tachypnea, tachycardia, and restlessness and confusion
Verify ventilator settings q1-2 hr and document same
Monitor chest radiograph results for presence of
Infiltrates indicating atelectasis
Diffuse haziness indicating pulmonary interstitial edema
Increased pulmonary interstitial edema and alveolar water by monitoring for presence of
Rales
Increased CVP, left atrial pressure, and/or PCWP
Hypoxemia
Increased respiratory rate, with retractions and nasal flaring in children
Notify physician for these abnormalities
If pulmonary interstitial edema occurs
Administer diuretics, morphine sulfate, and CPAP or PEEP and increase O_2 concentration as ordered
Monitor patient for response to therapy; notify physician if there is no response or poor response

Potential problems	Expected outcomes	Nursing activities
		See Standards: *Pulmonary edema* and *Positive end expiratory pressure* as appropriate
		If intubation and mechanical ventilation are necessary, see Standard: *Mechanical ventilation*
■ Respiratory insufficiency related to *pneumothorax, hemothorax, or pleural effusion*	■ Fully expanded lungs	■ Monitor for decreased breath sounds, decrease in chest tube drainage, bubbles in chest bottle, and signs/symptoms of hypoxia; notify physician of these abnormalities
		Maintain chest drainage system
		Chest tubes to water seal drainage and suction as per physician's order
		Milk chest tubes q1 hr while tubes are in place to facilitate drainage
		Be aware of chest radiograph results compatible with pneumothorax, hemothorax, or pleural effusion
		When chest tubes are removed
		Assist with chest radiograph if ordered
		Auscultate chest for equality of aeration
		Notify physician of any changes
		Apply an air-occlusive dressing to site
■ Respiratory insufficiency related to *thromboemboli*	■ Absence of pulmonary embolus and peripheral thromboembolus	■ Prevent by
		Providing for early, gradual ambulation as tolerated and as ordered
		Passive and active leg exercises
		Antithromboembolic stockings or Ace bandages
		Changing IV sites before they become inflamed and/or swollen
		Monitor for
		Sites of thrombus formation in deep leg veins, phlebitic IV sites
		Signs/symptoms of pulmonary embolus: sudden onset of chest pain, cyanosis, respiratory distress, diaphoresis, hypoxia
		Notify physician immediately for aforementioned signs/symptoms of pulmonary embolus
		If thromboemboli occur, see Standard: *Embolic phenomena*
■ Acid-base imbalance, which may be related to	■ Acid-base balance within normal limits	■ Prevent by
Metabolic acidosis associated with poor perfusion, tissue hypoxia, increased lactic acid production during CPB; (elevated levels are present in early postoperative period)	Blood gas levels within patient's normal limits, including pH Pa_{O_2} Pa_{CO_2} Base excess Total CO_2 Bicarbonate Other anions, cations that help to determine acid-base status	Administering fluids and electrolytes to keep fluid balance and serum electrolyte levels within normal limits
		Administering therapy to support cardiac output to achieve adequate peripheral perfusion, thereby minimizing anaerobic metabolism and acidosis
		Monitor serial arterial blood gas results for pH, Pa_{O_2}, Pa_{CO_2}, and bicarbonate levels; monitor lactic acid levels
		Note results not within normal limits and notify physician
		Monitor for etiological factors for acid-base imbalance
Metabolic alkalosis associated with many transfusions (citrate metabolized to bicarbonate), use of certain diuretics		If problem occurs
		Administer therapy as ordered to correct acid-base imbalance
		Administer therapy as ordered to provide for adequate oxygenation
		Administer therapy to correct etiological factors for the acid-base imbalance present

Potential problems	Expected outcomes	Nursing activities
■ Fluid imbalance	■ Fluid output is approximately two thirds of fluid intake in adults and one half of fluid intake in infants Weight gain per day is Less than 0.5 to 1 kg in adults Less than 200 g in children Less than 30 g in infants Urine output is at least 0.5 ml/kg/hour for adults and 1 to 2 ml/kg/hour for children and infants Adequate cardiac output with hemodynamic parameters within patient's normal limits	■ Prevent by Monitoring fluid intake and output q1 hr in the early postoperative period; particularly note the following IV intake Urine output for oliguria Chest tube drainage for hemorrhage NG tube drainage Monitoring insensible fluid loss, which is particularly high per kilogram of weight in neonates with little subcutaneous tissue Monitor hemodynamic parameters continuously—correlate systemic arterial BP, PAP, PCWP, CVP, P, peripheral perfusion, urine output, daily weight, and clinical signs of dehydration to determine adequacy of hydration, cardiac output In infants, monitor for fullness of fontanelle and for periorbital edema (in infants less than 20 months of age); both signs indicate systemic fluid engorgement Notify physician of significant abnormalities If fluid imbalance occurs Administer fluids or institute fluid restriction and diuretics as ordered Note patient's response to therapy employed, paticularly in terms of fluid and hemodynamic parameters
■ Electrolyte imbalance, which may include Hypokalemia associated with the use of Diuretics CPB machine Deep hypothermia Diuretic phase of renal failure K^+ shifts with acidosis/alkalosis NOTE: Significant total body depletion may exist in the presence of a normal serum K^+ level Hyperkalemia associated with decreased renal function Hypocalcemia related to multiple blood transfusions Immature calcium-regulating mechanisms in neonates	■ Serum electrolyte levels within normal limits Absence of signs and symptoms of electrolyte imbalance	■ Monitor For signs and symptoms of electrolyte imbalance Lab reports for serum K^+, Na^+, Cl^-, and Ca^{2+} levels Administer electrolyte replacement as ordered* If hyperkalemia occurs, administer therapy as ordered to decrease K^+ levels, which may include Peritoneal dialysis Potassium-binding resins (e.g., Kayexalate) Insulin and glucose K^+ should never be added to infusions that contain antiarrhythmic or cardiotonic agents, since increasing the rate of these medications would result in the patient receiving too much K^+, resulting in arrhythmias and possibly cardiac arrest High concentrations of K^+ should be avoided

*K^+ solutions should be clearly labeled to prevent accidental bolus administration.

Potential problems	Expected outcomes	Nursing activities
■ Renal failure, which may be related to Inadequate cardiac output and renal blood flow Renal capillary occlusion with microemboli	■ Indices of renal function within normal limits Urine output at least 0.5 ml/kg/hour in adults and 1 to 2 ml/kg/hour in children and infants After the early postoperative period, specific gravity indicates renal ability to concentrate Serum and urine electrolyte and creatinine levels within normal limits BUN levels within normal limits Urine pH, glucose, ketone, and protein levels within normal limits	■ Prevent by administering therapy to maintain adequate cardiac output and renal blood flow, including blood products, fluids, and cardiotonic agents Monitor Fluid intake and output q1 hr, noting imbalances Lab reports serially for BUN and urine and serum creatinine levels Urine glucose, ketones, protein, electrolyte and pH levels For adequate cardiac output Notify physician for any of these abnormalities If renal dysfunction/failure occurs, see Standard: *Acute renal failure*
■ Emboli, which may result from Thromboemboli related to Imperfections in the CPB machine gas exchange membrane, causing release of lipids, hemolysis of RBC Direct contact of RBC with O_2 Increased incidence in patients with cyanotic heart disease, particularly in the presence of a high Hct Calcium from resected valve Vegetations from resected valve Fat from sternotomy Air Disintegration of ball in ball-cage prosthetic valve, releasing fragments into circulation Disintegration of tissue valves (porcine and cadaver)	■ Adequate tissue perfusion Absence or resolution of emboli formation Absence of emboli in microcirculation	■ Prevention Heparin while patient is on CPB machine Hemodilution while patient is on CPB machine Maintenance of adequate systemic blood flow and perfusion with fluids and blood products, and cardiotonic/vasodilator medications administered as ordered Prevent phlebothromboemboli from occurring in lower extremities with Antiembolic stockings Passive or active ROM exercises Early ambulation Anticoagulation in patients with valve replacements as ordered (acetylsalicylic acid is often used with porcine valve replacement and warfarin with metal valve replacement; anticoagulation in patients with porcine valves is usually employed for approximately 3 months, although it is used for a longer period if atrial fibrillation or certain other complicating factors are present) Monitor for emboli, particularly myocardial, cerebral, pulmonary; also mesenteric, renal, splenic, and others; see Standard: *Embolic phenomena* for specific signs and symptoms If problem occurs Administer heparin continuously or intermittently as ordered Administer long-term warfarin if appropriate, as ordered (e.g., in patients with metal valve replacements) Administer fibrinolytic/enzyme therapy if ordered SEE STANDARD: *Embolic phenomena*

Potential problems	Expected outcomes	Nursing activities

■ Altered level of consciousness related to
Cerebral hypoxia and edema from decreased cardiac outout and/or hypoxemia
Cerebral microemboli (more common in children with cyanotic heart disease and high Hct)
Metabolic alterations from renal and/or hepatic damage
CNS depressant medications
Sleep deprivation, noise, sensory monotony of environment
Anxiety and fear
	■ Patient is alert and oriented and has normal neuromuscular function	■ Assess neurological status with vital signs, noting
		  Pupillary response
		  Spontaneous, purposeful movement of all extremities
		  Level of consciousness; note restlessness, disorientation
		  Response to commands
		  Response to touch (to painful stimuli if appropriate)
		  Spontaneous respiration
		Notify physician for abnormalities in these parameters
		If basic neurological examination is abnormal, perform further testing as appropriate
		  Response to pain
		  Reflexes
		    Extremity
		    Pupillary
		    Corneal
		  Visual and auditory disturbances
		Note signs of cerebral embolus, including
		  Unilateral weakness
		  Dysarthria
		  Aphasia
		Administer therapy to minimize the incidence of predisposing factors for altered level of consciousness
		  Administer therapy to augment cardiac output and cerebral blood flow if needed, as ordered
		  Administer therapy to alleviate cerebral edema (e.g., restriction of Na^+ and fluid intake, administration of steroids and/or osmotic diuretics, as ordered)
		  Correct metabolic abnormalities
		  Avoid or reduce dosage of drugs that produce CNS depression
		  Provide for rest periods and as much sleep as possible
		  Provide for meaningful sensory stimuli; reduce meaningless stimuli
		  Provide for psychological support and appropriate encouragement (see Problem, Patient/family's anxiety)
		Establish trusting confident relationship between doctor, nurse, and patient
		Spend time with, reassure, and comfort patient
		Explain procedures and what the patient will experience in simple terms
		Provide for and encourage increasing amounts of patient decision making and control in his/her care
		Monitor for more pronounced abnormalities such as visual and auditory hallucinations, paranoid delusions; notify physician if these occur
		Limit or reduce extraneous, monotonous noise in patient's environment as much as possible
		Provide for objects in environment that assist in reorientation of patient to surroundings; clock should be within patient's vision
		Administer medication to patient for pain regularly in the early postoperative period; administer sedatives if needed, as ordered (NOTE: Metabolism of narcotics may be decreased in the presence of chronic liver engorgement; reduced dosages may be necessary)
		Provide as much uninterrupted time for sleep as possible
		Build supportive relationship with family; mobilize their resources to encourage and assist patient during the recovery period
		Monitor for physiological abnormalities that predispose patient to altered level of consciousness, including

Potential problems	Expected outcomes	Nursing activities
		Infection Acid-base imbalance Hypoxia Cerebral emboli Medications Alcohol withdrawal Notify physician if these abnormalities occur Monitor for complications of cardiac surgery that predispose patient to abnormal psychological responses, including cardiac, respiratory, and/or renal failure Notify physician of abnormalities, and administer corrective/supportive therapy as ordered
■ Infection related to Sternotomy IV cutdown sites Prosthetic materials CPB Decreased lung compliance with atelectasis Mechanical ventilation Urinary tract infection from urethral catheter Some types of valves used for valve replacement are particularly prone to infection Damage to protein antibodies Early postoperative decrease in number and phagocytic activity of WBC Insertion of lines for CPB	■ Infection free Afebrile	■ Prevent by Being aware of length of time IV or arterial lines have been in place; remind physician if it has been more than 3 days or if site becomes inflamed Maintaining appropriate aseptic technique when administering IV fluids, changing IV bottles, giving medications, etc. Administering antibiotics as per physician's orders Applying povidone-iodine (Betadine) solution to sternotomy and chest tube site daily after dressing is removed Maintaining aseptic technique in handling urethral catheter; should be removed as soon as possible Administering respiratory care as in Problem, Respiratory insufficiency, to decrease potential for atelectasis, pneumonia Monitor Vital signs q½-2 hr until stable, with special attention to unusual fever spikes or hypothermia (in infants); notify physician for temperature over 101° F or less than 97° F (over 38.4° C or less than 36.2° C) For signs of sepsis: fever, chills, diaphoresis, altered level of consciousness For signs of localized wound infection; check sternotomy, chest tube sites, and all IV sites for redness, warmth, pain, edema, and drainage; report to physician For pulmonary infection, especially changes in character of sputum (note amount, color, consistency), fever, atelectasis; notify physician For signs of urinary tract infection: cloudy urine, dysuria, flank pain, persistent hematuria, foul smelling urine If problem occurs Administer antipyretics as ordered for elevated temperature (as fever increases, so does cardiac work); if patient is hypothermic warm him/her using heat lamps, warm blankets, Isolette, or overbed warmer Administer antibiotics as ordered Administer specific therapies as ordered to hasten resolution of infection, according to the organ system involved
■ Endocarditis, which may be related to secondary infection associated with multiple invasive lines, particularly in the early postoperative period	■ Absence or resolution of endocarditis	■ Prevent by Removing lines, catheters as soon as possible Administering prophylactic antibiotics as ordered in perioperative period Monitor for ECG abnormalities, including S-T segment elevation or depression Fever Positive blood cultures Petechiae on skin, mucous membranes

Potential problems	Expected outcomes	Nursing activities

		If severe endocarditis is suspected or occurs, monitor for signs of
		  Valvular dysfunction
		  Low cardiac output
		If endocarditis occurs, see Standard: *Endocarditis*

■ Pericarditis, which is related to direct surgical manipulation, trauma	■ Absence or resolution of postoperative pericarditis	■ Monitor for
		  ECG changes including S-T segment elevation and T wave abnormalities
		  Pericardial friction rub
		  Persistent chest discomfort, pain
		  Persistent fever
		If pericarditis occurs, see Standard: *Pericarditis*

■ Postcardiotomy syndrome, which may be related to
Hypersensitivity, immune response to pericardial injury
Signs and symptoms usually begin about 7 days postoperatively, although the syndrome may begin as early as 3 days postoperatively and as late as many months postoperatively
	■ Absence or resolution of postcardiotomy syndrome	■ Monitor for
		  Signs and symptoms of pericarditis, which may include ECG changes such as T wave abnormalities and/or S-T segment elevation
		  Pericardial friction rub
		  Persistence of chest discomfort, pain
		  Persistent fever or recurrent fever continuing after the first few postoperative days
		  General malaise
		  Arthralgia, joint pains
		  Pleurisy, pleural effusion, hemoptysis
		  Leukocytosis
		  Increased erythrocyte sedimentation rate
		Notify physician for any of these signs and symptoms
		If postcardiotomy syndrome occurs
		  Administer antipyretics and analgesics as ordered, usually aspirin
		  Administer steroids if ordered

■ Insufficient information for compliance with discharge regimen*	■ Patient/family has sufficient information to comply with discharge regimen
	Before discharge, patient/family
	  Verbalizes dietary management
	  Describes activity progression; identifies activities to avoid in first few weeks at home
	  Accurately performs specific procedures; describes precautions regarding special devices such as pacemaker
	  Accurately identifies medications and pertinent information
		■ Assess patient/family's understanding of disease process, follow-up plan of care, and discharge regimen
		Consult with physician regarding the rehabilitation plan
		Instruct patient/family in
		  Diet
		    Type of food to consume; foods to avoid (e.g., those high in cholesterol, saturated fat)
		    Sodium/salt restriction
		    Calorie restriction
		    After instruction, permit and encourage patient to do his/her own meal planning, selecting proper foods from the hospital menu, if possible
		  Fluid intake (restriction if appropriate)
		    Monitor for swelling of lower legs, with limitation of fluid intake if this occurs
		    Daily weight; notification of physician if weight gain is more than 4 to 5 pounds in 1 week or if marked ankle swelling is present
		    Avoidance of excessive eating and drinking of alcoholic beverages
		  Medications
		    Name of drug and purpose
		    Indications for use if drug is to be taken prn
		    Identification of

*If responsibility of critical care unit nurse includes follow-up care.

Potential problems	Expected outcomes	Nursing activities
		Dosage/number of pills and schedules
		Potential adverse side effects and how to minimize
		Avoidance of over-the-counter medications that can change the activity of medications prescribed
		Other precautions for each medication
		Assist patient in keeping a chart on which medications taken can be recorded
		Instruct mothers as to when (or if) to repeat medication if child vomits after swallowing it
		If chest pain (anginal pain) does not respond to antianginal medication, physician should be notified
		Avoidance of situations at home or work that elicit tense or angry feelings or marked fatigue
		Activity levels; patient should
		Consult physician before resuming more vigorous activities such as driving a car, lifting stuck windows, vacuuming
		Get plenty of rest, with 8 hours or so of sleep at night and spaced activities during the day, with rest periods in between
		Regular, moderate exercise
		Avoid prolonged periods of activity in very hot or cold temperatures
		Avoid undue straining with bowel movements; if this occurs, the patient may be instructed to add fiber to his/her diet; if straining is pronounced, physician should be notified; a stool softener may be ordered
		Encourage patient that chest movements associated with coughing, housework, driving a car may cause some discomfort for several weeks; in the first few weeks at home, a mild analgesic may be ordered
		Special care activities, followed by a return demonstration
		Suture line care
		Precautions with pacemaker if in situ (see Standard: *Pacemakers: temporary and permanent*)
		Other activities
	Indicates understanding of untoward signs and symptoms, including those which require medical attention	Describe indications for notification of physician (e.g., chest pain, fever, malaise, and other difficulties); include phone number and person to call in an emergency
	Accurately describes plan for follow-up care, including procedure for clinic visits	Describe plan for follow-up with cardiologist and, if needed, a visiting nurse, physical and/or occupational therapist, as ordered
		Discuss modifications of risk factors present
		Atherosclerosis
		Hyperlipidemia
		Glucose intolerance, diabetes
		Hypertension
		Type A personality (method of relaxation)
		Amelioration of job, home stress
		Smoking
		Obesity
		Discuss ways to prevent thromboemboli
		Provide opportunity for patient/family to ask questions and verbalize anxieties, fears regarding discharge regimen
		Assess patient/family's potential compliance with discharge regimen
		Provide information about and assistance in obtaining referral services for available community resources as appropriate

22 □ Vascular surgery: aneurysms

An aneurysm is a local dilatation of a weakened vessel wall. A true aneurysm involves a ballooning of the entire wall, whereas a false aneurysm involves a tear in the vessel lining that allows blood to collect in the lining and create a subsequent protrusion of the outer vessel wall.

Aneurysms most commonly occur in the aorta, although they are also found in the cerebral arteries, in the ventricle of the heart after a MI, and in other central and peripheral vessels.

The etiology of aneurysms may be classified as hereditary (e.g., congenital abnormalities, connective tissue abnormalities of the vessels, arteriovenous communications) or acquired (e.g., mycotic, syphilitic, traumatic, atherosclerotic, or dissecting lesions).

The atherosclerotic lesions involve intimal degeneration, subintimal proliferation, fibrosis and atrophy of the underlying media and associated weakening of the vessel wall. Calcification of the lining often develops as the fibrotic process continues. These lesions are often precursors of atherosclerotic aneurysms, which occur most often in the abdominal aorta between the origin of the renal arteries and the aortic bifurcation. Occasionally, the thoracic aorta, carotid arteries, and other vessels are involved.

A predisposing factor for aneurysm formation is hypertension. Hypertension adds to the mechanical pressure and force of turbulent blood flow against a weakened vessel wall and is thus associated with a greater tendency for aneurysm rupture and dissection.

Aortic aneurysms are classified into five major types according to location: thoracic-ascending, transverse, descending; thoracoabdominal, and abdominal.

Ascending thoracic aneurysms are located in the ascending portion of the thoracic aorta, which is the portion of the aorta closest to the heart.

Aneurysms of the transverse aortic arch involve the carotid, subclavian, and upper vertebral arteries. Aneuryms of the descending thoracic aorta are located in the proximal portion of the descending aorta.

Thoracoabdominal aneurysms extend from immediately above the diaphragm to the subdiaphragmatic aorta and are usually associated with reduced blood flow to the celiac, superior mesenteric, and renal arteries. Abdominal aneurysms are located below the renal arteries and above the bifurcation of iliac arteries.

Dissecting aneurysms involve progressive longtitudinal tearing of the media from the intima. If a rapid aortic dissection occurs, serious hemodynamic compromise results and may lead to cardiovascular collapse.

Most aneurysms are asymptomatic until they begin to leak, rapidly enlarge, or dissect. When any of these occur, the primary symptom is pain. Pain may develop as a result of the direct expansile process or as a result of hypoperfusion of an organ or an extremity (i.e., bowel ischemia).

Physical signs of aneurysms include a palpable pulsatile mass, pulse differences in the extremities, and evidence consistent with an intracranial, intrathoracic, or intra-abdominal mass.

Aneurysms may first be observed as masses on a radiograph. Conclusive diagnosis can be reached by ultrasonography and arteriography.

Medical management is employed when the patient is admitted. Hypertensive patients are treated with potent vasodilators to immediately lower the blood pressure. If possible, continuous pressure monitoring should be provided for such patients.

Surgery is performed if the aneurysm is compromising blood flow to distal or adjacent organs or is large enough to suggest that the risk of rupture is significant. Surgical repair can prevent extension of the aneurysm and reduce ischemic injury and the risk of rupture. Restoration of circulation to arteries and organs adjacent and distal to the aneurysm improves organ function. The aneurysm is either excised with a primary anastomosis or an interposition graft, or bypassed using a synthetic graft.

Hazards of surgery include hemorrhage and ischemic injury to the involved end organs during the surgical repair. Severe intraoperative ischemia can produce sloughing of mucosal cells and occasional infarction of the involved end organs.

Each type of aneurysm has unique potential preoperative and postoperative complications depending on the nature, location, and extent of the aneurysm and the difficulty of operative repair.

Mortality rates vary according to the location of the aneurysm. The lowest mortality rates are reported for aneurysms originating distal to the left subclavian artery. The risk increases for aneurysms of the ascending or transverse thoracic aorta where the carotid and coronary arteries and aortic valve are commonly involved. Surgical outcome is also determined by the patient's age, blood pressure abnormalities, and the degree of atherosclerosis present.

Postoperative nursing care is focused on achieving optimal hemodynamic stability. Therapy is directed toward preventing, monitoring for, and, if necessary, resolving problems associated with ischemic injury.

ASSESSMENT

1. If patient is known to have an aneurysm and presents with cardiovascular collapse, the aneurysm may be dissecting or have ruptured; obtain a brief history from patient or family while patient is prepared for emergency surgery
2. History, nature, presence, and severity of
   a. Palpitations, angina (aortic valve insufficiency, decreased coronary blood flow)
   b. Syncope (decreased carotid artery blood flow)
   c. Dyspnea (aneurysm compression of trachea, bronchus)
   d. Hoarseness (compression of recurrent laryngeal nerve)
   e. Abdominal pain (decreased mesenteric blood flow, aneurysm compression of abdominal organ)
   f. Bloody diarrhea (ischemic bowel)
   g. Hematuria (ischemic kidney)
   h. Painful, weak extremities (ischemia)
3. Previous and current medical therapy and prior surgery
4. Clinical signs and symptoms, including
   a. Deficits in circulation to extremities
      (1) Painful, weak extremities; presence of ischemic pain in one arm that is constant and nagging in character; pulsating mass present with decreased circulation distal to mass
      (2) Quality of pulses distal to aneurysm, noting fullness, pattern of filling, and occlusion pressure; note presence of edema
      (3) Capillary circulation of extremity distal to vascular problem—note color, relative temperature (warmth versus coolness), sympathetic discharge (clamminess versus dryness)
      (4) Impairment of nerve function secondary to ischemia of affected extremity
   b. Cardiac status
      (1) Note abnormalities in BP, P, and heart sounds and, if available, CVP and PAP; ECG, and presence of arrhythmias
      (2) Note signs of insufficient blood flow—an-

gina, palpitations (may also indicate aortic valve insufficiency)
   c. Pulmonary status, including
      (1) Rate and quality of respirations
      (2) Breath sounds
      (3) Arterial blood gas levels
      (4) Note signs of distress; dyspnea; paroxysmal cough (aneurysm may compress trachea, bronchus); hoarseness (compression of recurrent laryngeal nerve)
   d. Renal status
      (1) Presence of flank pain
      (2) Hematuria
      (3) Note abnormalities in baseline volume of urine and specific gravity
   e. GI status, including presence of
      (1) Abdominal pain (decreased mesenteric blood flow or compression of abdominial organs by aneurysm)
      (2) Bloody diarrhea (ischemic bowel)
      (3) Dysphagia (impingement on esophagus)
   f. Cerebral status
      (1) Level of consciousness, noting any abnormalities
      (2) Any episode of syncope (decreased carotid blood flow)
      (3) Presence of unequal pupils (compression of cervical sympathetic chain)
5. Weight
6. Results of lab and diagnostic tests, including
   a. Hgb, Hct, and platelet levels
   b. Coagulation studies
   c. WBC count
   d. Kidney function tests
   e. Liver function tests
   f. ECG
   g. Radiographs
   h. Arteriography
   i. Aortograpy
   j. Cardiac catheterization
   k. Ultrasound studies, as appropriate
7. Patient/family's knowledge regarding operative therapy
   a. What they have been told
   b. Their expectations
   c. Fears regarding surgery and the outcome
   d. Previous experiences with surgery, if any
8. Information and detail surgeon has provided patient/family about the need for surgery, the actual surgery to be done, and the expected outcomes

9. Patient/family's level of anxiety related to disease condition, accompanying signs and symptoms of circulatory insufficiency, hospitalization, and family role alterations associated with illness

GOALS

1. Reduction in patient/family's anxiety with provision of information, explanations
2. Hemodynamic stability—absence of hemorrhage; minimal postoperative bleeding; aneurysm repaired with no recurrence; adequate circulation distal to vascular repair
3. Patent vessel, graft
4. Respiratory function within normal limits
   a. Arterial blood gas levels within normal limits
   b. Full lung expansion with no atelectasis, pulmonary interstitial edema, or compressed bronchus
   c. Afebrile without atelectasis or pneumonia
5. Kidney function adequate for removal of body's nitrogenous waste products and maintenance of body fluid volume
6. Acid-base balance and electrolyte levels within normal limits
7. Absence of signs of mesenteric ischemia, infarction
8. Coagulation studies within normal limits; absence of emboli formation
9. Nervous system function within normal limits; no evidence of cerebral embolus, infarction
10. Spinal function and associated neuromuscular, autonomic, genitourinary function within normal limits; absence of paralysis
11. Patient/family verbalizes knowledge of discharge regimen, including precautions, medications, diet, and activity; patient/family able to describe follow-up plan, including where and when to go, who to see, and what specimens to bring

Potential problems	Expected outcomes	Nursing activities
Preoperative		
■ Patient/family's anxiety related to Disease process Hospitalization Therapeutic regimen Diagnostic tests planned Impending major surgery and associated risks Altered family roles Separation from family members Loss of job	■ Reduction in patient/family's anxiety with provision of information, explanations, and encouragement	■ Ongoing assessment of level of patient/family's anxiety Assess patient/family's knowledge and understanding of disease process, therapeutic regimen, anticipated diagnostic procedures, and anticipated surgery, if planned Explain in simple terms the nature of patient's circulatory problem and the symptoms patient is experiencing Explain in simple terms what patient will experience during certain diagnostic procedures Assist in preparing patient for procedures, which may include radiographs, ECG, cardiac catheterization with angiography and ultrasonography as appropriate Collaborate with physician and other health team members on teaching to be done When surgery is planned and the physician has discussed it with patient/family, assess their understanding of the information Reinforce the purpose and nature of the surgery and the expected outcomes Describe the perioperative experiences (adjust explanation according to patient's anxiety level and desire to know), including Preoperative Orient patient to (call chest physiotherapist, if available) 1. Coughing and deep breathing 2. Incentive spirometry 3. Chest physiotherapy Shave and light dinner NPO after midnight Medication for sleep if needed Morning bath/shower Preoperative medications Hospital gowns Care of valuables Ride to operating room Scrub suits, masks, and caps worn by operating room staff Anesthesia

Potential problems	Expected outcomes	Nursing activities
		Postoperative
		Waking up in the recovery room/intensive care unit
		1. Describe general environment (size of unit, room, etc.)
		2. Nurse always nearby
		3. Dull, continuous noises
		4. If anticipated, describe breathing tube that will be in place to ease patient's work of breathing and the load on the heart; explain that talking will not be possible while tube in place but that other means of communication will be possible
		5. NPO until breathing tube is removed
		Incision with bandage
		Intravenous, arterial lines
		If anticipated, chest tubes, bloody drainage expected
		ECG monitoring
		Medicine for discomfort, pain
		Policy for family visits
		Describe responsibility of patient for achieving a speedy recovery by taking an active role in coughing and deep breathing to keep lungs clear and so on
		As patient progresses
		Tubes, lines out
		Eating again
		Chest physiotherapy, deep breathing, and coughing
		Getting stronger, ambulation
		Home again
		Provide opportunity for and encourage questions and verbalization of fears, anxieties
		Reassure patient that nurse will be nearby at all times
		Provide calm, quiet environment
		Perform treatments in an unhurried manner, allowing rest periods between treatments
		Involve patient/family in planning for care
		Assess for reduction in level of patient/family's anxiety
■ Hemodynamic instability related to involvement of aortic valve *(ascending aortic aneurysm)*	■ Hemodynamic stability BP, P, CVP, PAP, urine output, peripheral circulation, and mentation are within patient's normal limits	■ Evaluate nature of pain, particularly location and severity
		Assess cardiovascular status at least q½-1 hr until stable, and monitor
		For changes in BP
		Pulses: palpate and auscultate, noting peripheral perfusion
		Heart sounds, noting murmurs
		CVP and PAP if available
		ECG, noting presence of arrhythmias, signs of left ventricular hypertrophy, myocardial ischemia
		For symptoms of ischemia; complaints of angina, palpitations
		Assess circulation to extemities and monitor for changes; note
		Presence of pain, particularly pain that is constant and nagging in character
		Presence of pulsating mass with decreased circulation distal to mass
		Evaluate pulses distal to pulsating mass, noting fullness, pattern of filling, occlusion pressure
		Evaluate capillary circulation of extremities distal to vascular problem; note color, relative temperature (warmth vs coolness), sympathetic discharge (clamminess vs dryness)

Potential problems	**Expected outcomes**	**Nursing activities**
		Monitor
		For impairment of nerve function secondary to ischemia of spinal cord and/or extremities
		For paralysis of nerves originating in the spine, which may result from compression of the aneurysm on the arteries feeding the spinal cord
		Assess signs/symptoms of impaired circulation to or compression of organs located along or distal to aneurysm and monitor for progression; evaluate the following
		Lungs
		Respiratory rate, quality of respirations, breath sounds; note decreased or absent sounds, presence of rales, rhonchi, or wheezing
		For signs of hemothorax
		For signs/symptoms of hypoxia
		For dyspnea, paroxysmal cough, hoarseness, hemoptysis
		Arterial blood gas results
		Chest radiograph results for upper airway compression
		Kidney
		For presence of flank pain, hematuria
		Volume of urine, specific gravity
		GI
		For abdominal pain
		For presence of bloody diarrhea
		Dysphagia
		Neurological
		Level of consciousness, mentation
		For presence of syncope, unequal pupil size
		For neurological abnormalities and weakness in the upper spine and upper extremity region
		Monitor lab results, noting abnormalities in
		Hgb, Hct, platelet levels, coagulation studies
		WBC counts
		Kidney function tests
		Liver function tests
■ Hemodynamic instability related to *dissecting aneurysm*	■ Aneurysm does not extend; remains stable in size Hemodynamic stability	■ Prevent progression of dissecting aneurysm by
		Administering intravenous vasodilators if ordered to lower BP; provide for continuous BP monitoring via an intraarterial line
		Administering diuretics and sedatives as ordered
		Maintaining a quiet, peaceful environment
		Monitor for
		Abrupt onset of severe pain, with localization depending on the organs involved
		Aortic diastolic murmur, which occurs with detachment of the aortic valve cusp
		Neurological symptoms, including syncope
		Chest radiograph results indicating widened aortic silhouette and mediastinum and, occasionally, a hemothorax
		ECG and cardiac enzymes to rule out MI
		Signs of left ventricular hypertrophy, particularly if patient is hypertensive
		Circulatory insufficiency of the organs involved
		Monitor for acute extension of a dissecting aneurysm, including sudden hypotension, extension of the area of pain, signs of aortic regurgitation, sudden drop in urine output, reduced peripheral circulation, sudden weakening or disappearance of peripheral pulses, altered mentation with sudden confusion, restlessness
		Notify physician for appearance of any of these abnormalities

Potential problems	Expected outcomes	Nursing activities
Postoperative		
■ Hemodynamic instability related to Hypotension associated with hypovolemia from hemorrhage Hypertension	■ Hemodynamic stability BP, P, CVP, PAP, urine output, peripheral circulation, and mentation are within patient's normal limits Absence of postoperative hemorrhage Hct and Hgb levels remain stable	■ Prevent by Administering fluids, blood products as ordered to maintain adequate intravascular volume and Hct Closely monitoring patient's hemodynamic response and Hct levels Monitor BP, P q½-1 hr until stable; note hypotension or hypertension, tachycardia For signs and symptoms of hemorrhage Hypotension, tachycardia Oliguria Falling CVP, PAP Cool, clammy, blanched extemities Altered mentation—restlessness, confusion Falling Hct levels Abdominal girth q2-4 hr until stable; note increasing size For tenseness of abdomen q2-4 hr until stable, then q4-8 hr Notify physician for these clinical abnormalities If hemorrhage occurs Administer blood and blood products as ordered, closely monitoring patient's vital signs, CVP, PAP, urine output and Hct levels If hypovolemia occurs, administer fluids as ordered, closely monitoring patient's hemodynamic response as before If hypertension occurs, administer diuretics, antihypertensives as ordered; potent intravenous antihypertensive medications should be given via an infusion pump with continuous monitoring of the arterial BP via an intra-arterial line
■ Myocardial ischemia with angina	■ Absence or early resolution of myocardial ischemia	■ Monitor for Chest pain ECG changes indicating ischemia—S-T segment elevation or depression, T wave inversion Notify physician if these abnormalities occur If angina occurs Administer antianginal medication as ordered, and monitor patient's response Monitor BP, P q15 min and prn during and immediately after acute anginal episode See Standard: *Angina pectoris*
■ MI	■ Absence of MI	■ Monitor for Chest pain unrelieved by antianginal medications Other signs/symptoms of MI Indigestion Shoulder, arm, or jaw pain ECG changes including S-T segment elevation or depression, T wave inversion and diagnostic Q waves Hemodynamic response to severe, unrelenting chest pain Notify physician of these abnormalities If problem occurs, monitor vital signs q¼-½ hr and prn until stable Administer supportive therapy as ordered (e.g., O_2, pain medication) SEE STANDARD: *Acute myocardial infarction*

Potential problems	Expected outcomes	Nursing activities
■ Vascular defect (aneurysm) recurs	■ Aneurysm does not recur Abdominal girth remains stable postoperatively Adequate circulation to aortic tributaries distal to vascular repair	■ Monitor 　Circulation distal to aneurysm repair, including pulses, color, capillary filling 　For occurrence of pain distal to repair 　Abdominal girths after repair of thoracoabdominal, abdominal aneurysms 　For compression of organs adjacent to aneurysm 　Results of serial chest, abdominal radiographs Notify physician of abnormalities in any of the aforementioned If vascular defect occurs, administer therapy as ordered To enhance circulation to lower extremities place patient in a reverse Trendelenburg position if ordered
■ Occlusion of peripheral vessel repair/graft, which may result from low BP and blood flow with circulatory stasis, clotting, and vessel occlusion	■ Patent vessel or graft Circulation distal to aneurysm is sufficient with full pulses, good color, and warmth in extremities	■ Prevent by 　Avoiding constricting clothing or apparatus and angulation at the groin or knee; avoid high Fowler's position 　Turning patient (or he/she turns) with leg straight and supported with pillows 　Applying antithromboembolic stockings as ordered in patients without severe peripheral circulatory insufficiency 　Assist with ROM, passive-assistive, and active-assistive exercises 　Assist in early ambulation as ordered Monitor 　Pulses distal to the repair; an ultrasound device (Doppler) may be needed for weak pulses 　Other circulatory parameters distal to repair, including color, temperature, and sensation
■ Respiratory insufficiency related to 　Pulmonary interstitial edema as a result of vigorous fluid administration 　Atelectasis 　Pulmonary infection 　Pneumonia 　Elevated diaphragm from abdominal surgery and associated distention, ileus 　Dyspnea due to compression of upper airway by aneurysm	■ Respiratory function within normal limits Arterial blood gas levels within patient's normal limits Breath sounds within normal limits; no adventitious sounds Auscultation and chest radiograph reveal full lung expansion without atelectasis, pulmonary interstitial edema, or compressed bronchus Afebrile, without pneumonia	■ Prevent by providing frequent chest physiotherapy 　While patient is on bed rest turn at least q2 hr 　Encourage deep breathing and coughing 　Administer humidified, oxygenated air as ordered 　Employ incentive spirometry and/or intermittent positive pressure breathing as ordered according to patient's clinical picture 　Employ tracheal suctioning as necessary Monitor 　Rate and quality of respirations q1-2 hr 　Secretions for amount, color, and consistency 　For decreased or absent breath sounds, rales, rhonchi, or wheezing 　For signs and symptoms of hypoxia 　For respiratory distress 　Temperature q1-2 hr for fever 　Arterial blood gas levels 　Chest radiograph results If problem occurs 　Emphasize direct chest physiotherapy to atelectatic areas 　Emphasize gravity drainage of involved pulmonary lobe(s) 　Assist with intubation if procedure becomes necessary 　Manage mechanical ventilation and PEEP if needed to maintain adequate gas exchange SEE STANDARDS: *Mechanical ventilation* 　　　　　　　*Positive end expiratory pressure*

Potential problems	Expected outcomes	Nursing activities

■ Kidney dysfunction related to
Preoperative renal ischemia in the presence of a renal artery aneurysm
Intraoperative renal ischemia associated with repair of a renal artery aneurysm
	■ Kidney function within normal limits and adequate to maintain BUN, creatinine, electrolyte levels, body fluid volume, and acid-base balance within normal limits	■ Prevent by
		  Administering fluids, blood, and blood products as ordered to maintain adequate cardiac output and kidney perfusion
		  Administering inotropic agents, if ordered, to increase renal blood flow and urine output
		  Administering diuretics, as ordered, closely monitoring urine output response
		Monitor
		  For signs of inadequate cardiac output, hypovolemia
		  Hypotension, tachycardia
		  Low CVP and PAP
		  Oliguria
		  Inadequate periperal circulation
		  For hematuria
		  Urine volumes and specific gravity q1 hr; note oliguria, high specific gravity
		  Daily weight for gain or loss
		  Arterial blood gas results for acid-base imbalance
		  Lab indices of renal function, including level of BUN, uric acid, creatinine, and electrolytes; serum and urine osmolality, urine creatinine and urine electrolytes
		Notify physician for abnormalities
		If kidney dysfunction or failure occurs, see Standard: *Acute renal failure*

■ GI dysfunction, ileus related to
Mesenteric infarction
Recurrence of abdominal aneurysm
	■ GI function within normal limits
	Bowel sounds within normal limits
	Absence of abdominal distention, rigidity, or other signs of mesenteric ischemia, infarction, or abdominal aneurysm
		■ Monitor
		  Abdominal girths q2-4 hr for increasing abdominal distention
		  Abdominal tenseness for increasing rigidity
		  Bowel sounds q4 hr for decreased or absent bowel sounds
		  For signs/symptoms of mesenteric infarction, including
		    Patient's complaints of discomfort, malaise
		    Temperature elevation
		    Bloody diarrhea (test for heme positive)
		    Elevated WBC count
		Notify physician of these clinical abnormalities
		If mesenteric infarction or recurrence of abdominal aneurysm occurs
		  Administer therapy as ordered, closely monitoring patient's response
		  Prepare patient for surgery if planned

■ CNS dysfunction related to
Ascending and *transverse thoracic aortic aneurysm* associated with deficient carotid artery blood flow
Arterial embolism associated with atherosclerosis, cholesterol plaques
	■ CNS function within normal limits
	Absence of confusion, disorientation, restlessness
	No evidence of cerebral embolus, infarction
		■ Monitor
		  Neurological status, level of consciousness on admission and serially thereafter
		  For signs of general cerebral ischemia, headache, confusion, disorientation, particularly in patients with a thoracic aneurysm
		  For delayed regaining of consciousness after anesthesia
		  For signs of cerebral embolism, infarction, particularly unilateral neurological deficiency, including weak limbs, ptosis of eyelid and/or side of mouth
		  Neurological function to extremities for abnormalities in sensation, movement, strength

Potential problems	Expected outcomes	Nursing activities
■ Emboli formation related to Frequent association of aneurysm with atherosclerosis Dislodgement of thrombus along with the aneurysm during surgery	■ Coagulation studies within normal limits Absence of emboli formation	■ Prevent by Assisting patient with ROM exercises and ambulation as ordered Applying antithromboembolic stockings as ordered Monitor for signs and symptoms of Pulmonary emboli and infarction Myocardial emboli and infarction Cerebral vascular emboli and infarction Renal emboli and infarction Mesenteric emboli and infarction If embolism and infarction occur, administer anticoagulation therapy as ordered SEE STANDARD: *Embolic phenomena*
■ Ischemic injury to spinal cord may occur, particularly during repair of *transverse, descending thoracic aneurysms* and dissecting thoracic aneurysms	■ Spinal function and associated neuromuscular, autonomic, genitourinary function within normal limits Absence of paralysis	■ Monitor for Impaired sensation Weakness Neuromuscular abnormalities Complete hemiplegia, paraplegia If problem occurs Evaluate for neuromuscular abnormalities, alterations in sensation q1-2 hr Reposition patient at least q2 hr Provide for skin care q2-4 hr Provide for adequate nutrition
■ Acid-base, electrolyte imbalances, including Metabolic alkalosis related to Upper GI tract fluid losses (NG tube) Hyperaldosteronism associated with Use of diuretics Hypovolemia Hyponatremia (use of intravenous fluids low in Na^+) Hypokalemia Hypochloremia Blood administration Citrate metabolized to bicarbonate, appearing several hours after administration Electrolyte imbalance, particularly hyponatremia, hypokalemia Respiratory acidosis, alkalosis	■ Acid-base balance within normal limits Electrolyte levels within normal limits	■ Prevent by Administering fluids, as ordered, based on fluid losses and consideration for variables that increase or decrease fluid requirements Administering electrolyte supplements as ordered based on losses in urine, stool, and drainage and on serum electrolyte levels Avoiding vigorous diuretic administration; if a brisk diuresis is necessary, administer careful electrolyte replacement as ordered Monitor Intake and output records for imbalances Serum and urine electrolyte levels For symptoms of fatigue, drowsiness, headaches, apathy, inattentiveness, restlessness, confusion, weakness Serial arterial blood gas levels for acid-base imbalance For respiratory acidosis/alkalosis by monitoring Pa_{CO_2} levels Vital signs q1-2 hr until stable Notify physician for abnormalities If problem occurs Monitor arterial blood gas levels q1-2 hr until stable Vital signs q1-2 hr until stable If electrolyte imbalance occurs Administer electrolytes as ordered Monitor for alleviation of signs/symptoms of electrolyte imbalance If respiratory acidosis occurs Administer therapy as ordered to increase alveolar ventilation Monitor arterial blood gas results q1-2 hr until stable for a decrease in Pa_{CO_2} levels to within patient's normal limits If respiratory alkalosis occurs Administer therapy to correct etiological factors as ordered Monitor arterial blood gas results q1-2 hr until stable for an increase in Pa_{CO_2} levels to within patient's normal limits If acid-base imbalance occurs and is related to the use of a certain diuretic, alter diuretic regimen as ordered

Potential problems	Expected outcomes	Nursing activities
■ Insufficient knowledge for compliance with discharge regimen*	■ Before discharge Patient/family verbalizes knowledge of discharge regimen, including precautions, medications, diet, and activity Patient/family is able to describe follow-up plan, including where and when to go, who to see, and what specimens to bring Patient/family accurately describes signs and symptoms requiring medical attention	■ Assess patient/family's understanding of discharge regimen, including dietary regimen, medications, activity modifications, and special precautionary measures Describe discharge regimen, including Medications—purpose, identification of, route, dosage, timing, frequency, and potential adverse effects Dietary regimen Activity progression; position modifications Avoidance of constricting clothing Avoidance of one position being maintained for more than 1 hour Monitoring circulation to affected extremity Instruct patient/family in specific measures according to residual impaired organ circulation and associated dysfunction Describe signs and symptoms requiring medical attention, depending on site of original aneurysm and outcome of surgery Discuss plan for follow-up visits with patient/family, including where and when to go, who to see, and what specimens to bring Provide opportunity for and encourage patient/family's questions and verbalization of anxiety regarding discharge regimen

*If critical care nurse is responsible for this type of follow-up care.

23 □ Embolic phenomena

An embolus has been defined as "a detached intravascular mass (solid or gaseous) that is carried by the blood to a site distant from its point of origin. Inevitably these lodge in vessels too small to permit their further passage, resulting in partial or complete occlusion of the vessel."*

An embolus may travel in either the venous or the arterial system. In rare cases an embolus may originate on the venous side but pass through a septal defect in the heart and become arterial (paradoxical embolus). Usually venous emboli that become clinically significant are lodged in the pulmonary circulation, causing varying degrees of respiratory compromise. Arterial emboli are more unpredictable in their ultimate destination, and because they potentially can obstruct a significant percentage of blood flow to one of several end organs (brain, kidney, bowel), their effects are usually more devastating.

Emboli may be composed of blood clots (thrombi), fat, air, calcium, amniotic fluid, fragments of tumors, and infected and foreign materials that enter the bloodstream and lodge in various end organs.

Thrombi are formed intravascularly by blood cells, platelets, and fibrin. They are the most common source of embolic phenomena. Factors predisposing the formation of thrombi include stasis of blood flow, injury to a blood vessel lining (e.g., sepsis, trauma), and a hypercoagulable state. The latter occurs in cancer patients, postoperative patients, and those suffering from chronic, debilitating diseases.

Fat emboli result from the release of fatty aggregates into the vascular system, the most common source of these being bone marrow in the setting of a fracture or operative procedure. Fat emboli travel until they reach a capillary bed, frequently in the lungs, where a reactive inflammatory process causes interstitial edema. A large embolus or shower of microemboli is capable of causing severe respiratory insufficiency.

Air emboli are usually introduced into the vascular system through catheters that have been inadvertently left open to air. Large amounts of air (1 cc/kg) are required intravenously before significant clinical findings become evident. A situation capable of producing such an effect is that in which a deep inspiration takes place in the presence of a large bore central venous catheter left open to air. The negative intrathoracic pressure may pull a bolus of air into the line, which can enter the venous circulation, flow to the lungs, and compromise pulmonary circulation in that area.

Arterial air emboli, on the other hand, require much less volume for disastrous effects. Air may be delivered into the arterial system at the beginning or end of CPB or hemodialysis or through various arterial monitoring lines.

Other less common sources of emboli include calcium from damaged heart valves, which may be released during surgical resection. Septic emboli originate from a nidus of intravascular infection such as a vegetation on a heart valve or an infected thrombus.

Amniotic emboli are contents of the amniotic sac that are forced into the systemic circulation by contractions during abortion or normal delivery. This sort of embolus is especially dangerous because of the intense systemic reaction that may result (i.e., shock, disseminated intravascular coagulation [DIC]).

Consideration of predisposing factors and careful attention to historical detail are important in formulating a diagnosis of embolic phenomena. Physical findings will vary, depending on the arterial or venous origin of the embolus and the organ systems involved. The significance of lab tests will likewise be determined by the location of the presumed embolus.

Therapeutic goals for embolic phenomena are the restoration of blood flow to affected systems and the prevention of further embolic events by removing or suppressing the source. In the case of thromboemboli, anticoagulation has been shown to effectively control the recurrence of such problems. Arterial emboli and large pulmonary emboli are often surgically removed in addition to their source being located and appropriately dealt with.

ASSESSMENT

1. History, presence, and nature of
   a. Physiological factors that predispose patient to the formation of blood clots, including
      (1) Stasis of blood flow as in prolonged immobility
      (2) Injury to a vessel lining as in trauma or sepsis

---

*From Robbins, S. L.: Pathologic basis of disease, Philadelphia, 1974, W. B. Saunders Co., pp. 334-335.

(3) Hypercoagulable state as in some cancers and in the immediate postoperative period following major surgery

(4) Obesity

b. Physiological factors that predispose patient to the formation of fat emboli

(1) Recent trauma to long bones, ribs (e.g., thoracic surgery, fracture), sternum (e.g., thoracic surgery)

(2) Metabolic/hematological abnormalities such as

(a) Diabetes, pancreatitis

(b) Severe infections, burns

(c) Carcinoma

(d) Leukemia, blood dyscrasias, sickle cell disease

c. Physiological factors that predispose patient to the formation of an air embolism

(1) Atrial, pulmonary artery, and/or central venous lines

(2) Hemodialysis therapy

(3) Recent cardiac surgery

d. Physiological factors that predispose patient to the formation of calcium emboli, including

(1) Recent cardiac surgery for valvular replacement

(2) Fracture or trauma of long bones, sternum, ribs

e. Physiological factors that predispose patient to the formation of septic emboli, including

(1) Any kind of infection, particularly systemic infection

(2) Local infections such as vegetations on heart valves

f. Physiological factors that predispose patient to the formation of amniotic fluid emboli, including

(1) Pregnancy, delivery

(2) Recent abortion

g. Presence of any kind of tumor that predisposes patient to emboli made of tumor fragments and also to hypercoagulability

2. Presence, nature, and extent of characteristic signs and symptoms of emboli (see more specific description in standard that follows) according to type and location

a. General restlessness, anxiety, dizziness

b. Fever

c. Respiratory distress

d. Signs and symptoms of hypoxia

e. Hemodynamic instability

f. Altered mental status concurrent with unilateral weakness, aphasia, fainting, and/or incontinence

g. Lower back pain with hematuria; note oliguria and/or pyuria

h. Lower abdominal discomfort; pain with bloody diarrhea

i. Pain in left upper quadrant of abdomen radiating to left shoulder; pleural friction rub

3. Results of lab and diagnostic tests, including

a. Doppler studies

b. Venograms, arteriograms

c. Scans (e.g., lung)

d. WBC count; ESR

e. Renal function tests

f. Myocardial enzyme levels

g. ECG

h. Arterial blood gas levels

i. Radiograph (e.g., chest)

4. Level of anxiety related to disease process, hospitalization, anticipated therapy, anticipated diagnostic procedures, altered family roles, and other factors

5. Patient/family's understanding of purpose of hospitalization, therapy planned, and, if appropriate, anticipated surgery, expected outcome, and perioperative experiences

GOALS

1. Reduction in patient/family's anxiety with provision of information, explanations, and encouragement

2. Absence or resolution of emboli

3. Resolution of organ dysfunction manifested by indices of organ function within normal limits

4. Hemodynamic stability

5. Absence or resolution of arrhythmias

6. Before discharge patient/family is able to

a. Accurately describe activity, dietary, and medication regimen

b. Identify signs and symptoms requiring medical attention

c. Accurately describe plan for follow-up care

Potential problems	Expected outcomes	Nursing activities
■ Patient/family's anxiety related to Hospitalization Disease process Therapeutic regimen Diagnostic procedures	■ Reduction in anxiety with provision of information, explanations, and encouragement	■ Assess level of patient/family's anxiety Assess level of understanding regarding disease process, therapy employed, and diagnostic procedures planned Explain relationship of disease process and rationale for various therapeutic interventions Explain in simple terms the diagnostic procedures anticipated and what the patient will experience Assist in preparation of patient for diagnostic procedures Provide opportunity for and encourage questions, verbalization of fears Assess reduction in patient/family's level of anxiety
■ Thromboemboli formation	■ Absence of/or resolution of embolus	■ Prevent thromboembolism by Applying antithromboembolic stockings without wrinkles or any tight areas that can cause hemostasis and clot formation; prevent constriction at joint areas by keeping the lower leg stockings 2 inches from the knee joint and ending the stocking or elastic bandage extending to the upper leg 2 inches below the groin Removing stockings/elastic bandage for 10 to 15 minutes q8 hr to allow for better superficial capillary filling, thereby preventing skin breakdown, and to correct any uneven pressure areas Enhancing lower extremity circulation with passive and active ROM exercises Repositioning patient at least q2 hr Elevating patient's legs with knees straight while patient is out of bed Positioning patient to avoid marked angulation at groin or knee Providing for early ambulation according to patient's toleration, as ordered Prevent injury to vessel lining by preventing local trauma, infection, or sepsis Do not massage or hold the leg muscles tightly Avoid prolonged bed rest Instruct patient not to cross feet at ankles Ambulate patient q1-2 hr unless contraindicated Minimize/prevent hypercoagulability by Discontinuing oral contraceptives and any medication that may cause hypercoagulability as ordered, particularly if surgery is planned Administering prophylactic low-dose heparin, if ordered, in certain high-risk patients, particularly if surgery is planned (persons over 60 years old, those in heart failure, persons with carcinoma or a history of thrombophlebitis and/or embolization) Administer stool softeners if ordered to limit straining at stool that could dislodge thromboemboli
■ Peripheral venous embolism	■ Absence of peripheral venous embolism Adequate peripheral blood flow	■ Monitor for Edema of lower extremity Painful swelling and tenderness on palpation in area of affected vein Pain when foot forcefully dorsiflexed (Homan's sign)

Potential problems	Expected outcomes	Nursing activities
		Palpable hard cordlike vein ("cord")
		Severe cramping of extremity
		Fever
		Results of venogram, if performed
		If any of these abnormalities occur, notify physician
		If peripheral venous embolism occurs
		Administer anticoagulation, using continuous or intermittent doses of sodium heparin during the acute period followed by a sodium warfarin compound in the subacute period as ordered
		Administer an analgesic if needed, as ordered
		Maintain patient on bed rest during acute period
		Keep edematous extremity elevated during acute period
		Avoid squeezing, massaging, or pressure against extremity where peripheral thrombus resides
		Avoid use of pillows
		Avoid gatching knees
		Instruct patient not to cross legs
		Reposition patient q1-2 hr
		Apply moist heat to affected area if ordered
		Use bed cradle over affected extremity
		Administer active and passive ROM exercises to *unaffected* extremities
		Apply antithromboembolic stockings to the unaffected extremity if ordered
		Monitor for mobilization of peripheral venous embolus; particularly note signs/symptoms of pulmonary embolus
■ Peripheral arterial embolism	■ Absence of peripheral arterial emboli Adequate circulation to extremities; color, pulses, skin temperature within normal limits	■ Monitor for
		Signs and symptoms of an arterial embolus and concurrent circulatory insufficiency to extremities, particularly noting tenderness, pain, blanching, decreased capillary filling, coolness, decreased to absent pulses in the affected area, q½-2 hr as needed
		Numbness and tingling
		Note circulation to tip of nose, pinnae of ears, fingers, and toes for infarction of tissue, which can become gangrenous
		Pulses that cannot be easily palpated
		Results of ultrasound (or Doppler) testing or noninvasive electrical impedance plethysmography
		Results of arteriogram, if performed
		Scaling and dryness of skin
		If any of these signs and symptoms occur, notify physician
		If peripheral arterial embolism occurs
		Administer anticoagulation with continuous or intermittent doses of sodium heparin as ordered
		Administer vasodilator medications if ordered
		Keep patient on bed rest during acute period; use of bed cradle; cotton blankets next to patient
		Avoid heating devices to or chilling of lower extremities
		Reposition patient q½-1 hr
		Avoid any one position for long periods of time
		Avoid raising lower extremity above level of heart
		Active and/or passive ROM exercises to extremities q2-4 hr unless contraindicated
		Apply antithromboembolic stockings to the unaffected extremity, if ordered
		Prepare patient for surgical removal of embolism, if planned

Potential problems	**Expected outcomes**	**Nursing activities**
		For cleansing use small amount of mild soap, rinse well, and dry gently but thoroughly; avoid vigorous rubbing; apply lanolin-base lotions; do not permit skin to remain wet
		Administer analgesic if needed, as ordered
		In the subacute period for both peripheral venous and arterial embolism
		Ambulation should start gradually, such as with a short walk q1-2 hr
		Legs should be elevated periodically throughout day, such as for 10 minutes q1-2 hr
		Remaining in one position for long periods (more than 1 to 2 hours) should be avoided
		Calf muscles should be periodically flexed when patient is sitting
		Apply antithromboembolic stockings
		Avoid extremes of temperature; keep extremities comfortably warm
		Patient should avoid
		Constricting clothing, including girdles, garter belts
		Leg crossing
		Smoking
		Rubbing, massaging legs

■ Pulmonary emboli with associated
Respiratory insufficiency
Hypoxia resulting from
Significant intrapulmonary shunting
Dyspnea associated with bronchoconstriction resulting from regional ischemia, pain, and anxiety
Exacerbation of pulmonary embolus, infarction
50% to 60% of the cross-sectional area of a major pulmonary artery must be occluded before significant cardiorespiratory symptoms are apparent
Signs and symptoms vary according to the size of the embolism and the patient's unique response
A small embolism may cause a mild tachycardia, mild dyspnea, unexplained wheezing, cough, tachypnea, and a mild temperature elevation
	■ Absence of or resolution of signs, symptoms of pulmonary embolus
	Adequate oxygenation and ventilation with Pa_{O_2} and Pa_{CO_2} levels within normal limits
	Respirations without distress; respiratory rate within normal limits
	Clear chest radiograph without atelectasis, pleural effusion, cardiac enlargement
	Cardiopulmonary stability
		■ Prevent by employing prophylactic measures to prevent emboli formation (see Problem, Peripheral venous embolism)
		Monitor for
		Restlessness, anxiety, fever, dizziness, faintness, or any unusual sensation in chest
		Respiratory distress: dyspnea, tachypnea, pleural and/or substernal pain that may be sharp or stabbing in nature; auscultation may reveal a pleural rub over the infarcted tissue, rales, wheezing with bronchoconstriction, pleural effusion, accentuation of the pulmonary component of the second heart sound
		Arterial blood gas levels for hypoxemia, hypercapnia or hypocapnia
		Signs of hypoxia: tachypnea, air hunger, anxiety, dyspnea, tachycardia, hypertension or hypotension
		Cardiovascular instability
		  Arrhythmias
		  Hypertension
		  Signs of reduced cardiac output—hypotension, tachycardia, angina, oliguria, peripheral vasoconstriction, and signs of venous congestion—jugular venous distention, elevated CVP measurements, presacral and peripheral edema
		ECG changes, including tall, peaked P waves in leads II, III, and a right atrial and ventricular strain pattern, right QRS axis shift, S-T segment and T wave changes in a massive pulmonary embolism; auscultation may reveal a right ventricular gallop rhythm, a systolic murmur, and a widely split S_2
		Lactic dehydrogenase, transaminase, and bilirubin levels; note elevation without concurrent serum glutamic-oxaloacetic transaminase elevation

Potential problems	Expected outcomes	Nursing activities

A moderate size embolism often presents with pleuritic chest pain, dyspnea, tachypnea; arterial blood gas analysis reveals hypoxemia and hypocapnia; cardiac compromise may result from a sympathetically induced tachycardia and from pulmonary hypertension (associated with local pulmonary vasoconstriction)

A massive embolism may produce marked dyspnea, air hunger, a feeling of impending doom, and occasionally hemoptysis, a marked tachycardia and hypotension and may progress to cardiovascular collapse

Serial chest radiograph results, particularly noting consolidation, atelectasis, dilated pulmonary arteries with decreased distal vascular markings, pleural effusions, elevated diaphragm, cardiac enlargements with a prominent right atrial border and/or right ventricular dilatation, a dilated superior vena cava

Results of arteriogram and/or lung scan if performed; prepare patient for these tests

Notify physician for any clinical abnormality

If pulmonary embolism occurs

Assess nature, severity of signs and symptoms

Administer therapy to attenuate the signs and symptoms (particularly chest pain, hypoxia) as ordered

Pain medication (e.g., morphine sulfate)

O$_2$ supplements

Chest physiotherapy

1. Monitor breath sounds q1-2 hr, noting decreased or absent sounds or the presence of rales, rhonchi, or wheezing
2. Monitor chest radiograph results for areas of consolidation; emphasize gentle chest physiotherapy to affected areas

A bronchodilator if ordered

Mechanical ventilation with PEEP, which may be necessary for adequate gas exchange

Position patient for comfort and to ensure optimal diaphragmatic excursion

Provide for psychological support

Monitor patient's progress, and institute therapy as ordered

Monitor

Serial chest radiograph results for resolution

Serial arterial blood gas results for adequate oxygenation, ventilation

For arrhythmias associated with pulmonary embolism; if significant incidence occurs, notify physician; provide for continuous monitoring of the ECG using cardiac monitor

For amelioration of dyspnea, pain, and anxiety with therapy

Administer anticoagulation therapy if ordered

Prepare patient for surgery if ordered, which may include

Surgical embolectomy, which is reserved for patients who achieve inadequate relief of signs and symptoms with medical therapy or when the embolus is very large, resulting in acute cardiopulmonary compromise

Insertion of a vena caval umbrella to trap emboli from the lower extremities

Plication of the large vein that is the source of recurrent emboli

■ Coronary embolus, MI

■ Absence of MI
Cardiac output within normal limits

■ Monitor for severe, crushing precordial or substernal chest pain (unrelated to movement); ECG changes—S-T elevation, followed by T wave inversion and finally Q waves; arrhythmias; hypotension and tachycardia; diaphoresis; cold, clammy skin; restlessness; anxiety; shortness of breath; faintness; indigestion; and elevated cardiac enzyme levels

If problem occurs, see Standard: *Acute myocardial infarction*

Potential problems	Expected outcomes	Nursing activities
■ Cerebral embolus, cerebrovascular infarct	■ Absence of cerebral embolus, infarct Mental status remains clear; patient oriented to time, place, and people	■ Monitor for Sudden dizziness Altered mental status progressing to coma, aphasia, dysphasia, seizures, unilateral weakness, paralysis, ptosis of eyelids, nystagmus, visual loss, ptosis of mouth, incontinence with concurrent elevated BP and bradycardia Notify physician for any of these abnormalities If problem occurs, institute therapy as ordered
■ Renal artery embolism, renal infarct	■ Absence of renal artery embolus, renal infarct Indices of renal function within normal limits	■ Monitor for costovertebral angle back pain, lower back pain, persistent hematuria, pyuria and/or oliguria, edema, and lab values indicating impaired renal function, embolism/infarction Monitor intake and output, for electrolyte imbalance and for acid-base imbalance very closely Notify physician of abnormalities Administer supportive therapy as ordered If renal failure occurs, see Standard: *Acute renal failure*
■ Mesenteric artery thrombosis, embolus; infarction of part of intestine	■ Absence of mesenteric artery thrombosis, embolus, or infarction of intestine Bowel function within normal limits	■ Monitor For fever and lower abdominal discomfort Pain and bloody diarrhea For shock—pallor, diaphoresis, cold and clammy extremities, tachycardia, hypotension Lab results including elevated WBC count, ESR, and lactic dehyrogenase Notify physician for any of these abnormalities If problem occurs Administer supportive therapy as ordered Prepare patient for arteriography and/or surgery if planned
■ Splenic artery thrombosis, embolus; splenic infarction	■ Absence of splenic artery thrombosis, embolus, and splenic infarction Splenic function, particularly regarding RBC destruction, within normal limits	■ Monitor for Signs and symptoms of a splenic infarction, including pain in the left upper quadrant of abdomen, which may radiate to left shoulder, and a pleural friction rub Lab values indicating an elevated WBC count or ESR; anemia Notify physician if any of these abnormalities occur Administer supportive therapy as ordered; prepare patient for arteriography and/or surgery if ordered

■ Fat embolism, including a diffuse shower of fat microemboli to various end organs; is commonly associated with
Trauma, particularly in presence of long bone fracture; signs and symptoms of diffuse shower of fat emboli occur 24 to 48 hours after traumatic injury
Infections such as
Osteomyelitis
Septicemia
Metabolic abnormalities such as
Diabetes
Acute pancreatitis
Alcoholism
	■ Absence of or resolution of fat emboli
	Respiratory, neurological, renal function within normal limits
	Absence of petechiae
		■ Carefully assess the patient's baseline
		Respiratory status, then repeat serially; note rate and ease of respirations
		Neurological status; level of consciousness
		Renal status—urine volume, specific gravity; a test for the presence of fat in urine may be ordered
		Prevent by
		Immobilizing fractures
		Monitoring for and administering therapy to prevent fluid and blood loss, dehydration, hypovolemia, and hemoconcentration
		Monitor for
		Signs and symptoms of fat embolism, particularly in patients with long bone fractures; signs and symptoms are primarily the result of diffuse shower of fat microemboli resulting in local circulatory insufficiency
		Signs and symptoms of fat emboli in the following organ systems
		Pulmonary
		  1. Dyspnea, tachypnea, signs of hypoxia, duskiness, bubbling rales
		  2. Chest radiograph often reveals diffuse haziness, in-

Potential problems	Expected outcomes	Nursing activities

Potential problems

Burns
Anesthesia
CPB
Fat emboli and petechiae impair microcirculatory flow, resulting in tissue hypoxia, anoxia, and hemorrhagic infarcts

Nursing activities

terstitial edema (inflammatory response to fat microemboli)
3. Arterial blood gas results may reveal hypoxemia
4. Signs of a sympathetic response to the hypoxia, particularly tachycardia
Cerebral: sudden development of urinary incontinence, abusiveness, restlessness, disorientation, irritability, delirium; occasionally neuromuscular dysfunction (e.g., twitching) and even convulsion and coma may occur
NOTE: Craniocerebral trauma should be ruled out in a trauma victim; compared to trauma, the cerebral fat embolism syndrome has a long lucid interval (18 to 24 hours), and when it does develop, confusion is more severe, deterioration is more rapid, and localizing signs are usually absent
Skin
1. Cyanosis
2. Petechiae (caused by endothelial damage of skin capillaries and/or thrombocytopenia); seen often on chest, upper arms, base of neck, in the axilla, and in the conjunctiva
Renal
1. Hematuria
2. Oliguria
Intestinal
1. Diarrhea
2. Abdominal discomfort
Gastric: hematemesis
Low-grade fever
Lab results indicating
Decreased Hgb, platelet levels
Free fat in urine; impaired kidney function
Fat globules in sputum
Elevated serum lipase level
Notify physician for any of these abnormalities
If fat embolism occurs, administer therapy as ordered, which may include
Humidified O_2
Chest physiotherapy q2-4 hr
Repositioning patient q1-2 hr
Intubation with mechanical ventilation
See Standard: *Mechanical ventilation*
PEEP may be required during mechanical ventilation; see Standard: *Positive end expiratory pressure*
Diuretics (osmotic diuretics for cerebral emboli)
Fluids to prevent hemoconcentration, shock, decreased capillary blood flow
Anticoagulation (usually sodium heparin) in intermittent doses or as a continuous infusion, as soon as fat embolic process is highly suspected, if ordered
Heparin if ordered; monitor for signs of bleeding, particularly in the trauma patient (observe and test skin, urine, sputum, emesis, feces for presence of blood)
Corticosteroids, if ordered, with a concurrent antacid or H_2 antagonist
Low molecular weight dextran if ordered; monitor closely for signs of fluid overload, CHF, pulmonary edema, and impaired renal function (oliguria)

Potential problems	Expected outcomes	Nursing activities

		Lytic enzymes and antibiotics if ordered
		Monitor
		  Arterial blood gas results for resolving hypoxemia, hypercapnia or hypocapnia, and acidosis
		  Chest radiograph results for resolution of pulmonary emboli and areas of atelectasis

■ Air embolus, which may be related to air entry through an arterial line, left atrial line, hemodialysis tubing	■ Absence of air in any line entering patient
	Absence of or resolution of large embolus in the heart or lungs or smaller air emboli in the coronary, pulmonary, carotid, renal, mesenteric, or peripheral arteries
	Absence of signs and symptoms of circulatory insufficiency and impaired function of the end organs
		■ Prevent by
		  Inserting lines into large central veins with patient in Trendelenburg position (if patient can tolerate this position)
		  Avoiding air entry while making connections in all tubings going to patient and in drawing blood samples
		  Ensuring the absence of air in fluid bag and tubing of all pressurized fluid infusions
		Monitor for
		  Air in tubings going to patient
		  Signs of ischemic tissue distal to arterial embolus
		  An arterial embolus in the cardiopulmonary system, manifested by hemodynamic instability
		  An arterial embolus in the brain; signs and symptoms may be similar to a stroke
		If venous air embolus is suspected, monitor BP, P, and level of consciousness
		If large venous air embolus is suspected
		  Immediately place patient in the left lateral position, with the head of the bed lowered; the head of the bed and the patient should not be elevated for any reason for 24 to 48 hours or as ordered; this position helps to keep the air in the right atrium, allows adequate pulmonary artery blood flow, and prevents the air from entering the cerebral circulation
		  Monitor pulmonary status closely; air may move into pulmonary artery, seriously impairing blood flow, oxygenation, and hemodynamic stability
		  Monitor serial arterial blood gas levels frequently during the acute period
		  If the aforementioned measures fail, assist in an emergency thoracotomy or direct needle aspiration in the right atrium if either of these procedures becomes necessary

■ Recurrent embolization	■ Absence of recurrent emboli
	Resolution of existent emboli
		■ Implement prescribed therapy to prevent further embolization
		Anticoagulants
		  Administer heparin intravenously, if ordered, either as a continuous drip or by intermittent IV or subcutaneous injections; a continuous intravenous infusion provides a consistent anticoagulant effect with a steady blood level; if subcutaneous heparin injections are given, do not massage injection site
		  Monitor site for hematoma formation
		  Doses are determined by APTT; monitor these levels
		  Administer warfarin, if ordered, for long-term anticoagulation; doses are determined by PT and clotting times (maintaining them at approximately 1½ to 2½ times the control values)
		  Anticoagulants are usually continued until the lung scan demonstrates further improvement and evidence of deep vein thrombosis subsides
		  For medications that the patient is receiving that enhance or diminish the activity of warfarin
		    Monitor chart for results of coagulation studies
		    Closely monitor patient for internal/external bleeding

Potential problems	Expected outcomes	Nursing activities

		If bleeding occurs
		  Protamine sulfate may be ordered to reverse the effects of heparin
		  Vitamin K may be ordered to block the action of warfarin
		Administer antiplatelet medications if ordered, which may include aspirin, dipyridamole (Persantine), or dextran
		Administer proteolytic enzymes if ordered
		Monitor for further thrombophlebitis; serially test legs for Homan's sign, pain, swelling, tenderness, erythema of extremity
		Monitor for recurrent thrombosis of or embolization to the pulmonary, cerebral, coronary, mesenteric, renal, or peripheral arteries
		Prepare patient for serial radiographs, scans as ordered
		Surgical therapy may be accomplished for
		  Large pulmonary emboli
		    Prepare patient for emergency surgery for removal of a large pulmonary embolus
		    This is usually reserved for patients with an associated significant reduction in cardiac output and hypoxemia
		  Recurrent emboli
		    Partial venous interruption of the vena cava, using an umbrella to filter out large emboli; this is usually reserved for patients in whom
		      1. Anticoagulation fails to prevent recurrent emboli or anticoagulation is contraindicated
		      2. Pulmonary emboli are producing severe cardiopulmonary compromise
		      3. Recurrent emboli occur in the presence of septic pelvic thrombophlebitis (as an adjunct to pulmonary embolectomy)
		    Plication of the femoral vein or vena cava, which helps to trap emboli in the femoral venous system; may be done for patients with
		      1. Mesenteric thrombi, emboli, and associated infarction of intestine
		      2. Splenic emboli, infarction
		      3. Renal artery emboli, infarction
		      4. Pulmonary emboli

■ Hemodynamic instability, which may be related to
  Hypotension, inadequate fluid replacement
  Hemorrhage
  Heart failure
  Arrhythmias
	■ Hemodynamic stability; BP, P within normal limits; other indices of adequate cardiac output within normal limits
	Absence or resolution of arrhythmias
		■ Prevent by administering fluids and blood products as ordered to maintain hemodynamic stability and adequate cardiac output
		Prevent arrhythmias by providing for
		  Adequate oxygenation
		  Pain relief
		  Comfort
		  Psychological support
		Monitor (q1 hr and prn until stable)
		  BP
		  Pulses for rate, quality
		  ECG—continuously if possible; if arrhythmias occur, note perfusion of and overall hemodynamic effect
		  CVP and PAP if available
		  For jugular venous distention
		  Urine output with specific gravity
		  Color for signs of reduced peripheral circulation
		  Mentation
		  Hgb, Hct levels

Potential problems	Expected outcomes	Nursing activities
		Coagulation studies
		Weight
		Notify physician for any clinical abnormalities
		If hypotension occurs
		Administer fluids as ordered, closely monitoring patient's hemodynamic response
		Administer an inotropic agent, if ordered, to increase the cardiac output of a compromised heart
		If hemorrhage occurs, monitor serial Hgb and Hct levels and administer blood and blood products as ordered
		If heart failure occurs, see Standard: *Heart failure*
		If arrhythmias occur, see Standard: *Arrhythmias*

■ Insufficient knowledge to comply with discharge regimen*	■ Before discharge patient/family is able to
	Describe regimen for medications
	Identify several precautionary measures to avoid bruising, inadvertent bleeding
	Describe exercises, accurately perform them, and describe precautions in activities
	Describe precautionary measures for specific discharge medications
	Describe several signs, symptoms requiring medical follow-up
		■ Assess patient/family's understanding of discharge regimen
		Instruct the patient/family in the following
		   Leg exercises that are designed to decrease venous stasis and enhance circulation
		   Medications, including their identification, route, dose, frequency, timing, and potential adverse effects
		   If warfarin sodium is ordered, take it at the same time every day
		   Not to take over-the-counter medications without consulting physician first
		   Foods that are high in vitamin K should be omitted altogether or eaten in a regular, consistent pattern (particularly yellow and green leafy vegetables); a list of these foods should be shared with patient/family
		   To tell dentist or any other doctor that he/she is receiving an anticoagulant medication
		   To report diarrhea, vomiting, or any febrile illness, which may indicate coagulation testing and require a temporary increment in the warfarin sodium dosage; review potential signs and symptoms requiring medical attention
		   To avoid bruises or falls and active "contact" activities
		   To report bruises that enlarge, cuts that do not stop bleeding, red or brown urine, red or dark brown stool, a nosebleed that does not stop with moderate pressure, flank or abdominal pain, headaches, unusual joint pain
		   When skin is cut, to apply direct pressure and maintain for several minutes until clotting occurs
		   Helpful guidelines to avoid accidents, including
		      Wearing gloves while gardening
		      Using electric shaver
		      Using soft bristle toothbrush (avoid using a Water Pik)
		      Using nonslip mat in bathtub
		      Avoiding use of oil in bath water
		      Hazards of going barefoot
		      Avoiding use of power tools, particularly those with blades
		   To avoid the following
		      Remaining in one position for a long time
		      Constricting clothing such as girdles, garter belts
		      Massaging or rubbing legs
		      Extremes of hot or cold; extremities should be kept dry and warm
		      Smoking
		   Patient should wear a medical alert bracelet and carry a card with

*If responsibility of critical care nurse includes such follow-up care.

Potential problems	Expected outcomes	Nursing activities
		patient's name, name of drug, and phone number of who to contact in an emergency
		Describe the follow-up plan of care, including when and where to go, who to see, and what specimens to bring; briefly explain the purpose and format of follow-up visits
		Provide opportunity for and encourage patient/family's questions
		Assess potential compliance of patient/family with discharge regimen

NEUROLOGICAL

24 □ Increased intracranial pressure

Intracranial pressure is the pressure exerted by the constituents of the brain, namely, the brain tissue, cerebrospinal fluid (CSF), and intravascular blood, which are contained within the rigid skull. The relationship between the cranial cavity and the contents largely determines the intracranial pressure (ICP). The normal volume ratios of the cranial cavity are brain tissue, 85%; CSF, approximately 10%; and intravascular blood volume, 2% to 11%. The expansion of one volume is at the expense of the other constituents (by subtracting from their volume), and the resulting alterations in volume and pressure eventually affect cerebral functioning and integrity and increase ICP.

ICP normally ranges from 110 to 140 mm H_2O or 0 to 10 mm Hg. Pressures above 200 mg H_2O or 15 mm Hg usually signify increased ICP. Compensatory mechanisms do occur when the volume of any one constituent increases in an effort to protect the brain against damage and interference with cerebral functioning. For instance, the growth of an intracranial mass may initiate a reduction in the volume of CSF and a lesser decrease in intracranial blood volume. As long as these fluids can be displaced, the ICP remains within normal limits. However, eventually a critical point is reached at which no further displacement is possible, and the ICP rises.

For adequate cerebral functioning a continual and effective blood supply, circulation, and perfusion are necessary. Cerebral blood flow is equal to the mean arterial pressure minus the intracranial pressure (Cerebral blood flow = MAP − ICP). Other factors such as vascular resistance and venous flow also affect the flow. The term *cerebral perfusion pressure (PP)* may also be used to determine the status of the cerebral circulation. Under normal conditions PP in cerebral vessels is approximately equal to the MAP. Any increase in intracranial pressure must be subtracted from the MAP in determining the effective PP; the resulting decrease in PP reduces cerebral blood flow. Cerebral blood flow ceases when ICP equals cerebral PP.

Two major problems associated with increased ICP are the nonuniform expansion of the brain and the interference with adequate blood supply. If the increased ICP significantly lowers the effective PP, resulting in decreased cerebral blood flow, two compensatory mechanisms are activated. In *autoregulation,* the cerebral vasculature compensates by altering vascular resistance through controlled vasodilation to maintain cerebral blood flow by decreasing arterial resistance. If ineffective, the further decrease in PP and cerebral blood flow causes Cushing's phenomenon to occur, possibly as a result of brain stem ischemia. In *vasomotor control,* the smooth muscle responds to altered arterial pressures of oxygen and, particularly, carbon dioxide. The CNS ischemic response produces a marked rise in systemic arterial pressure. Vasodilation also occurs in an attempt to improve cerebral blood flow. The prognosis of increased ICP can become worse if there is a complete loss of autoregulation or the development of vasoparalysis and cerebral edema. If ICP continues to increase and cannot be controlled or treated, the progression of cerebral pathology may culminate in herniation and irreversible brain damage or death.

Many processes can lead to or cause increased ICP. Among these are head trauma; brain tumors; cerebral hemorrhages, infarcts, infections, and abscesses; CSF overproduction, flow obstruction, or impaired absorption; metabolic disturbances; and toxic factors such as poisons and lead ingestion. The extent and progression of increased ICP and cerebral damage incurred vary with each individual. Some of the factors contributing to this variability include cerebral areas involved, preinsult functioning of cerebral tissue and circulation, effectiveness of collateral circulation, time period of increasing ICP (slow increase versus sudden pressure rise), effectiveness of compensatory mechanisms, amount and distribution of increased pressure and compression, and selective vulnerability of certain areas in the brain. The classical triad of symptomatology associated with increased ICP is headache, vomiting (with or without nausea), and papilledema. However, symptomatology may be varied, ranging from a single symptom to a myriad of symptoms. Many authorities propose that frequently the intracranial pressure has increased well above normal levels before clinical symptoms are evident. The advent of intracranial monitoring hopefully will improve the diagnosis of increased ICP and aid in early therapy to prevent cerebral damage.

ASSESSMENT

1. Onset, progression, duration, frequency, and specific description of neurological symptoms, including
   a. Headache: location, severity, association with specific activity/movement, time-related occurrence, any associated concurrent neurological symptoms
   b. Vomiting (with or without nausea), any projectile emesis, precipitating factors or associated symptoms, time-related patterns
   c. Papilledema; visual disturbances including diplopia, nystagmus, blurred vision, ocular palsies or impairments, pupillary changes
   d. Ataxia (severity, locality)
   e. Changes in behavior, including inattentiveness, irritability, personality changes, hallucinations
   f. Changes in level of consciousness (LOC) including forgetfulness, memory impairment, disorientation, confusion, sleepiness, or lethargy
   g. Motor/sensory dysfunctions
   h. Alterations in communication abilities
   i. Seizures
2. Previous head trauma incident; specific description of event, treatment, clinical course
3. Previous infection, particularly meningitis/encephalitis
4. Previous ingestion of poisons, toxins, or drug overdose
5. Previous symptomatology/treatment for increased ICP; neurological treatment or neurosurgical procedure
6. Medications taken for neurological status, including anticonvulsants, steroids, pain medications; effects and side effects of therapies
7. Presence of excessive thirst or urination
8. Presence of any medical problems and medications/treatments prescribed and followed
9. Patient's perceptions and reaction to diagnosis, therapeutic modalities and anticipated surgical intervention if planned
10. Presence of any alterations in body image; fears of permanent disability or deficit; altered roles in family, normal occupation, activities of daily living (ADL)
11. Baseline parameters status
    a. Neurological
    b. Respiratory
    c. Cardiovascular
    d. Metabolic
    e. Hydration
    f. Fluid/electrolyte
    g. Skin integument (rash, ecchymosis, open areas, edema)
    h. Urine output pattern
    i. Vital signs
    j. Weight
    k. Handedness (right or left)
12. Diagnostic test results, including
    a. Skull films
    b. Tomograms
    c. Computerized axial tomography (CAT)
    d. Cerebral angiography
    e. Pneumoencephalogram
    f. Electroencephalogram (EEG)
    g. Brain scan
    h. Lumbar puncture
13. Results of
    a. Serum electrolyte levels
    b. CSF determinations
    c. Urine analysis, culture, specific gravity, osmolality, electrolytes
    d. Arterial blood gases
    e. Clotting profile
    f. Serum anticonvulsant levels
    g. Hgb and Hct, platelet count, WBC count and differentiation
    h. Toxin screens
    i. Chest radiograph
    j. ECG

GOALS

1. Optimal neurological functioning
2. Optimal independence in ADL
3. Adequate alveolar ventilation and perfusion
4. Adequate cardiac output
5. Serum electrolytes and fluid balance within normal limits
6. Hgb and Hct stable and within normal limits
7. Acid-base balance within normal limits
8. Reduction in patient/family's anxiety with provision of information, demonstrations, support

9. Before discharge, patient/family is able to
   a. Describe medication, activity, exercise, and dietary regimens
   b. Describe any treatments/therapeutic measures prescribed
   c. Demonstrate safety measures and techniques; proper use of any equipment/devices prescribed
   d. Describe signs and symptoms requiring medical attention
   e. State necessary information regarding follow-up care

Potential problems	Expected outcomes	Nursing activities
■ Progressive increased ICP related to Further volume expansion Cerebral edema Loss of autoregulation Vasoparalysis Cerebral herniation	■ Absence or control of complications Control or resolution of increased ICP (if possible) Maximal neurological functioning	■ Establish neurological baseline and vital signs on admission; ongoing assessments of status and specific symptomatology/deficit q1 hr; monitor in particular extent and degree of Altered LOC Pupillary changes (size, equality, light reactivity) Motor/sensory system dysfunctions Ocular palsies/impaired extraocular movements Classical triad of increased ICP—headache, vomiting, papilledema Personality changes such as restlessness, irritability Ataxia Diplopia/nystagmus Dysphagia Alterations in communication abilities, speech quality Visual alterations For development of Cushing's phenomenon—increasing systolic BP with widening pulse pressure, decreasing pulse, and change in respiratory pattern In infants (if fontanelles are open, this allows greater area for brain expansion)—increased head circumference, bulging fontanelles, split sutures, irritability, somnolence, high-pitched cry, decreased feeding, sunsetting, nystagmus, vomiting Monitor for precipitating factors that may further increase cerebral edema and ICP such as hypoxia, hypercapnia, fever, hypotension, hypertension, myocardial damage, shock, Valsalva's maneuver; if controllable, institute measures to prevent such as Assist patient with positioning and turning; instruct patient not to hold breath Prevent constipation by establishing bowel regimen as individually warranted Avoid sharp angling of the neck, which can obstruct venous outflow Monitor for any signs/symptoms that could initiate factor development such as hypoventilation, infection, ECG abnormalities Maintain head of bed as ordered; frequently it is elevated to promote venous drainage and aid in decreasing ICP Administer medications/treatments as ordered; monitor effects and side effects; if patient is receiving steroids, monitor for side effects including GI bleeding, glycosuria Monitor and accurately record intake and output as ordered (frequently q1-2 hr); assess for any imbalance Monitor serum electrolytes, arterial blood gas values for any abnormalities Have emergency equipment and medications readily available, including Ventricular tap set and appropriate drill sets Osmotic diuretics

Potential problems	Expected outcomes	Nursing activities
		Notify physician immediately of any
		Change in baseline neurological status whether appearance of new deficit or increasing severity of prior symptomatology such as headache, restlessness, projectile vomiting
		Vital sign abnormality
		Presence/potential precipitating factor occurrence
		Fluid/electrolyte balance abnormality
		Arterial blood gas value abnormality
		Initiate and maintain hypothermia as ordered
		Prepare patient/family for any diagnostic tests/procedures necessary
		Monitor ICP values and waveforms if patient has intracranial monitoring line inserted
		Maintain patency/sterility of system
		Monitor effects of other treatments or therapies on ICP including coughing, turning, suctioning, chest physiotherapy
		Space therapies if possible to minimize increases in ICP
		Monitor neurological status correlated with ICP values and notify physician
		If ordered, assist physician with drainage of amount of CSF fluid to maintain ICP at specific level determined; record fluid amount drained each time; monitor effects on ICP value, correlation between neurological status and CSF drainage
		Hyperventilate patient as ordered by physician for specific ICP level increase
		Administer medications/treatments as ordered; monitor effects/side effects on status and ICP; frequently osmotic diuretics are ordered prn or as ongoing therapy
		Notify physician immediately of any increase in ICP/wave recording; frequently physician will specify maximal ICP levels
		Monitor ventricular drainage system or other external drain if patient has one inserted
		Prevent compression, kinking, pulling, or tension on tubing by proper positioning; if necessary, restrain patient's hands
		Maintain patency/sterility of system
		Maintain at specific level ordered by physician
		Measure and record pressure, amount, and quality of drainage as ordered
		Check dressing q1 hr; monitor for leakage around needle or catheter site, swelling/edema
		If patient is on ICP monitoring, record pressures and drain amount of fluid specified by physician to maintain pressure values
		Monitor neurological status correlated with fluid pressure/quantity
		Administer antibiotics as ordered
		Send CSF specimens as ordered and monitor results
		Monitor serum electrolytes as Na^+ values may decrease from loss of CSF by drainage
		Notify physician of results and replace fluids as ordered (frequently CSF fluid is ordered replaced milliliter for milliliter)
		Notify physician immediately of any change in neurological status; fluid pressure, amount/quality varying from norm specified or expected; nonpatency of system or abnormal lab values

Potential problems	Expected outcomes	Nursing activities
		Monitor for signs of epidural hematoma (potential complication of drain); see Standard: *Head trauma*, Problem Epidural hematoma
		If ordered, clamp tubing as specified by physician, maintaining precise time schedule and recording time, pressure, fluid drainage, amount/quality; notify physician immediately of any change in neurological status or signs of increased ICP; unclamp drain as per physician's standing or stat order
		After removal of ventricular drain by physician, monitor neurological status and vital signs frequently; drain site for bleeding, oozing, drainage/edema; monitor for signs of increased ICP
		See appropriate standard for identified etiology or surgical intervention planned, i.e.,
		Head trauma
		Meningitis/encephalitis
		Supratentorial craniotomy
		Infratentorial craniotomy
		Internalized shunting procedures
■ Presence of neurological signs/symptoms	■ Maximal neurological functioning Absence of complications	■ Establish baseline neurological assessment on admission with specific documentation of status; continue ongoing assessments as ordered; implement care plan based on individual needs/deficit
		Notify physician immediately of any increase in initial deficit, progression, increased severity of symtoms, or symptomatology/deficit appearance
Decreased LOC		Close observation; siderails at all times when patient is alone
		Reorient patient frequently to time, place, and person
		Have family bring familiar pictures, objects for bedside
		Reaffirm to family the relationship between patient's behavior and LOC and neurological condition
		Assess family's level of anxiety related to patient's decreased LOC
		Encourage family's verbalization of fears and concerns
		Support and realistically reassure family
		If patient becomes restless/combative, restrain as ordered by physician if absolutely necessary to protect from injury to self or others
		Explain reasons for restraints to family
		Check restraints frequently for proper placement; monitor effectiveness, skin integrity, and circulation
		Reapply q4 hr and prn
		Remove restraints as soon as possible
		If patient is not moving spontaneously
		Turn and position properly q2 hr
		Apply measures to aid in prevention of complications of immobility, including sheepskin or flotation pads to promote skin integrity maintenance; monitor skin surfaces frequently for signs of impaired circulation; massage skin and pad skin areas prone to irritation
Nausea/vomiting; possible dehydration		Assess frequency/degree, association with other neurological symptoms
		Monitor for any abnormality
		Accurately record intake and output as ordered
		State of hydration
		Presence/quality of gag, cough, swallowing reflexes
		Serum electrolytes
		Hct values

Potential problems	Expected outcomes	Nursing activities
		Administer medications as ordered; monitor effects; notify physician if control of nausea/vomiting is ineffective
		Notify physician if reflexes are decreased or absent
		Keep patient NPO
		Administer intravenous fluids/nasogastric feedings as ordered
		Frequent oral hygiene
Paresis or paralysis of extremity		Assess location/degree of weakness
		ROM exercises as ordered by physician; passive to active dependent on patient's status q2 hr
		Institute measures to prevent complications such as contractures, subluxations, wristdrop/footdrop; may include footboard, splint, sling, handrolls
		Obtain order for physical therapy referral as indicated
		Instruct and supervise patient/family in exercise program when status allows
Impaired sensation of extremity		Assess for nature, location/extent of impaired sensation
		Protect from injury and potential complications including abrasions, decubitus ulcers, burns
		Turn and position patient as necessary q2 hr
		Monitor skin integument q2 hr for any signs of impaired cirlation
		When status allows, assist and supervise patient in necessary safety measures required by deficit such as
		Testing of water temperature by nurse/family
		Avoiding use of heating pads or other temperature devices
Ataxia		Assess location/degree of ataxia
		Assist and supervise patient in ADL and ambulation as necessary
		Apply safety measures such as siderails while patient is in bed, safety belt for wheelchair
		Maintain safe environment
		Remove as many obstacles or objects that might cause falls as possible
		Obtain appropriate safety equipment
		Obtain physician's order for physical therapy referral as warranted
		Explain to patient/family reasons for assistance, special measures to promote safety
Headache		Assess location, degree, duration, and frequency of headache, association with any other neurological symptoms
		Maintain as quiet an environment as possible; prevent unnecessary disturbances
		Administer medication as ordered by physician (narcotics are usually not ordered)
		Monitor effectiveness
		Notify physician if headache persists
■ Fluid and electrolyte imbalance related to Increased ICP producing alterations in normal mechanism of production/release of antidiuretic hormone (ADH) Disruption/imbalances of normal hormonal control mechanism of salt and water balance	■ Fluid and electrolyte balance within normal or prescribed limits	■ Monitor and accurately record intake and output; urine specific gravity, osmolality as ordered (frequently q2 hr)
		Monitor for signs of dehydration or overhydration such as
		Poor skin turgor
		Dry mucous membranes
		Peripheral edema
		Excessive thirst
		Change in LOC
		Monitor for
		Abnormal vital signs, Hgb and Hct values
		Abnormal serum electrolyte/osmolality values, urine electrolyte values
		Weight alterations

Potential problems	Expected outcomes	Nursing activities
Osmotic diuretic medication administration Plasma hyponatremia—causes of hypo-osmolality include water intoxication, excess vasopressin (inappropriate ADH) either from overadministration of vasopressin or inappropriate secretion of ADH from cerebral injury or disease Plasma hypernatremia—causes of hyperosmolality include dehydration without coresponding loss of Na^+, impaired secretion of ADH from cerebral injury or disease		Temperature elevations Insensible fluid losses including respiratory, diaphoresis, secretions Presence/degree of nausea and vomiting; effectiveness of medications ordered Changes in neurological status Monitor for signs of decreased or increased production/release of ADH (or vasopressin) Decreased ADH; monitor for 　Hypernatremia 　Hyperosmolality 　Dehydration 　Diabetes insipidus—polyuria, polydipsia 　Cerebral dysfunction (usually occurs above 160 serum Na^+ level) including irritability, restlessness, hypertonicity, twitching, seizures, and nystagmus Increased ADH (inappropriate ADH); monitor for 　Hyponatremia 　Hypo-osmolality 　Overhydration 　Water retention/intoxication 　Cerebral dysfunction (usually occurs below 130 serum Na^+ level) including lethargy, inattention, slight confusion, nausea/vomiting Administer intravenous fluids, nasogastric feedings as ordered Administer medications as ordered; monitor effects and side effects; if patient is receiving steroids, monitor urine glucose and acetone levels as ordered Notify physician of any fluid imbalance or electrolyte abnormality, signs of cerebral dysfunction from ADH disorders If patient is receiving osmotic diuretics such as mannitol, urea, monitor 　Hourly urine output 　Serum electrolytes frequently for serious imbalances resulting from rapid diuresis of water and electrolytes 　For signs of congestive heart failure 　For dehydration or hypovolemia (may be masked) 　Notify physician of effects of therapy If po is allowed, maintain patient on fluid restriction or encouragement regimen as ordered by physician
■ Respiratory insufficiency related to CNS dysfunction Edema Cranial nerve dysfunction Pneumonia Atelectasis Pulmonary emboli Cerebral dysfunction may decrease or abolish the normal respiratory control mechanisms effected by chemoreceptors in aortic, carotid vessels and in the medulla	■ Patent airway Adequate alveolar ventilation and perfusion Arterial blood gas levels within patient's normal limits	■ Ongoing assessment of respiratory status q1 hr and prn; monitor for any abnormality/decline Respiratory rate, quality, and pattern Patency of upper airway and patient's ability to handle secretions Presence/strength of gag, cough, and swallowing reflexes Cranial nerve functioning, particularly presence/strength of nerves nine to twelve Skin color, nail beds, peripheral pulses, and skin warmth Breath sounds bilaterally for quality of aeration; signs of obstruction (rales, rhonchi) For signs of pulmonary edema (neurogenic may occur related to increased ICP) including tachycardia, dyspnea, wheezing, peripheral edema, weight gains, decreased urinary output Arterial blood gas values Chest radiograph results

Potential problems	Expected outcomes	Nursing activities

If cerebral dysfunction occurs in the brain stem, different respiratory abnormalities result, which may not be adequate to maintain adequate ventilation and perfusion

Area and respiratory pattern

Forebrain: posthyperventilation apnea

Internal capsule and basal ganglia: Cheyne-Stokes respirations

Midbrain: central neurogenic hyperventilation

Pons: apneustic

Medulla: ataxic, loss of automatic breathing

Respiratory acidosis can produce additional cerebral hypoxia and cerebral edema; both systemic hypoxia and hypercapnia can promote increased cerebral blood flow and cause a further increase in ICP by the increased volume of the blood compartment

- Hemodynamic instability

Expected outcomes

- BP, P, within patient's normal or prescribed limits

Nursing activities

Signs/symptoms of thrombophlebitis, pulmonary emboli

Maintain patent airway by

Turning and positioning to prevent obstruction or aspiration of secretions q2 hr and prn

Deep breathing and coughing q1 hr and prn (if allowed)

Suctioning prn

Adequate oxygenation and humidification as ordered

Chest physiotherapy/pulmonary toilet if warranted and not contraindicated by physician's order

If reflexes (gag, cough, swallowing) are decreased or absent, keep patient NPO as ordered by physician; when reflexes are stronger and patient is started on po, stay with patient for initial feedings, monitor swallowing effectiveness, and assess for any signs of choking/nasal regurgitation

Apply antithromboembolic stockings or Ace bandages as ordered; reapply every shift and prn; and monitor for constriction/looseness, condition of skin

Instruct and supervise patient in performing leg exercises and ROM exercises as status and physician's order allow

Increase activity level/progression when allowed

Notify physician immediately of any change in respiratory/neurological status or signs of complication potential/occurrence

If respiratory problem occurs, assist with emergency measures to maintain patent airway and adequate ventilation

Administer medications/treatments as ordered; monitor effects and side effects

Monitor neurological status closely as both hypoventilation/hyperventilation may increase ICP

SEE STANDARD: *Mechanical ventilation*

Explain procedures and reasons for equipment/respiratory assistance to patient/family; provide reassurance and support

Establish alternate means of communication as needed

If embolism occurs, see Standard: *Embolic phenomena*

- Monitor BP as ordered for any variance from minimal or maximal acceptable level specified by physician

Administer medications as ordered to maintain BP level; monitor effects and side effects

Notify physician immediately of BP variance or ineffectiveness of medications

Monitor for

Hypotension—signs of bleeding, falling Hgb levels

Hypertension—signs of Cushing's phenomenon

Alterations in neurological status

Monitor and record pulse rate and quality as ordered; notify physician immediately if patient suddenly develops symptoms of bradycardia

ECG monitoring as warranted

Monitor serum electrolyte values for any abnormalities, particularly in K^+

Administer medications as ordered; monitor effects and side effects

Potential problems	Expected outcomes	Nursing activities
■ Fever related to Infection Disruption in normal temperature regulation by hypothalamus from increased ICP	■ Normal body temperature	■ Prevent precipitating factors such as urinary retention, pulmonary congestion-aspiration Maintain strict sterile technique for procedures such as catheterization, endotracheal/tracheostomy tube care/management Monitor Temperature as ordered and prn for any fever IV sites frequently for any signs of redness, tenderness, phlebitis WBC count (may be falsely elevated if patient is receiving steroids) For possible drug reactions, presence of skin rash For signs of meningitis For alterations in neurological status; fever may increase ICP Notify physician immediately of any temperature elevation/signs of infection Monitor possible infection sources, including urine and sputum cultures, chest radiograph results, CSF determinations Administer medications/treatments as ordered; monitor effects and side effects Maintain hypothermia blanket as ordered; institute measures to prevent complications of therapy; monitor effects and side effects If infection occurs, monitor for resolution or progression If problem occurs, see Standard: *Meningitis/encephalitis*
■ Seizures	■ Absence or control of seizures	■ Prevention of precipitating factors in seizure occurrence including fever, hypoxia, H_2O intoxication, electrolyte disturbances Notify physician of potential/presence of any factors Seizure precautions (if indicated) Padded siderails up at all times when patient is alone Bed height at lowest level Padded tongue blade and airway at bedside Emergency medications and equipment readily available Close observation and supervision Administer anticonvulsant medications as ordered; monitor effects and side effects, serum anticonvulsant levels If seizure occurs, monitor and record seizure activity; notify physician SEE STANDARD: *Seizures*
■ GI bleeding related to CNS factors Stress Steroid administration	■ Absence or resolution of GI bleeding	■ Monitor vital signs q2-4 hr; Hgb and Hct; Hematest of stools three times a week; Hematest of aspirate, emesis, and urine for any abnormalities Obtain order for antacid administration as soon as patient able to take po Monitor for signs of GI bleeding, including abdominal tenderness/distention, hypotension, sudden tachycardia Notify physician immediately if any abnormality occurs If problem occurs, see Standard: *Acute upper gastrointestinal bleeding*
■ Patient/family's anxiety related to Limited understanding of clinical problem, diagnostic procedures, therapeutic measures Threat of continued neurological deficit	■ Patient/family's behavior demonstrates decreased anxiety with provision of information	■ Ongoing assessment of level of anxiety Encourage patient/family's verbalization of questions, fears, concerns Collaborate with physician in providing realistic information and reassurance appropriate to level of understanding Explain relationship between condition and clinical symptoms, status, course Explain reasons/necessity for frequent assessments Explain and prepare patient/family for treatments, diagnostic

Potential problems	Expected outcomes	Nursing activities
		tests/procedures, therapeutic measures, anticipated operative intervention (if planned) Collaborate medical plan of care and nursing care plan if expected prognosis is known If complete recovery is expected, reassure patient/family If partial recovery is expected, support and encourage verbalization of fears, angers, questions; see problem, Continued presence of neurological deficit
■ Continued presence of neurological deficit Patient/family's fears, anxiety, anger related to deficit and possible alterations in lifestyle	■ Maximal neurological functioning* Maximal independence in ADL (within capabilities) Patient/family verbalizes concerns	■ Assess patient's specific neurological deficit Collaborate with physician regarding prognosis, possible degree of recovery Implement individualized plan of care based on patient's needs and deficits Assist as needed in ADL Monitor potential for independent functioning and obtain equipment to maximize function and promote safety Obtain orders for appropriate referrals such as physical, speech, occupational therapy; social service Encourage verbalization of patient/family's fears, anxieties, and other reactions—level and degree Answer questions realistically Encourage their participation in care planning, implementation, evaluation, and decision making Realistically reassure and support patient/family Reinforce any gains or independence patient achieves Plan, instruct, demonstrate, supervise, and evaluate patient/family's demonstration of needed information/skills for maximal independent functioning such as Measures to prevent complications Assistance necessary—type, amount, degree Proper use of therapeutic devices/equipment Monitor level of achievement toward maximizing potentials and independence; means to promote as "normal" a life-style as possible
■ Insufficient knowledge to comply with discharge regimen†	■ Patient/family demonstrates or verbalizes understanding of discharge regimen Patient/family accurately describes medication, activity, and dietary regimens	■ Assess patient/family's level of understanding of neurological problem and therapy received Explain relationship between patient's neurological status and therapies prescribed If present, explain relationship of increased ICP occurrence to head injury, toxin exposure or drug overdose; explore with patient/family measures to prevent recurrence of condition, importance of controlling precipitating factors Instruction of patient/family regarding required information/skills so that before discharge patient/family is able to Describe medication regimen Name and purpose Route, dosage, frequency, times Side effects Special precautions necessary including drugs, foods, beverages contraindicated or regulated in quantity; factors potentiating/decreasing effects or side effects; physical restrictions; safety measures Describe dietary regimen Describe activity regimen, exercise program Describe and demonstrate any special therapeutic measures prescribed

*If responsibility of critical care nurse includes this stage of care.

†If responsibility of critical care nurse includes such follow-up care.

Potential problems	Expected outcomes	Nursing activities
	Patient/family describes means to achieve maximal independence in ADL, promote safety, and prevent complications	Describe and demonstrate proper use of equipment or therapeutic devices Reasons for using Time, method, and duration of use Precautions/safeguards Necessary maintenance (type, frequency) Measures to promote optimal functioning, upkeep/duration
	Patient/family describes signs/symptoms requiring medical attention	Describe signs/symptoms of neurological status requiring medical care
	Patient/family describes follow-up care regimen	Describe plan for follow-up care, including purpose of appointment, when and where to go, who to see, what to expect

25 □ Head trauma

The causes of head trauma are multiple and include motor vehicle accidents, falls, and gunshot and stab wounds. Head injuries may be penetrating or nonpenetrating wounds. Cerebral trauma may result in a wide range of pathology, diversity, and complexity from a mild injury with spontaneous, complete recovery to massive brain injury with irreversible damage culminating in cerebral death. Factors influencing the variable pathological consequences include patient's age and prior status; force, duration, location, and nature of the injury; adequacy of emergency on-the-scene treatment; and functioning of other bodily systems. Common cerebral damage produced by head trauma includes contusions, concussion, skull fractures, epidural hematomas, intracerebral hematomas/hemorrhages, subdural hematomas, cranial nerve injury, and metabolic injury of neurons and brain cells (see Table 3 for specifics of the most frequent pathologies). Brain injury may occur at the time of initial trauma insult or develop days to weeks later.

Priorities of treatment and management of head trauma include maintenance of adequate airway; adequate pulmonary ventilation and perfusion; treatment of shock; prevention/control of metabolic disturbances, which cause cerebral damage that exceeds the direct traumatic effects on neuron functioning; and control of increased ICP and cerebral edema. Cerebral edema is a frequent complication of head injury, possibly due to an alteration in the blood-brain barrier and paralysis of autoregula-

tion. Any patient with head trauma should initially be handled as having a potential cervical cord injury until this is ruled out.

A complete assessment is necessary to establish if there are any other injuries or complicating factors. If multiple trauma is the case, priority focuses on the injury that is most immediately life threatening (see Standard: *Multiple trauma*). Complications of head injury that commonly occur and that must be controlled (especially since they can mimic head injury signs/symptoms) include respiratory acidosis, cerebral fat embolism, dehydration/water intoxication, and pneumonia. Injuries in other body areas may have indirect effects on CNS functioning and may increase the progression and extent of cerebral damage. Direct cardiac damage or excessive blood loss and shock may affect the vascular system and produce cerebral hypoxia and injury. Respiratory acidosis from chest injury, pulmonary hemorrhage, and aspiration or other ventilatory problems may produce cerebral hypoxia and damage. The head injury itself frequently causes a depression of respiratory drive and promotes development of respiratory acidosis.

Head trauma requires critical observations, assessments, recognition, and prompt interventions to prevent development/progression of cerebral damage, complications, and irreversibility of pathology. No head injury can be treated "lightly," for even a seemingly insignificant head trauma incident may progress or may be masking significant and severe cerebral damage or potential for damage. The treatment of head injury (see Table 3) may be medical management, immediate emergency surgical intervention, or elective surgical procedures. Surgical intervention is usually necessary for severe depressed skull fractures; hematomas; hemorrhages; persistent or recurrent rhinorrhea, otorrhea, or meningitis. Many head trauma patients, with proper nursing and medical management/interventions, can recover fully or achieve the highest possible degree of recovery within the limitations of their residual deficit.

Table 3. Common cerebral pathology

Type	Clinical manifestation	Clinical course/management
Concussion Occurs most frequently with blunt, nonpenetrating minor head injury (patients who do not regain consciousness usually have severe damage; those who regain consciousness after trauma but then become unconscious usually require immediate surgery for evacuation of clot/hemorrhage, relief of massive cerebral swelling)	Transient loss of consciousness, which is immediate and of varying duration (from seconds to hours) Depression/suppression of reflexes Transient cessation of respiration Brief period of bradycardia and hypotension	Usually resolves spontaneously and rapidly Vital signs quickly return to normal Reflexes start returning Slow regaining of consciousness through successive levels/stages Patient may remain amnesic of injury but usually regains full recovery awareness of present situation Frequently duration of amnesia is indicative of concussion severity
Skull fracture Pathological considerations involve Site and potential severity of brain damage Pathways for influx of bacteria/air, efflux of CSF Depression—location and extent	May have drowsiness, headache, confusion, numbness and weakness of legs with Babinski's sign present, temporary blindness Basal skull fractures frequently manifest cranial nerve dysfunctions particularly olfactory, optic, oculomotor, trigeminal, trochlear, facial. and auditory If underlying meninges are torn or basal fracture passes through posterior wall of nasal sinus, bacteria or air may enter the cranial cavity with resulting meningitis, abscess, or air within ventricles Fractures of base of skull with dural tear Rhinorrhea (anterior fossa) Otorrhea (posterior fossa)	Depressed skull fractures become significant when underlying dura is lacerated by bone fragments or brain is compressed Surgical reelevation is usually done if fracture depression is greater than one half of skull thickness Persistence or recurrence of rhinorrhea, otorrhea, or meningitis usually requires surgical repair
Contusion Occurs most often with closed blunt injury Bruising of brain, disruption of brain tissue Coup lesion—directly below site of impact Contrecoup lesion—opposite side of brain from impact	Variable, depending on location, degree, effects on brain integrity/functioning; amount of cerebral edema; increased ICP	Mild contusions frequently resolve spontaneously Severe contusions frequently require surgical intervention to correct pathology and to decrease edema/ICP

ASSESSMENT

1. Specific description of head trauma occurrence/sequelae, including
   a. Time
   b. Nature of, such as fall, blow, car accident; if blow, instrument involved; if fall, object or distance struck
   c. Area/side of head involved, force, and duration
   d. Patient status at time of trauma and afterward, including any loss of consciousness (when,

Table 3. Common cerebral pathology—cont'd

Type	Clinical manifestation	Clinical course/management
Intracerebral hematoma/hemorrhage Frequently occurs with penetrating or open head wounds	Variable, depending on size, location, progression, amount of cerebral edema and increased ICP Focal signs of damage common (see Table 4, Standard: *Supratentorial craniotomy*) If subarachnoid hemorrhage is present, see Standard: *Subarachnoid hemorrhage*	If amenable to surgical evacuation supratentorial craniotomy or infratentorial craniotomy is done See Standards: *Supratentorial craniotomy; Infratentorial craniotomy*
Subdural hematoma May be acute or chronic *Epidural hematoma* Clot is usually produced by temporal or parietal fracture crossing groove containing middle meningeal artery and lacerating or rupturing the artery Bleeding is usually arterial, rapid, and forceful Enlarging clot pushes medially, causing a shift of brain tissue toward the tentorial opening, or notch; progresses to displacement of the uncal portion of temporal lobe through the notch, called *uncal or tentorial herniation*	See Standard: *Subdural hematoma* *Syndrome of uncal herniation* Early third nerve stage: oculomotor (third) nerve compressed at point where it exits from midbrain by uncus pushing through notch, producing dilating ipsilateral pupil that reacts sluggishly to light Late third nerve stage: midbrain dysfunction from rapid encroachment on brain stem by herniating hippocampal gyrus; may exhibit stupor or coma, decreased or absent oculovestibular responses, contralateral hemiparesis and Babinski's sign (from cerebral peduncle compression on herniation side) progressing to ipsilateral as opposite cerebral peduncle is compressed Midbrain–upper pons stage: opposite pupil dilates and fixes; sustained hyperventilation, bilateral decerebrate rigidity	See Standard: *Subdural hematoma* Immediate surgical evacuation of epidural hematoma in early stages of uncal herniation is necessary to prevent progression of syndrome

length, recovery period); headache (location, severity, concurrent neurological symptoms); nausea/vomiting (severity, amount); confusion; agitation/irritability; seizures (onset, progression, type, locality, length, postictal status)

e. Patient awareness/amnesia of incident, events prior/following; last event patient remembered

f. Cuts, abrasions, swelling, ecchymosis, skull deformity, or scalp damage (location, severity)

g. Amount of bleeding or other drainage from injury

h. Cerebrospinal leak from nose (rhinorrhea) or ear (otorrhea)—location, duration, frequency, amount, association with any other symptoms or certain activities (such as bending over, coughing, sneezing)

i. Neurological status at time of injury and following trauma

j. Treatment, emergency procedures administered

k. Other injuries or signs/symptoms of trauma areas (see Standard: *Multiple trauma*)

2. Onset, duration, progression, frequency, and specific description of neurological symptoms, particularly

a. Alterations in LOC, including forgetfulness, drowsiness, irritability, agitation

b. Changes in behavior or personality including fatigability, insomnia, nervous instability

c. Headache

d. Nausea/vomiting

e. Alterations in motor/sensory abilities

f. Pupillary alterations, impaired extraocular movements

g. Visual disturbances including field cuts, photophobia, diplopia, nystagmus, decreased vision

h. Cranial nerve dysfunctions

i. Dizziness/ataxia

j. CSF leak from nose or ear

k. Nuchal rigidity, neck movement limitation

l. Decrease in communication abilities

m. Incontinence

n. Neurological status from trauma occurrence to admission; any fluctuations in status

3. Previous seizures—exact description including onset, progression, type, locality, length, aura, incontinence

a. Postictal status; any injury incurred

b. Presence of any precipitating factors such as fever, emotional upset

c. Frequency of seizures

d. If multiple seizures, whether seizure activity is varied or similar

e. If patient is receiving anticonvulsants, whether prescribed regimen has been adhered to

4. Previous neurological treatment or neurosurgical procedure

5. Medications taken for neurological problem such as anticonvulsants, steroids, pain medications; effects of medications on clinical course/status

6. Presence of alcohol or drug abuse

7. Presence of any medical problems and medications/treatments prescribed and followed

8. Patient's perceptions and reaction to trauma occurrence, diagnosis, therapeutic modalities, anticipated surgical intervention (if planned)

9. Presence of any alterations in body image; fears of permanent disability or deficit; altered role in family, normal occupation/performing ADL

10. Baseline parameters status

a. Neurological

b. Respiratory/pulmonary

c. Cardiovascular

d. Metabolic

e. Renal

f. Hydration

g. Hemodynamic

h. Fluid and electrolyte

i. Other injury

j. Vital signs

k. Weight

l. Urine output pattern

m. Handedness (right or left)

11. Diagnostic test results including

a. CAT

b. Cerebral angiography

c. Skull radiographs

d. Cervical spine radiographs

e. Chest radiographs

f. Abdominal radiographs

g. EEG

h. Lumbar puncture

i. Pneumoencephalogram

j. Brain scan

12. Results of

a. Serum electrolyte levels

b. Hgb and Hct, platelet count, WBC count with differential

c. Arterial blood gas levels

d. Clotting profile

e. CSF determinations

f. Serum drug/alcohol levels

g. Anticonvulsant drug levels

h. Blood typing and cross matching

i. Urine analysis, gravity, culture, osmolality, electrolytes

j. ECG

GOALS

1. Maximal neurological functioning
2. Maximal independence in ADL
3. Adequate alveolar ventilation and pefusion
4. Adequate cardiac output
5. Serum electrolyte levels and fluid balance within normal limits
6. Hgb and Hct stable and within normal limits

7. Acid-base balance within normal limits

8. Infection free

9. Absence or resolution of CSF leak

10. Reduction in patient/family's anxiety with provision of information, demonstrations, support

11. Before discharge patient/family is able to

a. Describe medication, activity, exercise, and dietary regimens

b. Demonstrate safety measures and techniques; proper use of any equipment/therapeutic devices prescribed

c. Describe signs and symptoms requiring medical attention

d. State necessary information regarding follow-up care

Potential problems	Expected outcomes	Nursing activities
■ Increased ICP/decline in neurological status related to Hematoma Hemorrhage Skull fracture Cerebral edema Vasospasm Concussion/contusion	■ Absence of complications Maximal neurological functioning Control or resolution of increased ICP (if possible)	■ Establish neurological baseline and vital signs on admission; ongoing assessments of status and specific symptomatology/deficit q1 hr; in particular, monitor extent and degree of LOC (arousal and content components) alterations, especially subtle changes Change in personality, behavior, mental abilities Pupillary changes (size, equality, light reactivity); impaired extraocular movements, ocular palsies Appearance of or increase in restlessness, agitation, irritability, headache, nausea/vomiting Motor/sensory system dysfunctions Cranial nerve dysfunctions Decline in communication abilities Decline in visual abilities including diplopia, nystagmus Alterations in vital signs especially development of Cushing's phenomenon Alterations in reflex status Abnormal posturing; decerebrate/decorticate to stimuli or spontaneously Monitor q1-2 hr For any CSF leakage—location, amount, quality For any bloody head drainage—location, amount For any swelling, edema, bulging of cranium—location, degree For any ecchymosis, open areas, tenderness, bone depression/protrusion For any signs/symptoms of subdural hematoma, intracranial hemorrhage, embolism, or cerebral infarction; for specifics see Standards: *Subdural hematoma; Supratentorial craniotomy; Embolic phenomena* Avoid precipitating factors of increased ICP such as hypoxia, hypercapnia, fever, Valsalva's maneuver Assist patient with positioning Instruct patient not to hold breath, blow nose vigorously, or reach for bedside articles (if there is CSF leak or skull fracture of sinus, instruct patient not to blow nose) Monitor for any signs/symptoms that could initiate development of factors such as hypoventilation/constipation

Potential problems	Expected outcomes	Nursing activities
		Notify physician of factor presence/potential
		Administer intravenous fluids, medications/treatments as ordered; monitor effects and side effects
		Maintain head gatch and activity (usually bedrest) as ordered
		Accurately record intake and output as ordered (frequently q2 hr); monitor for any imbalance; notify physician if imbalance occurs
		Monitor serum electrolytes, complete blood count, and arterial blood gas levels for any abnormalities; notify physician if any abnormality occurs
		Notify physician immediately of any change in neurological status, vital signs, signs/symptoms of cerebral complications
		Prepare patient for any diagnostic tests/procedures ordered
		If surgery is necessary, see appropriate standard, i.e., *Subdural hematoma; Supratentorial craniototmy; Infratentorial craniotomy*
		Assist with emergency measures/treatments as necessary
		If patient has ICP line inserted, monitor values and waveforms
		Maintain patency/sterility of system
		Monitor effects of other therapies on ICP including coughing, turning, chest physiotherapy, suctioning
		Space therapies if possible to minimize increases in ICP
		Monitor neurological status correlated with ICP values and notify physician
		If ordered, assist physician with drainage of CSF amount to maintain ICP at specific level determined; record fluid amount drained each time; monitor effects on ICP value, correlation between neurological status and CSF drainage
		Hyperventilate patient as ordered by physician for specific ICP level increase
		Administer medications/treatments as ordered; monitor effects and side effects on status and ICP; frequently osmotic diuretics are ordered prn or as ongoing therapy
		Notify physician immediately of any increase in ICP/wave recording; frequently physician will specify maximal ICP limit
		SEE STANDARD: *Increased intracranial pressure*
■ Epidural hematoma	■ Absence or resolution of uncal herniation (by prompt clot evacuation) Maximal neurological functioning	■ See Problem, Increased ICP/decline in neurological status, for specific activities
		In addition in particular monitor for
		History of brief episode of loss of consciousness followed by a lucid interval progressing to unconsciousness (from hematoma enlargement and impending/actual uncal herniation)
		Subtle change in LOC including slightly more restless, agitated, or irritable behavior; thought content slightly impaired; patient slightly more difficult to arouse
		Increase in headaches, nausea/vomiting
		Change in vital signs especially development of hypertension, bradycardia, altered respiratory rate and quality
		Dilating ipsilateral pupil, which reacts sluggishly to light (from third cranial nerve dysfunction); cardinal early sign of uncal herniation
		Notify physician immediately of any change in neurological status/vital signs; dilating ipsilateral pupil warrants immediate surgical evacuation of clot
		Administer emergency medications and treatments as ordered (osmotic diuretics are frequently ordered)
		Prepare patient for surgery as ordered
		For postoperative specifics see Standard: *Supratentorial craniotomy* or *Infratentorial craniotomy*

Potential problems	Expected outcomes	Nursing activities

■ Depressed LOC, restlessness/agitation	■ Safe patient environment Absence of injury complications	■ Close observation—siderails up at all times when patient is alone
		Maintain as quiet an environment as possible, reducing excessive external stimuli to a minimum
		Establish baseline and continue ongoing assessments of LOC and reflex status monitoring
		  For signs of restlessness/agitation, noting degree, frequency, extent
		  Components of consciousness—arousal and content
		  Presence/quality of reflexes including corneal, gag, cough, swallowing; if reflexes are decreased or absent, institute preventive measures such as protecting cornea with eye drops; lid taping/closure; suctioning equipment at bedside
		Monitor for other possible causes of restlessness such as bladder/abdominal distention, headache, hypoxia
		  Notify physician if any of the aforementioned occurs
		  Administer medications/treatments as ordered; monitor effects
		Reorient patient frequently to time, place, person, head trauma occurrence, and necessity of hospitalization
		Apply restraints as ordered by physician if this is only alternative to protect patient from injury
		  Explain to patient/family reasons for restraints
		  Reassure family of necessity for restraints and the relationship between patient's behavior and head trauma
		  Check restraints frequently for proper placement; monitor effectiveness, skin integrity, and circulation
		  Reapply q4 hr and prn
		  Frequently reevaluate need for continuing restraints
		Notify physician immediately if there is a sudden appearance or increase in degree of prior restlessness, irritability, agitation, and/or headache or change in reflex/cranial nerve status

■ Shock	■ Absence or resolution of shock Adequate cardiac output Hemodynamic stability	■ Monitor for
		  Hypotension, tachycardia, diaphoresis, oliguria, skin warmth, elevated temperature q1 hr and prn
		  Abnormal respiratory rate and quality, arterial blood gas values
		  Falling Hgb/Hct values
		  Decreasing CVP q1 hr (if available)
		  Any ECG abnormality/arrhythmia
		  Any external signs of bleeding and note location, amount, force, duration; apply external pressure to control bleeding; assist physician with any procedures and note effects
		Notify physician of any abnormality
		  Administer medications/treatments as ordered
		  Monitor blood transfusions; note effects
		  Monitor for resolution/progression of problem; if shock persists, the cause is usually not the head injury (unless a massive open bleeding head wound is present); monitor for other possible trauma sources including chest, abdomen
		SEE STANDARD: *Multiple trauma*

Potential problems	Expected outcomes	Nursing activities
■ Respiratory insufficiency related to CNS dysfunction Edema Cranial nerve dysfunction Pneumonia Atelectasis Pulmonary emboli	■ Patent airway Normal respiratory rate and pattern Adequate alveolar ventilation and perfusion Arterial blood gas levels within patient's normal limits	■ Ongoing assessment of respiratory status q1 hr and prn; monitor for any abnormality/decline Respiratory rate, quality, and pattern Patency of upper airway and patient's ability to handle secretions Presence/strength of gag, cough, and swallowing reflexes Cranial nerve functioning, particularly presence/strength of ninth to twelfth nerves Skin color, nail beds, peripheral pulses, and skin warmth Breath sounds bilaterally for quality of aeration, signs of obstruction (rales, rhonchi) For signs of pulmonary edema (neurogenic may occur related to head injury) including tachycardia, dyspnea, wheezing, peripheral edema, weight gains, decreased urinary output Arterial blood gas values Chest radiograph results Signs/symptoms of thrombophlebitis, pulmonary emboli Maintain patent airway by Turning and positioning to prevent obstruction or aspiration of secretions q2 hr and prn Deep breathing and coughing q1 hr and prn (if allowed) Suctioning prn (check with physician before nasotracheal suctioning to determine potential for basilar skull fracture) Adequate oxygenation and humidification as ordered Chest physiotherapy/pulmonary toilet if warranted and not contraindicated by physician's order If reflexes (gag, cough, swallowing) are decreased or absent, keep patient NPO as per physician's order; when reflexes are stronger and patient is started on po, stay with patient for initial feedings; monitor swallowing effectiveness and assess for any signs of choking/nasal regurgitation Apply antithromboembolic stockings or Ace bandages as ordered; reapply every shift and prn; monitor for constriction/looseness, condition of skin Instruct and supervise patient in performing leg exercises and ROM exercises as status and physician's order allow Increase activity level/progression when allowed Notify physician immediately of any change in respiratory/neurological status or signs of complication potential/occurrence If respiratory problem occurs, assist with emergency measures to maintain patent airway and adequate ventilation Administer medications/treatments as ordered, monitoring effects and side effects Monitor neurological status closely as both hypoventilation and hyperventilation may increase ICP See Standard: *Mechanical ventilation* Explain procedures and reasons for equipment/respiratory assistance to patient/family; reassure and support Establish alternate means of communication as needed If embolism occurs, see Standard: *Embolic phenomena*

Potential problems	Expected outcomes	Nursing activities

■ Fluid and electrolyte imbalance related to Cerebral trauma commonly producing positive balance of Na⁺ and H₂O—salt retention from overproduction of aldosterone; water retention from overproduction of ADH or vasopressin
 	
Osmotic diuretic medication administration
	■ Fluid and electrolyte balance within normal or prescribed limits	■ Monitor and accurately record intake and output, urine specific gravity, osmolality as ordered (frequently q2 hr)
		Monitor for signs of dehydration/overhydration such as
		  Poor skin turgor
		  Dry mucous membranes
		  Peripheral edema
		  Excessive thirst
		  Change in LOC
		Monitor for
		  Abnormal vital signs, Hgb/Hct values
		  Weight alterations
		  Abnormal serum/urine electrolyte values, particularly Na⁺, K⁺
		  Abnormal serum/urine osmolalities
		  Temperature elevations
		  Insensible fluid losses including respiratory, diaphoresis, secretions
		  Presence/degree of nausea and vomiting; effectiveness of medications ordered
		  Changes in neurological status
		Monitor for signs of increased production/release of ADH (inappropriate ADH), including
		  Hyponatremia
		  Hypo-osmolality
		  Overhydration
		  Water retention/intoxication
		  Cerebral dysfunction
		Administer intravenous fluids, nasogastric feedings as ordered
		Administer medications as ordered; monitor effects and side effects; if patient is receiving steroids, monitor urine glucose and acetone levels as ordered
		Notify physician of any fluid imbalance or electrolyte abnormality; signs of cerebral dysfunction from ADH disorder
		If patient is receiving osmotic diuretics such as mannitol, urea, monitor
		  Hourly urine output
		  For signs of congestive heart failure
		  For serious imbalances from rapid diuresis of H₂O and electrolytes
		  For dehydration or hypovolemia (may be masked)
		  Notify physician of effects of therapy
		If patient is allowed po, maintain fluid restriction or encouragement regimen as ordered by physician

■ Seizures related to Head injury
  Irritative effect of blood
  Cerebral edema
  Cerebral ischemia
	■ Absence or control of seizures	■ Prevention of precipitating factors in seizure occurrence including fever, hypoxia, H₂O intoxication, electrolyte disturbances; notify physician of potential/presence of any of these factors
		Seizure precautions (if indicated)
		  Padded siderails up at all times when patient is alone
		  Bed height at lowest level
		  Padded tongue blade and airway at bedside
		  Emergency medications and equipment readily available
		  Close observation and supervision
		Administer anticonvulsant medication as ordered; monitor effects and side effects, serum anticonvulsant levels
		If seizure occurs, monitor and record seizure activity; notify physician; see Standard: *Seizures*

Potential problems	Expected outcomes	Nursing activities
■ CSF leakage related to Skull fracture Tearing/laceration of meninges from bone fragments or stress Penetrating or open head wounds	■ Absence or resolution of CSF leak	■ If there is basilar skull fracture, avoid nasotracheal suctioning or any nasal treatments Monitor for any signs of CSF leak particularly rhinorrhea (with anterior fossa fractures) and otorrhea (posterior fossa fractures) If CSF leak occurs, try to collect specimen and test for presence of glucose (result positive if CSF) Monitor site, amount, and quality of drainage Notify physician immediately Administer medications/treatments as ordered Monitor for persistence/resolution of CSF leak Monitor for signs/symptoms of meningitis; if problem occurs, see Standard: *Meningitis/encephalitis* If CSF leak/meningitis is persistent or recurrent, surgical intervention is usually performed; see Standard: *Supratentorial craniotomy* for postoperative specifics
■ Infection related to Skull fracture Penetrating or open head wounds Other sources of infection	■ Absence or resolution of infection	■ Keep patient's hands from any open head wounds, CSF leak sites Prevent precipitating factors such as urinary retention, pulmonary congestion/aspiration Maintain strict sterile technique for procedures such as wound irrigations, dressing changes, catheterization, endotracheal/ tracheostomy tube care/management Monitor Temperature q2-4 hr for any elevation IV sites frequently for any signs of redness, tenderness, phlebitis Wounds for any signs of redness, bulging, tenderness, drainage quantity/quality Neurological status and vital signs for any decline/abnormality For any signs of meningitis WBC count (may be falsely elevated if patient is receiving steroids) Notify physician of any signs of infection If signs of infection are present Administer medications/treatments as ordered; monitor effects and side effects Monitor wound culture results Monitor for other possible infection sources if warranted, including urine and sputum cultures, chest radiograph results, CSF determinations Institute measures if possible to promote resolution of infection source Monitor for resolution/progression of infection If problem occurs, see Standard: *Meningitis*
■ Presence of neurological deficit	■ Absence of complications Maximal neurological functioning	■ On admission establish and implement nursing care plan based on individual needs and specific deficit present; ongoing assessments of effectiveness of interventions Institute measures to promote optimal muscular tone, functioning, and maintenance; skin integrity; and circulation Prevent complications such as contractures, footdrop/wristdrop, decubiti by measures such as sheepskin/air mattress, footboard, handrolls/splints, ROM exercises from active to passive as status allows, frequent turning, and proper positioning Keep skin clean, dry, and pressure free; monitor skin integrity, circulation, and potential pressure sites q2 hr and prn Obtain orders for appropriate referrals/equipment such as physical/occupational therapy

Potential problems	Expected outcomes	Nursing activities
■ Patient/family's fear, anxiety, anger related to Limited understanding of diagnostic tests/procedures Head trauma occurrence Presence of neurological deficit or potential development/worsening	■ Patient/family's behavior indicates decreased anxiety with provision of information Patient/family verbalizes fears, angers, concerns	■ Ongoing assessment of level of anxiety and other reactions Encourage patient/family's verbalization of questions, fears, anger Collaborate with physician in providing realistic information and reassurance appropriate to level of understanding Explain relationship between pathology and clinical symptoms, status, course Explain anticipated treatments, therapeutic measures, and clinical course/prognosis (if known) Explain and prepare patient/family for diagnostic tests or procedures, operative intervention if planned Explain reasons for frequent monitoring of neurological status and vital signs If patient/family expresses anger regarding head trauma (especially if it was induced by violence), encourage them to express feelings and support them in dealing with stages and reactions and accepting reality of present situation Obtain appropriate referrals such as religious personnel, social service
■ Posttraumatic nervous instability/psychiatric disorders Patient/family's anxiety, anger related to presence This posttraumatic syndrome frequently occurs and usually lessens or disappears over a period ranging from months to years Persistent amnesia of trauma incident, headache, impaired memory capabilities, fatigability, and insomnia are common symptoms	■ Patient/family verbalizes concerns Patient/family's behavior indicates decreased anxiety with provision of information	■ Ongoing assessment of patient behavior, signs/symptoms, patient/family's anxiety Explain relationship of behavior, signs/symptoms to head trauma Reassure patient/family that status will gradually improve with time Establish plan of care and instruct family in appropriate interventions based on individual patient needs such as Maintain calm, quiet, supportive environment Reduce environmental/emotional stresses, external stimuli as much as possible Repeat explanations frequently and simply Support and reassure patient in progression of recovery according to individual rate of recovery; avoid "pushing" or "demand pressuring" Avoid taxing mental energies Reorient patient to reality and circumstances of present and past experiences; have family bring in familiar pictures, objects Assist and support patient in gradually returning to "normal" life-style, role, ADL Assist patient in judgments, perceptions, reorientation to space and time, etc., as needed Protect patient from self-injury as needed Encourage patient/family to maintain support, patience; encourage family acceptance of behavior by reinforcing pathological causes
■ GI bleeding related to CNS factors Stress Steroid administration	■ Absence or resolution of GI bleeding	■ Monitor vital signs q2-4 hr, Hgb and Hct, stools for Hematest three times a week, Hematest of aspirate, emesis and urine for any abnormalities Obtain order for antacid administration as soon as patient is able to take po Monitor for signs of GI bleeding including abdominal tenderness/distention, hypotension, sudden tachycardia Notify physician immediately if any abnormality occurs; if problem occurs, see Standard: *Acute upper gastrointestinal bleeding*

Potential problems	Expected outcomes	Nursing activities
■ Dizziness when activity increase initiated	■ Control of dizziness Patient ambulates safely	■ When patient increases activity level, monitor vital signs and assess for dizziness Gradually increase head gatch level Have patient dangle legs at side of bed for short periods Assist/supervise patient in getting out of bed and ambulating as needed Provide rest periods between activities to gradually increase activity tolerance levels/strengths
■ Continued presence of neurological deficit Patient/family's fears, anxiety, anger related to deficit and possible alterations in lifestyle	■ Maximal neurological functioning* Maximal independence in ADL (within capabilities) Patient/family verbalizes concerns	■ Assess patient's specific neurological deficit; collaborate with physician regarding prognosis, expected degree of recovery Implement individualized plan of care based on patient's needs and deficits Assist as needed in ADL Monitor potential for independent functioning, and obtain equipment to maximize function and promote safety Obtain orders for appropriate referrals such as physical, speech, occupational therapy, and social service Encourage verbalization of patient/family's fears, anxieties, and other reactions—level and degree Answer questions realistically Encourage patient/family's participation in care planning, implementation, evaluation, and decision making Realistically reassure and support patient/family Reinforce any gains or independence that patient achieves Plan, instruct, demonstrate, supervise, and evaluate patient/family's demonstrations of needed information/skills for maximal independent functioning such as Measures to prevent complications Assistance necessary—type, amount, degree Proper use of therapeutic devices/equipment Monitor level of achievement toward maximizing potentials and independence; means to promote as "normal" a life-style as possible
■ Insufficient knowledge to comply with discharge regimen†	■ Patient/family demonstrates or verbalizes understanding of discharge regimen	■ Assess patient/family's level of understanding of neurological problem and therapy received Explain relationship between patient's neurological status and therapies prescribed If factors/circumstances in head trauma can be controlled, explain to patient/family relationship of factors to head trauma and importance of controlling them to prevent recurrence of trauma; some individual factors may include alcohol intake, drug ingestion, safety precautions/measures, safety devices/equipment; obtain appropriate referrals and counseling services as needed Instruction of patient/family regarding required information and skills so that before discharge patient/family is able to Describe medication regimen
	Patient/family accurately describes medication, activity, and dietary regimens	Name and purpose Route, dosage, frequency, times Side effects Special precautions necessary, including drugs, foods, beverages contraindicated or regulated in quantity; factors potentiating/decreasing effects or side effects; physical restrictions; safety measures

---

*If responsibility of critical care nurse includes this stage of care.
†If responsibility of critical care nurse includes such follow-up care.

Potential problems	Expected outcomes	Nursing activities
		Describe dietary regimen
		Describe activity regimen, exercise program
		Describe and demonstrate any special therapeutic measures prescribed
	Patient/family describes means to achieve maximal independence in ADL, promote safety, and prevent complications	Describe and demonstrate proper use of equipment or therapeutic devices
		Reasons for using
		Time, method, and duration of use
		Precautions/safeguards
		Necessary maintenance (type, frequency)
		Measures to promote optimal functioning, upkeep/duration
	Patient/family describes signs/symptoms requiring medical attention	Describe signs/symptoms of neurological status requiring medical care
	Patient/family describes follow-up care regimen	Describe plan for follow-up care including purpose of appointment, when and where to go, who to see, what to expect

26 □ Subarachnoid hemorrhage

The subarachnoid space lies between the pia mater and the arachnoid membranes. The brain and spinal cord are suspended in CSF, which fills the subarachnoid space surrounding them. A subarachnoid hemorrhage (SAH) occurs when blood escapes from a cerebral artery to the subarachnoid space. Etiologies of SAH include head trauma, rupture of an intracranial aneurysm, bleeding from arteriovenous malformations, and hemorrhage into brain tumors.

Diagnosis of a subarachnoid hemorrhage is suspected from the patient's history and presenting signs and symptoms. Confirmation is usually obtained by performing a lumbar puncture. Significant findings confirming a SAH include an elevation of CSF pressure (often greater than 300 mm H_2O); presence of blood on an atraumatic tap; a high CSF erythrocyte count on the first and last specimens; and/or xanthochromic appearance of the spinal fluid. The protein content of the CSF may be elevated above normal levels due to the presence of cells.

Signs and symptoms of SAH may range from a minimal to a severe neurological deficit. Some of the factors affecting the symptomatology variability include type of pathology, size and extent of the bleeding, areas involved in the bleeding, presence and degree of vaso-spasm, and/or hydrocephalus. Signs/symptoms that frequently occur with SAH include

1. Headache—usually sudden, severe, and associated with activity
2. Alteration in consciousness—patient may have brief loss of consciousness and then become alert or drowsy
3. Mental dysfunctions such as confusion, apathy, restlessness, irritability
4. Meningeal irritation from blood in the spinal fluid, possibly with irritation of nerve roots, resulting in irritability, photophobia, nuchal rigidity (neck stiffness and resistance to passive motion), and fever
5. Nausea/vomiting
6. Focal neurological signs such as motor weakness, sensory disturbances, speech disorders, seizures, visual disturbances, and diplopia

On admission the immediate goal of therapy is to prevent further hemorrhage and promote recovery of neurological functioning. The therapeutic intervention decided on for the future depends on the cause of the SAH. Surgical intervention may be performed for some patients, whereas for others medical treatment is preferable. The following assessment and standard apply to any patient with a SAH, regardless of the cause or possible future surgical intervention.

ASSESSMENT

1. Onset, duration, progression, and specific description of neurological symptoms, including
   a. Headache
   b. Nuchal rigidity
   c. Alterations in LOC
   d. Changes in behavior or personality
   e. Changes in motor/sensory functioning
   f. Communication deficits
   g. Nausea/vomiting
   h. Visual disturbances
   i. Pupillary changes; ptosis of eyelid
   j. Seizures
2. Previous head trauma or injury—exact description of incident, clinical course, treatment, sequelae
3. Previous neurological treatment or neurosurgical procedure; medications taken, effects on clinical course/status
4. Presence of any medical problems and medications/treatments employed
5. Patient's perceptions and reaction to diagnosis and treatment modalities
6. Presence of any alterations in body image; fear of permanent disability or deficit; altered role in family, normal occupation, performance of ADL
7. Baseline parameters status
   a. Neurological
   b. Respiratory
   c. Cardiac
   d. Circulatory and vascular
   e. Metabolic
   f. Hydration/nutritional
   g. Vital signs
   h. Weight
   i. Handedness (right or left)
8. Diagnostic test results, including
   a. CAT
   b. Lumbar puncture
   c. Cerebral angiography
   d. Brain scan
   e. EEG
9. Results of
   a. Serum electrolyte levels
   b. Hgb and Hct, platelet count
   c. Clotting profile
   d. Anticonvulsant drug levels
   e. CSF determinations
   f. Urinalysis, culture, gravity, osmolality
   g. ECG
   h. Chest radiograph
   i. Arterial blood gas levels

GOALS

1. Maximal neurological functioning
2. Optimal independence in ADL within physical limitations (when allowed)
3. Adequate alveolar ventilation
4. Serum electrolytes and fluid balance within normal limits
5. Hgb and Hct stable within normal limits
6. Acid-base balance within normal limits
7. Infection free
8. Reduction in patient/family's anxiety with provision of information, demonstrations, support
9. Before discharge patient/family is able to
   a. Describe medication, activity, exercise, and dietary regimens
   b. Demonstrate safety measures and techniques; proper use of any equipment, therapeutic devices
   c. Describe any special precautions/measures to decrease rebleeding potential (especially if SAH is the result of head trauma)
   d. Describe signs and symptoms requiring medical attention
   e. State necessary information regarding follow-up care

Potential problems	Expected outcomes	Nursing activities
■ Rebleeding Greatest potential for rebleeding is usually 1 to 2 weeks after initial bleed	■ Absence or resolution of rebleeding Absence of complications Minimal external stimulation	■ Establish neurological baseline and vital signs on admission Follow physician's policy/orders regarding minimization of external stimuli; may include Single, quiet, dark room Absolute bed rest Feeding, turning, and bathing patient Limitation of visitors to immediate family; certain number, time period Minimization of patient's verbalization

Potential problems	Expected outcomes	Nursing activities
		Head of bed elevated at degree specified (usually 15 to 20 degrees)
		Siderails in position when patient is alone
		No smoking in patient's room or by patient
		Restriction or no use allowed of telephone, television, radio
		Restriction of coffee/tea, very hot/cold foods
		No rectal temperatures or treatments
		Prevent constipation by establishing bowel regimen when patient is admitted
		Assess patient's normal elimination pattern, food likes, aids in elimination
		Obtain necessary orders from physician such as stool softeners, laxatives
		Accurately record bowel movements, amount, consistency
		Monitor neurological status and vital signs as ordered and prn, especially for changes in
		LOC
		Motor and sensory functioning
		Behavior or personality
		Pupil equality, size, reaction; extraocular movements; ptosis
		Visual abilities including acuity, diplopia, nystagmus, photophobia
		Presence/extent of headache, nausea or vomiting, nuchal rigidity
		Communication abilities
		Cranial nerve functioning
		Monitor for factors that could increase anxiety/agitation such as bladder and abdominal distention; notify physician if not resolved
		Administer medications as ordered; monitor effect and side effects
		Sedation is usually ordered for patient
		Notify physician of effectiveness; monitor serum drug levels
		Caution family to avoid discussing condition, potential complications, or prognosis with patient
		Notify physician immediately of any change in neurological status or vital signs
■ Increased ICP related to Hematoma formation Hydrocephalus Cerebral edema from vasospasm Ischemic infarction/ rebleeding	■ Absence or resolution of increased ICP	■ Avoid precipitating factors in increased ICP such as hypoxia, hypercapnia, fever, Valsalva's maneuver
		Assist patient in positioning and turning
		Instruct patient not to hold breath, blow nose vigorously, or reach for bedside articles
		Monitor for any signs/symptoms that could initiate development of factors such as hypoventilation, constipation
		Notify physician potential/presence of any factors
		Maintain head gatch and bed rest as ordered
		Monitor neurological status and vital signs as ordered and prn (see Problem, Rebleeding: monitor neurological status and vital signs [nursing activities] for specifics)
		Administer medications, treatments, and intravenous fluids as ordered; monitor effects and side effects
		Accurately record intake and output; monitor for any imbalance
		Monitor serum electrolyte levels, complete blood count, arterial blood gas values for any abnormalities
		Notify physician of any change in neurological status or vital signs or of abnormal fluid balance/lab values
		If problem occurs, see Standard: *Increased intracranial pressure*

Potential problems	Expected outcomes	Nursing activities

■ Presence of neurological deficit	■ Absence of complications
	  Maximal neurological functioning
		■ On admission establish and implement nursing care plan based on individual needs and specific deficit present
		  Implement interventions based on needs/deficit such as
		    Diplopia: provide and institute alternating eye patch
		    Headache: provide quiet environment; medicate as per physician's order; monitor effects and notify physician if measures are ineffectual
		    Restricted activity/movement: turn and position properly q2 hr; use sheepskin or air mattress; monitor skin and bony prominences frequently for any abnormalities
		    Weakness or paralysis: maintain proper limb alignment to prevent footdrop, subluxation/contractures; measures may include footboard, splints, sling, handrolls, ROM exercises if allowed
		    Communication deficits: establish alternate means of communication if possible
		  Ongoing assessments and evaluations of neurological status and effectiveness of interventions
		  Notify physician of any signs/symptoms of complications

■ Hypertension	■ BP within normal or prescribed limits	■ Maintain minimal amount of external stimuli/emotional stress
		  Monitor and record BP as ordered (usually q1-2 hr)
		  Administer medications as ordered; monitor effects, side effects, and relevant serum level values
		  Notify physician immediately of any increase in BP above specified maximal level

■ Seizures	■ Absence or control of seizures	■ Prevention of precipitating factors in seizure occurrence, including fever, hypoxia, H_2O intoxication, electrolyte disturbances
		  Notify physician of potential/presence of any factors
		  Seizure precautions (if indicated)
		    Padded siderails up at all times when patient is alone
		    Bed height at lowest level
		    Padded tongue blade and airway at bedside
		    Emergency medications and equipment readily available
		    Close observation and supervision
		  Administer anticonvulsant medications as ordered; monitor effects and side effects, serum anticonvulsant levels
		  If seizure occurs, monitor and record seizure activity; notify physician; see Standard: *Seizures*

■ Fluid and electrolyte imbalance	■ Fluid and electrolyte balance within normal limits	■ Monitor and accurately record intake and output, urine specific gravity as ordered
		  Monitor for signs of dehydration or overhydration such as
		    Poor skin turgor
		    Dry mucous membranes
		    Peripheral edema
		    Excessive thirst
		    Change in LOC
		  Monitor for
		    Abnormal vital signs, Hgb/Hct values
		    Abnormal serum electrolyte values
		    Weight alterations
		    Temperature elevations
		    Insensible fluid losses including respiratory, diaphoresis, secretions
		    Presence/degree of nausea and vomiting; effectiveness of medications ordered

Potential problems	Expected outcomes	Nursing activities
		Administer IV fluids, NG feedings as ordered
		Administer medications as ordered; monitor effects and side effects; if patient is receiving steroids, monitor urine glucose and acetone levels four times a day
		Notify physician of any fluid imbalance or electrolyte abnormality
■ Respiratory insufficiency related to CNS dysfunction Pneumonia Atelectasis Pulmonary emboli	■ Patent airway Adequate alveolar ventilation Normal respiratory rate and quality Arterial blood gas levels within patient's normal limits	■ Ongoing assessment of respiratory status q2 hr and prn Assess and monitor for any abnormality/decline Respiratory rate, quality, and pattern Patency of upper airway and patient's ability to handle secretions Skin color, nail beds, peripheral pulses, and skin warmth Presence/strength of gag, cough, and swallowing reflexes Breath sounds bilaterally for quality of aeration; signs of obstruction (rales, rhonchi) Arterial blood gas values Chest radiograph results Signs/symptoms of thrombophlebitis, pulmonary emboli, pulmonary edema Maintain patent airway by Turning and positioning to prevent obstruction or aspiration of secretions q2 hr Deep breathing, gentle suctioning, and coughing prn if not contraindicated by physician's orders Adequate oxygenation and humidification as ordered Apply antithromboembolic stockings or Ace bandages as ordered; reapply every shift and prn; monitor for constriction/looseness, condition of skin Instruct and supervise patient in performing leg exercises (if allowed by physician) Increase activity level/progression when allowed Notify physician immediately of any change in respiratory/neurological status If problem occurs, assist with emergency measures to maintain patent airway and adequate ventilation; see Standard: *Mechanical ventilation* If emboli occur, see Standard: *Embolic phenomena*
■ Infection	■ Absence or resolution of infection	■ Prevent precipitating factors such as urinary retention, pulmonary congestion/aspiration Maintain strict sterile technique for procedures such as catheterization; endotracheal/tracheostomy tube care, management, suctioning Monitor Temperature (usually ordered orally) q4 hr and prn for any elevation IV sites frequently for any signs of redness, tenderness/phlebitis For potential infection sources including pulmonary, urinary, exposure to infection sources WBC count (may be falsely elevated if patient is receiving steroids) If temperature elevation or sign of infection occurs, notify physician and culture possible infections sources Monitor sputum/urine cultures, chest radiograph results, CSF cultures Continue accurate recording of intake and output; monitor for dehydration/overhydration

Potential problems	Expected outcomes	Nursing activities
		Institute measures to promote resolution of infection source if possible Administer medications and treatments as ordered If CSF infection occurs, see Standard: *Meningitis/encephalitis*
■ GI bleeding related to CNS factors Stress Steroid administration	■ Absence or resolution of GI bleeding	■ Monitor vital signs q2-4 hr, Hgb and Hct, stools for Hematest three times a week; Hematest of aspirate, emesis, and urine for any abnormalities Obtain order for antacid administration as soon as patient able to take po Monitor for signs of GI bleeding including abdominal tenderness/distention, hypotension, sudden tachycardia Notify physician immediately if any abnormalities occur If problem occurs, see Standard: *Upper gastrointestinal bleeding*

■ Patient/family's anxiety related to
Fear of disability/death
Uncertain prognosis
Potential/presence of deficit
	■ Minimal emotional stress
	Family verbalizes fears/concerns away from patient
		■ Ongoing assessment of patient/family's level of anxiety
		Reduce external stimuli and stress factors to patient
		   Explain to family reasons for avoiding stress
		   Instruct family not to question patient or discuss stressful issues
		Collaborate with physician in determining amount, depth, and quality of information he/she wants patient to know
		   Provide patient with only the information physician has determined to give
		   Reinforce to family information physician has provided
		Collaborate with physician in providing realistic information and reassurance to family
		   Encourage verbalization of fears and concerns
		   Answer questions appropriate to level of understanding
		If patient is to undergo surgical intervention, see Standard: *Supratentorial craniotomy,* but check with physician regarding what specific information and preparation of patient is allowed (physician may not want any done or only minimal to avoid preoperative stress)
		If patient is being treated conservatively, is progressing toward plans of discharge, and is stable
		   Encourage verbalization of fears/concerns
		   Answer questions appropriate to level of understanding
		   Provide time and support
		   Ongoing assessment of level of anxiety; potential for independent functioning in ADL; and reactions to hospitalization, diagnosis/treatments

■ Continued presence of neurological deficit
Patient/family's fears, anxiety, anger related to deficit and possible alterations in life-style
	■ Maximal neurological functioning*
	Maximal independence in ADL (within capabilities)
	Patient/family verbalizes concerns
		■ Assess patient's specific neurological deficit
		Implement individualized plan of care based on patient's needs and deficits
		   Assist as needed in ADL
		   Monitor potential for independent functioning and obtain equipment to maximize function and promote safety
		   Obtain orders for appropriate referrals such as physical, speech, occupational therapy; social service
		Encourage verbalization of patient/family's fears, anxieties, and other reactions—level and degree
		   Answer questions realistically
		   Encourage their participation in care planning, implementation, evaluation, and decision making
		   Realistically reassure and support patient/family

*If responsibility of critical care nurse includes this stage of care.

Potential problems	Expected outcomes	Nursing activities
		Reinforce any gains or independence patient achieves
		Plan, instruct, demonstrate, supervise, and evaluate patient/family's verbalization/performance of needed information/skills for maximal independent functioning such as
		Measures to prevent complications
		Assistance necessary—type, amount, degree
		Proper use of therapeutic devices/equipment
		Monitor level of achievement toward maximizing potentials and independence; means to promote as "normal" a life-style as possible
■ Insufficient knowledge to comply with discharge regimen*	■ Patient/family demonstrates or verbalizes understanding of discharge regimen	■ Assess patient/family's level of understanding of neurological problem and therapy received
		Explain relationship between patient's neurological status and therapies prescribed
		If appropriate, explain relationship between head injury occurrence and SAH
		Encourage patient/family to discuss means, measures, alterations, precautions to decrease potential for head injury recurrence
		Explain safety precautions to prevent head injury recurrence
		Instruct patient/family regarding required information and skills so that before discharge patient/family is able to
	Patient/family describes medication, activity, and dietary regimens	Describe medication regimen
		Name and purpose
		Route, dosage, frequency, times
		Side effects
		Special precautions necessary including drugs, foods, beverages contraindicated or quantity regulated; factors potentiating/decreasing effects or side effects; physical restrictions; safety measures
		Describe dietary regimen
		Describe activity regimen, exercise program
		Describe and demonstrate any special therapeutic measures prescribed
	Patient/family describes and demonstrates means to achieve maximal independence in ADL, promote maximal safety, and prevent complications	Describe and demonstrate proper use of equipment or therapeutic devices
		Reasons for using
		Time, method, and duration of use
		Precautions/safeguards
		Necessary maintenance (type, frequency)
		Measures to promote optimal functioning, upkeep/duration
	Patient/family describes signs/symptoms requiring medical attention	Describes signs/symptoms of neurological status requiring medical care
	Patient/family describes follow-up care regimen	Describes plan for follow-up care including purpose of appointment, when and where to go, and who to see, what to expect

*If responsibility of critical care nurse includes such follow-up care.

27 □ Subdural hematoma

A subdural hematoma is a collection of blood, which may be mixed with blood pigments and proteins, that accumulates in the subdural space (area where the dura and arachnoid membranes meet). Subdural hemorrhage is usually a consequence of head trauma. The hemorrhages are mainly venous in origin so bleeding and accumulation are slower compared to epidural hemorrhages. The common sources of subdural bleeding are cortical hemorrhagic contusions involving tearing of the arachnoid and lacerations or tears of the dura. Approximately one third of hemorrhages result from rupture of bridging veins. Subdural hemorrhage is most common over the lateral and upper aspects of the hemispheres and in the temporal regions. The hematomas may be unilateral or bilateral.

Subdural hematomas are more common in the elderly (especially if cortical atrophy is present, allowing a larger area in the subdural space for accumulation), alcoholics, and patients receiving anticoagulant therapy. Etiology is unknown in approximately one tenth of hematoma occurrence.

The two main types or classifications of subdural hematoma are acute and chronic.

An *acute* subdural hematoma is usually associated with a severe head injury. Frequently the hematoma is accompanied by cerebral contusion and laceration. The most frequent symptoms are headaches, drowsiness, confusion, slowness in thinking, and sometimes agitation. The symptoms worsen progressively, and in later stages hemiparesis or focal signs may occur. Acute subdural hematomas are rapidly evolving because they mainly involve tearing of bridging veins, and symptoms result from direct compression of the brain by the fresh, expanding clot. The bleeding may cease when the ICP rises, compressing the veins, so the progression of symptoms is usually not as rapid as with an epidural hematoma. Rarely a subdural hematoma may occur in the posterior fossa causing symptoms of headache, vomiting, dysphagia, cranial nerve palsies, and anisocoria (pupil inequality).

In patients with *chronic* subdural hematoma the traumatic etiology is often more obscure—the injury may have been so slight that the person is unaware or has forgotten the incident. The bleeding usually spreads thinly and widely over the hemisphere for a period extending from weeks to months. The blood clot organizes and then becomes encased by fibrous membranes. As red cells hemolyze and blood proteins disintegrate, the osmotic pressure rises, resulting in fluid entrance into the hematoma and producing an enlargement of the hematoma and increased compression of brain tissue. This stage of membrane formation around the hematoma usually occurs within 4 to 8 weeks after the initial insult. The common symptoms frequently occurring weeks after the injury include headache, diffuse mental changes, personality changes, confusion, and occasionally seizures and hemiparesis. The symptoms frequently fluctuate from day to day, possibly due to alterations in the delicate balance between compensation and decompensation of neural and vascular structures around the tentorial notch.

The diagnosis of subdural hematoma is frequently suspected based on the patient's history, clinical status and symptoms, and past or recent head injury. Treatment of a subdural hematoma is surgical—burr holes are placed over the appropriate brain lobe and the clot is evacuated. Surgical evacuation can prevent further progression of neurological deterioration from cerebral compression and displacement.

ASSESSMENT

1. Previous head injury or trauma—exact description of incident, clinical course, treatment, sequelae
2. Presence of external physical signs of head injury including ecchymosis, swelling, lacerations—location, severity, duration
3. Onset, progression, frequency, duration, fluctuations, and specific description of neurological symptoms, including
   a. Headache
   b. Mental changes
   c. Personality changes
   d. Alterations in LOC
   e. Alterations in communication abilities
   f. Motor weakness
   g. Sensory disturbances
   h. Nausea/vomiting
   i. Ataxia
   j. Pupillary changes
   k. Visual deficits/alterations
   l. Seizures
4. Previous neurological treatment or neurosurgical

procedure; medications taken, effects on clinical course/status
5. Presence of any potentially related medical problems especially blood dyscrasias, emboli, alcoholism, hypertension; medications taken, particularly anticoagulants; therapies employed
6. Patient's perceptions and reaction to diagnosis, treatment modalities, surgical intervention
7. Presence of any alterations in body image; fears of permanent disability or deficit; altered role in family, normal occupation, performing ADL
8. Baseline parameters status
   a. Neurological
   b. Respiratory
   c. Circulatory and vascular
   d. Cardiac
   e. Metabolic
   f. Hydration/nutritional
   g. Vital signs
   h. Weight
   i. Handedness (right or left)
9. Diagnostic test results, including
   a. CAT
   b. Cerebral arteriograpy
   c. Skull radiographs
   d. Tomography
   e. EEG
   f. Brain scan
   g. Lumbar puncture
10. Results of
    a. Serum electrolyte levels
    b. Hgb and Hct, platelet count

c. Clotting profile
d. Arterial blood gas levels
e. Anticonvulsant drug levels
f. Type and cross matching
g. Urinalysis, osmolality, gravity, culture
h. ECG
i. Chest radiograph
j. If indicated; alcohol levels, liver/renal function tests, lung scan/thrombophlebitis studies

GOALS

1. Maximal neurological functioning
2. Optimal independence in ADL
3. Serum electrolytes and fluid balance within normal limits
4. Hgb and Hct stable within normal limits
5. Acid-base balance within normal limits
6. Burr hole sites well-healed and infection free
7. Reduction in patient/family's anxiety with provision of information, demonstrations, support
8. Before discharge patient/family is able to
   a. Describe medication, activity, exercise, and dietary regimens
   b. Demonstrate safety measures and techniques; proper use of any equipment, therapeutic devices
   c. Describe any special precautions/measures to aid in prevention of hematoma recurrence
   d. Describe signs and symptoms requiring medical attention
   e. State necessary information regarding follow-up care

Potential problems	Expected outcomes	Nursing activities
Preoperative		

■ Increased ICP/decline in neurological functioning related to suspected/confirmed subdural hematoma	■ Absence/resolution of increased ICP
	Maximal neurological functioning
		■ Establish neurological baseline and vital signs on admission
		Prevent precipitating factors in increased ICP such as hypoxia, hypercapnia, fever, Valsalva's maneuver
		  Monitor for any signs/symptoms that could initiate development of factors such as hypoventilation, constipation
		  Assist patient with positioning; instruct patient not to hold breath
		  Notify physician of potential/presence of any factors
		Monitor neurological status and vital signs as ordered and report any change to physician immediately, especially
		  Subtle alteration in LOC, personality, mental abilities; may have drowsiness, inattentiveness, forgetfulness, confusion, withdrawal, etc.
		  Appearance of or increase in restlessness, agitation, irritability
		  Appearance of or increase in headache, nausea/vomiting (severity, frequency, duration)

Potential problems	Expected outcomes	Nursing activities
		Decline in motor, sensory, or communication abilities/functioning
		Pupillary changes, decreased visual abilities
		Alterations in vital signs
		Appearance of or increased ataxia
		Fluctuations in status; monitor specific symptomatology onset, progression, duration, appearance of or increased headache
		Maintain activity level and head gatch as ordered
		Monitor for any imbalance/abnormality; notify physician if any imbalance/abnormality occurs
		Intake and output
		Serum electrolytes
		Hgb and Hct
		Arterial blood gas levels
		Temperature
		Administer medications/treatments as ordered; monitor effects and side effects
		Establish and record neurological baseline immediately before surgery (if possible) to provide for comparison postoperatively
■ Restlessness and agitation	■ Safe patient environment Absence of injury complications	■ Close observation; siderails up at all times when patient is alone
		Monitor for other possible causes of restlessness/agitation such as abdominal/bladder distention, headache, hypoxia
		Notify physician if any of the aforementioned occurs
		Administer analgesics, comfort measures, treatments as ordered
		Monitor for signs/degree of restlessness and agitation; notify physician immediately regarding sudden appearance or increase in degree
		Reorient patient to reality—time, place, and person; reasons for hospitalization, treatments
		Reduce external stimuli to minimum, maintaining room as quiet and dark as feasible
		Apply restraints as per physician's order if this is only alternative to protect patient from self-injury; before applying restraints, try explanations and reasons for necessary care, orders, procedures to patient
		If restraints are necessary
		Explain to patient/family reasons for restraints
		Reassure family of necessity for restraints and of relationship between patient's behavior and pathology
		Check restraints frequently for proper placement; monitor effectiveness, skin integrity, and circulation
		Reapply q4 hr and prn
		Frequently reevaluate need for continuing restraints
■ Seizures	■ Absence or control of seizures	■ Prevention of precipitating factors in seizure occurrence including fever, hypoxia, H_2O intoxication, electrolyte disturbances
		Notify physician of potential/presence of any factors
		Seizure precautions (if indicated)
		Padded siderails up at all times when patient is alone
		Bed height at lowest level
		Padded tongue blade and airway at bedside
		Suctioning and O_2 equipment readily available
		Emergency medications available
		Close supervision and observation
		Administer anticonvulsant medications as ordered; monitor effects, side effects, and serum drug levels
		If seizure occurs, monitor and record seizure activity; notify physician; see Standard: *Seizures*

Potential problems	Expected outcomes	Nursing activities
■ Presence of neurological deficit	■ Absence of complications Maximal neurological functioning	■ On admission establish and implement nursing care plan based on individual needs and specific deficit present Ongoing assessments and evaluations of effectiveness of interventions
■ Patient/family's anxiety related to Limited understanding of diagnostic tests, procedures, anticipated surgery, postoperative course Potential/presence of neurological deficit; fears of disability or worsened deficit	■ Patient/family's behavior indicates decreased anxiety with provision of information	■ Ongoing assessment of level of anxiety, knowledge base, and understanding Encourage patient/family's verbalization of questions and fears; collaborate with physician in providing realistic information and reassurance appropriate to level of understanding Explain relationship between symptoms and neurological problems—reasons for therapies Explain and prepare patient for procedures, tests, preoperative routines If hair is to be shaved, assess anxieties regarding hair loss and possible altered body image; save hair if patient desires; provide information on means to deal with hair loss, such as wigs Explain postoperative care anticipated, including routines, setting, monitoring equipment, IVs, drains, length of stay, visiting policy Explain reasons for frequent neurological assessments and vital sign monitoring Instruct patient in deep breathing and leg exercises; evaluate patient's performance Provide time needed for support and instruction of patient/family Notify unit where patient will be after surgery of any special problems or items patient needs such as Eyeglasses: for vision, to evaluate visual fields/acuity Dentures: for patient comfort, to evaluate facial symmetry If language barrier is present: an effort should be made to have interpreter available postoperatively

Postoperative

■ General immediate postoperative complications	■ Absence or resolution of complications	■ Monitor for recovery from anesthesia; notify physician if patient is not recovered in expected time period Monitor for recovery from any special measures induced during surgery such as hypotension/hypothermia Monitor for signs/symptoms of potential complications including hypovolemia, shock, hypostatic pneumonia, pulmonary emboli, thrombophlebitis, abdominal ileus, nausea/vomiting, oliguria/urinary retention Notify physician immediately of any signs/symptoms of complication Administer medications and treatments as ordered Monitor effects and side effects and for resolution or progression of complication See appropriate standard for identified complication such as *Embolic phenomena; Shock*
■ Increased ICP/neurological deficit; appearance of deficit related to Edema Hemorrhage Hematoma Air formation	■ Absence or resolution of increased ICP Maximal neurological functioning Absence or resolution of complications	■ Establish neurological baseline postoperatively and compare to preoperative baseline; notify physician immediately if there is any decrease in status Neurological assessments and vital signs as ordered (usually q15 min until stable, q30 min until stable, then q1-2 hr) Monitor Closely LOC, pupils (size, equality, light reactivity, and ocular movements); motor/sensory systems; communication

Potential problems	Expected outcomes	Nursing activities
		abilities and speech quality; BP, P, respiratory rate, pattern and quality; for any abnormality/decline
		For any increase in headache, nausea/vomiting above usual postoperative expectation
		Notify physician immediately of any change in neurological status or vital signs
		See Problem, Increased ICP (preoperative) for all other activities and more detailed neurological assessments as status allows
		Maintain patency of subdural drain if present
		See Problem, Nonpatent subdural drain
■ Nonpatent subdural drain Potential reaccumulation of subdural hematoma	■ Patent subdural drain Absence/resolution of hematoma accumulation	■ Frequent neurological assessments and vital signs as ordered; notify physician of any change in status
		Maintain head position as ordered by physician; patient is frequently kept flat for 2 to 3 days postoperatively to aid in prevention of reaccumulation
		Prevent pulling, tension, or compression of tubing by
		Properly securing and positioning tubing
		Assisting patient with positioning
		Restraining patient as per physician's order if absolutely necessary (first try explanations of reasons, dangers of pulling)
		Monitor frequently
		Patency of drainage tubing, ensuring that it is kink/compression free
		Bottle or collection apparatus for position maintenance as ordered
		Amount and quality of drainage; record accurately
		Drain site for intactness; any oozing or bleeding/bulging around site; fluid leakage/swelling
		If dressing is in place, check for any leakage of blood or other fluid
		Any correlation between amount of drainage and neurological status; if physician orders tubing clamped, maintain specific interval schedule ordered and closely monitor correlations
		Notify physician immediately if drain is not patent or oozing/leakage occurs at site
		Have new equipment needed for drainage change
		Assist physician with procedure
		When subdural drain is removed by physician
		Record total output and quality
		Send specimens as ordered and monitor results
		Monitor drain site for any oozing, fluid leakage/bulging
		Monitor for any signs of reaccumulation
■ Leakage or infection at burr hole sites	■ Burr hole sites sealed, well-healed, and infection free	■ Restraints applied as per physician's order if necessary to prevent patient touching burr hole sites
		Monitor
		Burr hole sites for any leakage, drainage (amount, quality); edema; redness; or exudate
		Temperature q4 hr and prn for any elevation
		WBC count (may be falsely elevated if patient is receiving steroids)
		Administer antibiotics as ordered; monitor effects and side effects
		Notify physician if any abnormality occurs
		Monitor culture results of exudate
		Assist physician with treatments/suturing of site

Potential problems	Expected outcomes	Nursing activities

■ Fluid and electrolyte imbalance	■ Fluid and electrolyte balance within normal limits	■ Monitor and accurately record intake and output, urine specific gravity as ordered
		Monitor for signs of dehydration or overhydration such as
		    Poor skin turgor
		    Dry mucous membranes
		    Peripheral edema
		    Excessive thirst
		    Change in LOC
		Monitor for
		    Abnormal vital signs, Hgb/Hct values
		    Abnormal serum electrolyte values
		    Weight alterations
		    Temperature elevations
		    Insensible fluid losses including respiratory, diaphoresis, secretions
		    Presence/degree of nausea or vomiting; monitor effectiveness of medications ordered
		Administer IV fluids as ordered
		Administer medications as ordered; monitor effects and side effects; if patient is receiving steroids, monitor urine glucose and acetone levels four times a day
		Notify physician of any fluid imbalance or electrolyte abnormality

■ Seizures	■ Absence or control of seizures	■ See problem, Seizures (preoperative)

■ Thrombophlebitis/pulmonary emboli
May be related to withdrawal of anticoagulation therapy patient was previously receiving
	■ Absence or resolution of thrombophlebitis/pulmonary emboli	■ Apply antithromboembolic stockings or Ace bandages as ordered; reapply every shift and prn; monitor for constriction/looseness, condition of skin
		Instruct and supervise patient in leg exercises, ROM exercises
		Increase activity level/progression when allowed
		Explain to patient/family the reasons why anticoagulants are being withheld
		Monitor q4 hr and prn
		    Respiratory rate, quality, and pattern for any dyspnea, tachypnea
		    Breath sounds bilaterally for quality of aeration, signs of obstruction
		    Extremities for increase in warmth/girth, tenderness, Homan's sign
		    Vital signs for tachycardia, hypotension
		    For patient complaints of chest pain, leg cramps, increasing anxiety/apprehension
		    If indicated, serial measurements of both calves and thighs daily in same spot
		Notify physician immediately if any abnormalities occur
		Prepare patient/family for any diagnostic procedures ordered
		If problem occurs, see Standard: *Embolic phenomena*

■ GI bleeding related to CNS factors Stress Steroid administration	■ Absence or resolution of GI bleeding	■ Monitor vital signs q2-4 hr, Hgb and Hct; stools for Hematest three times a week; Hematest of aspirate, emesis, and urine for any abnormalities Obtain order for antacid administration as soon as patient able to take po Monitor for signs of GI bleeding, including abdominal tenderness/distention, hypotension, sudden tachycardia Notify physician immediately if any abnormalities occur If problem occurs, see Standard: *Upper gastrointestinal bleeding*

Potential problems	Expected outcomes	Nursing activities
■ Continued presence of neurological deficit Patient/family's fears, anxiety, anger related to deficit and possible alterations in life-style	■ Maximal neurological functioning* Maximal independence in ADL (within capabilities) Patient/family verbalizes concerns	■ Assess patient's specific neurological deficit Implement individualized plan of care based on patient's needs and deficits Assist as needed in ADL Monitor potential for independent functioning and obtain equipment to maximize function and promote safety Obtain orders for appropriate referrals such as physical, speech, occupational therapy, social service Encourage patient/family's verbalization of fears, anxieties, and other reactions—level and degree Answer questions realistically Encourage their participation in care planning, implementation, evaluation, and decision making Realistically reassure and support patient/family Reinforce any gains or independence patient achieves Plan, instruct, demonstrate, supervise, and evaluate patient/family's verbalization/performance of needed information/skills for maximal independent functioning such as Measures to prevent complications Assistance necessary—type, amount, degree Proper use of therapeutic devices/equipment Monitor level of achievement toward maximizing potentials and independence; means to promote as "normal" a life-style as possible
■ Insufficient knowledge to comply with discharge regimen†	■ Patient/family demonstrates or verbalizes understanding of discharge regimen	■ Assess patient/family's level of understanding of neurological problem and therapy received Explain relationship between patient's neurological status and therapies prescribed If appropriate, explain relationship between head injury occurrence and subdural hematoma; other contributing factors Encourage patient/family to discuss means, measures, alterations, precautions to decrease potential for head injury recurrence; if patient is alcoholic, secure appropriate resources for assistance in dealing with problem Explain safety precautions to prevent/minimize falls Instruct patient/family regarding required information/skills so that before discharge patient/family is able to
	Patient/family accurately describes medication, activity, and dietary regimen	Describe medication regimen Name and purpose Route, dosage, frequency, times Side effects Special precautions necessary including drugs, foods, and beverages contraindicated or quantity regulated; factors potentiating/decreasing effects/side effects; physical restrictions; safety measures Describe activity regimen, exercise program Describe dietary regimen Describe and demonstrate any special therapeutic measures prescribed; safety precautions
	Patient/family describes means to achieve maximal independence in ADL, promote safety, and prevent complications	Describe and demonstrate proper use of equipment or therapeutic devices Reasons for using Time, method, and duration of use Precautions/safeguards

*If responsibility of critical care nurse includes this stage of care.
†If responsibility of the critical care nurse includes such follow-up care.

Potential problems	Expected outcomes	Nursing activities
		Necessary maintenance (type, frequency)
		Measures to promote optimal functioning, upkeep, duration
	Patient/family describes signs/symptoms requiring medical attention	Describe signs/symptoms of neurological status requiring medical care
	Patient/family describes follow-up care regimen	Describe plan for follow-up care including purpose of appointment, when and where to go, who to see, what to expect

28 □ Supratentorial craniotomy

Supratentorial craniotomy is a surgical procedure in which the cranium is incised above the tentorium (fold of the dura mater that separates the cerebral cortex from the cerebellum and brain stem). This type of operative approach is frequently performed in adults, since approximately two thirds of cerebral conditions requiring surgical intervention are located above the tentorium. The pathological conditions for which a supratentorial craniotomy may be performed are numerous. They commonly include complete or partial removal of a brain tumor or arteriovenous malformation, clipping or wrapping of an intracerebral aneurysm, excision of abscess, evacuation of clot, elevation of depressed skull fractures, tissue biopsy, and temporal lobectomy for seizure control. Whatever the pathological entity involved, a supratentorial craniotomy may be performed to correct or attempt to control the potential presence or progression of cerebral damage, disturbance, or impaired functioning.

The diverse pathological conditions warranting operative therapy manifest widely variable neurological symptoms ranging from no symptoms or subtle signs to a sudden cerebral herniation syndrome. Many factors influence the presence, extent, type, and progression of neurological symptoms exhibited. These factors include location and area of pathological conditions, onset of pathological conditions (slow growing versus abrupt onset); effectiveness of compensatory mechanisms; effects on ICP, cerebral blood flow, and cerebral edema; effects on CSF dynamics; extent of displacement and compression of cerebral tissue; invasion of other areas; and extent and degree of cerebral damage. Some common neurological signs manifested by the myriad of pathological conditions include headache, vomiting, altered LOC, mental changes, visual defects, seizures, and papilledema.

There are some common focal neurological signs occurring with pathology in specific lobes of the brain (see Table 4). The signs are not absolute indicators of pathology location, but their presence would increase the probability of certain areas as suspected pathological sites. In some instances, a strong correlation does exist between the area involved in pathology and the clinical signs manifested. However, symptoms alone from a certain focal area of the cerebral cortex cannot be absolutely equated with the functions distributed to that area. The brain is a complex structure whose normal functioning depends on many associative areas, integrative areas, feedback systems, and interrelationships. Dysfunction in one cerebral area may produce a wide range of signs from the physiological and pathological effects on other areas and overall cerebral functioning. In general, supratentorial motor and sensory functioning are manifested and effected on the opposite side of the body from the hemisphere. The right cerebral hemisphere controls motor and sensory functioning of the left side of the body; the left hemisphere controls functioning of the right side of the body. The term *contralateral* refers to the opposite body side from the hemisphere involved in the pathological condition; for instance, a right frontal tumor may result in left arm/leg weakness or paralysis (contralateral motor signs, that is, opposite to side of hemisphere pathological condition). The term *ipsilateral* refers to the same body side as the hemisphere involved, for instance, right hemisphere pathology producing signs that are manifested on the right side of the body (ipsilateral signs). The dominant hemisphere for the majority of the population is thought to be the left; speech center functions also are usually located on this side. Frequently invasive treatments or tests are performed in the nondominant hemisphere (usually right), if feasible, to minimize damage or interference with functioning.

ASSESSMENT

1. Onset, duration, progression, and specific description of neurological symptoms, especially any alterations in
   a. LOC
   b. Behavior or personality
   c. Motor system
   d. Sensory system
   e. Pupils and extraocular movements
   f. Visual abilities
   g. Communication skills
2. Presence or history of headache including location, severity, frequency, duration, precipitating factors or time-related occurrence, association with other neurological symptoms; nausea/vomiting including frequency, severity, time-related factors
3. Previous seizures—exact description including onset, progression, type, locality, length, aura, incontinence
   a. Postictal status; any injury incurred
   b. Presence of any precipitating factors such as fever, emotional upset
   c. Frequency of seizures
   d. If multiple seizures, any variation in seizure activity or similar episodes

Table 4. Common focal signs of lobe pathology

Frontal lobe damage
1. Mental changes such as personality changes, impaired memory, lack of initiative, mood changes
2. Motor weakness or spastic paralysis on contralateral side
3. Presence of sucking and grasping reflexes
4. Expressive (Broca's) aphasia if dominant hemisphere is involved (left hemisphere for most people)
5. Seizures—jacksonian or generalized motor
6. Agraphia
7. Apraxia

Temporal lobe damage
1. Visual field defect of upper contralateral quadrant
2. Auditory illusions and hallucinations
3. Personality changes—psychotic behavior
4. Seizures—psychomotor or generalized
   a. Dreamy state—"unicinate epilepsy"
   b. May have auditory hallucinations alone or with visual, gustatory hallucinations
   c. Masticatory movements
   d. Disturbances in time perception
5. In dominant hemisphere involvement (usually left)
   a. Receptive (Wernicke's) aphasia
   b. Difficulty in tests of verbal material presented through auditory sense
6. In nondominant hemisphere involvement
   a. Difficulty judging spatial relationships
   b. Difficulty in tests of nonverbal material presented through visual sense

Parietal lobe damage
1. Sensory disturbances
   a. Loss of two-point discrimination
   b. Loss of ability to judge size and shape of objects (astereognosis)
   c. Hypoesthesia/paresthesia—contralateral side
   d. Impairment or loss of position sense
2. Motor weakness—contralateral side
3. Homonymous hemianopia or visual inattention
4. Seizures—sensory type
5. Inattentiveness
6. Impaired memory
7. If dominant lobe involvement
   a. Language disorders, especially alexia
   b. Gerstmann's syndrome
      (1) Difficulty writing (agraphia)
      (2) Difficulty doing math (acalculia)
      (3) Finger agnosia
      (4) Right/left confusion
   c. Apraxia—ideomotor
8. If nondominant hemisphere involvement
   a. Memory loss
   b. Neglect of one half of body (anosognosia)
   c. Dressing apraxia

Occipital lobe damage
1. Homonymous hemianopia—contralateral
2. Visual illusions and hallucinations
3. Cortical blindness
4. Visual agnosia—cannot name or identify use of object seen
5. Defects in visual perceptions with loss of topographic memory
6. Loss of color perception

e. If patient is receiving anticonvulsants, whether prescribed regimen has been adhered to
4. Medications taken for neurologicial problem such as anticonvulsants, steroids, pain medications; effects and side effects of drug therapies
5. Previous neurological treatment or neurosurgical procedure
6. Presence of any medical problems and medications/ treatments prescribed and followed
7. Patient's perceptions and reaction to diagnosis, therapeutic modalities, anticipated surgical intervention
8. Presence of any alterations in body image; fears of permanent disability or deficit; altered roles in family, normal occupation, performing ADL; fears of tumor regrowth or recurrence of pathological condition
9. Baseline parameters status
   a. Neurological
   b. Respiratory
   c. Cardiovascular
   d. Hydration
   e. Vital signs
   f. Weight
   g. Handedness (right or left)
   h. Urine output pattern
10. Diagnostic test results, including
    a. CAT
    b. Cerebral angiography
    c. Skull radiographs
    d. Brain scan
    e. EEG
    f. Pneumoencephalogram
    g. Lumbar puncture
11. Results of
    a. Serum electrolyte levels

b. Hgb and Hct, platelet count, WBC count and differentiation
c. Type and cross matching
d. Urinalysis, culture, specific gravity, osmolality, electrolytes
e. Arterial blood gas levels
f. Clotting profile
g. Anticonvulsant drug levels
h. CSF determinations
i. Chest radiograph
j. ECG

GOALS

1. Optimal neurological functioning
2. Optimal independence in ADL
3. Adequate alveolar ventilation
4. Serum electrolytes and fluid balance within normal limits
5. Hgb and Hct stable within normal limits
6. Acid-base balance within normal limits
7 Incision well-healed
8. Infection free
9. Reduction in patient/family's anxiety with provision of information, demonstrations, support
10. Before discharge patient/family is able to
    a. Describe medication, activity, exercise, and dietary regimens
    b. Demonstrate safety measures and techniques; proper use of any equipment/therapeutic devices prescribed
    c. Describe signs and symptoms requiring medical attention
    d. State necessary information regarding follow-up care

Potential problems	Expected outcomes	Nursing activities
Preoperative		
■ Patient/family's anxiety related to Limited understanding of diagnostic tests, procedures, anticipated surgery, postoperative course Potential/presence of neurological deficit; fears of disability or worsened deficit	■ Patient/family's behavior indicates decreased anxiety with provision of information	■ Ongoing assessment of level of anxiety, knowledge base, and understanding Encourage patient/family's verbalization of questions and fears; collaborate with physician in providing realistic information and reassurance appropriate to level of understanding (if surgery is to be performed for aneurysm, physician may allow provision of only limited information; see Standard: *Subarachnoid hemorrhage* if this occurs) Explain relationship between symptoms and neurological problem; reasons for therapies Explain and prepare patient for procedures, tests, preoperative routines

Potential problems	Expected outcomes	Nursing activities
		If hair is to be shaved, assess anxieties regarding hair loss and possible altered body image; save hair if patient desires; provide information on means to deal with hair loss, such as wigs
		Explain anticipated postoperative care including routines, setting, monitoring equipment, IVs, drains, length of stay, visiting policy
		Explain reasons for frequent neurological assessments and vital sign monitoring
		Instruct in deep breathing and leg exercises; evaluate patient's performance
		Provide time needed for support and instruction of patient/family
		Notify unit where patient will be after surgery of any special problems or items patient needs such as
		Eyeglasses: for vision; to evaluate visual fields/acuity
		Dentures: for patient comfort; to evaluate facial symmetry
		If language barrier is present: an effort should be made to have interpreter available postoperatively
■ Increased ICP with possible development or worsening of neurological deficit	■ Absence of complications Maximal neurological functioning	■ Establish neurological baseline and vital signs on admission; ongoing assessments as ordered of status and specific symptomatology, monitoring especially for extent and degree of Headache Nausea/vomiting Altered LOC Mental changes such as disorientation, impaired memory Pupillary changes Visual defects Papilledema Motor/sensory system dysfunctions Communication ability deficits Personality changes such as restlessness, irritability, apathy Avoid precipitating factors in increased ICP such as hypoxia, hypercapnia, fever, Valsalva's maneuver Assist patient with positioning and turning; instruct patient not to hold breath Prevent constipation by establishing bowel regimen as individually warranted; ensure that patient has bowel movement preoperatively Monitor for any signs/symptoms that could initiate factor development such as hypoventilation Notify physician of potential/presence of any factors Maintain head gatch and activity as ordered Administer medications and treatments as ordered; monitor effects and side effects Accurately record intake and output; monitor for any imbalance Monitor serum electrolyte levels for any abnormalities Notify physician immediately of any change in neurological status, vital signs, or abnormal fluid/electrolyte balance If problem occurs, see Standard: *Increased intracranial pressure*
■ Presence of neurological deficit	■ Absence of complications	■ On admission establish and implement nursing care plan based on individual needs and specific deficit present Ongoing assessments and evaluations of effectiveness of interventions Establish neurological baseline immediately preoperatively to provide for comparison postoperatively

Potential problems	**Expected outcomes**	**Nursing activities**

■ Seizures	■ Absence or control of seizures	■ Prevention of precipitating factors in seizure occurrence including fever, hypoxia, H_2O intoxication, electrolyte disturbances
		Notify physician of potential/presence of any factors
		Seizure precautions (if indicated)
		  Padded siderails up at all times when patient is alone
		  Bed height at lowest level
		  Padded tongue blade and airway at bedside
		  Emergency medications and equipment readily available
		  Close observation and supervision
		Administer anticonvulsant medications as ordered; monitor effects and side effects, serum anticonvulsant levels
		If seizure occurs, monitor and record seizure activity; notify physician
		SEE STANDARD: *Seizures*

Postoperative

■ General postoperative complications immediately after surgery	■ Absence or resolution of complications	■ Monitor for
		  Recovery from anesthesia; notify physician if patient has not recovered in expected time period
		  Potential hypovolemia, shock, hypostatic pneumonia, pulmonary emboli, thrombophlebitis, abdominal ileus, nausea/vomiting, oliguria/urinary retention
		  Recovery from any special measures induced during surgery such as hypotension/hypothermia
		Notify physician immediately of any signs/symptoms of complication
		  Administer medications and treatments as ordered
		  Monitor effects and side effects
		  Continue monitoring for resolution or progression of complication
		See appropriate standard for identified complication such as *Embolic phenomena; Shock*

■ Increased ICP/increased neurological deficit/appearance related to
Edema
Hemorrhage
Hematoma formation
	■ Absence or control of increased ICP
	Maximal neurological functioning
		■ Establish neurological baseline postoperatively and compare to preoperative baseline
		See Problem, Increased ICP (preoperative) for all specific activities
		In addition, monitor
		  Neurological assessments and vital signs as ordered and prn (usually q15 min until stable, q30 min until stable, q1 hr until stable, and then q2 hr)
		  Particularly LOC; pupil size, equality, and reactivity; extraocular movements; motor and sensory systems; communication abilities and speech quality; respiratory rate, pattern, and quality; BP and P for any abnormalities
		  For any increase in headache, nausea/vomiting above usual postoperative expectation
		  For signs of epidural hematoma (see Standard: *Head trauma*, Problem, Epidural hematoma)
		  For more detailed and specific assessments as patient's status allows
		  Head dressing with neurological assessments for any bleeding or oozing, elevation in surgical site or edema in other sites, unusual constriction or looseness
		Maintain head gatch as ordered (usually elevated to promote venous drainage)
		If Hemovac (or other drainage collection apparatus) is used
		  Prevent any tension or pulling on drainage tubing by proper positioning of patient and securing of drainage tubing; if

Potential problems	Expected outcomes	Nursing activities

necessary, restrain patient's hands to prevent pulling or tension of tubing (first try explanations of reasons necessary/purposes of drain)

Maintain Hemovac as per physician's order such as suction or gravity drainage (if frontal sinus is incised intraoperatively, suction is usually avoided postoperatively)

Monitor
And accurately record amount and quality of drainage; notify physician immediately if amount is more than expected or quality differs from normal
Functioning of system
Drain site for any oozing or bleeding around area
For patency of drain and intactness
Notify physician of any signs of drainage malfunctioning

When drain is removed by physician, monitor
And accurately record output
Drain site for oozing, bleeding, or edema
Results of any specimens obtained

Notify physician immediately of any decline in neurological status from preoperative status, or change in status or vital signs postoperatively; of any increase in symptoms or worsening deficit

Administer medications/treatments as ordered; monitor effects and side effects

Prepare patient/family for any diagnostic tests/procedures ordered

- Respiratory insufficiency related to
  CNS dysfunction
  Pneumonia
  Atelectasis
  Pulmonary emboli

- Patent airway
  Adequate alveolar ventilation and perfusion
  Normal respiratory rate and quality
  Arterial blood gas levels within patient's normal limits

- Ongoing assessments of respiratory status q2 hr and prn; monitor for any abnormality/decline
  Respiratory rate, quality, and pattern
  Patency of upper airway and patient's ability to handle secretions
  Skin color, nail beds, peripheral pulses, and skin warmth
  Presence/strength of gag, cough, and swallowing reflexes
  Breath sounds bilaterally for quality of aeration; signs of obstruction (rales, rhonchi)
  Arterial blood gas values
  Chest radiograph results
  Signs/symptoms of thrombophlebitis, pulmonary emboli, pulmonary edema

Maintain patent airway by
Turning and positioning to prevent obstruction or aspiration of secretions q2 hr and prn; (if bone flap has been removed, patient may not be permitted to lie on one side of head)
Deep breathing and coughing q1 hr and prn (if allowed)
Suctioning prn (if frontal sinus was incised intraoperatively, nasal suctioning is usually contraindicated)
Adequate oxygenation and humidification as ordered
Chest physiotherapy/pulmonary toilet if warranted and not contraindicated by physician's order

Apply antithromboembolic stockings or Ace bandages as ordered; reapply every shift and prn; monitor for constriction/looseness, condition of skin

Instruct and supervise patient in performing leg exercises, ROM exercises

Increase activity level/progression when allowed

Notify physician immediately of any change in respiratory/neurological status or signs of complication potential/occurrence

Potential problems	Expected outcomes	Nursing activities
		If problem occurs, assist with emergency measures to maintain patent airway and adequate ventilation Administer medications/treatments as ordered; monitor effects and side effects See Standard: *Mechanical ventilation;* if emboli occur, see Standard: *Embolic phenomena*

■ Fluid and electrolyte imbalance	■ Fluid and electrolyte balance within normal limits	■ Monitor and accurately record intake and output, urine specific gravity as ordered
		Monitor for signs of dehydration or overhydration such as
		  Poor skin turgor
		  Dry mucous membranes
		  Peripheral edema
		  Excessive thirst
		  Change in LOC
		Monitor for
		  Abnormal vital signs, Hgb/Hct values
		  Abnormal serum electrolyte values (retention of Na^+ from increased aldosterone effect with increased release of ADH frequently occurs postoperatively, resulting in decreased serum Na^+ values)
		  Weight alterations
		  Temperature elevations
		  Insensible fluid losses including respiratory, diaphoresis, secretions
		  Presence/degree of nausea/vomiting; effectiveness of medications ordered
		  Presence/quality of bowel sounds for any abnormality
		Administer IV fluids, NG feedings as ordered
		Administer medication as ordered; monitor effects and side effects; if patient is receiving steroids, monitor urine glucose and acetone levels four times a day
		Notify physician of any fluid imbalance or electrolyte abnormality

■ Headache/incisional pain	■ Absence or control of pain	■ Administer pain medications as ordered; monitor effects and side effects Notify physician if medication is not effective Monitor dressing for increased tightness/constriction Maintain environment at quietest level possible

■ Seizures	■ Absence or control of seizures	■ See Problem, Seizures (preoperative), for all activities
		In addition
		  Phenytoin (Dilantin) is frequently ordered postoperatively; if given IV, monitor ECG for any abnormalities, BP for any hypotension
		  Prevent, if possible, exposure to potential fever sources, since elevated temperature can precipitate seizure activity
		  Monitor and report to physician signs of other factors predisposing patient to postoperative seizures such as hypoxia, hypoglycemia, H_2O intoxication, hyperventilation
		  Administer medications/treatments as ordered; monitor effects and side effects; monitor appropriate lab test results

■ Hypotension or hypertension	■ BP within patient's normal or prescribed limits	■ Monitor
		  BP as ordered for any abnormality
		  For signs of hypovolemia/hypervolemia
		  For signs of shock
		  Neurological status for any decline q1-2 hr
		Maintain BP at level ordered by physician by administration of prn medications ordered
		  Monitor effects and side effects

Potential problems	Expected outcomes	Nursing activities
		Notify physician if medication regimen is not resulting in desired BP level
		Notify physician immediately of any abnormality
■ Infection	■ Infection free Incision well-healed	■ Keep patient's hands from operative site/drain
		Maintain sterility of head dressing/drainage apparatus
		Administer antibiotics as ordered; monitor effects and side effects (frequently ordered postoperatively prophylactically)
		Monitor
		Temperature as ordered and prn for any elevation
		Dressing/incision site q2 hr for any signs of redness, tenderness, bulging, separation, or drainage (amount and quality)
		If drainage apparatus is present, monitor amount and quality for any abnormality
		Neurological status and vital signs for any decline/abnormality
		IV sites frequently for any signs for redness, tenderness, phlebitis
		WBC count (may be falsely elevated if patient is receiving steroids)
		For any signs/symptoms of meningitis
		Notify physician immediately of any signs/symptoms of infection
		Administer medications/treatments as ordered
		Monitor wound culture results
		Monitor for other possible infection souces if warranted, including urine, sputum, chest radiograph results, CSF determinations
		Monitor for resolution/progression of infection
		If problem occurs, see Standard: *Meningitis/encephalitis*
■ GI bleeding related to CNS factors Stress Steroid administration	■ Absence or resolution of GI bleeding	■ Monitor vital signs q2-4 hr, Hgb and Hct, stools for Hematest three times a week; Hematest of aspirate, urine, and emesis for any abnormalities
		Obtain order for antacid administration as soon as patient able to take po
		Monitor for signs of GI bleeding including abdominal tenderness/distention, hypotension, sudden tachycardia
		Notify physician immediately if any abnormality occurs
		If problem occurs, see Standard: *Acute upper gastrointestinal bleeding*
■ Continued presence of neurological deficit Patient/family's fears, anxiety, anger related to deficit and possible alterations in lifestyle	■ Maximal neurological functioning* Maximal independence in ADL (within capabilities) Patient/family verbalizes concerns	■ Assess patient's specific neurological deficit; collaborate with physician regarding prognosis, possible degree of recovery
		Implement individualized plan of care based on patient's needs and deficits
		Assist as needed in ADL
		Monitor potential for independent functioning and obtain equipment to maximize function and promote safety
		Obtain orders for appropriate referrals such as physical, speech, occupational therapy; social service
		Encourage verbalization of patient/family's fears, anxieties, and other reactions—level and degree
		Answer questions realistically
		Encourage their participation in care planning, implementation, evaluation, and decision making
		Realistically reassure and support patient/family

*If responsibility of critical care nurse includes this stage of care.

Potential problems	Expected outcomes	Nursing activities
		Reinforce any gains or independence patient achieves Plan, instruct, demonstrate, supervise, and evaluate patient/family's verbalization/performance of needed information/skills for maximal independent functioning such as 　Measures to prevent complications 　Assistance necessary—type, amount, degree 　Proper use of therapeutic devices/equipment Monitor level of achievement toward maximizing potentials and independence; means to promote as "normal" a life-style as possible
■ Insufficient knowledge to comply with discharge regimen*	■ Patient/family demonstrates or verbalizes understanding of discharge regimen	■ Assess patient/family's level of understanding of neurological problem and therapy received Explain relationship between patient's neurological status and therapies prescribed 　If cerebral pathological condition was caused by head injury or trauma, explore with patient/family measures to decrease injury recurrence potential and importance of controlling factors precipitating head injury Instruct patient/family regarding required information and skills so that before discharge patient/family is able to
	Patient/family accurately describes medication, activity, and dietary regimens	Describe medication regimen 　Name and purpose 　Route, dosage, frequency, times 　Side effects 　Special precautions necessary including drugs, foods, beverages contraindicated or quantity regulated; factors potentiating/decreasing effects or side effects; physical restrictions; safety measures Describe dietary regimen Describe activity regimen, exercise program Describe and demonstrate any special therapeutic measures prescribed
	Patient/family describes means to achieve maximal independence in ADL, promote safety, and prevent complications	Describe and demonstrate proper use of equipment or therapeutic devices 　Reasons for using 　Time, method, and duration of use 　Precautions/safeguards 　Necessary maintenance (type, frequency) 　Measures to promote optimal functioning, upkeep/duration
	Patient/family describes signs/symptoms requiring medical attention	Describe signs/symptoms of neurological status requiring medical care
	Patient/family describes follow-up care regimen	Describe plan for follow-up care including purpose of appointment, when and where to go, who to see, what to expect

*If responsibility of critical care nurse includes such follow-up care.

29 □ Infratentorial craniotomy

Infratentorial craniotomy is a surgical procedure in which the cranium is incised below the tentorium (fold of the dura mater that separates the cerebral cortex from the cerebellum and brain stem). The areas below the tentorium that may be involved in pathological conditions are numerous. Tumors, hemorrhages, and clots may reside in the midbrain, pons, medulla, fourth ventricle, cerebellum, and cerebellar pontine angle (particularly acoustic neurinomas and meningiomas). Infratentorial craniotomies are usually longer and more complex because of a less accessible operative site, the difficult positioning required, the need to avoid many vital structures in the infratentorial area such as respiratory and reticular activating system, the frequent presence of increased ICP, the frequent compression of additional areas by displacements from original pathological site, and so on. In general, recovery from infratentorial craniotomy takes longer than recovery after supratentorial craniotomy.

The symptoms manifested when a pathological condition exists in the brain stem, cerebellum, or fourth ventricle vary with each individual. Some of the factors contributing to this variability include size, location, rate of growth, quality, and extent of tumor or clot; effectiveness of compensatory mechanisms; location, amount and degree of compression of other cerebral structures; effects on ICP, CSF dynamics. There are frequently occurring symptoms associated with certain areas of the brain stem, cerebellum, and fourth ventricle (Table 5). The presence of these symptoms does not pinpoint the original site of the pathological condition in all cases, since the dysfunction could be caused by compression or displacement from another area.

A pathological condition in the brain stem commonly produces cranial nerve dysfunctions by an interference with the nuclei or processes for effecting cranial nerve function. Cranial nerve nuclei located within the brain stem include hypoglossal (XII), spinal accessory (XI), glossopharyngeal (IX), and vagus (X) in the medulla; trigeminal (V), abducens (VI), facial (VII), and acoustic (VIII) in the pons; and oculomotor (III) and trochlear (IV) in the midbrain.

Unilateral lesions of the cerebellum produce signs on the same side of the body as the lesion (ipsilateral) due to the double pathway–crossing mechanism of cerebellar output. The signs of cerebellar dysfunction are due to a loss of the usual cerebellar influences, resulting in centers released from normal modulating controls. Incoordination, impaired balance, and disorders of equilibrium and gait are common signs of cerebellar dysfunction. Clinical signs may also include hypotonia, decomposition of movement, asthenia (muscles tire easily), adiadochokinesia (impaired ability to perform alternating repetitive movements rapidly), tremor (usually intention), dysmetria (inability to stop at desired point), ataxia, scanning speech or dysarthria, and nystagmus.

Pathological disorders in the fourth ventricle, either from a primary source or as a result of compression from another area, commonly produces hydrocephalus. This CSF accumulation, from overproduction or interference with normal reabsorption and circulation may increase the ICP. Further increases in ICP may result in additional damage by displacement and compression. Herniation syndromes, both upward through the tentorial notch and downward through the foramen magnum, may occur with infratentorial lesions. Frequently a burr hole is placed, either preoperatively or intraoperatively, in the lateral ventricle for relief of increased ICP by insertion of a ventriculostomy drain for ventricular fluid drainage. This external ventricular drainage system may be left in place for a period of time postoperatively to relieve the pressure and also provide a parameter for assessing the amount of pressure and fluid within the ventricular system. If long-term hydrocephalus is a problem, an internalized shunting mechanism will usually be inserted.

Other considerations in infratentorial pathophysiology relate to the functioning of important vital structures and systems. The medulla has centers for vomiting, respiration, vasomotor control, and the swallowing reflex. The vagal system is composed of reflexes normally utilized for protection and compensation, including the carotid sinus reflex, carotid body reflex, and cough, gag, and swallowing reflexes. Damage or compression of these vital centers may obliterate normal protective mechanisms and further increase the potential for cerebral damage or death. The brain stem contains a reticular formation composed of multiple neurons and fibers, which are involved with consciousness and wakefulness. Interference with this reticular activating system can result in altered LOC and various stages of coma.

Table 5. Common symptoms of brain stem lesions

Medulla

Hypoglossal nerve (XII) damage, producing a lower motor neuron paralysis on ipsilateral side; initially fasciculations of tongue may occur followed by atrophy; on protrusion the tongue deviates to paralyzed side

Corticospinal tract of pyramid (motor) and medial lemniscus (discriminative general senses) damage, producing an upper motor neuron paralysis and a loss of position and muscle and joint sense, impaired tactile discrimination, and loss of vibratory sense on contralateral side of body (lesion interrupts tracts above level of decussation)

Spinothalamic tract damage, producing loss of senses of pain and temperature on opposite side of body

Spinal trigeminal tract and nucleus damage, producing loss of senses of pain and temperature on same side of face and in nasal and oral cavities

Vagal, glossopharyngeal, and spinal portions of accessory nerves damage, producing dysphagia, hoarseness, and loss of gag reflex on same side

Midbrain

Weber's syndrome: damage to oculomotor nerve (III) on same side, producing ptosis; diplopia; external strabismus; dilated pupil; inability to gaze up, down, and in; corticospinal tract damage producing upper motor neuron paralysis of contralateral side

Corticobulbar and corticoreticular fiber damage, producing lower facial expression weakness on opposite side

Benedikt syndrome: damage to oculomotor nerve (III), producing lower motor neuron paralysis of extraocular muscles and dilated pupil on ipsilateral side; red nucleus and fibers of superior cerebellar peduncle damage, producing signs of cerebellar damage on contralateral side; spinothalamic tract and medial lemniscus damage, resulting in loss of senses of pain and temperature and discriminative senses on opposite side of body

Pons

Abducens nerve (VI) damage, producing an inability to abduct eye to same side as lesion and horizontal diplopia (which worsens when patient attempts to gaze toward side of lesion)

Corticospinal fibers and medial lemniscus damage, producing a contralateral upper motor neuron paralysis and loss of discriminative senses (position, muscle and joint, vibration)

Medial longitudinal fasciculus damage, producing a disturbance of conjugate horizontal eye movements (abduction and adduction)

Trigeminal nerve (V) damage, producing loss of sensation on ipsilateral side of face, forehead, nasal and oral cavities; absence of corneal sensation and reflex; lower motor neuron paralysis of muscles of mastication with chin deviating to lesion side when mouth is opened

Lateral lemniscus damage, producing a decrease in hearing that is more pronounced on opposite side

Pontocerebellar fibers interrupted, producing cerebellar signs on same side

Cerebellopontine angle

Acoustic nerve (VIII) damage, producing tinnitus followed by progressive deafness on same side as lesion; abnormal labyrinthine responses including tilting and rotating of the head with chin pointing to lesion side

Cerebellar peduncle damage, producing coarse intention tremor, ataxic gait, dysmetria on lesion side

Spinal trigeminal tract damage, producing loss of senses of pain and temperature on ipsilateral side of face, oral cavity, and nasal cavity

Spinothalamic tract damage, producing loss of pain and temperature on contralateral side of body

Facial nerve (VII) injury, producing lower motor neuron paralysis of muscles of facial expression (Bell's palsy) and loss of taste on anterior two thirds of tongue ipsilaterally

ASSESSMENT

1. Onset, progression, frequency, duration, and specific description of neurological symptoms, including
   a. Cranial nerve dysfunctions
   b. Cerebellar signs; disturbances of balance and coordination
   c. Headache—location, severity, association with specific activity/movement, time-related pattern or occurrence, any associated concurrent neurological symptoms
   d. Nausea/vomiting
   e. Papilledema
   f. Pupillary alterations; impaired extraocular movements
   g. Visual disturbances including diplopia, blurred vision, nystagmus, field defects
   h. Hearing defects including diminished or loss of hearing, tinnitus, vertigo
   i. Motor/sensory dysfunctions
2. Medications taken for neurological problem such as steroids, antiemetics, pain medications; effects and side effects of therapies
3. Previous head trauma or injury; specific description of incident, treatment, clinical course

4. Previous neurological treatment or neurosurgical procedure
5. Presence of any medical problems and medications/treatments prescribed and followed
6. Patient's perceptions and reaction to diagnosis, therapeutic modalities, anticipated surgical intervention
7. Presence of any alterations in body image; fears of permanent disability or deficit; altered roles in family, normal occupation, performing ADL; fears of tumor regrowth or recurrence of pathological condition
8. Baseline parameters status
   a. Neurological
   b. Respiratory
   c. Cardiovascular
   d. Hydration
   e. Urine output pattern
   f. Vital signs
   g. Weight
   h. Handedness (right or left)
9. Diagnostic test results including
   a. CAT
   b. Cerebral angiography
   c. Pneumoencephalogram
   d. Skull radiographs
   e. Brain scan
   f. Lumbar puncture
   g. Ventriculogram
   h. Hearing acuity testing
10. Results of
    a. Serum electrolyte levels
    b. Hgb and Hct, platelet count, WBC count with differentiation

c. Type and cross matching
d. Urinalysis, culture, specific gravity, osmolality, electrolytes
e. Arterial blood gas levels
f. Clotting profile
g. CSF determinations
h. Chest radiograph
i. ECG

GOALS

1. Optimal neurological functioning
2. Optimal independence in ADL
3. Adequate alveolar ventilation and perfusion
4. Adequate cardiac output
5. Serum electrolytes and fluid balance within normal limits
6. Acid-base balance within normal limits
7. Hgb and Hct stable within normal limits
8. Incision well-healed
9. Infection free
10. Reduction in patient/family's anxiety with provision of information, demonstrations, support
11. Before discharge patient/family is able to
    a. Describe medication, activity, exercise, and dietary regimens
    b. Demonstrate safety measures and techniques; proper use of any equipment/therapeutic devices prescribed
    c. Describe signs and symptoms requiring medical attention
    d. State necessary information regarding follow-up care

Potential problems	Expected outcomes	Nursing activities
Preoperative		
■ Patient/family's anxiety related to Limited understanding of diagnostic tests, procedures, anticipated surgery, postoperative course Potential/presence of neurological deficit; fears of disability or worsened deficit	■ Patient/family's behavior indicates decreased anxiety with provision of information	■ Ongoing assessment of level of anxiety, knowledge base, and understanding Encourage patient/family's verbalization of questions and fears; collaborate with physician in providing realistic information and reassurance appropriate to level of understanding Explain relationship between symptoms and neurological problem; reasons for therapies Explain and prepare for procedures, tests, preoperative routines If hair is to be shaved, assess anxieties regarding hair loss and possible altered body image; save hair if patient desires; provide information on means to deal with hair loss, such as wigs

Potential problems	Expected outcomes	Nursing activities
		Explain anticipated postoperative care including routines, settings, monitoring equipment, IVs, drains, length of stay, visiting policy
		Explain reasons for frequent neurological assessments and vital sign monitoring
		Instruct in deep breathing and leg exercises; evaluate patient's performance
		Provide time needed for support and instruction of patient/family
		Notify unit where patient will be after surgery of any special problems or items patient needs such as
		Eyeglasses: for vision; to evaluate visual fields/acuity
		Dentures: for patient comfort; to evaluate facial symmetry
		If language barrier is present: an effort should be made to have interpreter available postoperatively
■ Increased ICP with possible development or worsening of neurological deficit	■ Absence of complications Maximal neurological functioning	■ Establish neurological baseline and vital signs on admission; ongoing assessments as ordered of status and specific symptomatology, especially monitoring for extent and degree
		Headache
		Nausea/vomiting
		Visual problems such as diplopia, blurred vision, nystagmus, field defects
		Hearing defects such as diminished or loss, tinnitus, vertigo
		Cranial nerve dysfunctions
		Cerebellar disturbance signs such as ataxia, tremor, falling to one side, hypotonia, disorders or equilibrium, incoordination, dizziness, vertigo, dysarthria, muscle weakness/fatigability
		Presence/quality of gag, cough, and swallowing reflexes
		Papilledema
		Altered LOC
		Motor/sensory system dysfunctions
		Pupil size, equality, light reactivity; extraocular movements
		Balance and coordination
		Communication ability deficits
		Avoid precipitating factors in increased ICP such as hypoxia, hypercapnia, fever, Valsalva's maneuver
		Assist patient with positioning and turning; instruct patient not to hold breath
		Prevent constipation by establishing bowel regimen as individually waranted; ensure that patient has bowel movement preoperatively
		Monitor for any signs/symptoms that could initiate factor development such as hypoventilation
		Notify physician of potential/presence of factors
		Maintain head gatch and activity as ordered
		Administer medications and treatments as ordered; monitor effects and side effects
		Accurately record intake and output; monitor for any imbalance
		Monitor serum electrolytes for any abnormalities
		Notify physician immediately of any change in neurological status, vital signs, or abnormal fluid/electrolyte balance
		If problem occurs, see Standard: *Increased intracranial pressure*
■ Presence of neurological deficit	■ Absence of complications	■ On admission establish and implement nursing care plan based on individual needs and specific deficit present
		Ongoing assessments and evaluations of effectiveness of interventions
		Establish neurological baseline immediately preoperatively to provide for comparison postoperatively

Potential problems	Expected outcomes	Nursing activities
■ Ataxia—impaired balance and coordination	■ Ambulates safely with assistance	■ Assess degree, location, and extent of ataxia Assist and supervise patient in ADL and ambulation Apply safety measures such as siderails while patient is in bed, safety belt in wheelchair Maintain safe environment 　Remove as many obstacles or objects with the potential for causing falls as possible 　Obtain appropriate safety equipment Explain to patient/family reasons for assistance, special measures to promote safety

Postoperative

Potential problems	Expected outcomes	Nursing activities
■ General immediate postoperative complications	■ Absence or resolution of complication	■ Monitor for 　Recovery from anesthesia; notify physician if patient has not recovered in expected time period 　Potential hypovolemia, shock, hypostatic pneumonia, pulmonary emboli, thrombophlebitis, abdominal ileus, nausea/vomiting, oliguria/urinary retention 　Recovery from any special measures induced during surgery such as hypotension/hypothermia Notify physician immediately of any signs/symptoms of complication Administer medications and treatments as ordered Monitor effects and side effects Continue monitoring for resolution or progression of complication See appropriate standard for identified complication such as *Embolic phenomena; Shock*
■ Increased ICP related to 　Edema 　Hematoma 　CSF obstruction 　Possible upward or downward cerebral herniation from increased ICP	■ Absence or control of increased ICP 　Maximal neurological functioning	■ Establish neurological baseline postoperatively and compare to preoperative baseline See Problem, Increased ICP (preoperative), for all specific activities In addition, monitor 　Neurological assessments and vital signs as ordered and prn (usually q15 min until stable, q30 min until stable, and then q1 hr) 　Particularly LOC; pupil size, equality, and reactivity; extraocular movements; motor and sensory systems; communication abilities and speech quality; respiratory rate, pattern, and quality; BP and P for any abnormalities 　For any increase in headache, nausea/vomiting above usual postoperative expectation 　For any sudden appearance or increase in diplopia, nystagmus, ataxia, cerebellar dysfunctions, cranial nerve dysfunctions 　For more detailed and specific assessments as patient's status allows 　Operative site q1-2 hr for any signs of bleeding, bulging, or tenseness Maintain head gatch as ordered (usually elevated 30 to 45 degrees Accurately record intake and output q1-2 hr; monitor for signs of dehydration/overhydration; see Problem, Fluid and electrolyte imbalance Avoid hyperflexion or extension of neck 　Support head when turning or lifting patient 　Frequently neck collar may be ordered; maintain in proper position

Potential problems	Expected outcomes	Nursing activities

If pillow is allowed, position with type to avoid aforementioned (such as horseshoe)

Notify physician immediately of any decline in neurological status from preoperative baseline or change in status or vital signs postoperatively; of any increase in symptoms or worsening deficit

Administer medications/treatments as ordered; monitor effects and side effects

Prepare patient/family for any diagnostic tests/procedures ordered

If ventricular drainage system is continued postoperatively

Prevent any compression, kinking, pulling, or tension on tubing by proper positioning of patient; if necessary restrain patient's hands to prevent pulling or tension of tubing (first try explanations of necessary reasons/purposes for drain)

Monitor drainage system q1 hr for patency; fluid should be fluctuating in tubing or draining into collection apparatus

Maintain sterility of system

Maintain at specific level ordered by physician

Measure and record as ordered pressure, amount, and quality of drainage; notify physician if variable from norm specified; (physician will usually specify acceptable ranges of pressure and amount)

Notify physician immediately of any cloudiness of CSF

Check dressing q1 hr; monitor for any leakage around drain site, swelling, or edema

Monitor neurological status correlated with fluid pressure/quantity

If patient is on ICP monitoring, record pressures and drain fluid amount specified by physician's order to maintain pressure values; monitor effects of certain treatments on ICP such as coughing, turning, and suctioning; space activities if possible to minimize increases in ICP

Administer antibiotics as ordered; monitor effects and side effects

Send CSF specimens as ordered and monitor results

Monitor serum electrolyte levels as Na^+ values may decrease from loss of CSF by drainage; notify physician of results and replace fluid as ordered (frequently CSF fluid is ordered replaced milliliter for milliliter)

Monitor for signs of epidural hematoma (see Standard: *Head trauma*, Problem, Epidural hematoma) and meningitis (see Standard: *Meningitis/encephalitis*)—both potential problem complications of ventricular drainage

If ordered, clamp tubing as specified by physician, such as may be ordered when coughing and turning patient

Notify physician immediately of any change in neurological status; fluid pressure, amount or quality abnormality; nonpatency of system; or abnormal lab values

If clamping schedule is ordered, clamp tubing as specified, maintaining precise time schedule and recording of time, pressure, fluid drainage amount/quality; notify physician of any change in neurological status or signs of increased ICP; unclamp drain as per physician's standing or stat order

After removal of ventricular drain by physician, monitor neurological status and vital signs frequently; burr hole sites for oozing, bleeding, drainage/edema; for signs of increased ICP; have emergency ventriculostomy set, medications readily available; report to physician immediately any ab-

Potential problems	Expected outcomes	Nursing activities
		normality/decline; if internal shunting procedure is necessary, see Standard: *Internalized shunting procedures*
■ Respiratory insufficiency related to CNS dysfunction Edema Cranial nerve dysfunction Pneumonia Atelectasis Pulmonary emboli	■ Patent airway Adequate alveolar ventilation and perfusion Normal respiratory rate and quality Arterial blood gas levels within patient's normal limits	■ Ongoing assessment of respiratory status q1 hr and prn; monitor for any abnormality/decline Respiratory rate, quality, and pattern Patency of upper airway and patient's ability to handle secretions Presence/strength of gag, cough, and swallowing reflexes Cranial nerve functioning, particularly presence/strength of nerves IX to XII Skin color, nail beds, peripheral pulses, and skin warmth Breath sounds bilaterally for quality of aeration; signs of obstruction (rales, rhonchi) Arterial blood gas values Chest radiograph results Signs/symptoms of thrombophlebitis, pulmonary emboli, pulmonary edema Maintain patent airway by Turning and positioning to prevent obstruction or aspiration of secretions q2 hr and prn Deep breathing and coughing q1 hr and prn (if allowed) Suctioning prn Adequate oxygenation and humidification as ordered Chest physiotherapy/pulmonary toilet if warranted and not contraindicated by physician's order Apply antithromboembolic stockings or Ace bandages as ordered; reapply every shift and prn; monitor for constriction/looseness, condition of skin Instruct and supervise patient in performing leg exercises, ROM exercises Increase activity level/progression when allowed Notify physician immediately of any change in respiratory/neurological status or signs of complication potential/occurrence If patient electively remains intubated postoperatively, see Standard: *Mechanical ventilation* (this is frequently done if surgery was performed near or in medulla, edema was found intraoperatively or is anticipated postoperatively, or severe cranial nerve dysfunctions are expected) Explain procedures and reasons for equipment/respiratory assistance to patient/family; reassure and support Establish alternative means of communication When patient is extubated, closely monitor respiratory/neurological status and vital signs If respiratory problem occurs, assist with emergency measures to maintain patent airway and adequate ventilation Administer medications/treatments as ordered; monitor effects and side effects See Standard: *Mechanical ventilation* If emboli occur, see Standard: *Embolic phenomena*
■ Cranial nerve dysfunction	■ Absence of complications	■ Ongoing assessments of cranial nerve functioning—presence, strength, and quality—q1-2 hr Specifically monitor any symptoms of dysfunction Notify physician of any increase in cranial nerve dysfunction Monitor for improvement or decline Plan and implement individualized care based on patient's status; make ongoing assessments and evaluations of effectiveness of interventions

Potential problems	Expected outcomes	Nursing activities
Oculomotor (III) Trochlear (IV) Abducens (VI) Nystagmus, ptosis, decreased extraocular movements, diplopia		Monitor pupil size, equality, and reactivity; extraocular movements Monitor for ptosis/nystagmus—degree/extent If diplopia occurs, apply alternating eye patch
Trigeminal (V) Loss of facial sensation		Monitor facial sensation If decreased, protect from injury by removal of sharp objects on pillow, pads for cushioning

Trigeminal (V) and facial (VII)
  Loss of corneal reflex
		Monitor for presence/strength of corneal reflex bilaterally
		If decreased or absent
		  Obtain order for protective eyedrops and lubricants
		  Tape eyelid on affected side shut to prevent corneal abrasion, which may occur due to inability to close eyelid

Facial (VII)
  Decreased facial muscle strength/facial expression
  Facial weakness/paralysis
  Patient/family's anxiety related to body image from distortion of mouth
		Monitor for facial weakness/asymmetry
		If present, determine patient's chewing ability
		  Assess patient's food likes and preferences
		  Assist patient in diet selection within chewing capabilities
		  Have patient chew on unaffected side
		  Stay with patient during mealtimes, assessing and evaluating chewing abilities and diet appropriateness
		Monitor for facial droop, which may cause drooling of saliva from affected side
		  Excellent oral hygiene
		  Frequent removal of secretions
		  Instruct and supervise in facial exercises
		  If patient has dentures, assess if refitting is necessary and obtain order for appropriate referral
		Assess level of patient's anxiety and altered body image related to facial nerve weakness, droop/drooling from mouth
		If speech is impaired from facial weakness/paralysis, establish alternate means of communication
		Encourage patient's verbalization of fears, concerns, feelings, since decreased facial strength may inhibit normal facial expression conveyance

Acoustic (VIII) Decreased hearing		Assess hearing loss Obtain hearing aid if patient possesses one and insert it Speak to patient from unaffected side; assess volume level necessary Face patient when speaking If hearing loss is bilateral, establish alternate means of communication such as magic slate, pad, word board

Disturbance of balance and equilibrium		Assess degree of ataxia and location (may be more pronounced falling to one side)
		Determine measures necessary for safety and implement such as
		  Assist patient in getting out of bed
		  Assist in ambulation
		  Maintain safe environment by removing obstacles
		  Assess for nystagmus
		  Obtain equipment to help patient toward independence, instructing and supervising in use
		  Obtain order for physical therapy consultation
		  Reassure and support patient, praising frequently for progress achieved

Dizziness		Have patient move slowly and cautiously when changing position Dangle for 5 to 10 minutes before standing Assist in ambulation and activities as needed

Potential problems	Expected outcomes	Nursing activities

Glossopharyngeal (IX)
Vagus (X)
    Decreased or absent gag, swallowing, and cough reflexes
    Dysphagia/aspiration
    Nasal, dysarthric speech
		Assess presence and quality of gag, cough, and swallowing reflexes; ability to handle secretions
		If reflexes are absent/diminished, maintain interventions to prevent complications
		    Suction prn
		    Position to prevent obstruction or aspiration of secretions
		    Keep patient NPO
		    Administer IV fluids/NG feedings as ordered; monitor NG tube for patency and proper placement; nasogastric feedings for absorption/retention
		    Frequent oral hygiene
		    Explain necessity for NG or IV feedings, reasons NPO
		If gag reflex is adequate, start po fluids slowly as per physician's order
		    Stay with patient at mealtimes, monitoring swallowing ability and effectiveness
		    Assess foods patient tolerates best and assist with diet selection
		    Continually assess for any choking/nasal regurgitation
		Assess for nasal speech and hoarseness; obtain order for speech consultation if indicated; if dysarthria is a problem, establish alternate means of communication
		Reassure and support patient/family; encourage verbalization and answer questions

Hypoglossal (XII) Decreased tongue strength		Assess for tongue position and muscle strength; monitor for any deviation or tongue tremor (location and degree) Provide for frequent oral hygiene Instruct and supervise patient in exercise programs for strengthening
Spinal accessory (XI) Impaired/absent shoulder shrug and head turning to side		Assess ability to shrug shoulder, turn head, and bend forward Assist with ADL as needed Place objects within field of head turning capability and vision Instruct and supervise in exercise program

■ Cardiac arrhythmia related to
    Vagal stimulation
    Brain stem edema
	■ Normal sinus rhythm
	Absence or control of arrhythmia
	Adequate cardiac output
		■ Monitor
		    ECG recording for any abnormality
		    Vital signs including apical and radial pulse q1 hr
		    Serum electrolyte levels for any abnormality
		    Adequacy of cardiac output and perfusion
		Avoid vagal stimulation such as Valsalva's maneuver, neck vein compression
		Notify physician of any arrhythmia or abnormality
		    Administer medications/treatments as ordered
		    Monitor for resolution or progression of ECG abnormality
		    Notify physician if therapy is not effective
		SEE STANDARD: *Arrhythmias*

■ Fluid and electrolyte imbalance related to
    Ventricular fluid loss
    CNS pathology
    Medications administered
	■ Fluid and electrolyte balance within normal limits	■ Monitor and accurately record intake and output, urine specific gravity q1-2 hr; if there is ventricular drainage, record and report amount
		Monitor for signs of dehydration or overhydration such as
		    Poor skin turgor
		    Dry mucous membranes
		    Peripheral edema
		    Excessive thirst
		    Change in LOC
		Monitor for
		    Abnormal vital signs, Hgb/Hct values
		    Abnormal serum electrolytes

Potential problems	Expected outcomes	Nursing activities

Weight alterations

Temperature elevations

Insensible fluid losses including respiratory, diaphoresis, secretions

Presence/degree of nausea and vomiting; effectiveness of medications ordered

Presence/quality of bowel sounds for any abnormality

Monitor for signs of fluid imbalance, which may occur due to decreased or increased production/release of ADH (vasopressin); either condition can occur postoperatively

Decreased ADH: monitor for

  Hypernatremia

  Hyperosmolality

  Dehydration

  Diabetes insipidus: polyuria, polydipsia

  Alterations in LOC such as irritability, increased muscle tone, hyperactive reflexes, muscle twitching, convulsions, decerebrate rigidity

Increased ADH (inappropriate ADH): monitor for

  Hyponatremia

  Hypo-osmolality

  Overhydration

  H_2O retention/intoxication

  Nausea/vomiting

  Apathy, muscle twitching, irritability, disorientation

Administer IV fluids, NG feedings as ordered

Administer medications as ordered; monitor effects and side effects; if patient is receiving steroids, monitor urine glucose and acetone levels four times a day

Notify physician of any fluid imbalance or electrolyte abnormality, any signs of ADH disorder

Administer medications/treatments as ordered

Maintain intake at specific level ordered

Monitor hourly intake and output

Explain to patient reasons for fluid restriction or encouragement; plan oral intake based on regimen ordered assessing fluid preferences

---

■ Infection

■ Infection free
Incision well-healed

■ Keep patient's hands from operative site/drain

Maintain sterility of head dressing/drainage apparatus

Monitor

  Temperature as ordered and prn for any elevation

  Dressing, incision site, drainage site q2 hr for any signs of redness, tenderness, bulging, separation, or drainage (amount and quality)

  If ventricular drain is present, monitor CSF amount and quality for any abnormality

  Neurological status and vital signs for any decline/abnormality

  IV sites frequently for any signs of redness, tenderness, phlebitis

  WBC count (may be falsely elevated if patient is receiving steroids)

  For any signs/symptoms of meningitis

Administer antibiotics as ordered; monitor effects and side effects (frequently ordered prophylactically postoperatively)

Notify physician immediately of any signs/symptoms of infection

Administer medications/treatments as ordered

Potential problems	Expected outcomes	Nursing activities
		Monitor wound culture results, CSF determinations Monitor for other possible infection sources if warranted including urine, sputum, chest radiograph results Monitor for resolution/progression of infection If problem occurs, see Standard: *Meningitis/encephalitis*
■ GI bleeding related to CNS factors Stress Steroid administration	■ Absence or resolution of GI bleeding	■ Monitor vital signs q2-4 hr, Hgb and Hct, stools for Hematest three times a week; Hematest of aspirate, urine, and emesis for any abnormalities Obtain order for antacid administration as soon as patient able to take po Monitor for signs of GI bleeding including abdominal tenderness/distention, hypotension, sudden tachycardia Notify physician immediately if any abnormality occurs; if problem occurs, see Standard: *Upper gastrointestinal bleeding*
■ Cerebellar dysfunction Ataxia, loss of balance and coordination	■ Patient ambulates safely with assistance Patient performs ADL safely with maximal possible independence	■ Monitor cerebellar functioning Establish and implement plan of care based on individual needs and specific deficit Focus plan of care on maintaining safety while promoting maximal possible independence Involve patient/family in planning care and decision making Encourage verbalization by patient/family; answer questions realistically; reassure and support gains/realistic goals Instruct and evaluate patient/family in necessary information and skills required to deal with problem/deficit, such as Safety precautions Exercise program Special equipment Assistance needed (type, amount, degree)
■ Continued presence of neurological deficit Patient/family's fears, anxiety/anger related to deficit and possible alterations in lifestyle	■ Maximal neurological functioning* Maximal independence in ADL (within capabilities) Patient/family verbalizes concerns	■ Assess patient's specific neurological deficit Collaborate with physician regarding prognosis, possible degree of recovery Implement individualized plan of care based on patient's needs and deficits Assist as needed in ADL Monitor potential for independent functioning and obtain equipment to maximize function and promote safety Obtain orders for appropriate referrals such as physical, speech, occupational therapy; social service Encourage verbalization of patient/family's fears, anxieties, and other reactions—level and degree Answer questions realistically Encourage their participation in care planning, implementation, evaluation, and decision making Realistically reassure and support patient/family Reinforce any gains or independence patient achieves Plan, instruct, demonstrate, supervise, and evaluate patient/family's verbalization/performance of needed information/skills for maximal independent functioning such as Measures to prevent complications Assistance necessary—type, amount, degree Proper use of therapeutic devices/equipment Monitor level of achievement toward maximizing potentials and independence; means to promote as "normal" a life-style as possible

*If responsibility of critical care nurse includes this stage of care.

Potential problems	Expected outcomes	Nursing activities
■ Insufficient knowledge to comply with discharge regimen	■ Patient/family demonstrates or verbalizes understanding of discharge regimen*	■ Assess patient/family's level of understanding of neurological problem and therapy received Explain relationship between patient's neurological status and therapies prescribed If cerebral pathology was caused by head injury or trauma, explore with patient/family measures to decrease potential injury recurrence, importance of controlling factors precipitating head injury Instruct patient/family regarding required information/skills so that before discharge patient/family is able to

	Patient/family accurately describes medication, activity, and dietary regimens	Describe medication regimen
		    Name and purpose
		    Route, dosage, frequency, times
		    Side effects
		    Special precautions necessary including drugs, foods, beverages contraindicated or quantity regulated; factors potentiating/decreasing effects or side effects; physical restrictions; safety measures
		Describe dietary regimen
		Describe activity regimen, exercise program
		Describe and demonstrate any special therapeutic measures prescribed

	Patient/family describes and demonstrates means to achieve maximal independence in ADL, promote safety, and prevent complications	Describe and demonstrate proper use of equipment or therapeutic devices Reasons for using Time, method, and duration of use Precautions/safeguards Necessary maintenance (type, frequency) Measures to promote optimal functioning, upkeep/duration Describe and demonstrate safety precautions in performing ADL
	Patient/family describes signs/symptoms requiring medical attention	Describe signs/symptoms of neurological status requiring medical care
	Patient/family describes follow-up care regimen	Describe plan for follow-up care including purpose of appointment, when and where to go, who to see, what to expect, what specimens to bring

*If responsibility of critical care nurse includes such follow-up care.

30 □ **Internalized shunting procedures**

Internalized shunt insertions are usually performed when the patient's clinical status demonstrates an enlargement of part or all of the ventricular system of the brain. *Hydrocephalus*, or "water on the brain," is a term commonly used to denote this ventricular enlargement produced by an overproduction of cerebrospinal fluid (CSF) or obstruction of CSF flow. Increased intracranial pressure (ICP) frequently results from the CSF accumulation and retention. Internalized shunt insertion does not correct the original condition that is producing the overproduction or obstruction but rather removes and diverts the excessive CSF away from the brain in an effort to decrease the dilated and enlarged ventricular size and diminish the increased ICP. The shunting devices commonly inserted consist of a catheter placed in a lateral ventricle, a reservoir for fluid accumulation, a one-way valve to maintain flow out of the ventricle, and a catheter to transfer the CSF to the internal jugular vein, heart, or peritoneum. Shunt insertion is frequently done in the right lateral ventricle, since the right hemisphere is the nondominant side for the majority of the population. The purpose of the shunt insertion and functioning is to remove the excess CSF from the ventricles and transfer the fluid to other circulatory pathways, thereby reducing or eliminating the degree of hydrocephalus within the brain.

HYDROCEPHALUS

Two types of hydrocephalus are commonly identified. *Communicating* hydrocephalus results from increased production of CSF with normal absorptive rate or impairment of CSF absorption back into the circulating blood. It may also occur as the result of a block in the CSF pathways distal to the foramina of Magendie and Luschka. In this situation fluid reaches the subarachnoid space but does not circulate over the surface of the brain and is therefore not reabsorbed in sufficient quantities to prevent ventricular dilatation. *Noncommunicating* hydrocephalus is due to blockage in the CSF pathway between formation in the ventricular system and proximal to the foramina of Magendie and Luschka.

Three common processes that cause hydrocephalus either singly or in combination include

1. Overproduction of CSF from choroid plexus papillomas and other tumors; also associated with the condition known as *pseudotumor cerebri.*
2. Obstruction of normal CSF flow (most common cause of hydrocephalus). The blockage or obstruction of the CSF results in accumulation of the fluid and ventricular dilatation. Common sites of obstruction include the foramina of Monro (frequently from third ventricular tumors); aqueduct of Sylvius (frequently from congenital or inflammatory obliterations, brain stem lesions); fourth ventricle foramina (frequently from displacement of medulla by lesions, congenital malformations, or meningeal fibrosis); and subarachnoid pathways (frequently from congenital malformations, inflammation, hemorrhage, or adhesions in subarachnoid space).
3. Impaired or failed absorption at arachnoid villi and granulations. Absorption problem as a primary cause of hydrocephalus is rare but can occur when the blood breakdown products from a SAH flow to the arachnoid villi where they then impair absorption of CSF.

Many etiologies can produce the process that causes hydrocephalus including tumors, infections, hemorrhages, congenital malformations, and adhesions. Hydrocephalus may also occur as a postoperative complication; especially following posterior fossa operations and shunting procedures for previously diagnosed hydrocephalus (whether initial shunt insertion, revision, or removal of a shunt system or component). The extent and degree of hydrocephalus or ventricular dilatation depends on many factors. These factors affecting the clinical variability include primary/secondary causes of hydrocephalus; duration, progression, and location of pathological condition; and compensatory mechanisms and effectiveness. Hydrocephalus is a clinical syndrome whose causes are numerous, variable, and frequently unknown.

Normal pressure hydrocephalus is a clinical syndrome usually characterized by dementia, gait apraxia, and urinary incontinence. Enlargement of the cerebral ventricles is present but ICP is not increased. Diagnostic procedures demonstrate accumulation of CSF in the lateral ventricles, indicating impairment/failure of normal CSF circulation. Controversy exists as to whether normal pressure hydrocephalus should or can be treated surgically.

ASSESSMENT

1. Onset, progression, duration, frequency, and specific description of neurological symptoms, including
   a. Headache
   b. Nausea/vomiting
   c. Changes in behavior/personality
   d. Changes in mental abilities
   e. Pupillary/visual alterations including diplopia, ocular palsies, nystagmus, blurred vision, papilledema
   f. Alterations in LOC
   g. Changes in motor/sensory functioning
   h. Difficulty ambulating; ataxia; falls
   i. Incontinence
   j. Alterations in communication abilities
   k. Seizures
2. Previous history of head trauma/injury, congenital anomalies, delayed growth and development milestones, CNS infections
3. Previous neurological treatment or neurosurgi-

cal procedure; medications taken and effects on clinical course and status

4. If prior shunt insertion was performed
   a. Number, type, placement, and duration of previous shunt systems
   b. Effects on clinical status
   c. Complications both immediate and long-term; if shunt malfunction occurred, cause and treatment/surgical intervention
   d. Any special therapeutic measures prescribed to promote shunt functioning such as pumping of shunt system valve or reservoir, shunt taps by physician
   e. Follow-up care regimen of shunt insertion and clinical course
5. Presence of any medical problems and medications/treatments prescribed and followed
6. Patient's perceptions and reaction to diagnosis, treatment modalities, surgical interventions
7. Presence of any alterations in body image; fears of shunt insertion, functioning/malfunctioning; fears of permanent disability or deficit; altered role in family, normal occupation/performing ADL
8. Baseline parameters status
   a. Neurological
   b. Respiratory
   c. Cardiovascular
   d. Hydration/nutritional
   e. Metabolic
   f. Skin integument
   g. Infection
   h. Vital signs
   i. Weight
   j. Urine output pattern
   k. Handedness (right or left)
9. Diagnostic test results, including
   a. CAT
   b. Skull radiographs
   c. Lumbar puncture
   d. Cisternal puncture, isotope cisternography
   e. Subdural taps
   f. Brain scan, isotopic scanning
   g. Pneumoencephalogram
   h. Ventriculogram
   i. Shunt injections and scanning
   j. Cerebral angiography
10. Results of
   a. Serum electrolyte levels
   b. Hgb and Hct, platelet count, WBC count with differentiation
   c. Type and cross matching
   d. CSF determinations
   e. Urinalysis, culture, specific gravity, osmolality, electrolytes
   f. Arterial blood gas levels
   g. Clotting profile
   h. Anticonvulsant drug levels
   i. Chest radiograph
   j. ECG

GOALS

1. Optimal neurological functioning
2. Optimal independence in ADL
3. Serum electrolyte levels and fluid balance within normal limits
4. Hgb and Hct stable within normal limits
5. Incisions well-healed without any external protrusion of shunt system
6. Shunt system patent and functioning
7. Infection free
8. Reduction in patient/family's anxiety with provision of information, demonstrations, support
9. Before discharge patient/family is able to
   a. Describe medication, activity, exercise, and dietary regimens
   b. Demonstrate safety measures and techniques; proper use of any equipment/therapeutic devices prescribed
   c. Demonstrate and describe any special therapeutic measures; shunt care, maintenance, or treatments prescribed
   d. Describe signs and symptoms requiring medical attention
   e. State necessary information regarding follow-up care

Potential problems	Expected outcomes	Nursing activities
Preoperative		
■ Patient/family's anxiety related to Limited understanding of diagnostic tests, procedures, antici-	■ Patient/family's behavior indicates decreased anxiety with provision of information	■ Ongoing assessment of level of anxiety, knowledge base, and understanding Encourage patient/family's verbalization of questions and fears; collaborate with physician in providing realistic information and reassurance appropriate to level of understanding

Potential problems	Expected outcomes	Nursing activities
pated surgery, post-operative course Potential/presence of neurological deficit; fears of disability or worsened deficit		Explain relationship between symptoms and neurological problem; reasons for therapies Explain and prepare for procedures, tests, preoperative routines If hair is to be shaved, assess anxieties regarding hair loss and possible altered body image; save hair if patient desires; provide information on means to deal with hair loss, such as wigs Explain anticipated postoperative care including routines, setting, monitoring equipment, IVs, drains, length of stay, visiting policy Explain reasons for frequent neurological assessments and vital sign monitoring Instruct in deep breathing and leg exercises; evaluate patient's performance Provide time needed for support and instruction of patient/family Notify unit where patient will be after surgery of any special problems or items patient needs such as Eyeglasses: for vision; to evaluate visual fields/acuity Dentures: for patient comfort; to evaluate facial symmetry If language barrier is present: an effort should be made to have interpreter available postoperatively
■ Increased ICP with possible development or worsening of neurological deficit/symptomatology	■ Absence of complications Maximal neurological functioning	■ Establish neurological baseline and vital signs on admission; ongoing assessments, as ordered, of status and specific symptomatology; especially monitor extent and degree of Headache Nausea/vomiting Papilledema Mental changes such as disorientation, impaired memory Personality changes such as irritability, restlessness, apathy Pupillary changes and ocular palsies, particularly abducens nerve (VI) dysfunction Blurred vision; diplopia; nystagmus Incontinence Alterations in LOC Difficulty ambulating, ataxia Alterations in motor/sensory functioning Alterations in communication abilities, speech quality In infants: increased head circumference, bulging fontanelles, split sutures, irritability, somnolence, high-pitched cry, decreased feeding, sun-setting, nystagmus, vomiting Avoid precipitating factors in increased ICP such as hypoxia, hypercapnia, fever, Valsalva's maneuver, sharp angling of neck (may block venous outflow) Assist patient with positioning and turning; instruct patient not to hold breath Prevent constipation by establishing bowel regimen as individually warranted; ensure that patient has bowel movement preoperatively Monitor for any signs/symptoms that could initiate factor development such as hypoventilation Notify physician of potential/presence of precipitating factors Maintain head gatch and activity as ordered Administer medications and treatments as ordered; monitor effects and side effects Accurately record intake and output; monitor for any imbalance

Potential problems	Expected outcomes	Nursing activities
		Monitor serum electrolyte levels for any abnormalities Notify physician immediately of any change in neurological status, vital signs, or abnormal fluid/electrolyte balance If problem occurs, see Standard: *Increased intracranial pressure*
■ Presence of neurological deficit	■ Absence of complications	■ On admission establish and implement nursing care plan based on individual needs and specific deficit present Ongoing assessments and evaluations of effectiveness of interventions Establish neurological baseline immediately preoperatively to provide for comparison postoperatively
■ Seizures	■ Absence or control of seizures	■ Prevention of precipitating factors in seizure occurrence including fever, hypoxia, H_2O intoxication, electrolyte disturbances Notify physician of potential/presence of any factors Seizure precautions (if indicated) Padded siderails up at all times when patient is alone Bed height at lowest level Padded tongue blade and airway at bedside Emergency medications and equipment readily available Close observation and supervision Administer anticonvulsant medications as ordered; monitor effects and side effects, serum anticonvulsant levels If seizure occurs, monitor and record seizure activity; notify physician SEE STANDARD: *Seizures*
■ Skin breakdown	■ Skin integument intact	■ Ongoing assessments of skin integument and intactness q2 hr and prn Prevent skin breakdown by instituting measures such as Turn and position q2 hr Change head position frequently; utilize pillows to prevent pressure areas Monitor all skin areas frequently; massage, rub, apply protective lubricants and lotions as needed Keep skin clean and dry Obtain devices to prevent skin breakdown such as sheepskin, air mattress, padding Notify physician immediately of any signs/symptoms of skin abrasion, decreased skin circulation Administer medications and treatments as ordered; monitor effects and side effects Notify physician of results, resolution/progression
■ Nausea/vomiting	■ Control of nausea/vomiting Absence of complications	■ Initial assessment of presence, extent, duration of nausea/vomiting; ongoing assessments as ordered and prn Prevent aspiration by Suctioning equipment readily available Monitor closely presence/quality of gag, cough, and swallowing reflexes; keep patient NPO if decreased or absent If nausea/vomiting occurs, turn patient on side and position properly; suction prn Notify physician immediately of presence, new appearance, or increased severity of nausea/vomiting Keep patient NPO as ordered Administer medications/treatments as ordered; monitor effects and side effects Administer IV fluids as ordered Accurately record intake and output Monitor neurological status closely; assess for any associated neurological symptoms or vital sign changes preceding, concurrent with, or following nausea/vomiting

Potential problems	Expected outcomes	Nursing activities

Postoperative
■ General immediate post-operative complications
	■ Absence or resolution of complication	■ Monitor for
		   Recovery from anesthesia; notify physician if patient has not recovered in expected time period
		   Potential hypovolemia, shock, hypostatic pneumonia, pulmonary emboli, thrombophlebitis, abdominal ileus, nausea/vomiting, oliguria/urinary retention
		   Recovery from any special measures induced during surgery such as hypotension/hypothermia
		Notify physician immediately of any signs/symptoms of complication
		Administer medications and treatments as ordered
		Monitor effects and side effects
		Continue monitoring for resolution or progression of complication
		See appropriate standard for identified complication such as *Embolic phenomena; Shock*

■ Increased ICP/increased neurological deficit/appearance related to
  Shunt obstruction/malfunction
  Hematoma/air formation
  Edema
	■ Absence or control of increased ICP
	Maximal neurological functioning
		■ Establish neurological baseline postoperatively and compare to preoperative baseline
		See Problem, Increased ICP (preoperative), for all specific activities
		In addition, monitor
		   Neurological assessments and vital signs as ordered (usually q15 min until stable, q30 min until stable, q1 hr until stable, and then q2 hr)
		   Particularly LOC; pupil size, equality, and reactivity; extraocular movements, motor and sensory systems; communication abilities and speech quality; respiratory rate, pattern, and quality; BP, P; cranial nerve functioning; cerebellar functioning for any abnormality/decline
		   For any increase in headache, nausea/vomiting above usual postoperative expectations
		Maintain head level position as ordered (frequently flat or small degree of elevation)
		Notify physician immediately of any decline from preoperative baseline or change in neurological status or vital signs postoperatively
		   If shunt pumping is ordered by physician, pump as specifically ordered including location, frequency, and duration; maintain schedule regimen and recording of pumping, effects and side effects
		   Prepare patient/family for any diagnostic procedures/tests ordered
		Monitor for shunt functioning (see Problem, Shunt obstruction/malfunction)

■ Shunt obstruction/malfunction
One of the greatest problems associated with procedure, clinical prognosis, and outcomes; patients frequently require repeated surgical interventions either immediately or over a period of years to correct the shunt malfunction
	■ Absence or resolution of shunt obstruction/malfunction
	Shunt patent and functioning
		■ Ongoing assessments as ordered of neurological status, vital signs and monitoring for signs/symptoms of increased ICP
		Monitor sites of shunt system placement q2 hr and prn
		   For any signs of redness, tenderness, fluid collection, bulging, edema, skin opening/protrusion of shunt system components
		   For any signs of CSF "tracking" or accumulation/cranial depression
		   Dressings for any signs of bleeding or other drainage
		Maintain head position as ordered by physician; patient is frequently kept flat for 1 to 2 days to prevent too rapid decompression or potential accumulation of subdural hematoma/air formation

Potential problems	Expected outcomes	Nursing activities

Common causes of shunt malfunction include
Malposition of the catheters
Detachment of the shunt system components
Infection of shunt system (see Problem, Infection of shunt system/insertion site)
Plugging or obstruction of shunt system
		Position patient as ordered to prevent compression of shunt tubing; frequently patient may only be allowed to lie on one side of head
		Explain to patient/family reasons for bed and head positions ordered
		Increase head gatch as specifically ordered by physician
		   Monitor neurological status, vital signs, shunt site/functioning with head elevations
		   Monitor for any headache, nausea/vomiting, dizziness; notify physician if any of these occur
		Activity progression as ordered; monitor closely for any ataxia
		Notify physician immediately of any change in neurological status, vital signs or any signs/symptoms of shunt malfunctioning
		   Administer medications/treatments as ordered; monitor effects and side effects
		   Explain and prepare patient/family for any diagnostic tests or procedures ordered
		   Assist physician with any procedures or tests necessary such as shunt taps, CSF specimen collections
		If problem occurs, see Standard: *Subdural hematoma*

■ Fluid and electrolyte imbalance	■ Fluid and electrolyte balance within normal limits	■ Monitor and accurately record intake and output, urine specific gravity as ordered
		Monitor for signs of dehydration or overhydration such as
		   Poor skin turgor
		   Dry mucous membranes
		   Peripheral edema
		   Excessive thirst/urine output
		   Change in LOC
		Monitor for
		   Abnormal vital signs, Hgb/Hct values
		   Abnormal serum electrolyte values
		   Weight alterations
		   Temperature elevations
		   Insensible fluid losses including respiratory, diaphoresis, secretions
		   Presence/degree of nausea and vomiting; effectiveness of medications ordered
		Assess presence and quality of bowel sounds especially if peritoneal shunt system has been placed
		   Keep NPO as per physician's order
		   Begin fluids slowly when allowed
		   Monitor for signs/symptoms of paralytic ileus, abdominal tenderness/distention, peritonitis
		   Monitor abdominal site and dressing if peritoneal shunt is in place
		   Notify physician immediately of any signs/symptoms of abdominal obstruction or infection
		Administer IV fluids, NG feedings as ordered
		Administer medications as ordered; monitor effects and side effects; if patient is receiving steroids, monitor urine glucose and acetone levels four times a day
		Notify physician of any fluid imbalance or electrolyte abnormality

Potential problems	Expected outcomes	Nursing activities
■ Infection of shunt system/ insertion sites	■ Infection free Incision sites well-healed	■ Keep patient's hands from operative sites Administer antibiotics as ordered; monitor effects and side effects (frequently ordered prophylactically postoperatively) Monitor shunt insertion and system placement site frequently for Intactness of suture line and containment of shunt system Any signs of edema, bulging, redness, tenderness Any drainage; note amount, quality Any signs of CSF "tracking" or accumulation Any signs of abdominal distention, ileus, pain, peritonitis if peritoneal shunt is in place Monitor Temperature q4 hr and prn for any elevation (commonly low grade or spikes) Neurological status and vital signs for any decline/abnormality WBC count (may be falsely elevated if patient is receiving steroids) For any general systemic complaints For any signs/symptoms of meningitis Notify physician immediately of any signs/symptoms of suspected shunt infection Administer medications and treatments as ordered; monitor effects and side effects Explain and prepare patient/family for any diagnostic tests or procedures ordered Assist physician with procedures such as shunt tap, lumbar puncture Monitor results of CSF determinations and cultures If problem occurs, see Standard: *Meningitis/encephalitis*
■ Seizures	■ Absence or control of seizures	■ See Problem, Seizures (preoperative), for all activities
■ GI bleeding related to CNS factors Stress Steroid administration	■ Absence or resolution of GI bleeding	■ Monitor vital signs q2-4 hr; Hgb and Hct; stools for Hematest three times a week; Hematest of aspirate, emesis, and urine for any abnormalities Obtain order for antacid administration as soon as patient able to take po Monitor for signs of GI bleeding including abdominal tenderness/distention, hypotension, sudden tachycardia Notify physician immediately if any abnormalities occur; if problem occurs, see Standard: *Upper gastrointestinal bleeding*
■ Continued presence of neurological deficit Patient/family's fears, anxiety, anger related to deficit and possible alterations in lifestyle	■ Maximal neurological functioning* Maximal independence in ADL (within capabilities) Patient/family verbalizes concerns	■ Assess patient's specific neurological deficit; collaborate with physician regarding prognosis, possible degree of recovery Implement individualized plan of care based on patient's needs and deficits Assist as needed in ADL Monitor potential for independent functioning and obtain equipment to maximize function and promote safety Obtain orders for appropriate referrals such as physical, speech, occupational therapy; social service Encourage patient/family's verbalization of fears, anxieties, and other reactions—level and degree Answer questions realistically Encourage their participation in care planning, implementation, evaluation, and decision making

*If responsibility of critical care nurse includes this stage of care.

Potential problems	Expected outcomes	Nursing activities
		Realistically reassure and support patient/family
		Reinforce any gains or independence patient achieves
		Plan, instruct, demonstrate, supervise, and evaluate patient/family's verbalization/performance of needed information/skills for maximal independent functioning such as
		Measures to prevent complications
		Assistance necessary—type, amount, degree
		Proper use of therapeutic devices/equipment
		Monitor level of achievement toward maximizing potentials and independence; means to promote as "normal" a life-style as possible
■ Insufficient knowledge to comply with discharge regimen*	■ Patient/family demonstrates or verbalizes understanding of discharge regimen	■ Assess patient/family's level of understanding of neurological problem and therapy received
		Explain relationship between patient's neurological status and therapies prescribed
		Describe reasons for shunt insertion, purpose of shunt, expected effects, type of shunt inserted, and mechanism of action; common problems occurring, short- or long-term; diagrams or pictures may enhance explanations
		Instruct patient/family regarding required information and skills so that before discharge patient/family is able to
	Patient/family accurately describes medication, activity, and dietary regimens	Describe medication regimen
		Name and purpose
		Route, dosage, frequency, times
		Side effects
		Special precautions necessary including drugs, foods, beverages contraindicated or quantity regulated; factors potentiating/decreasing effects or side effects; physical restrictions; safety measures
		Describe dietary regimen
		Describe activity regimen, exercise program
		Describe and demonstrate any special therapeutic measures prescribed such as shunt pumping (when, where, how)
	Patient/family describes means to achieve maximal independence in ADL, promote safety, and prevent complications	Describe and demonstrate proper use of equipment or therapeutic devices
		Reasons for using
		Time, method, and duration of use
		Precautions/safeguards
		Necessary maintenance (type, frequency)
		Measures to promote optimal functioning, upkeep/duration
	Patient/family describes signs/symptoms requiring medical attention	Describe signs/symptoms of neurological status requiring medical care; signs/symptoms of shunt malformation, obstruction/infection
	Patient/family describes follow-up care regimen	Describe plan for follow-up care including purpose of appointment, when and where to go, who to see, what to expect, what charting or recorded data to bring

*If responsibility of critical care includes such follow-up care.

31 □ Carotid endarterectomy

Carotid endarterectomy is an operative procedure in which a plaque is removed from an artery and a graft is performed, using either synthetic substances or a graft from the patient's own body. The purposes of the operation are to restore normal circulation to the brain and to prevent the development of a stroke and irreversible neurological damage. Plaques may occur in numerous arteries within the cerebral circulatory system. Commonly they form in the internal and external carotid arteries, vertebral arteries, and the innominate, common carotid, and subclavian arteries. Plaques narrow the lumen of the vessel and restrict blood flow. If uncorrected, the obstruction of blood flow eventually results in thrombosis and occlusion.

Controversy exists regarding the benefits of carotid endarterectomy procedures, but most authorities recommend operative intervention if the plaque can be surgically removed and if the patient has experienced transient ischemic attacks (TIA). Several studies have documented that, if untreated, one third of patients who have experienced a TIA will develop a severe neurological deficit within 5 years. Carotid endarterectomy may be the procedure of choice if the plaque is accessible for removal and if the occlusion can be surgically corrected.

TIA refers to the onset and disappearance of a neurological deficit within 24 hours due to a temporary disruption of blood supply to the brain. Usually recovery is complete within a few minutes to hours. The signs and symptoms and extent of recovery after this disturbance of the blood supply to a local area of the brain depend on how quickly and effectively the individual's collateral blood supply can provide adequate circulation and perfusion to the area. There are some typical signs and symptoms that occur with TIA, depending on the artery that is involved (see Table 6).

ASSESSMENT

1. History of any previous TIA
   a. Exact description of symptomatology including onset, duration, progression, and resolution (time and extent of recovery)
   b. Frequency of occurrence
   c. Whether episodes of TIA are of similar symptomatology or of variable symptoms or degree
   d. Precipitating factors in attacks such as activity, sharp angling of neck, rapid position change
2. Presence of any residual neurological deficit—specific description
3. Presence of medical factors prominent in stroke-prone profile such as cardiac abnormalities, hypertension, diabetes, hyperlipidemia; medications/treatments prescribed and followed
4. Presence of other factors identified in stroke-prone profile such as family history, smoking, gout, platelet aggregation, oral contraceptive use, obesity
5. Medications taken for neurological problem such as anticoagulants, vasodilators
6. Previous neurological treatment or neurosurgical procedure
7. Patient's perceptions and reaction to diagnosis, treatment modalities, surgical intervention
8. Presence of any alterations in body image; fears of permanent disability or deficit; altered roles in family, normal occupation, performance of ADL
9. Baseline parameters status
   a. Neurological
   b. Vital signs including BP recording on both arms in lying and standing positions
   c. Cardiac; circulatory and vascular
   d. Respiratory/pulmonary
   e. Handedness (right or left)
   f. Weight
   g. Hydration
10. Diagnostic test results, including
    a. Cerebral angiography   c. EEG
    b. Thermogram   d. CAT
11. Results of
    a. Serum electrolyte levels
    b. Hgb and Hct, platelet count
    c. Clotting profile
    d. Arterial blood gas levels
    e. ECG
    f. Chest radiograph
    g. Urinalysis, gravity, culture
    h. Type and cross matching

GOALS

1. Optimal neurological functioning
2. Optimal independence in ADL
3. Adequate alveolar ventilation

Table 6. Transient ischemic attacks

Carotid arterial system

The classical history consists of a swift onset of contralateral weakness or numbness of arms or legs, dysphasia (difficulty in speaking or understanding) if the dominant hemisphere is involved (for about 80% of the population the left hemisphere is the dominant), and impaired vision of the eye on the side of diminished carotid blood flow

1. Internal carotid: typically the patient experiences fleeting blindness of one eye, known as *amaurosis fugax*
2. On physical examination there may be evidence of arterial disease such as decreased pulsation in carotid artery or bruit over the carotid artery

Middle cerebral artery

1. Contralateral paralysis or weakness of side, limb, face—worse in upper extremities
2. Impairment of sensation—numbness or hypoesthesia
3. Blindness in one half of visual field (hemianopia)
4. Dysphasia
5. Inability to recognize persons and things (agnosia)

Anterior cerebral artery

1. Contralateral paralysis or weakness of lower extremities
2. Mental change—impaired judgment and insight
3. Clumsiness in walking
4. Grasping and sucking reflexes on opposite side
5. Incontinence

Posterior cerebral artery

1. Inability to recognize or comprehend written words (alexia)
2. Mental change with memory impairment
3. Blindness in one half of visual field
4. Inability to recognize people and things
5. Weakness or paralysis of cranial nerve III (oculomotor)

Vertebrobasilar artery system

1. Impaired sense of touch on the face
2. Vertigo—dizziness, sensation of revolving movement
3. Vomiting
4. Difficulty swallowing (dysphagia)
5. Loss of muscle coordination on same side as paralysis or weakness
6. Weakness or paralysis of all limbs
7. Stammering and inability to articulate (dysarthria)
8. Double vision (diplopia) and visual field defects or blindness
9. Temporary loss of consciousness (syncope)
10. "Drop attacks"—falling due to sudden loss of postural tone without loss of consciousness
11. Contralateral loss of pain and temperature sensations

4. Adequate cardiac output
5. Artery involved remains patent after operative procedure
6. Serum electrolyte levels within normal limits
7. Hgb and Hct stable within normal limits
8. Fluid balance within normal limits
9. Incision well-healed
10. Infection free
11. Reduction in patient/family's anxiety with provision of information, demonstrations, support
12. Before discharge patient/family is able to
    a. Describe medication, activity, exercise, and dietary regimens
    b. Demonstrate safety measures and techniques; proper use of any equipment, therapeutic devices if prescribed
    c. Identify, if present, risk factors of patient and importance of controlling or eliminating to decrease potential for recurrent plaque formation
    d. Describe signs and symptoms requiring medical attention
    e. State necessary information regarding follow-up care

Potential problems	Expected outcomes	Nursing activities
Preoperative ■ Development of neurological deficit; possibility of stroke	■ Maintenance of neurological functioning Absence of complications	■ Establish neurological baseline and vital signs on admission; ongoing assessments as ordered and prn Assess and immediately notify physician if patient experiences any TIAs Instruct patient to inform nurse immediately if TIA occurs; reassure and reemphasize the importance and necessity of patient reporting any symptoms of a TIA

Potential problems	Expected outcomes	Nursing activities
		Monitor episode for exact description of symptoms, onset, progression, location, duration, resolution time period, frequency
		Monitor vital signs as ordered and prn
		Monitor for any precipitating factors enhancing TIA occurrence, and institute measures to control factors if possible
		Maintain BP in prescribed range ordered by physician by administration of standing and prn medications ordered for BP control
		Administer medications/treaments as ordered
		Explain reasons for therapy to patient/family
		Monitor effects and side effects
		Monitor clotting profile results
		Notify physician immediately of any neurological deficit development
		Prepare patient/family for any tests or procedures ordered
		Assess and document neurological status and vital signs immediately preoperatively to provide baseline for comparison postoperatively
■ Presence of neurological deficit on admission	■ Maximal neurological functioning Absence of complications	■ On admission establish and implement nursing care plan based on individual needs and specific deficit present
		Ongoing assessments and evaluations of effectiveness of interventions
		Monitor neurological status frequently; notify physician of any change in status
		Monitor and document preoperatively specific deficit patient has to provide for comparison postoperatively
■ Patient/family's anxiety related to Limited understanding of diagnostic tests and procedures Anticipated surgery Lack of knowledge regarding expected postoperative course Fears of disability or worsened deficit	■ Patient/family's behavior indicates decreased anxiety with provision of information	■ Ongoing assessment of level of anxiety, knowledge base, and understanding
		Encourage patient/family's verbalization of questions and fears; collaborate with physician in providing realistic information and reassurance appropriate to level of understanding
		Explain relationship between neurological problem and symptoms; reasons for therapies
		Explain and prepare for tests, procedures, preoperative routines
		If patient is receiving anticoagulation therapy, medication will usually be stopped 24 to 48 hours before surgery; explain reasons for medication cancellation
		Explain anticipated postoperative care including setting, routines, monitoring equipment, ECG recording, IVs, neck dressing, length of stay, visiting policy
		Explain reasons for frequent neurological assessments and vital sign monitoring
		Instruct in deep breathing, leg exercises; evaluate patient's performance
		Provide time needed for support and instruction of patient/family
		Notify unit where patient will be after surgery of any special problems or items patient needs such as
		Eyeglasses: for patient vision; to evaluate visual abilities
		Dentures: for patient comfort; to evaluate facial symmetry
		Communication problems: if a language barrier is present, an effort should be made to have interpreter available postoperatively; if communication deficit is present, assess what aids or measures have assisted patient in improving abilities to communicate

Potential problems	Expected outcomes	Nursing activities
Postoperative		

■ General immediate post-operative complications	■ Absence or resolution of complications	■ Monitor for
		  Recovery from anesthesia; notify physician if patient has not recovered in expected time period
		  Signs/symptoms of hypovolemia, shock, hypostatic pneumonia, pulmonary emboli, thrombophlebitis, abdominal ileus, nausea/vomiting, oliguria/urinary retention
		  Recovery from any special measures induced during surgery such as hypotension/hypothermia
		Notify physician immediately of any signs/symptoms of complication
		Administer medications and treatments as ordered
		Monitor effects and side effects
		Continue monitoring for resolution or progression of complication
		See appropriate standard for identified complication such as *Embolic phenomena; Shock*

■ Neurological deficit related to decreased cerebral blood flow	■ Maintenance or improvement of neurological status from preoperative baseline	■ Establish neurological baseline postoperatively and compare to preoperative baseline status; ongoing neurological assessment and vital sign monitoring q15 min until stable, q30 min until stable, and then q1 hr
		Monitor for any abnormalities in LOC; motor and sensory functioning; pupil size, equality, and light reactivity; extraocular movements; cranial nerve functioning; and communication system
		Notify physician immediately of any worsening of preoperative neurological deficit/status, new deficit appearance, or significant change in vital signs
		  Administer medications and treatments as ordered; monitor effects and side effects
		  Maintain BP in specific range ordered by physician
		  Prepare patient/family for any tests or procedures ordered
		  Continue monitoring neurological status closely for improvement/resolution of deficit or worsening
		Explain to patient necessity for frequent assessments and reasons for specific tests being done
		Monitor for more detailed and specific neurological assessments as patient's status allows

■ Lack of patency of artery operated on related to
  Hematoma
  Occlusion
  Bleeding
  Embolus
	■ Artery patent and functioning normally
	  External pulses easily palpable and strong
		■ Monitor with onging neurological assessments and vital signs; see Problem, Neurological deficit, for specific activities
		  Appropriate external pulses for presence, strength, quality, and bilateral symmetry
		  If operation was performed on internal carotid arteries, palpate temporal pulses bilaterally; if vertebral artery was operated on, palpate radial pulses bilaterally
		  For any correlations between external pulse status and neurological status; BP levels and neurological status
		  For any decline in neurological status
		  Operative site for any bleeding, swelling, or hematoma development; record amount, quality, and degree
		Notify physician immediately if external pulse is absent or diminished or hyperpulse develops; of any abnormality in operative site and/or any decrease in neurological status or correlations with signs/symptoms of abnormalities
		  Administer medications and treatments as ordered; monitor effects and side effects
		  Maintain BP within specific range ordered by physician
		  Prepare patient/family for any tests ordered
		  Continue monitoring for resolution or progression of abnormality

Potential problems	Expected outcomes	Nursing activities

■ Hypotension related to Carotid sinus manipulation Distensibility of carotid artery after removal of plaque	■ BP within patient's normal or prescribed limits	■ Maintain head of bed at degree ordered Monitor and record BP as ordered and prn Maintain BP at specific level ordered by physician
		  Administer and titrate prn medications ordered by physician to maintain BP level; monitor effects and side effects; notify physician if not effective for control
		  If prn medication not ordered for maintaining BP, notify physician immediately if BP above or below specified level
		  Monitor for any correlation between BP levels and neurological status; notify physician if occurs

■ Bleeding, hematoma, or swelling at operative site	■ BP, P within normal limits Surgical site free of bleeding, swelling, or hematoma Hgb and Hct stable	■ Monitor
		  Ongoing neurological assessments for any decline in neurological status
		  BP and P as ordered for any abnormalities or deviations from specified acceptable range
		  Surgical site for any bleeding, swelling, or hematoma (amount, quality, degree)
		  For any decrease in Hgb/Hct levels
		  For any signs of hypovolemia, bleeding, shock
		  Clotting profile if indicated
		 Notify physician immediately of any abnormalities of operative site, signs/symptoms of bleeding
		  Administer medications/treatments as ordered; monitor effects and side effects
		  Assist physician with procedures such as resuturing

■ Respiratory insufficiency related to Vagal nerve (X) edema or manipulation Shift of trachea Pneumonia Atelectasis Pulmonary emboli	■ Patent airway Normal respiratory rate and quality Adequate alveolar ventilation Arterial blood gas levels within patient's normal limits	■ Ongoing assessment of respiratory status q1 hr and prn Assess and monitor for any abnormality
		  Respiratory rate, quality, and pattern
		  Patency of upper airway and patient's ability to handle secretions
		  Position of trachea
		  Operative site for any bleeding, swelling, or hematoma development
		  Breath sounds bilaterally for quality of aeration; signs of obstruction (rales, rhonchi)
		  Presence/strength of gag, cough, and swallowing reflexes
		  Skin color, nail beds, peripheral pulses, and skin warmth
		  Arterial blood gas values
		  Chest radiograph results
		  Signs/symptoms of thrombophlebitis, pulmonary emboli, pulmonary edema
		 Maintain patent airway by
		  Turning and positioning to prevent obstruction or aspiration of secretions q2 hr and prn
		  Deep breathing and coughing q1 hr and prn
		  Suctioning prn
		  Adequate oxygenation and humidification as ordered
		  Chest physiotherapy/pulmonary toilet if warranted and not contraindicated by physician's order
		 Apply antithromboembolic stockings or Ace bandages as ordered; reapply every shift and prn; monitor for constriction/looseness, condition of skin
		 Instruct and supervise patient in leg exercises, ROM exercises
		 Increase activity level/progression when allowed
		 Notify physician immediately of any change in respiratory/neurological status or signs/symptoms of complication occurrence or potential

Potential problems	Expected outcomes	Nursing activities
		If problem occurs, assist with emergency measures to maintain patent airway and adequate ventilation See Standard: *Mechanical ventilation* If emboli occur, see Standard: *Embolic phenomena*
■ Difficulty swallowing related to edema, bleeding, or manipulation around glossopharyngeal (IX) and vagus (X) nerves	■ Gag reflex present and strong bilaterally Patient swallows without difficulty	■ Monitor patient's gag reflex and swallowing ability q1-2 hr and prn Ongoing assessments of presence/quality Notify physician immediately if any decrease in gag reflex or swallowing difficulty develops Explain necessity for frequent assessments and interventions to patient Encourage verbalization of fears and answer questions Reassure patient that reflexes will return; explain relationship between surgery and diminished reflex ability Keep patient NPO until gag and swallowing reflexes return to normal Suction secretions prn Start po fluids as per physician's order when reflexes are strong; stay with patient when initially beginning po fluids Reassess presence/quality of reflexes
■ Hoarseness from edema of recurrent laryngeal nerve/intubation	■ Absence or resolution of hoarseness Voice tone and strength normal	■ Monitor patient's voice for signs of hoarseness Notify physician if hoarseness develops or progresses Administer medications and treatments as ordered; monitor effects and side effects Obtain order for throat lozenges Reassure patient that hoarseness will resolve Explain relationship between surgery and hoarseness Encourage patient to rest voice until hoarseness resolves Continue monitoring voice until tone and strength are normal
■ Fluid and electrolyte imbalance Oliguria or retention	■ Fluid and electrolyte balance within normal limits Voiding is satisfactory	■ Administer IV fluids, medications as ordered; monitor effects and side effects Monitor Accurate recording of intake and output, urine specific gravity as ordered For any signs of urine retention or oliguria Presence/degree of nausea or vomiting; effectiveness of medications ordered Quality of bowel sounds; start po fluids as per physician's order when warranted Abnormal vital signs, Hgb/Hct values Abnormal serum electrolyte values Temperature elevations Signs of dehydration or overhydration Neurological status for any decline in LOC Notify physician of any fluid imbalance or electrolyte abnormality Administer medications/treatments as ordered; monitor effects and side effects

Potential problems	Expected outcomes	Nursing activities
■ Arrhythmia related to Preexisting cardiac abnormalities Carotid sinus manipulation intraoperatively Vagal nerve (X) edema or manipulation intraoperatively	■ Absence or control of arrhythmia	■ Monitor Bedside ECG recording for any abnormalities Pulse rate and quality for bradycardia/tachycardia, irregularity; if indicated compare apical pulse rate to radial pulse and assess for perfusion irregularities For patient complaints of chest pain/discomfort, angina, arm pain, and radiation Notify physician immediately of any abnormality Administer medications and treatments as ordered; monitor effects and side effects If problem is not resolved, see appropriate standard, e.g., *Arrhythmia; Angina; Acute myocardial infarction*
■ Dizziness when head gatch is elevated Potential orthostatic hypotension	■ Patient can sit, stand, and ambulate without dizziness	■ Gradually elevate head of bed when physician's order permits Check BP frequently Monitor for any signs of dizziness or headache Slowly raise head of bed if BP is stable and patient is without dizziness until head is fully elevated Have patient dangle at side of bed for 5 to 10 minutes before assisting patient out of bed Initially assist patient and supervise until patient can ambulate safely and independently If problem occurs with hypotension or dizziness, notify physician Maintain head gatch at level that supports normal BP and prevents dizziness Slowly and gradually increase gatch level and activity progression within tolerance limits
■ Infection	■ Infection free Incision well-healed	■ Keep patient's hands away from operative site Monitor Temperature as ordered and prn for any elevation Incision site for any signs of redness, tenderness, swelling, separation, or drainage (amount and quality) Graft site, if present, for any abnormalities Notify physician of any signs of infection Administer medications/treatments as ordered; monitor effects and side effects Monitor wound culture results Monitor for other possible infection souces if warranted including sputum, urine, chest radiograph results Monitor WBC counts for elevations; if elevated, monitor serially for resolution or progression
■ Continued presence of neurological deficit Patient/family's fears, anxiety, anger related to deficit and possible alterations in life-style	■ Maximal neurological functioning* Maximal independence in ADL (within capabilities) Patient/family verbalizes concerns	■ Assess patient's specific neurological deficit Implement individualized plan of care based on patient's need and deficits Assist as needed in ADL Monitor potential for independent functioning and obtain equipment to maximize function and promote safety Obtain orders for appropriate referrals such as physical, speech, occupational therapy, social service Encourage verbalization of patient/family's fears, anxieties, and other reactions—level and degree Answer questions realistically Encourage their participation in care planning, implementation, evaluation, and decision making

*If responsibility of critical care nurse includes this stage of care.

Potential problems	Expected outcomes	Nursing activities
		Realistically reassure and support patient/family
		Reinforce any gains or independence patient achieves
		Plan, instruct, demonstrate, supervise, and evaluate patient/family's verbalization/performance of needed information/skills for maximal independent functioning such as
		Measures to prevent complications
		Assistance necessary—type, amount, degree
		Proper use of therapeutic devices/equipment
		Monitor level of achievement toward maximizing potentials and independence; means to promote as "normal" a life-style as possible
■ Insufficient knowledge to comply with discharge regimen*	■ Patient/family demonstrates or verbalizes understanding of discharge regimen	■ Assess patient/family's level of understanding of neurological problem and therapy received
		Explain relationship between patient's neurological status and therapies prescribed
		If present, explain relationship of patient's risk factors to plaque formation and importance of controlling/eliminating factors to decrease potential for recurrent plaque formation
		Instruction of patient/family regarding required information/skills so that before discharge patient/family is able to
	Patient/family accurately describes medication, activity, and dietary regimens	Describe medication regimen
		Name and purpose
		Route, dosage, frequency, times
		Side effects
		Special precautions necessary including drugs, foods, beverages contraindicated or quantity regulated; factors potentiating/decreasing effects or side effects; physical restrictions; safety measures
		Describe activity regimen, exercise program
		Describe dietary regimen
		Describe and demonstrate any special therapeutic measures prescribed
	Patient/family describes and demonstrates means to achieve maximal independence in ADL, promote safety, and prevent complications	Describe and demonstrate proper use of equipment or therapeutic devices
		Reasons for using
		Time, method, and duration of use
		Precautions/safeguards
		Necessary maintenance (type, frequency)
		Measures to promote optimal functioning, upkeep/duration
	Patient/family describes signs/symptoms requiring medical attention	Describe signs/symptoms of neurological status requiring medical care
	Patient/family describes follow-up care	Describe plan for follow-up care including purpose of appointment, when and where to go, who to see, what to expect

*If responsibility of the critical care nurse includes such follow-up care.

32 □ Transphenoidal hypophysectomy (pituitary tumors)

The pituitary gland (hypophysis) is a small gland located in the sella turcica at the base of the brain. A circular fold of dura mater, the *diaphragm sella,* forms the roof of this fossa and contains an opening through which the pituitary stalk (infundibulum) passes. The pituitary stalk is the connecting pathway between the pituitary gland and the hypothalamus. The pituitary gland contains two lobes: the anterior lobe, known as the *adenohypophysis;* and the posterior lobe, or *neurohypophysis*.

The pituitary gland is the principal regulator of most of the glands of internal secretion by its own secretion of many important hormones. Pituitary secretion is controlled mainly by signals transmitted from the hypothalamus. Secretion from the anterior lobe is regulated by neurosecretory substances secreted by the hypothalamus. Posterior lobe secretion is controlled by nerve fibers originating in the hypothalamus and terminating in the posterior lobe.

The hormones secreted by the anterior pituitary (adenohypophysis) stimulate target organs and glands. Some of the major hormones include human growth hormone (HGH); adenocorticotropic hormone (ACTH); thyrotropin (TSH); gonadotropic hormones—follicle-stimulating hormone (FSH); luteinizing hormone (LH); luteotropic hormone (LTH); melanocyte-stimulating hormone (MSH); and prolactin.

The posterior lobe (neurohypophysis) is a storage area for the neurosecretory system of the hypothalamus that includes the supraoptic and paraventricular nuclei. The axons of these nuclei travel from the hypothalamus through the supraoptic hypophyseal tract of the stalk to storage areas in the posterior lobe. The two main hormones secreted and transported by these nuclei are antidiuretic hormone (ADH), also known as vasopressin, and oxytocin. The main function of ADH is the control of water reabsorption by the kidneys, which is effected by altering the permeability of the renal tubules. The release of ADH from the posterior lobe is controlled by a feedback regulatory mechanism that senses and responds to the plasma osmotic pressure. Normally this mechanism functions to maintain a normal range of osmolality and osmotic pressure. Hypothalamic osmoreceptors monitor the serum osmolality and respond to changes in the normal range by either stimulating or suppressing the release of ADH from the posterior lobe storage cells in an attempt to restore the osmolality to a normal level as given in the following:

Dehydration: hyperosmolality results in stimulation of ADH release to promote kidney reabsorption of water.

Overhydration: hypo-osmolality results in suppression of ADH release to promote kidney excretion of water through urinary diuresis.

PITUITARY TUMORS

Since the pituitary gland secretes many important hormones, patients with lesions of the gland frequently have endocrine dysfunctions or symptoms of dysfunctions. The anatomical relationship of the pituitary gland to the optic chiasm is important in the consideration of pituitary tumors and their effects. The optic chiasm lies just above the anterior portion of the diaphragm sella. At the optic chiasm the fibers from each nasal retina (which carry temporal vision) cross over to join the fibers from the temporal retina (carrying nasal vision) of the other eye. The two sets of fibers then form the optic tract. Compression of the optic chiasm by a pituitary tumor produces various types of visual defects. The type of visual defect depends on the position of the chiasm in relation to the pituitary gland and the direction of growth of the tumor. If the tumor grows beyond the sella, the optic nerve may be compressed, producing optic atrophy and eventual loss of vision in the affected eye.

Pituitary tumors are located mainly in the anterior lobe (adenohypophysis). Their expansion and growth may erode surrounding bone; cause atrophy or distortion of the optic nerves, chiasm, or tracts; or produce pressure on the hypothalamus or impinge on the third ventricle. The pituitary tumors arising in the anterior lobe are usually benign and slow growing. The majority are adenomas, which frequently are partly cystic. They may cause hypofunctioning of the gland or secretion of abnormally high amounts of pituitary hormones.

Common signs and symptoms

1. Visual loss or failure: visual field defects—more than one half of patients with pituitary adenomas receive medical attention due to the occurrence of this symptom
   a. Frequently the visual loss involves a partial or complete bitemporal hemianopia that has developed gradually; the superior quadrants of the visual fields are usually affected first
   b. In cases of long-standing visual disorder, some degree of optic atrophy is present
2. Headache
3. Endocrine syndromes
   a. Hypopituitary signs—may include impotency, amenorrhea, loss of body hair; hypothyroidism and adrenal insufficiency may also be present
   b. Hormone-secreting pituitary tumors
      (1) Prolactin-secreting pituitary tumors—patient may have galactorrhea, amenorrhea
      (2) Human growth hormone–secreting pituitary tumors—patient may have gigantism and acromegaly
      (3) Adrenocorticotropin-secreting pituitary tumors—patient may have Cushing's syndrome
4. Ocular palsies may occur if the cavernous sinus is compressed
5. Rarely patient may have seizures, rhinorrhea, diabetes insipidus, hypothermia/somnolence

The treatments for pituitary tumors are numerous and include radiotherapy, medical management by drug regimens, and surgical removal. The two available surgical approaches are craniotomy or transphenoidal hypophysectomy. The transphenoidal hypophysectomy is a more recently perfected approach and is frequently the preferable choice. The following standard focuses on care postoperatively following this approach.

ASSESSMENT

1. Onset, duration, progression, and specific description of neurological symptoms, particularly
   a. Visual loss or defect
   b. Alterations in pupil size, equality, and reaction; extraocular movements
   c. Headache
   d. Nausea/vomiting
   e. Diplopia, nystagmus
   f. Ataxia
   g. Seizures
2. Presence of any endocrine problems or signs/symptoms of dysfunction such as
   a. Impotence
   b. Amenorrhea
   c. Loss of body hair
   d. Galactorrhea
   e. Gigantism, acromegaly
   f. Cushing's syndrome
   g. Diabetes insipidus (polyuria, polydipsia)
   h. Hypothyroidism
   i. Adrenal insufficiency
   j. Excessive weight gain
   k. Intolerance to cold
3. Medications taken for neurological/endocrine problem such as steroids, hormonal replacement, anticonvulsants, and pain medications
4. Previous neurological treatment or neurosurgical procedure
5. Presence of any alterations in body image; fears of permanent disability or deficit; altered role in family, normal occupation/performance of ADL; fears of tumor regrowth
6. Patient's perceptions and reaction to diagnosis, treatment modalities, surgical intervention
7. Presence of any other medical problems and medications/treatments prescribed and followed
8. Baseline parameters status
   a. Neurological
   b. Endocrine
   c. Metabolic
   d. Vital signs
   e. Weight
   f. Visual ability
   g. Hydration, urine output and pattern
9. Diagnostic test results, including
   a. Skull radiographs
   b. Tomograms of sella
   c. CAT
   d. Pneumoencephalogram
   e. Lumbar puncture
   f. EEG
   g. Cerebral angiography
   h. Visual field studies
   i. Endocrine studies such as HGH, prolactin, plasma ACTH, thyroid-stimulating hormone, hydrocortisone and ketosteroids, urine for gonadotropic hormone
10. Results of
    a. Serum electrolyte levels
    b. Type and cross matching
    c. Hgb and Hct, platelet count

d. Urinalysis, specific gravity, osmolality, electrolytes
e. Thyroid, pituitary/adrenal function tests if indicated
f. Clotting profile if indicated

GOALS

1. Optimal neurological functioning
2. Optimal independence in ADL
3. Serum electrolyte levels within normal limits
4. Hgb and Hct stable within normal limits
5. Fluid balance within normal limits—diabetes insipidus controlled
6. Acid-base balance within normal limits
7. Incision healed without CSF leak
8. Infection free
9. Endocrine function controlled within normal limits

10. Reduction in patient/family's anxiety with provision of information, demonstrations, support
11. Before discharge patient/family is able to
    a. Describe medication, activity, and dietary regimens
    b. Describe any special therapeutic measures such as recording and balancing fluid intake/output; urine testing of glucose and acetone, specific gravity; weight recording
    c. Demonstrate safety measures and techniques; proper use of any equipment, therapeutic devices
    d. Describe, if present, relationship between neurological problem and endocrine dysfunction
    e. Describe signs/symptoms requiring medical attention
    f. State necessary information regarding follow-up care

Potential problems	Expected outcomes	Nursing activities
Preoperative		
■ Decreased vision Visual loss/visual field defect	■ Maximal independence in ADL Safety of patient	■ Monitor visual ability; assess acuity, field cut, color loss Specifically monitor and document baseline visual loss/field defects Monitor for any increase in visual loss and notify physician if this occurs Promote independent functioning in ADL by Placing within patient's field of vision objects such as food, telephone, hygiene items Tell patient location of objects Have patient turn head to compensate for visual defects Obtain eyeglasses if patient has pair and uses them to improve visual ability Promote patient safety Assist with activities as needed to maintain safety Place call light within field of vision; inform patient of location Assist with ambulation as needed Siderails up if necessary to prevent falls
■ Patient/family's anxiety related to Limited understanding of diagnostic tests and procedures Anticipated surgery Lack of knowledge regarding expected postoperative course Fears of disability or worsened deficit	■ Patient/family's behavior indicates decreased anxiety with provision of information	■ Ongoing assessment of level of anxiety, knowledge base, and understanding Encourage patient/family's verbalization of questions and fears; collaborate with physician in providing realistic information and reassurance appropriate to level of understanding Explain relationship between neurological problem and symptoms, endocrine disorders; reasons for therapies Explain and prepare for tests, procedures, preoperative routines Explain anticipated postoperative care including setting, routines, monitoring equipment, IVs, Foley catheter, nasal packing, visiting policy, length of stay Explain reasons for frequent neurological assessments and vital sign monitoring Instruct in mouth breathing, leg exercises; evaluate patient's performance Provide time needed for support and instruction of patient/family

Potential problems	Expected outcomes	Nursing activities
		Notify unit where patient will be after surgery of any special problems or items patient needs such as
		Eyeglasses: for patient vision; to evaluate visual fields/acuity
		Visual field defect: notify unit of specific deficit as this could prevent having patient restricted to viewing wall postoperatively if bed selection can be flexible and chosen appropriately
		If language barrier is present: an effort should be made to have interpreter available postoperatively

Postoperative

Potential problems	Expected outcomes	Nursing activities
■ General immediate postoperative complications	■ Absence or resolution of complication	■ Monitor for
		Recovery from anesthesia; notify physician if patient has not recovered in expected time period
		Signs/symptoms of hypovolemia, shock, hypostatic pneumonia, pulmonary emboli, thrombophlebitis, abdominal ileus, nausea/vomiting, oliguria/urinary retention
		Recovery from any special measurements induced during surgery such as hypotension/hypothermia
		Notify physician immediately of any signs/symptoms of complication
		Administer medications and treatments as ordered
		Monitor effects and side effects
		Continue monitoring for resolution or progression of complication
		See appropriate standard for identified complication such as *Embolic phenomena; Shock*
■ Increased ICP/potential neurological deficit related to Hemorrhage Hematoma Edema	■ Absence or resolution of increased ICP Maximal neurological functioning	■ Establish neurological baseline postoperatively and compare to preoperative baseline; notify physician immediately if there is any decrease in status
		Neurological assessments and vital signs as ordered and prn (usually q15 min four times, q30 min four times, then q1 hr); monitor particularly
		Pupil size, equality, and light reactivity—both direct and consensual; extraocular movements; visual acuity and fields
		LOC; motor and sensory functioning; communication abilities
		For any increase in headache, nausea/vomiting above usual postoperative expectation
		Notify physician immediately of any change in neurological status or vital signs
		Administer medications and treatments as ordered; monitor effects and side effects
		Prepare patient/family for any tests or procedures ordered
		If increased ICP occurs see Standard: *Increased intracranial pressure*
■ Excessive bloody nasal drainage	■ Normal amount of nasal drainage Absence or resolution of excessive amount	■ Prevent by
		No nasal treatments or suctioning
		Ice bag to nose as per physician's order
		Keep patient's hands from nose/packing; restrain if absolutely necessary as per physician's order
		Instruct patient to not use toothbrush for 10 days
		Provide oral hygiene q2 hr and prn
		Monitor
		Amount of bloody drainage on packing/oozing from nose; notify physician if above usual expectation
		For falling Hgb/Hct levels
		For hypotension, tachycardia
		Notify physician of any abnormality

Potential problems	Expected outcomes	Nursing activities

■ CSF leak	■ Absence or resolution of CSF leak	■ Instruct patient to not blow nose or sneeze (if preventable); explain reasons why it is necessary to avoid these
		Assist physician with lumbar puncture, which may be done to decrease potential for CSF leak
		  Explain procedure to patient
		  Send CSF specimens as per physician's order; monitor results
		Monitor
		  Amount and type of nasal drainage; if quality is suspicious (clear), obtain specimen and test for glucose (result usually positive for sugar if specimen is CSF); monitor for CSF "circle" on bed linen
		  For complaints of severe, continuous headache
		  Temperature as ordered for any elevation
		  For signs of meningitis
		Notify physician immediately of any signs/symptoms of CSF leak (headache, fever, clear nasal drainage/positive dextrose result)
		  Administer medications as ordered; monitor effects and side effects
		  Monitor CSF culture results
		  Monitor WBC count (may be falsely elevated if patient is receiving steroids)
		If meningitis occurs, see Standard: *Meningitis/encephalitis*

■ Fluid and electrolyte imbalance
 	
  Diabetes insipidus*
	■ Fluid and electrolyte balance within normal or prescribed limits
	  Diabetes insipidus controlled
		■ Monitor
		  Hourly intake and output accurately and record on graph sheet
		  Specific gravity q1 hr or with each voiding
		  Notify physician immediately of any increased output or decreased specific gravity deviating from levels specified by physician's order that establishes fluid balance maintenance
		  Daily weights or as ordered for any alterations, particularly weight loss
		  For signs of polydipsia
		  Serum electrolytes for any abnormalities particularly hyponatremia, hyperglycemia
		  Urine glucose and acetone determinations as ordered
		  Presence/degree of nausea and vomiting; effectiveness of medications ordered
		  Hgb and Hct values for any abnormalities
		Administer IV fluids as ordered
		If problem occurs, notify physician immediately
		  Administer medications as ordered; monitor effects and side effects; frequently vasopressin may be ordered; insulin coverage for glucose and acetone determinations
		  Maintain intake at specific level ordered
		  Monitor results of urine osmolality/electrolytes, serum osmolality values
		  If patient is taking po fluids, determine fluid preferences and offer these frequently if po is encouraged by physician
		  Explain to patient relationship between surgery and diabetes insipidus

---

*Diabetes insipidus is characterized by polyuria and polydipsia. Specific gravity frequently falls to 1.000 to 1.005. Urine output rises well above the fluid intake. Restriction of intake, which in the normal functioning body mechanism would stimulate release of ADH from the pituitary gland (in response to hyperosmolality) and end diuresis, does not occur in patients with diabetes insipidus. This disruption of normal stimulation of ADH secretion mechanism is related to surgical manipulation or edema near the hypothalamus or supraoptic hypophyseal tract.

Potential problems	Expected outcomes	Nursing activities
■ GI bleeding related to CNS factors Stress Steroid administration	■ Absence or resolution of GI bleeding	■ Monitor vital signs q2-4 hr, Hgb and Hct; stools for Hematest three times a week; Hematest of aspirate, emesis, and urine for any abnormalities Obtain order for antacid administration as soon as patient able to take po Monitor for signs of GI bleeding including abdominal tenderness/distention; hypotension, sudden tachycardia Notify physician immediately if any abnormality occurs If problem occurs, see Standard: *Acute upper gastrointestinal bleeding*
■ Continued presence of decreased vision Visual loss/visual field defect	■ Maximal independence in ADL Safety of patient	■ See Problem, Decreased vision (preoperative), for nursing activities Collaborate with physican regarding prognosis for recovery or improvement in vision (physician may have expectations for prognosis based on operative findings) Provide realistic information and reassurance to patient/family Encourage verbalization of anxieties and fears if visual loss is permanent Assess level of anxiety related to potential altered body image/role Support patient/family in verbalizing concerns, anger Instruct patient/family in measures to promote maximal independence and safety Obtain orders for appropriate referrals such as social service, vocational training
■ Insufficient knowledge to comply with discharge regimen*	■ Patient/family demonstrates or verbalizes understanding of discharge regimen	■ Assess patient/family's level of understanding of neurological problem and therapy received Explain relationship between patient's neurological status and therapies prescribed If endocrine symptoms or dysfunctions are present, explain relationship to neurological status and reasons, importance, and necessity of complying with hormonal replacement medication regimen Instruction of patient/family regarding required information and skills so that before discharge patient/family is able to
	Patient/family describes medication, activity, and dietary regimens	Describe medication regimen Name and purpose Route, dosage, frequency times Side effects Special precautions necessary, including drugs, foods, beverages contraindicated or quantity regulated; factors potentiating/decreasing effects or side effects; physical restrictions; safety measures Describe dietary regimen Describe activity regimen, exercise program
	Patient/family describes special therapeutic measures	Describe and demonstrate any special therapeutic measures prescribed such as Accurate monitoring, recording, and graphing of intake and output Monitoring and recording urine specific gravity, glucose, and acetone determinations Maintenance of intake and output at prescribed level by adjustment of fluid intake, utilization of medications ordered prn Weight monitoring and recording

*If the responsibility of the critical care nurse includes such follow-up care.

Potential problems	Expected outcomes	Nursing activities
		Describe and demonstrate any visual therapeutic devices, techniques/measures prescribed
	Patient/family describes signs/symptoms requiring medical attention	Describe signs/symptoms of neurological status requiring medical care; signs of endocrine/metabolic status requiring care if present
	Patient/family describes follow-up care regimen	Describe plan for follow-up care including purpose of appointment, when and where to go, who to see, what to expect, what recorded information, charts, and specimens to bring

33 □ Seizures

A seizure can be basically described as a sudden, excessive, disorderly discharge of cerebral neurons that produces an intermittent derangement of the nervous system. For a variety of reasons certain neve cells may fire or discharge an excessive amount of sudden impulses, resulting in electrical disturbances in the brain and instigating seizure occurrence. This abnormal discharge activity commonly results in disturbances of sensation, loss of consciousness or psychic function, motor disturbances, convulsive movements, or varied combinations of symptoms.

A seizure indicates that the nervous system has been affected by disease disturbance. Most authorities propose that an isolated seizure is a symptom of an underlying pathological condition, and they suggest that the term *epilepsy* be restricted to describing recurrent or repeated seizure occurrence. Subdivisions of epilepsy include *primary* (recurrent seizures of unknown cause) and *secondary* (recurrent seizures from a known cause).

Seizures may be caused by a variety of pathological conditions including brain tumors, trauma, clots; meningitis and encephalitis; electrolyte disorders; alcohol and drug overdose/withdrawal; metabolic disorders; uremia; overhydration; toxic substances; and cerebral anoxia. Seizures are also a major potential complication of various neurosurgical procedures. In the majority of seizure disorders the cause of the recurrent seizure activity is unknown; this type is termed *idiopathic epilepsy*.

Seizures have been classified in various ways according to site, EEG correlates, symptomatology, therapy responses, and so on. Some common types of seizures that nurses frequently encounter include generalized seizures such as grand mal and petit mal; minor motor seizures such as akinetic and myoclonic; and focal seizures such as psychomotor, jacksonian, focal somatic sensory, and focal visual. Status epilepticus denotes a series of seizures occurring without complete recovery between attacks or a continuing seizure attack usually lasting longer than 30 minutes. See Table 7 for common seizure types and clinical signs/presentation.

The treatment of seizures is aimed at determining and removing the cause if possible; effective anticonvulsant drug control (either short-term or long-term, depending on necessity); prevention of precipitating factors; and promotion and regulation of physical and mental hygiene. A complete workup will be done on most patients to determine if there is an underlying pathological cause that can be corrected or controlled. In some cases the cause of the seizure symptomatology may be surgically removed, such as with a brain tumor or clot. Other pathological conditions causing seizures may be controlled by medical management and treatment, such as metabolic or electrolyte disturbances and renal dysfunctions.

ASSESSMENT

1. Specific description of any previous seizure, including
   a. Time of first occurrence
   b. Frequency of seizures; any increase in seizure activity
   c. Onset, duration, progression, type, locality, length of seizure

Table 7. Types of seizures: common clinical signs and presentation

GENERALIZED

Grand mal *(tonic clonic)*

Frequently preceded by aura, loss of consciousness

Tonic phase: jaw snapped shut; frequently tongue biting; respiratory muscles caught in tonic spasm—cyanosis of skin and mucous membranes; pupils dilated and unreactive; frequently incontinence; usual length is 10 to 15 seconds

Clonic phase: generalized trembling progressing to violent muscle contractions of entire body; eye rolling; tachycardia; excessive salivation; facial grimacing; profuse diaphoresis; respirations jerky; usual length from 1 to 2 minutes

Postictal: loss of consciousness persists from minutes to hours; pupils begin to react; muscle relax and breathing becomes quiet and regular; patient awakens, usually startled and confused, and then falls asleep

Patient may remember aura but not seizure occurrence; may have headache, muscle stiffness, and fatigue following seizure

Petit mal *(absence attacks)*

Consists of sudden, brief episode of interruption of consciousness in which patient seems to be daydreaming, staring and is motionless and stops in middle of conversation

May have brief period of eyelid fluttering, clonus of facial muscles/fingers

Automatisms—lip smacking and chewing—are common

Postural tone may be decreased or increased but usually patient does not fall

Patient may or may not be aware of attacks

MINOR MOTOR

Akinetic

Momentary lapse of consciousness; loss of postural tone

Myoclonic

Sudden onset of brief muscle contractions/jerks

FOCAL *(from lesion in certain area of cerebral cortex)*

Psychomotor *(commonly from temporal lobe involvement)*

Aura: frequently hallucination or perceptual illusion

Behaves in confused manner and is amnesic of this

Hallucinations: usually visual and auditory; infrequently olfactory

Illusions/distortion of perceptions

Psycognitive states: increased reality/familiarity (déjà vu) or unfamiliarity/strangeness

Automatisms: lip smacking, sucking/chewing movements or repetition of inappropriate acts

May proceed to tonic spasms

Jacksonian *(frequently from lesion of frontal lobe)*

Tonic contraction of fingers/face/foot on one side, which may spread to involve the entire same side and progress to clonic movements

Eye and head turning/deviation usually to side opposite irritative focus (looking at convulsing side)

May have sensory signs

May progress to grand mal

Somatic sensory

Numbness and tingling initially of lips, fingers, and toes; then spreads

Visual

Visual sensations of darkness/spots

Visual hallucinations

---

d. Any aura, incontinence, eye/head deviation, tongue biting, mouth frothing, chewing-sucking movements, eye rolling, pupillary status

e. Respiratory status and skin color

f. Postictal status; any injury incurred

g. Patient amnesic or aware of seizure, events prior and following

h. If patient has been receiving anticonvulsant drugs, whether schedule has been adhered to

i. Presence of any precipitating factors such as fever, emotional/physical stress

j. Whether seizures were associated with any other symptoms such as headaches, nausea/vomiting

k. If multiple seizures, any variation in activity or similarity of episodes

2. Onset, duration, and progression of any other neurological symptoms; if present whether there is any association between symptom appearance and seizure occurrence

3. Previous head trauma or injury; specific description and details

4. Previous toxin ingestion or exposure such as metals, carbon monoxide
5. Previous infectious process such as meningitis, encephalitis
6. Previous drug/alcohol abuse or withdrawal
7. Presence of congenital anomaly, delayed growth and development milestones, birth injury
8. Previous metabolic, electrolyte, or renal disturbances; any anoxic episodes
9. Medications taken for neurological problem such as anticonvulsants, steroids
10. Previous neurological treatment or neurosurgical procedure
11. Presence of any medical problems; medications/treatments prescribed and followed
12. Presence and degree of any physical/emotional stress
13. Nutritional habits and dietary regimen
14. Patient's perceptions and reactions to diagnosis, treatment modalities; level of anxiety related to hospitalization
15. Level of patient/family's knowledge of seizure disorder, treatments, medication regimens, precipitating factors, and so on if seizures are not new occurrence
16. Presence of any alterations in body image; fears of permanent disability or deficit; altered role in family, normal occupation/performance of ADL; restrictions due to disorder; "stigma" reactions
17. Baseline parameters status
    a. Neurological
    b. Seizure history
    c. Respiratory
    d. Metabolic
    e. Renal
    f. Fluid/electrolyte
    g. Cardiovascular
    h. Nutritional
    i. Emotional
    j. Vital signs
    k. Weight
    l. Handedness (right or left)
    m. Growth and developmental level
    n. Associated congenital anomalies
18. Diagnostic test results, including
    a. EEG
    b. CAT

c. Cerebral angiograpy
d. Brain scan
e. Skull radiographs
f. Lumbar puncture
g. Psychological testing
19. Results of
    a. Serum electrolyte levels
    b. Serum Ca^{2+} and phosphorus levels, BUN levels
    c. Anticonvulsant drug levels
    d. Amino acid screen
    e. Alcohol/drug levels
    f. Toxin screens
    g. Urine specific gravity, osmolality, analysis, culture, electrolytes
    h. Serum osmolality
    i. Hgb and Hct, platelet count, WBC count and differentiation
    j. Clotting profile
    k. Arterial blood gas levels
    l. Chest radiograph
    m. ECG

GOALS

1. Optimal neurological functioning
2. Optimal seizure control and safety maintenance
3. Optimal independence in ADL within safety restrictions/limitations
4. Adequate alveolar ventilation
5. Serum electrolyte levels within normal limits
6. Acid-base balance within normal limits
7. Fluid balance within normal range
8. Hgb, Hct, and platelets stable within normal limits
9. Anticonvulsant drug levels within therapeutic range
10. Reduction in patient/family's anxiety with provision of information, demonstrations, support
11. Before discharge patient/family is able to
    a. Describe medication, activity, and dietary regimens
    b. Describe safety measures, necessary restrictions, safety techniques
    c. Describe methods to maintain seizure threshold
    d. Describe appropriate interventions if seizure occurs at home
    e. Describe signs and symptoms requiring medical attention
    f. State necessary information regarding follow-up care

Potential problems	**Expected outcomes**	**Nursing activities**
■ Recurrence of seizure	■ Seizure control Absence of complications	■ Assess seizure history of patient on admission (see Assessment No. 1 for specifics); establish baseline neurological status and vital signs

■ Assess seizure history of patient on admission (see Assessment No. 1 for specifics); establish baseline neurological status and vital signs

If patient frequently has aura prior to seizure, instruct patient to call nurse immediately if aura occurs; stress importance of patient notifying nurse and ensure that call light is within patient's reach

Close observation and supervision

Seizure precautions (especially if potential grand mal); may include

Padded tongue blade and airway at bedside

Bed height at lowest level

Padded siderails up at all times when patient is alone

Call light within easy reach

Suction and O_2 equipment readily available

Emergency medications and respiratory assistance equipment readily available

Plastic eating utensils and dishes; no straws

No smoking by patient when unsupervised

Instruct patient to call nurse immediately if "focal" seizure occurs; stress importance of notifying and reasons why

Administer anticonvulsants as ordered

Monitor effects and side effects

Monitor serum anticonvulsant levels; other tests ordered for evaluation of therapeutic dosage levels

Prevention of precipitating factors including

Hypoxia: monitor respiratory rate, quality and pattern; adequacy of alveolar ventilation and perfusion; for any signs of hypoventilation or other abnormalities

Hyperventilation: encourage patient to breathe slowly and deeply; reassure and support

Hypoglycemia: assess patient's food preferences and assist in selection of well-balanced meals; monitor for signs/symptoms of hypoglycemia including decreased serum glucose levels, restlessness, weakness, faintness

Overhydration: monitor and accurately record intake and output; monitor for any signs/symptoms of fluid imbalance

Electrolyte disorders: monitor serum electrolytes including Ca^{2+}; phosphorus, BUN levels for any abnormalities

Hyperthermia: protect patient from possible sources of infection; monitor temperature for any elevation q4 hr and prn; maintain sterile technique as warranted; institute and maintain hypothermia blanket as ordered

Metabolic disorder: monitor amino acid screen for any abnormalities; monitor for signs/symptoms of disturbances

Extreme fatigue: provide rest periods between activity; encourage good night's sleep

Emotional stress: try to minimize stressful situations; consistently reassure and support

Notify physician immediately if any precipitating factors occur or potential is present

Administer medications and treatments as ordered

Monitor effects and side effects

Monitor for resolution or progression of factor

If seizure occurs, stay with patient and call for help (see Problems, Patient self-injury during seizure and Respiratory distress during seizure, for specific problems occurring with seizures)

Potential problems	Expected outcomes	Nursing activities

		Monitor
		  Seizure activity for onset, progression, type, focus, and duration
		  Pupil size, equality, and reactivity
		  For eye/head deviation; gaze preference
		  For chewing/sucking movements, eye rolling, mouth frothing
		  For presence of aura or incontinence
		Notify physician of seizure and specific description
		  Administer medications as ordered; monitor effects and side effects
		  Accurately record specific description of seizure and medications administered; effects on seizure activity
		Monitor postictal status q15 min or as ordered, including
		  LOC
		  Vital signs
		  Neurological status
		  Patient's awareness or amnesia of seizure occurrence; events prior to and following
		  Presence of headache, muscle soreness, or stiffness

▪ Patient self-injury during seizure	▪ Absence or control of injury
	Absence of complications
		▪ Stay with patient
		  If jaws are not clenched, insert tongue blade to prevent possible tongue biting
		  If patient is wearing dentures, remove if possible, if jaws are not clenched
		  Protect patient's head by placing pillow, other soft object, or hands under head
		  Loosen any tight or restrictive clothing
		  Do not attempt to restrain patient as this may result in limb fractures
		  Move dangerous objects, sharp furniture away from patient
		  When seizure ceases, remain with patient; inform patient about what has happened; reassure and support
		  Monitor for any signs of injury such as cuts, bruises; notify physician if any occurred and administer therapy as ordered

▪ Respiratory distress during seizure	▪ Patent airway
	Normal respiratory rate and pattern
	Adequate alveolar ventilation
		▪ Maintain patent airway
		  Turn and position patient on side to prevent aspiration
		  Position head to maintain airway
		  Insert airway if needed
		  Suction secretions as needed
		  Administer O_2 prn
		Monitor respiratory status
		  Period of apnea
		  Color of skin and mucous membranes
		  Respiratory rate, pattern, and quality
		  Vital signs
		If respiratory distress continues, call for emergency equipment and notify physician
		  Assist with emergency measures to maintain patent airway and adequate alveolar ventilation
		  Administer medications and treatments as ordered; monitor effects and side effects
		  If unresolved, see Problem, Respiratory insufficiency, for specific activities

Potential problems	Expected outcomes	Nursing activities
■ Patient/family's anxiety related to potential or actual seizure occurrence	■ Patient/family verbalizes fears	■ Ongoing assessment of level of anxiety Encourage verbalization of fears, anxieties, and questions Collaborate with physician in providing realistic information and reassurance appropriate to level of understanding 　Explain, if present, relationship between seizures and underlying pathology 　Explain routines, precautions, and medication regimens; reaffirm that medication control of seizures requires time to determine adequate regimen 　Explain reasons for frequent monitoring of neurological status and vital signs 　Explain and prepare for treatments, tests, therapeutic measures 　Provide continuing time, support, and explanations 　Reassure that patient does not have to become upset about "losing control"
■ Status epilepticus Status epilepticus is a medical emergency and must be controlled to prevent potential cerebral anoxia, damage, and ischemia The EEG during status epilepticus usually demonstrates extreme discharging by the neurons of the reticular activating system and cerebral cortex	■ Absence of complications Resolution or control of status epilepticus	■ Monitor initially same activities as in Problems, Recurrence of seizure; Patient self-injury during seizure; and Respiratory distress during seizure Notify physician immediately of recurrent seizures without full recovery or of a prolonged single seizure Have emergency equipment and medications readily available 　Intubation equipment and mechanical ventilator will usually be needed due to further respiratory depression from medications administered 　Medications commonly administered intravenously include diazepam (Valium), phenytoin (Dilantin), phenobarbital, and paraldehyde Monitor vital signs, respiratory and neurological status, seizure activity q5 min or as ordered Monitor ECG recording for any abnormalities Assist physician with administration of emergency medications; monitor for effectiveness of seizure control and side effects including 　Phenytoin (Dilantin): monitor for hypotension, cardiovascular collapse, arrhythmias 　Diazepam (Valium): monitor for respiratory depression, hypotension, cardiac arrest 　Phenobarbital: monitor for respiratory depression, cumulative effect, prolonged coma, delayed action Continue monitoring neurological status and vital signs q1 hr or as ordered; monitor for any signs of seizure activity and notify physician immediately if recurs Monitor 　Anticonvulsant drug levels for therapeutic range maintenance 　Serum electrolytes including Ca^{2+}, glucose, phosphorus for any abnormalities Control precipitating factors in seizure occurrence whenever possible including hypoxia, hyperventilation, hyperthermia

Potential problems	Expected outcomes	Nursing activities
■ Status epilepticus: respiratory insufficiency related to Medication administration CNS pathology	■ Patent airway Normal respiratory rate and quality Adequate alveolar ventilation and perfusion Arterial blood gas values within patient's normal limits	■ Ongoing assessments of respiratory status q1-2 hr and prn; monitor for any abnormality/decline Respiratory rate, quality, and pattern Patency of upper airway and patient's ability to handle secretions Skin color, nail beds, peripheral pulses, and skin warmth Breath sounds bilaterally for quality of aeration, signs of obstruction (rales, rhonchi) Presence/strength of gag, cough, and swallowing reflexes Arterial blood gas values Chest radiograph results For signs/symptoms of thrombophlebitis, pulmonary emboli, pulmonary edema Monitor neurological status frequently, particularly LOC, seizure activity, focal deficits Maintain patent airway by Turning and positioning to prevent obstruction or aspiration of secretions q2 hr and prn Artificial airway if needed Suctioning prn Chest physiotherapy/pulmonary toilet q2 hr if not contraindicated Adequate oxygenation and humidification as ordered Apply antithromboembolic stockings or Ace bandages as ordered; reapply every shift and prn; monitor for constriction/looseness, condition of skin Notify physician immediately of any decline in respiratory status, neurological status, or seizure control Assist with emergency measures to maintain patent airway and adequate ventilation See Standard: *Mechanical ventilation* Administer medications and treatments as ordered; monitor effects and side effects When seizure control is achieved and respiratory effects of medications are eliminated, monitor For improvement in LOC Respiratory status, adequacy of ventilation and perfusion
■ Status epilepticus: fluid and electrolyte imbalance	■ Fluid and electrolyte balance within normal limits	■ Monitor and accurately record intake and output, urine specific gravity, and osmolality as ordered Monitor for signs of dehydration or overhydration such as Poor skin turgor Dry mucous membranes Peripheral edema Change in LOC Monitor for Abnormal vital signs, Hgb/Hct values Abnormal serum electrolyte values, particularly glucose, Ca^{2+}, and phosphorus levels (disorders may potentiate or prolong status occurrence) Insensible fluid losses including respiratory, diaphoresis, secretions Weight alterations Acute renal failure if status is result of anoxia; see Standard: *Acute renal failure* Monitor temperature q2 hr and prn for any elevation as fever can potentiate seizures If elevation occurs, notify physician immediately Monitor and culture possible sources Institute and maintain hypothermia blanket as ordered

Potential problems	Expected outcomes	Nursing activities
		Administer IV fluids and medications as ordered; if patient is receiving steroids, monitor urine glucose and acetone levels four times a day Notify physician immediately of any fluid imbalance or electrolyte abnormality Administer medications and treatments as ordered Monitor for resolution or progression of abnormality and notify physician of results

■ Status epilepticus: family's fears and anxiety related to patient in status epilepticus	■ Family verbalizes fears	■ Encourage verbalization of fears and concerns
		 Collaborate with physician in providing realistic information and reassurance to family
		 Explain
		   Pathology and relationship to present status
		   Reasons for medications and treatments; importance of controlling seizures
		   Reasons patient's LOC/respiratory functioning is depressed
		   Reasons for certain therapies and mechanical assistance at this time
		   Anticipated course and prognosis
		 Ongoing support of family; provide time, explanations, and reassurance

■ Continued potential or presence of seizure activity
 Patient/family's anxiety and fears related to
 Lack of knowledge
 Threat of seizure
 Altered life-style and restrictions
	■ Patient/family verbalizes concerns*
	 Patient/family demonstrates or verbalizes required knowledge and skills
		■ Ongoing assessments of patient/family's level of anxiety
		   Encourage verbalization of fears, concerns, anger related to potential continuation of seizure disorder
		   Collaborate with physician in providing realistic information and reassurance based on expected prognosis
		   Encourage patient/family's verbalization and questions regarding restrictions imposed by threat of potential seizure and effects on life-style; restrictions of prior activities or job responsibilities may include revocation of driver's license, constant supervision for certain activities, restriction on using electrical equipment at home/job
		   Assess patient/family's reactions to restrictions and alterations; effects on usual life-style and responsibilities, role, and ADL
		 Explore ways patient/family can cope with condition; capabilities to maximize potential for independent functioning within confines of necessary safety precautions
		 Stress importance of and support and encourage patient/family in accepting seizure disorder reality and adopting positive attitude toward coping; monitor reactions, acceptance level, degree of control expected
		   Reaffirm that although there is no cure for seizure disorder, a nearly "normal" life can continue by adherence to control measures and regimens
		   Reinforce that potential for maximal control of seizure disorder and independence is promoted by acquisition of knowledge and skills; implementation and adherence to prescribed regimens, precaution; and confidence in dealing and coping with disorder
		 Assess and monitor level of understanding of seizure disorder and needed information and skills
		   Promote collaboration of patient/family and health team in achieving maximal control, independence, positive attitude, and as "normal" a life-style as possible

*If responsibility of critical care nurse includes this stage of care.

Potential problems	Expected outcomes	Nursing activities
		Provide facts and realistic information to correct fallacies and misconceptions including dealing with "stigma" misperceptions
		Obtain orders for appropriate referrals such as social service, vocational training, National Epilepsy Foundation
		Stress variability of achieving seizure control with each individual
		Reassure and support patient/family
		Instruct, demonstrate, and evaluate patient/family's knowledge acquisition and performance in needed information/skills such as
		What seizure is; reason for occurrence if related to pathology
		Knowledge of seizure disorder
		Patient's own specific seizure manifestations; if aura is present, what to do if occurs
		Identification of precipitating factors and importance of controlling; includes excessive fatigue, poor nutrition, electrolyte imbalance, fever, emotional stress/strain
		Verbalization of means to control precipitating factors; appropriate actions to take if precipitating factors occur
		Provision of realistic facts and information, correction of fallacies and myths
		Necessary interventions if seizure occurs including airway maintenance, safety measures, monitoring and recording of specific activity
		Restrictions necessitated by seizure disorder including dietary, activity, alcohol intake, seizure precautions
		Importance of good oral hygiene
		Explain and reinforce to patient/family
		Necessary reasons for restrictions
		Theats/dangers of noncompliance
		Necessity of wearing medical alert identification
		Explore with patient/family alternate means/measures to maintain as "normal" a life-style as possible
		Promote maintenance of usual routines, activities, and relationships within limits of restrictions
		Means to deal with other family members, friends, social occasions
		Avoidance of overdependence and overprotection within the family and outside the family
■ Insufficient knowledge to comply with discharge regimen*	■ Patient/family demonstrates or verbalizes understanding of discharge regimen	■ Assess patient/family's level of understanding of neurological problem and therapy received
		Explain relationship between patient's neurological status and therapies prescribed
		Importance of and identification of means to maintain seizure threshold
		Specific disorder; restrictions necessary
		Reasons and importance of compliance to control seizure; prevention of precipitating factors
		Instruction of patient/family regarding required information and skills so that before discharge patient/family is able to
	Patient/family accurately describes medication, activity, and dietary regimens	Describe medication regimen
		Name and purpose
		Route, dosage, frequency, times
		Side effects

*If the responsibility of the critical care nurse includes such follow-up care.

Potential problems	Expected outcomes	Nursing activities
		Special precautions necessary including drugs, foods, alcohol contraindicated or quantity regulated; factors potentiating/decreasing effects or side effects; physical restrictions; safety measures
		Measures to promote effectiveness and minimize side effects
		Blood tests required; reasons and importance
		Scheduling of regimen to enhance compliance
		Times when medication addition/adjustment may be needed
		If patient is to adjust own regimen: when, how often, effectiveness
		Describe dietary regimen
		Describe activity regimen, exercise program
		Describe and demonstrate any special therapeutic measures prescribed
	Patient/family describes means to achieve maximal independence in ADL, promote safety, and prevent complications	Describe restrictions, precautions, control of precipitating factors
		Describe proper interventions, observations/recording if seizure occurs
	Patient/family describes signs/symptoms requiring medical attention	Describe signs/symptoms of seizure disorder/control requiring medical attention
	Patient/family describes follow-up care regimen	Describe plan for follow-up care including purpose of appointment, when and where to go, who to see, what to expect, specimens to bring, charting or recording to bring

34 □ Meningitis/encephalitis

Meningitis and encephalitis are common infectious processes of the CNS, which may occur as a primary disease or a secondary complication of neurosurgery, certain diagnostic procedures, trauma, ear/sinus infections, systemic infections, and so on. A large variety of bacteria and viruses can be responsible for the primary infections of the CNS.

MENINGITIS

Bacterial meningitis (leptomeningitis) is mainly an infection of the pia mater and arachnoidea and the fluid in the space they enclose. The subarachnoid space is continuous around the brain, spinal cord, and optic nerves. An infective organism that enters the subarachnoid space can extend and spread throughout the entire space and reach the ventricles of the brain. The effect of bacteria in the subarachnoid space is to cause an inflammatory response in the pia mater, arachnoidea, CSF, and ventricles. Blood vessels become engorged and may rupture or thrombose. The subarachnoid exudate is increased by the irritative effects of the bacteria, which promote vascular congestion and increased capillary permeability. The exudate accumulation may spread into cranial and spinal nerves or obstruct the normal flow route of the CSF, resulting in the development of hydrocephalus. Secondary encephalitis and neuronal degeneration may occur if the brain surface adjacent to the meninges becomes involved.

Bacteria enter the CNS through two major routes: hematogenous spread (emboli of bacteria or infected thrombi) or spread from cranial structures (ears, sinuses, cranial trauma). A small proportion of infections are iatrogenic, having been introduced by lumbar puncture needles. Factors that promote the bloodstream invasion by the bacteria to reach the meninges are not fully known but may include a preceding viral infection of the upper respiratory tract or lung. The disruption of the normal blood-brain barrier may contribute to the entry of bacteria into the subarachnoid space. Skull fractures and dural tears from head trauma may promote meningitis development. Occasionally, a brain abscess may infect the meninges if it ruptures into the subarachnoid space or ventricles.

The early clinical manifestations of bacterial meningitis are signs of meningeal irritation. These include fever, severe headache, nuchal rigidity, generalized convulsions, and altered LOC. Two signs that are frequently present are Kernig's (inability to completely extend the legs) and Brudzinski's (forward flexion of head causes hip and knee flexion response). Focal signs of cerebral damage and cranial nerve abnormalities may occur with meningitis due to the various bacteria involved and diversity of stages. A diagnosis of bacterial meningitis is suspected from the clinical signs and confirmed by examination of the CSF. Features of the CSF usually include pleocytosis, elevated spinal fluid pressure, elevated protein levels, and decreased glucose content. Cultures and gram stains of the CSF usually identify the infective organism, and treatment of meningitis consists of antibiotic administration. Some cases may be caused by a mixture/combination of organisms, and administration of multiple antibiotic drugs may be required. The resolution of the inflammatory process and degree of recovery depend largely on the stage at which the infection is controlled, with potential complete recovery greatest in the early stages. If the meningitis continues, the chances for further progression of inflammation and resulting cerebral damage increase.

Aseptic meningitis is a term used to describe a clinical symptomatology entity that can be produced by a variety of infective agents, the majority of which are viral. Common symptoms are fever, headache, and other signs of meningeal irritation. Photophobia and pain with ocular movements commonly occur, whereas Kernig's and Brudzinski's signs are usually absent. The common viruses involved are enteroviruses, mumps, and herpes simplex (type 2). Many times the specific virus cannot be isolated. Data that may assist in the differential diagnosis of viral meningitis include immunizations, past infectious diseases, family outbreaks, animal bites, recent travel, epidemic outbreaks, and seasonal/geographical distributions. Viral meningitis is usually benign and lasts 1 to 2 weeks with complete recovery afterward.

ENCEPHALITIS

Encephalitis is a syndrome characterized by an acute febrile state; signs of meningeal involvement; and signs/symptoms of dysfunction of the cerebrum, brain stem, or cerebellum. It is usually caused by a viral infection. The onset of neurological signs is commonly preceded by a prodromal illness of a few days' duration with fever, headache, malaise, aches, sore throat, nausea, and vomiting resulting from organism invasion. Within the CNS viral infections cause inflammation that can involve the cortex, white matter, meninges, and so on. The resultant pathologic condition may include destruction of neurons, demyelination, diffuse edema, hemorrhage, and necrosis.

The main types of encephalitis are caused by arboviruses, acute herpes simplex (type 1), animal bites, infectious mononucleosis, and aftermaths of prophylactic inoculations. A variety of pathological effects can result from the viral infection due to variations in susceptibility of nervous tissue areas and the diversity of viral organisms. Invasion of the CNS usually occurs by the hematogenous (blood) and peripheral nerve (retrograde axoplasmic spread) pathways. The neurological dysfunctions may include weakness, aphasia, ataxia, involuntary movements, myoclonic jerks, ocular palsies, nystagmus, facial weakness, and coma.

Patients with herpes simplex, in addition to signs of acute encephalitis, usually manifest signs that include bizarre behavior, olfactory/gustatory hallucinations, temporal lobe seizures, and anosmia. The frontal and temporal lobes are frequently affected.

Herpes zoster (shingles) produces an acute inflammatory reaction in spinal or cranial sensory ganglia, the posterior grey matter of the spinal cord, and adjacent meninges. Clinical signs include rash, pain, palsies, itching, and burning or tingling sensations.

The prognosis of viral encephalitis is widely variable and frequently unpredictable during its early clinical course. The death and morbidity rates vary greatly, and residual neurological deficits occur in about one fifth of patients postencephalitis. In some cases the virus may not be isolated, whereas in others an antiviral agent may not be available or effective for an identified virus.

ASSESSMENT

1. Onset, progression, frequency, duration, and specific description of neurological symptoms, including
   a. Headache
   b. Nuchal rigidity
   c. Fever
   d. Alterations in LOC
   e. Changes in behavior or personality
   f. Alterations in motor/sensory abilities
   g. Alteration in communication abilities
   h. Ocular palsies, photophobia, nystagmus, ptosis
   i. Cranial nerve palsies
   j. Alterations in visual abilities, hearing acuity
   k. Kernig's/Brudzinski's signs
   j. Seizures
   m. Medullary symptoms: vomiting, tachyardia, respiratory difficulties, arrhythmias
2. Recent preceding viral illness or infectious disease; past history of disease, rash
3. Recent inoculations, immunizations, exposure to infection/viral disease
4. Recent travel, insect bites, contact with animal, bites
5. Family outbreaks, geographical outbreaks, work/social contacts; exposure to or presence of infection/disease
6. Previous head trauma or injury: incident; clinical course, treatment, sequelae; any skull fracture, dural tear, CSF leak
7. Previous/present ear, sinus infections or recurrent infections
8. Previous ingestion of poisons, drug overdose, toxin exposure
9. Previous neurological treatment or neurosurgical procedure; medications taken, effects on clinical course/status
10. Presence of any medical problems and the therapy employed; risk factors that have been identified as contributing to the development of meningitis/encephalitis include debilitation, alcoholism, diabetes mellitus, long-term radiation therapy, immunosuppressive therapy, immunoglobulin deficiency, reticuloendothelial system malignancies, and renal failure
11. Patient's perceptions and reaction to diagnosis, disease progression, treatment modalities
12. Presence of any alterations in body image; fears of permanent disability or deficit; altered role in family, normal occupation, performance of ADL
13. Baseline parameters status
    a. Neurological
    b. Respiratory/pulmonary
    c. Cardiovascular
    d. Metabolic
    e. Renal
    f. Hydration/nutritional
    g. Fluid/electrolyte
    h. Infection
    i. Vital signs
    j. Temperature
    k. Weight
    l. Handedness (right or left)
14. Diagnostic test results, including
    a. Lumbar puncture
    b. Skull radiographs
    c. EEG
    d. CAT
    e. Cerebral angiography
    f. Brain scan
    g. Brain biopsy
15. Results of
    a. CSF determinations
    b. Serum electrolyte levels
    c. Hgb, Hct, platelet count, WBC count/differential
    d. Sedimentation rate
    e. Urinalysis, culture, osmolality, gravity
    f. Amino acid screen
    g. Antibody detection
    h. Clotting profile
    i. Arterial blood gas levels
    j. Anticonvulsant drug levels
    k. Toxin screens
    l. C and S including blood, sputum, urine, nasal secretions, wound/sinus drainage, CSF
    m. ECG
    n. Chest radiograph

GOALS

1. Maximal neurological functioning
2. Optimal independence in ADL
3. Resolution of acute infectious process; infection free systemically, in CSF, and in specific bodily systems
4. Afebrile, normal blood values
5. Adequate alveolar ventilation and perfusion
6. Serum electrolyte levels and fluid balance within normal limits
7. Hgb and Hct stable within normal limits

8. Acid-base balance within normal limits
9. Seizures controlled
10. Reduction in patient/family's anxiety with provision of information, demonstrations, support
11. Before discharge patient/family is able to
    a. Describe medication, activity, exercise, and dietary regimens

b. Demonstrate safety measures and techniques; proper use of any equipment, therapeutic devices prescribed
c. Describe signs and symptoms requiring medical attention
d. State necessary information regarding follow-up care

Potential problems	Expected outcomes	Nursing activities
■ Increased ICP Decline in neurological status related to acute infection—swelling, inflammatory process/hydrocephalus	■ Absence or resolution of signs of increased ICP Maximal neurological functioning	■ Avoid precipitating factors in increased ICP such as hypoxia, hypercapnia, fever, Valsalva's maneuver Assist patient with positioning and turning Instruct patient not to hold breath, blow nose vigorously, or reach for bedside articles Monitor for any signs and symptoms that could initiate development of factors such as hypoventilation, constipation Notify physician of potential/presence of any factors Establish baseline and ongoing assessments of neurological status and vital signs q1 hr; monitor especially LOC Headache locality/severity Motor, sensory, and communication systems functioning/deficits Cranial nerve functioning Visual abilities and functioning; field cuts, photophobia, nystagmus, ptosis Auditory system functioning Nausea/vomiting Kernig's/Brudzinski's signs Ataxia, myoclonic jerks Reflex status Pupil size, equality; direct and consensual light responses; extraocular movements Behavior and personality alterations (in infants decreased feeding, high-pitched cry) Posturing spontaneously or stimuli response, decerebrate/decorticate Administer medications, treatments, and IV fluids as ordered; monitor effects and side effects Maintain head gatch/bed rest as ordered Accurately record intake and output; monitor for any imbalance Monitor serum electrolytes, complete blood count, arterial blood gas values for any abnormalities Notify physician of any change in neurological status, vital signs, or abnormal fluid balance/lab values Initiate and maintain hypothermia as ordered If patient has ICP line inserted, monitor values and waveforms Maintain patency/sterility of system Monitor effects of other treatments or therapies on ICP including coughing, turning, chest physiotherapy, suctioning Space therapies if possible to minimize increases in ICP Monitor neurological status correlated with ICP values and notify physician If ordered, assist physician with drainage of CSF fluid amount to maintain ICP at specific level determined; record fluid amount drained/time; monitor effects on ICP value, correlation between neurological status and CSF drainage Hyperventilate patient as ordered by physician for specific ICP level increase

Potential problems	Expected outcomes	Nursing activities
		Administer medications/treatments as ordered; monitor effects and side effects on status and ICP; frequently osmotic diuretics are ordered prn or as ongoing therapy
		Monitor ventricular drainage system or other external drain if patient has one inserted
		Prevent compression, kinking, pulling, or tension on tubing by proper positioning; if necessary, restrain patient's hands to prevent pulling or tension of tubing (first try explanations of reasons/purposes for drain)
		Maintain patency/sterility of system
		Maintain at specific level ordered by physician
		Measure and record as ordered pressure, amount and quality of drainage
		Check dressing q1 hr; monitor for leakage around needle or catheter site, swelling/edema
		If patient is on ICP monitoring, record pressures and drain fluid amount specified by physician's order to maintain pressure values
		Monitor neurological status correlated with fluid pressure/quantity
		Administer antibiotics as ordered
		Send CSF specimens as ordered and monitor results
		Monitor serum electrolytes as Na^+ values may decrease from loss of CSF by drainage; notify physician of results and replace fluids as ordered (frequently CSF fluid is ordered replaced milliliter for milliliter)
		Monitor for signs of epidural hematoma (potential complication of drain); see Standard: *Head trauma,* Problem, Epidural hematoma
		Notify physician immediately of any change in neurological status; fluid pressure, amount/quality varying from norm specified or expected; nonpatency of system or abnormal lab values
		If ordered, clamp tubing as specified by physician maintaining precise time schedule and recording time, pressure, fluid drainage amount/quality; notify physician of any change in neurological status or signs of increased ICP; unclamp drain as per physician's standing or stat order
		After removal of ventricular drain by physician, monitor neurological status and vital signs frequently; drain site for bleeding, oozing, drainage/edema; for signs of increased ICP; have emergency ventriculostomy set/medications available
		SEE STANDARD: *Increased intracranial pressure*
		If internalized shunting procedure is necessary, see Standard: *Internalized shunting procedures*
▪ Infection progression	▪ Resolution of infection Maximal neurological functioning	▪ Ongoing assessments of neurological status and vital signs q1 hr and prn (see Problem, Increased ICP: avoiding precipitating factors in increased ICP and establishing baseline and ongoing assessments of neurological status and vital signs (nursing activities)
		Maintain strict isolation procedures/precautions as warranted by specific pathogen
		Post procedure on door of patient's room
		Restrict visitors
		Instruct/supervise visitors in correct procedures
		Maintain strict sterile procedure where required

Potential problems	Expected outcomes	Nursing activities
		Monitor
		Temperature q1-2 hr and prn
		Skin integument frequently for presence/extent of rash, petechiae, open skin areas
		Culture results and drug sensitivities of CSF, urine, sputum, blood specimens
		For signs of toxemia/septicemia including decreased LOC, hypotension
		WBC counts for elevations (may be falsely elevated if patient is receiving steroids)
		Drug levels
		IV sites frequently for any signs of redness, tenderness/phlebitis
		Administer
		Antipyretic medications as ordered
		Cooling blankets as ordered; institute measures to prevent complications of hypothermia
		Tepid sponges as ordered
		Antibiotic medications at precise time ordered
		Frequent skin and oral hygiene
		Assist physician with treatments/diagnostic procedures
		Anticipate frequent lumbar punctures; explain necessity to patient/family
		Monitor pressure levels of CSF with each lumbar puncture; correlation with neurological status
		Monitor CSF specimen results including cultures, protein glucose, cell counts for resolution/progression of infectious process
		Notify physician immediately of any change in neurological status, abnormal lab values, signs of complications, or appearance of new culture pathogen/drug resistance
■ Depressed/altered LOC, restlessness, agitation/irritability	■ Safe patient environment Absence of injury complications	■ Close observation; siderails up at all times when patient is alone
		Maintain as quiet an environment as possible, reducing excessive external stimuli to minimum
		Provide rest periods between activities
		Dark room
		Establish baseline and continue ongoing assessments of LOC and reflex status; monitor
		For signs of restlessness/agitation; note degree, frequency, extent
		Components of consciousness—arousal and content
		Presence/quality of reflexes including corneal, gag, cough, swallowing; if reflexes are absent or decreased, institute preventive measures such as protecting cornea with eyedrops, lid taping/closure; suctioning equipment at bedside
		Monitor for other possible causes of restlessness such as bladder/abdominal distention, headache, hypoxia
		Notify physician if any of these occurs
		Administer analgesics, comfort measures, treatments as ordered
		Reorient patient frequently to time, place, person; reasons for hospitalization; pathology and relationship to symptoms
		Have family bring familiar objects, pictures to aid in orientation
		Continually reassure patient
		Support family; reaffirm frequently relationship between LOC and pathology

Potential problems	Expected outcomes	Nursing activities
		Apply restraints as per physician's order if this is only alternative to protect patient from injury
		Explain to patient/family reasons for restraints
		Reassure family of restraint necessity; relationship between patient's behavior and pathology
		Check restraints frequently for proper placement; monitor effectiveness, skin integrity, and circulation
		Reapply q4 hr and prn
		Frequently reevaluate need for continuing restraints
		Notify physician immediately of sudden appearance or increase in prior restlessness, irritability, agitation, headache, or change in reflex status/neurological functioning
■ Presence of neurological symptoms/deficit	■ Absence of complications Maximal comfort	■ On admission establish and implement care plan based on individual needs and specific symptoms/deficit present
		Institute measures to promote maximal comfort and prevent complications; common symptoms/deficits include
		Headache: maintain quiet, dark environment; ice bag, analgesics as ordered
		Nuchal rigidity: reposition frequently, supporting with pillows for comfort; massage and apply lotion
		Vomiting: keep NPO; turn slowly and carefully; prn medication as ordered
		Motor deficit: ROM, turn and reposition properly to promote optimal muscular tone, functioning, maintenance, and circulation; sheepskin, air mattress, handrolls, splints, etc.
		Sensory deficit: hypoalgesia/hyperalgesia—monitor skin integument frequently; administer frequent skin care to keep skin clean and dry; change linen frequently; if rash is present, keep skin free of friction, apply lubricants to decrease itching, medications prn; if aches/pains, neuritis are present, administer medications as ordered
		Communication deficits: evaluate and implement effective alternate means of communication such as magic slate, word board, pictures if feasible
		Visual deficits: if field cut, approach patient and place objects within visual field abilities; if diplopia is present, use alternating eye patch; if photophobia is present, keep room dark and provide glasses for patient
		Auditory deficits: approach patient from greater hearing side; establish alternate means of communication
		Cranial nerve dysfunctions/decreased reflexes:measures to prevent complications such as corneal abrasions, aspiration
		Reflex status alteration: hyporeflexia/hyperreflexia—protect from injury
		Altered LOC: prevention and control of hazards of immobility; promotion of safety maintenance
		Ongoing assessments and evaluations of patient status/effectiveness of interventions; readjust plan based on status alterations
		Collaborate with physician regarding anticipated prognosis for extent of recovery from deficit (if known); provide realistic information and reassurance
		Assist as needed with ADL
		Provide frequent rest periods between activities
		Provide explanations to patient/family for specific interventions; even if full recovery from deficit is expected, complication prevention must be instituted from admission to promote optimal recovery and functioning

Potential problems	Expected outcomes	Nursing activities
■ Seizures	■ Absence or control of seizures	■ Prevention of precipitating factors in seizure occurrence including fever, hypoxia, H_2O intoxication, electrolyte disturbances Notify physician of potential/presence of any factors Seizure precautions for any patient with suspected meningitis/encephalitis Padded siderails up at all times when patient is alone Bed height at lowest level Padded tongue blade and airway at bedside Suction and O_2 equipment readily available Emergency medications/equipment readily available Close supervision and observation Administer anticonvulsant medications as ordered; monitor effects, side effects, serum anticonvulsant levels If seizure occurs, monitor and record seizure activity; notify physician; see Standard: *Seizures*
■ Fluid and electrolyte imbalance	■ Fluid and electrolyte balance within normal limits	■ Monitor and accurately record intake and output, urine specific gravity as ordered Monitor for signs of dehydration or overhydration such as Poor skin turgor Dry mucous membranes Peripheral edema Excessive thirst Change in LOC Monitor for Abnormal vital signs, Hgb/Hct values Abnormal serum electrolyte values Weight alterations Temperature elevations Insensible fluid losses including respiratory, diaphoresis, secretions Presence/degree of nausea or vomiting, emesis quality; monitor effectiveness of medications ordered Presence/quality of gag, cough, and swallowing reflexes; if depressed, keep patient NPO and notify physician Administer IV fluids, NG feedings as ordered Administer medications as ordered; monitor effects and side effects if patient is receiving steroids, monitor urine glucose and acetone levels four times a day If po is allowed and tolerated, assist patient with diet selection within chewing capabilities, food likes, and nutritionally well-balanced meals Notify physician of any fluid imbalance or electrolyte abnormality
■ Respiratory insufficiency related to CNS dysfunction Pneumonia Atelectasis Pulmonary emboli	■ Patent airway Adequate alveolar ventilation and perfusion Normal respiratory rate and quality Arterial blood gas levels within patient's normal limits	■ Ongoing assessment of respiratory status q2 hr and prn; monitor for any abnormality/decline Respiratory rate, quality, and pattern Patency of upper airway and patient's ability to handle secretions Skin color, nail beds, peripheral pulses, and skin warmth Presence/strength of gag, cough, and swallowing reflexes Breath sounds bilaterally for quality of aeration; signs of obstruction (rales, rhonchi) Arterial blood gas values Chest radiograph results Signs/symptoms of thrombophlebitis, pulmonary emboli, pulmonary edema

Potential problems	Expected outcomes	Nursing activities

		Maintain patent airway by
		    Turning and positioning to prevent obstruction or aspiration of secretions q2 hr and prn
		    Deep breathing and coughing q1 hr and prn
		    Suctioning prn
		    Adequate oxygenation and humidification as ordered
		    Chest physiotherapy/pulmonary toilet if warranted and not contraindicated by physician's order
		Apply antithromboembolic stockings or Ace bandages as ordered; reapply every shift and prn; monitor for constriction/looseness, condition of skin
		Instruct and supervise patient in performing leg exercises, ROM exercises
		Increase activity level/progression when allowed
		Notify physician immediately of any change in respiratory/neurological status or signs of complication potential/occurrence
		If problem occurs, assist with emergency measures to maintain patent airway and adequate ventilation
		    Administer medications and treatments as ordered; monitor effects and side effects
		    Explain procedures and reasons for equipment/respiratory assistance to patient/family; reassure and support
		    Establish alternate means of communication as needed
		See Standard: *Mechanical ventilation*
		If emboli occur, see Standard: *Embolic phenomena*

■ Bradycardia	■ Absence or resolution of bradycardia	■ Monitor and record pulse rate and quality with neurological assessments; assess for any correlation between pulse rate/quality and neurological status Monitor serum electrolyte values; especially note hypokalemia/hyperkalemia Notify physician immediately if patient develops pulse rate less than 60 Administer medications and treatments as ordered; monitor effects and side effects

■ Bowel/bladder dysfunction	■ Urinary output adequate
	No bladder distention
	Normal bowel elimination
		■ Assess patient's prior elimination patterns: usual voiding pattern, bowel pattern, problems, dietary/medication measures for elimination
		Monitor
		    Accurate recording of intake and output
		    For any signs/symptoms of urinary retention, overflow voiding, or residual; notify physician if any of these occurs and administer medications/treatments as ordered; monitor effects and side effects
		    Bowel movements (amount, consistency, frequency)
		    Bowel sounds, presence/quality; signs/symptoms of paralytic ileus
		Establish and implement individualized bowel regimen based on patient's needs, pattern, previous measures, preferences/effectiveness
		    Involve patient in planning
		    Obtain orders for administration of stool softeners, cathartics, enemas as needed
		    Assess effectiveness of regimen; readjust as needed
		    When patient is allowed po, assist in food selection to promote bowel elimination

Potential problems	Expected outcomes	Nursing activities
■ GI bleeding related to CNS factors Stress Steroid administration	■ Absence or resolution of GI bleeding	■ Monitor vital signs q2-4 hr, Hgb and Hct; stools for Hematest three times a week; Hematest of aspirate, emesis, and urine for any abnormalities Monitor for signs of GI bleeding including abdominal distention, tenderness; hypotension, sudden tachycardia Obtain order for antacid administration as soon as patient is able to take po Notify physician of any abnormalities; if problem occurs, see Standard: *Upper gastrointestinal bleeding*
■ Patient/family's anxiety, fears, anger related to Limited understanding of disease, diagnostic tests/procedures Presence of neurological deficit or potential continuation, development, worsening Possible alterations in life-style	■ Patient/family's behavior indicates decreased anxiety with provision of information Patient/family verbalizes fears, angers, concerns	■ Ongoing assessments of level of anxiety Encourage patient/family's verbalization of questions, fears, concerns Collaborate with physician in providing realistic information and reassurance appropriate to level of understanding Explain relationship between pathology and clinical symptoms, status, course Explain anticipated treatments, therapeutic measures, and clinical course prognosis (if known) If prognosis is unknown, explain reasons why course is obscure Provide continuing time, support, and explanations to patient/family; maintain calm, accepting attitude of their reactions to lengthy disease course, undetermined prognosis Support family's acceptance of patient's behavior alterations by reinforcing the pathological causes Explain and prepare patient/family for all diagnostic tests/procedures Involve patient/family in decision making, care planning, participation, and evaluation As status improves, promote patient progression from dependent to independent functioning Slowly and progressively increase activity as status and tolerance levels allow Stress any positive gains or improvements in status Encourage participation in diversional interests/activities Encourage verbalization of family/patient's perceptions of possible alterations in life-style; means to promote as "normal" a life-style as possible Obtain appropriate referrals such as religious personnel, counseling services Evaluate for reduction in level of anxiety
■ Continued presence of neurological deficit Patient/family's fears, anxiety, anger related to deficit and possible alterations in life-style	■ Maximal neurological functioning* Maximal independence in ADL (within capabilities) Patient/family verbalizes concerns	■ Assess patient's specific neurological deficit Collaborate with physician regarding prognosis, possible degree of recovery Implement individualized plan of care based on patient's needs and deficits Assist as needed in ADL Monitor potential for independent functioning and obtain equipment to maximize function and promote safety Obtain orders for appropriate referrals such as physical, speech, occupational therapy; social service Encourage verbalization of patient/family's fears, anxieties, and other reactions—level and degree Answer questions realistically

*If responsibility of critical care nurse includes this stage of care.

Potential problems	Expected outcomes	Nursing activities
		Encourage their participation in care planning, implementation, evaluation, and decision making
		Realistically reassure and support
		Reinforce any gains or independence patient achieves
		Plan, instruct, demonstrate, supervise, and evaluate patient/family's verbalization/performance of needed information/skills for maximal independent functioning such as
		Measures to prevent complication
		Assistance necessary—type, amount, degree
		Proper use of therapeutic devices/equipment
		Monitor level of achievement toward maximizing potentials and independence; means to promote as "normal" a life-style as possible
■ Insufficient knowledge to comply with discharge regimen*	■ Patient/family demonstrates or verbalizes understanding of discharge regimen	■ Assess patient/family's level of understanding of neurological problem and therapy received
		Explain relationship between patient's neurological status and therapies prescribed
		If pathological condition is related to factors such as head trauma, toxin exposure/drug overdose, explain relationship and importance of patient/family controlling identified individual factors to prevent disease recurrence
		Instruction of patient/family regarding required information/skills so that before discharge patient/family is able to
	Patient/family accurately describes medication, activity, and dietary regimens	Describe medication regimen
		Name and purpose
		Route, dosage, frequency, times
		Side effects
		Special precautions necessary including drugs, foods, beverages contraindicated; factors potentiating/decreasing effects/side effects; physical restrictions; safety measures
		Describe activity regimen, exercise program
		Describe dietary regimen
		Describe and demonstrate any special therapeutic measures prescribed
	Patient/family describes means to achieve maximal independence in ADL, promote safety, and prevent complications	Describe and demonstrate proper use of equipment or therapeutic devices
		Reasons for using
		Time, method, and duration of use
		Precautions/safeguards
		Necessary maintenance (type, frequency)
		Measures to promote optimal functioning, upkeep/duration
	Patient/family describes signs/symptoms requiring medical attention	Describe signs/symptoms of neurological status requiring medical care
	Patient/family describes follow-up care regimen	Describe plan for follow-up care including purpose of appointment, when and where to go, who to see, what to expect

*If responsibility of critical care nurse includes such follow-up care.

35 □ Myasthenia gravis (including thymectomy)

Myasthenia gravis is a neuromuscular weakness that primarily involves the skeletal muscles. Its onset may be precipitous or insidious, and it usually progresses slowly following the initial onset of symptoms. Clinical features of myasthenia gravis include exhaustion of muscle strength and paresis in response to repetitive or constant activity/stimulation.

Myasthenia gravis is a disease that is unpredictable in course and prognosis and is frequently characterized by periods of remissions and exacerbations. The voluntary muscles commonly involved in the weakness are

1. Extraocular—ocular palsies, drooping eyelid, and intermittent diplopia (most commonly affected)
2. Facial expression—altered mobility/expression
3. Mastication—difficulty chewing
4. Swallowing—dysphagia
5. Speech—dysarthria
6. Jaw
7. Neck

If muscular involvement of the limbs and trunk is present, the proximal muscles are affected more than the distal. Myasthenia gravis may range from mild ocular involvement to severe muscular involvement including the diaphragm, intercostal muscles, and abdominal and external sphincters. The common clinical manifestations of myasthenia gravis are usually a fluctuating ocular, facial, and bulbar palsy. Muscular weakness of the bulbar cranial nerves may produce dysphagia, dysarthria, dyspnea, facial drooping, and jaw weakness. Two life-threatening symptoms of myasthenia gravis are dyspnea and dysphagia, which frequently occur in crisis situations and increase the potential threat of aspiration and acute respiratory failure.

The cause of myasthenia gravis is unknown, but the defect is generally presumed to occur at the neuromuscular junction. Multiple theories of etiology have been advanced, but to date no single one has been firmly established. Proposed theories of etiology include the following:

1. Decreased formation/release of acetylcholine
2. Increased formation/release of acetylcholinesterase
3. Muscle fiber defect of motor end plate
4. Marked reduction of acetylcholine receptors in the muscle end plates

5. Autoimmune response—most popular theory to date due to
   a. Frequent association of thymic hyperplasia and thymoma in myasthenia gravis patients
   b. A high percentage of myasthenia gravis patients have thyrotoxicosis and other autoimmune disorders (e.g., rheumatoid arthritis, lupus erythematosis, and polymyositis)
   c. Frequent presence of antiacetylcholine antibody (against acetylcholine receptor) in postsynaptic membrane—immunological reaction to destroy the receptor

The diagnosis of myasthenia gravis is suspected based on the clinical history of signs/symptoms. Myasthenia gravis is highly suspect in patients with a clinical history of muscle weakness developing after repetitive or consistent activity and partial strength restoration after rest. Some muscle weakness may be present at all times but is usually made worse by activity. Confirmation of myasthenia gravis is attempted by use of a variety of diagnostic tests including electromyogram, edrophonium chloride (Tensilon) test, neostigmine test, curare test, and immunological studies.

The medical management of myasthenia gravis includes medication therapy control utilizing anticholinesterases and corticosteroids. Surgical intervention, or thymectomy, is performed in some cases of myasthenia gravis. Recently, plasma-electrophoresis has been utilized as a therapeutic modality for patients with myasthenia gravis.

Thymectomy consists of removal of the thymus gland, either by a sternal-split or transcervical approach. Thymectomy is usually performed if a thymoma is present, which occurs in approximately one fifth of myasthenia gravis patients. Hyperplasia of the thymic gland is found in a large number of remaining patients. Thymectomy is also frequently performed in cases of bulbar myasthenia gravis that are poorly responsive to medical therapy/management. Postoperatively, remission or an improvement in clinical status may not occur immediately. Following thymectomy the patient may still require medical management with medication regimens, but the amount of medications may be decreased and/or effectiveness of medication control may be enhanced. The surgery is considered successful if less ongoing medication is required and less supplementary medication is needed during periods of stress such as infection and menses. Surgical results are most successful in patients who have had myasthenia gravis for a shorter time period (1 to 2 years).

ASSESSMENT

1. Onset, duration, progression, and description of neuromuscular symptoms, especially
   a. Ocular—impaired extraocular movements/palsies, drooping eyelid/ptosis, diplopia, weakened eyelid closure
   b. Facial weakness/alterations in facial expression
   c. Difficulty chewing; choking/nasal regurgitations
   d. Difficulty swallowing (dysphagia)
   e. Alterations in speech abilities, voice tone, quality; nasal and dysarthric speech
   f. Jaw weakness
   g. Neck weakness
   h. Muscle weakness of trunk or limbs, motor functioning
   i. External sphincter weakness—bowel/bladder
   j. Dyspnea
2. Time-related presence, extent, severity of neurological symptoms
   a. Association with activity—type, extent, length
   b. Association with time of day, fatigue
   c. Fluctuations in symptomatology
3. Presence of any precipitating factors in symptomatology occurrence such as infection, emotional upset, stress
4. Previous clinical course of disease (if prior diagnosis)
   a. Disease management/control
   b. Adequacy of treatment/control
   c. Any "crisis" occurrences—when, type, duration, treatment, any precipitating factors; postcrisis status
   d. Any previous intubation/tracheotomy—when, type, duration, status after procedure
5. Medications taken for neurological problem including anticholinesterases, corticosteroids
   a. Dosage, frequency, schedule
   b. Length of time medication taken
   c. Effects and side effects
   d. Alterations in regimen—if on demand schedule what factors necessitate medication adjustment; effectiveness of demand scheduling

6. Previous neurological treatment or neurosurgical procedure
7. Presence and degree of any physical/emotional stress
8. Nutritional habits and dietary regimen
9. Activity regimen and sleep habits
10. Presence of any alterations in body image; fears of permanent disability or deficit; altered role in family, normal occupation/performance of ADL; restrictions due to myasthenia gravis
11. Level of anxiety related to hospitalization; if patient was previously hospitalized, reactions, coping mechanisms, etc.
12. Level of patient/family's knowledge of myasthenia gravis—medications, precipiating factors, treatments, potential complications, and so on
13. Presence of any medical problems; medications/treatments prescribed and followed
14. Baseline parameters status
    a. Neurological
    b. Myasthenia gravis disease history, course
    c. Respiratory
    d. Cardiac; circulatory and vascular
    e. Metabolic
    f. Nutritional
    g. Hydration
    h. Emotional
    i. Weight
    j. Vital capacity
    k. Inspiratory force/forced expiratory volume
15. Diagnostic test results, including
    a. Electromyography
    b. Edrophonium chloride (Tensilon), neostigmine/curare tests
    c. Tomography
    d. Thyroid function tests
    e. Pulmonary function tests
    f. Immunological studies
16. Results of
    a. Serum electrolyte levels
    b. Hgb and Hct, platelet count
    c. Serum Ca^{2+} level
    d. Arterial blood gas levels
    e. Urine output, specific gravity, osmolality, urinalysis
    f. Chest radiograph
    g. ECG
    h. Clotting profile
    i. Cultures if indicated—sputum, urine
    j. Parathyroid hormone levels if indicated

GOALS

1. Optimal neurological functioning
2. Optimal independence in ADL within safety restrictions, tolerance levels/limitations
3. Adequate alveolar ventilation and perfusion
4. Adequate cardiac output
5. Acid-base balance within normal limits
6. Fluid balance within normal range
7. Serm electrolyte levels within normal limits
8. Hgb, Hct, and platelets stable and within normal limits
9. Medication regimen control at optimal management level of disease
10. Infection free
11. If thymectomy is performed, incision well-healed, without signs of infection
12. Reduction in patient/family's anxiety with provision of information, explanations, demonstrations, support
13. Before discharge patient/family is able to describe
    a. Medication regimen
    b. Activity regimen
    c. Dietary regimen
    d. Safety measures, necessary restrictions/precautions, safety techniques
    e. Methods to promote optimal disease control/management
    f. Appropriate interventions if complication, crisis occurs at home
    g. Demonstrate any special therapeutic measures prescribed
    h. Signs and symptoms requiring medical attention
    i. Necessary information regarding follow-up care

Potential problems	Expected outcomes	Nursing activities
Medical management		
■ Muscle weakness Increased muscle weakness with fatigue	■ Optimal muscle strength	■ Establish baseline and continue ongoing assessments as ordered and prn of
		Neurological status: monitor
		Muscle strength of all groups with repetitive activity; establish specific testing modalities and record on flow sheet q2-4 hr and prn
		Ability to raise/lower eyelids completely; location/degree of ptosis if present
		Facial (cranial nerve VII) muscular strength bilaterally
		Extraocular movements; presence, degree, and location of ocular palsies, nystagmus, diplopia
		Presence/quality of chewing and swallowing abilities; foods manageable, ability to handle secretions; signs and symptoms of dysphagia
		Presence/quality of gag and cough reflexes
		Speech quality and ability; degree of dysarthria if present
		Cranial nerve functioning
		Respiratory status: monitor for any abnormality/decline
		Vital signs including respiratory rate, quality/pattern
		Bilateral breath sounds for signs of obstruction/decreased aeration (rales, rhonchi, etc.)
		Strength of diaphragmatic and intercostal muscles
		Presence/quality of cough, gag, and swallowing reflexes
		Presence, amount/quality of secretions and saliva and ability to handle secretions
		For any signs/symptoms of dysphagia, dyspnea (at rest or exertional), dysarthria
		Vital capacity measurement q2-4 hr and prn using same spirometer, proper position, and recording technique; inflate cuff if tracheostomy tube is in place; if jaw weakness due to facial muscle involvement is present, prevent air leak while using mouthpiece; position in sitting position for measurement if feasible
		Maintain flow sheet recording of vital capacities
		Serial arterial blood gas levels
		Chest radiograph results

Potential problems	Expected outcomes	Nursing activities
		Close observation—place patient close to nurse's station

Avoid precipitating factors in myasthenic crisis such as emotional upset, physical stress, infection, constipation

Develop care plan based on individual patient needs/status—involve patient/family in planning

    Assess adjustments in ADL regimen that patient has made and adapt to hospital setting

    Ongoing evaluations of effectiveness of interventions

    If muscle weakness/paralysis is present, prevent complications by measures including turning, positioning, ROM exercises, coughing, deep breathing

Always anticipate and be prepared for sudden worsening in neurological/respiratory status especially aspiration/respiratory failure

    Suctioning equipment, O_2, airway at bedside

    Emergency ventilation, intubation, mechanical ventilator, medications readily available

Administer anticholinesterases, corticosteroids, and other medications as ordered at precise time specified

    Prevent or minimize GI side effects by giving with small amount of food or after meals (if mealtime is flexible); medications such as atropine may also be ordered to minimize side effects

    Monitor and record on flow sheet muscle strength status related to medication

        Effects and side effects

        Duration

        Peak action effect (usually optimal 1 to 2 hours after medication)

        Minimal action effect (usually 3 to 4 hours after medication)

    Assess patient's evaluation of strength and motor ability related to medication regimen

    Monitor vital capacity measurements and relate to medication time effects

    If patient experiences worsening of symptoms, notify physician immediately as this may be sign of overdosage or ineffective medication regimen

    Plan activities around peak effect levels of medications, arranging for meal consumption 45 minutes to 1 hour after medication; plan treatments and major activities early in the day

Prevent overexertion or greater than usual fatigue

    Provide uninterrupted rest periods between activities

    Space activities to correlate with peak effects of medication

    Provide calm, quiet, supportive environment

    Minimize physical stress by maintaining activity within tolerance limitation levels

    Minimize emotional stress; See Problem, Patient/family's anxiety

Notify physician immediately of any decline in neurological or respiratory status; any decrease in vital capacity below minimal acceptable level individually specified

Potential problems	Expected outcomes	Nursing activities

■ Bulbar cranial nerve (V, VII, IX, X, XII) dysfunction/weakness
Facial (VII)
Trigeminal (V)
  Decreased facial muscle strength/facial expression
  Difficulty chewing
  Inability to close eyelid
  Decreased/absent corneal reflex
Glossopharyngeal (IX)
Vagus (X)
Hypoglossal (XII)
  Decreased or absent swallowing, gag, and cough reflexes
  Dysphagia/aspiration
  Dyspnea/respiratory failure
  Dysarthria
	■ Absence or resolution of dysfunction
	Absence of complications
		■ Assess chewing ability; assist patient in diet selection within chewing capabilities; instruct patient to chew on unaffected side; stay with patient during mealtime
		Assess facial droop; provide excellent oral hygiene, frequent removal of secretions
		If ability to completely close eyelids is decreased/absent, obtain order for protective drops, maintain eyelid closure, and monitor for any signs of corneal irritation/abrasion
		Encourage verbalization of patient's fears, concerns, and feelings since decreased facial strength may inhibit normal facial expression conveyance
		Assess level of patient's anxiety/altered body image related to facial nerve weakness, droop/drooling from mouth
		Monitor presence/strength of swallowing, gag, and cough reflexes; ability to handle secretions and po
		Schedule meals when strength is maximum; stay with patient at mealtimes; monitor swallowing effectiveness
		Assess for any choking/nasal regurgitation
		Avoid fluids that enhance saliva production such as milk
		Assess foods that patient tolerates best and assist with diet selection
		If any impairment in swallowing, gag, or cough reflexes is present, keep patient NPO and notify physician; suction secretions prn; prevent aspiration by positioning, maintaining patent airway; and closely monitor respiratory status/functioning; see Problem, Respiratory insufficiency
		If dysarthria is a problem, establish alternate means of communication; evaluate effectiveness and readjust prn; see Problem, Altered communication ability

■ Respiratory insufficiency/arrest related to weakness or paralysis of respiratory muscles due to
Pneumonia
Atelectasis
Aspiration
Dyspnea/dysphagia
	■ Patent airway
	Adequate alveolar ventilation
	Normal respiratory rate and quality
	Clear breath sounds
	Arterial blood gas levels within patient's normal limits
		■ Ongoing assessment of neurological and respiratory status q2 hr and prn; see Problem, Muscle weakness
		Assess and monitor for any abnormality/decline
		  Patency of upper airway and patient's ability to handle secretions
		  Skin color, nail beds, peripheral pulses, and skin warmth
		  For signs/symptoms of thrombophlebitis, pulmonary emboli, pulmonary edema, dyspnea/dysphagia
		Maintain patent airway by turning and positioning to prevent obstruction or aspiration of secretions q2 hr and prn; deep breathing, coughing, and suctioning prn; chest physiotherapy; adequate oxygenation and humidification as ordered
		Apply antithromboembolic stockings or Ace bandages as ordered; reapply every shift and prn; monitor for constriction/looseness, condition of skin
		Instruct and supervise patient in leg exercises, ROM exercises
		Prevent precipitating factors in respiratory failure; patient is especially vulnerable if either of the following is present
		  Severe dysphagia—ongoing monitoring of swallowing reflex, keep patient NPO if necessary to prevent potential aspiration
		  Respiratory tract infection—protect from potential infection sources; vigorous suctioning, chest physiotherapy to maintain patent airway; position for proper ventilation/lung expansion
		Notify physician immediately of any change in respiratory/neurological status or development of potential complication

Potential problems	Expected outcomes	Nursing activities
		If respiratory problem occurs, assist with emergency measures and procedures to maintain patent airway and ventilation; see Standard: *Mechanical ventilation* When neurological/respiratory status improves, begin to slowly wean patient for short periods of time Wean periods at peak medication time effectiveness Stay with patient; reassure and support frequently Reaffirm that ventilator assistance will not be withdrawn until patient can breathe independently Assess patient/family's reactions to respiratory problem occurrence/experience Progressively increase activity; monitor effects on neurological/respiratory status and notify physician of results; limit activity to tolerance level
▪ Crisis—worsening of muscle weakness with potential respiratory failure/aspiration Myasthenic—sudden worsening in status; drug regimen ineffective for unknown reasons Cholinergic—worsening in status from overdose of myasthenic drugs	▪ Resolution of crisis Absence of complications	▪ Prevent precipitating factors in crisis such as infection, emotional crisis, constipation Careful observations and frequent assessments of neurological/respiratory status Administer medications and treatments as ordered at precise time; monitor Effects by flow sheet record; correlate medication time specifics on graded muscle strength; cranial nerve functioning; swallowing, gag, and cough reflexes Presence/degree of dysphagia, dyspnea, dysarthria Respiratory status Vital capacities Side effects Monitor for signs/symptoms of crisis Common manifestations of both myasthenic and cholinergic (present in either type) Increased skeletal muscular weakness Anxiety, restlessness Dyspnea, dysphagia, dysarthria Differentiating signs of crisis type Myasthenic: ocular palsies, ptosis, diplopia development/worsening Cholinergic: fasciculations/fine twitching; abdominal cramps and diarrhea, nausea/vomiting; increased secretions including salivation, sweating, lacrimation, bronchial; blurred vision; most ominous sign is increased weakness 1 hour after medication instead of expected improvement Notify physician immediately of any signs/symptoms of crisis Assist with emergency measures and procedures to maintain patent airway and ventilation Assist physician with tests (usually edrophonium chloride [Tensilon] test done to differentiate crisis type) and have emergency medications available (i.e., atropine, prostigmine) in anticipation of worsened crisis; if patient is in myasthenic crisis, status usually improves with edrophonium chloride (Tensilon) injection (positive test result) and if in cholinergic crisis, status worsens Assessments/interventions common to either crisis Maintain patent airway and adequate ventilation, mechanical ventilator as ordered; see Problem, Respiratory insufficiency/arrest Monitor respiratory status and vital capacity q1 hr

Potential problems	Expected outcomes	Nursing activities
		Monitor neurological status q1 hr including muscle strength grading; cranial nerve functioning; swallowing, cough, and gag reflexes; presence/extent of dysphagia, dyspnea, dysarthria
		Accurate recording of intake and output
		Administer IV fluids/NG feedings as ordered
		Bed rest; prevent complications of immobility by turning and positioning, ROM exercises, skin care, etc.
		Establish alternate means of communication if ability is altered
		Explain all tests, procedures, measures to patient/family and necessary reasons
		Explain reasons why medications are being withheld, anticipated restarting time, and course
		Provide rest periods between activity to prevent fatigue or overexertion
		When medication regimen is restarted, continue to closely monitor effects/side effects, neurological/respiratory status
		When activity progression is allowed, slowly increase to tolerance levels
		As status improves, promote patient assuming independence in appropriate activities
		Slowly wean from dependent position/role
		Encourage self-participation in care, decisions, medication evaluation; assist as needed in ADL
		Continually provide explanations, support, reassurance, understanding to patient/family throughout crisis period/duration
		Try to assign individual nurse to consistently care for patient
		Encourage verbalization/other means of communication of patient/family's fears, angers, concerns, depression; help them to cope with crisis threat and promote positive attitude that status will improve
		Maintain calm, consistent, and supportive attitude/environment
		Specific interventions in myasthenic crisis
		Maintain endotracheal/tracheostomy tube in proper position, patency, and with proper care techniques; mechanical ventilator as ordered
		Chest physiotherapy and pulmonary toilet; vigorous regimen to maintain patent airway and adequate ventilation
		Strict sterile technique maintained when necessary including suctioning, catheterization
		See Problem, Respiratory insufficiency/arrest, and Standard: *Mechanical ventilation* for more specifics
		Specific interventions in cholinergic crisis
		Monitor for GI signs/symptoms—presence, degree/frequency
		Administer medications ordered; monitor effects/side effects and notify physician of results
		Frequent and scrupulous skin care to prevent complications of increased secretions from sweating, diarrhea, lacrimation, etc.; keep skin clean, dry, and intact; monitor all surfaces frequently for integument maintenance

■ Fluid and electrolyte imbalance	■ Fluid and electrolyte balance within normal limits	■ Monitor
		  Vital signs, Hgb and Hct for any abnormality
		  Serum electrolytes for any abnormality
		  Weight determinations as ordered

Potential problems	Expected outcomes	Nursing activities
		Accurate recording of intake and output; urine specific gravity as ordered
		Insensible fluid losses including respiratory, diaphoresis, secretions
		For presence, degree of nausea/vomiting; administer medications and notify physician if ineffectual
		For presence/degree of dysphagia, difficulty chewing, nasal regurgitation; keep NPO if severe dysphagia is present
		For signs of dehydration/overhydration such as poor skin turgor, peripheral edema, dry mucous membranes, excessive thirst, change in LOC
		Administer IV fluids, NG feedings as ordered
		Notify physician of any fluid/electrolyte abnormality; if ordered
		Monitor and record hourly intake and output
		Maintain intake at specific amount ordered
		Send specimens and monitor results
■ Altered communication ability related to Cranial nerve dysfunction Motor paralysis Endotracheal/tracheostomy tube insertion	■ Alternate means of communication established	■ Monitor communication abilities
		If ability is altered, establish alternate means of communication based on individual patient needs/status such as writing tablet, word or letter board, eye-blinking system
		Convey alternate means to other staff and family, assisting prn in effective use
		Anticipate patient's needs
		Establish means for patient to quickly/easily get nurse's attention
		Encourage staff/family to speak to patient even if he/she is unable to respond
		Evaluate effectiveness of alternate means of communication with patient/family
		Involve patient/family in planning care; reevaluate/readjust alternate means as necessary
		Try to find means that are least physically, mentally, and emotionally taxing to the patient
		Accept frustrations the patient frequently experiences from altered ability and resulting depression; try to minimize frustrations by anticipating needs, constant supervision, having the same nurse provide care
■ Bowel/bladder dysfunction	■ Adequate urine output Absence of bladder distention Normal bowel elimination	■ Monitor
		Accurate recording of intake and output
		Patient's prior elimination pattern—usual voiding, bowel problems, dietary/medication measures
		For any signs/symptoms of urinary retention, overflow voiding, or residual; notify physician if problem occurs and administer medications, treatments as ordered; monitor effects and side effects; intermittent catheterization may be ordered
		Bowel movements (amount, consistency, frequency)
		Bowel sounds, presence/quality; signs/symptoms of paralytic ileus
		Establish and implement individualized bowel regimen based on patient's needs, pattern, prior measures
		Involve patient in planning bowel regimen program, time for elimination/treatments based on patient's preference and effectiveness
		Obtain physician's orders for stool softener, cathartics, enemas as needed
		When patient is allowed po, assist in food selection to promote bowel elimination
		Assess effectiveness of bowel regimen; reevaluate and readjust prn

Potential problems	Expected outcomes	Nursing activities
■ GI bleeding related to CNS factors Stress Steroid administration	■ Absence or resolution of GI bleeding	■ Monitor vital signs, Hgb and Hct; stools for Hematest three times a week; Hematest of aspirate, emesis, and urine for any abnormality Monitor for signs of GI bleeding including abdominal tenderness, pain, distention; hypotension, sudden tachycardia Obtain order for antacid administration as soon as patient able to take po Notify physician of any abnormalities; if any abnormalities occur, see Standard: *Acute upper gastrointestinal bleeding*
■ Complications of corticosteroid therapy	■ Absence or resolution of complications	■ Monitor for any complications of corticosteroid therapy, especially GI irritation Development or exacerbation of diabetes mellitus Increased susceptibility to infection Psychoses, behavioral changes Hypokalemia Hypertension Osteoporosis Acne Moon face Ongoing assessments and implementation of measures to prevent complications; instruction of patient/family in monitoring and preventing such as Control of GI irritation; see Problem, GI bleeding Prevent exposure to sources of infection Prevent potential osteoporosis by ROM exercises, encouraging activity within fatigue limitations when allowed; notify physician of any complaints of bone, radicular pain and monitor bone radiograph results Careful and frequent skin cleansing to decrease acne occurrence/potential Report immediately any mental, emotional/behavioral changes Monitor urine determinations of glucose and acetone, serum glucose levels, signs/symptoms of diabetes Monitor serum electrolytes for hypokalemia; BP q2 hr and prn for hypertension Notify physician of any abnormality Monitor neurological/respiratory status frequently; be aware of danger of exacerbation of weakness that may occur usually between 4 to 10 days of treatment initiation but must be monitored for from day 1 Report immediately any signs/symptoms of exacerbation If exacerbation occurs, see Problem, Crisis
■ Infection	■ Absence or resolution of infection	■ Prevent precipitating factors such as urinary retention, pulmonary congestion/aspiration Maintain strict sterile technique for procedures such as catheterization; endotracheal/tracheostomy tube care management, suctioning; ventilator maintenance Monitor Temperature q4 hr and prn for any elevation IV sites frequently for any signs of redness, tenderness/phlebitis For potential infection sources including pulmonary, urinary, exposure to infection sources WBC count (may be falsely elevated if patient is receiving steroids)

Potential problems	Expected outcomes	Nursing activities
		If temperature elevation or sign of infection occurs, notify physician and culture possible infection sources Monitor sputum/urinary cultures, chest radiograph results Continue accurate recording of intake and output; monitor for dehydration/overhydration Institute measures to promote resolution of infection source if possible Administer medications/treatments as ordered; monitor effects
■ Patient/family's anxiety related to lack of understanding of diagnostic tests, treatments, disease process, therapeutic interventions	■ Patient/family's behavior indicates decreased anxiety with provision of information	■ Ongoing assessment of level of anxiety and knowledge base/understanding of patient/family Collaborate with physician in providing realistic information to patient/family Provide information relevant to level of understanding Explain all diagnostic tests, procedures, therapeutic interventions, regimens, and necessary reasons Explain relationship between symptoms and disease process Explain reasons for frequent neurological assessments, vital signs and vital capacity monitoring Encourage patient/family's verbalization of questions, fears, concerns Provide time and support Answer questions realistically Assess patient/family's comprehension and acceptance of information Explain and continually reinforce that optimal medication control and determination take time to achieve and require frequent reevaluations, readjustments, and periods of medication withdrawal to best control disease and potential crisis occurrence Explain relationship between medication regimen and status; peak and minimal effect times Explain relationship between fatigue/time of day and status If crisis occurs, explain reasons for procedures, treatments, tests Continually support, provide explanations, answer questions Reinforce that cause of crisis occurrence many times is unknown, but that patient/family will be taught preventive measures to try to decrease potential for crisis and appropriate information/interventions for identification and management of crisis if it occurs See Problem, Patient/family's fears, anger, depression
■ Patient/family's fear, anger, depression related to disease Alteration in body image/life-style Dependency; threat of disease crisis Fear of home care management	■ Patient/family verbalizes fear, anger, depression* Patient/family verbalizes required care	■ Ongoing assessments of level of anxiety, knowledge base of disease/problems, and other reactions Collaborate with physician regarding disease prognosis/control in promoting patient/family's acceptance of disease and regarding necessity of patient/family's knowledge acquisition and implementation to promote optimal control and potential independent functioning Encourage verbalization of patient/family's fears and reactions Provide time and support; accept reactions and stage of emotions Reassure patient/family that reactions and behavior are "normal" in confrontation with disease Reassure patient/family that depression, frustration, anger, fear are natural reactions and occur frequently

*If responsibility of critical care nurse includes this stage of care.

Potential problems	Expected outcomes	Nursing activities
		Assess patient/family's strengths/weaknesses in disease confrontation, potential for coping with acceptance, management of disease threat, and attitude
		Support patient/family with calm, reassuring, and accepting manner
		Assess patient/family's normal life-style, occupation, interests, living situation
		Implement plan of care and intervention based on individualized patient status, patient/family's needs and potentials
		Encourage patient/family's participation in care and decisions regarding short-term and long-term goals
		Monitor patient/family's potential for achieving maximal independence in ADL
		Obtain orders for appropriate referrals such as physical and occupational therapy, social service
		Obtain appropriate equipment to promote maximal independence in ADL and safety maintenance
		Encourage patient's maximal independence in ADL within capabilities/limitations; readjust interventions as status progresses from dependent to independent functioning
		Reinforce any gains patient achieves
		Promote patient/family's acceptance of disease and realities
		Reaffirm that best control potential occurs with patient/family's knowledge of disease, problems, and appropriate management
		Reaffirm that reactions are normal experiences but that patient/family's acceptance of disease and positive attitude toward control/management may enhance maximal independence and as "normal" a life-style as feasible
■ Insufficient knowledge to comply with discharge regimen*	■ Patient/family verbalizes and demonstrates necessary information and skills to comply with discharge regimen	■ Assess patient/family's level of understanding of neurological problem and therapies received
		Explain relationship between patient's neurological status and therapies prescribed
		Assess alterations in usual life-style necessitated by individual patient's status, severity/control of disease
		Try to promote as normal a life-style as possible by collaboration with patient/family and other health team members in planning regimens such as medications, activity
		Involve patient/family to maximal degree possible in planning, decision making, establishing regimen schedules
		Continually reassure and support patient/family that they will be provided with needed knowledge, skills, information to optimally cope with/manage disease and problems
		Collaborate with physician in providing realistic information and reassurance regarding control potential, prognosis, disease process
		Promote positive aspects of medication adjustments, demand schedule regimens
		Continually assess patient/family's potential for assuming responsibility in control/management of disease; promote strengths and abilities to cope and assume control
		Reaffirm that patient/family can best control disease by maximal knowledge acquisition/implementation
		Encourage patient/family's participation in assessing home situation, necessary alterations; decisions regarding home care and management

*If responsibility of critical care nurse includes such follow-up care.

Potential problems	Expected outcomes	Nursing activities
		Instruct and evaluate patient/family's acquisition/demonstration of necessary information and skills to comply with discharge regimen and promote maximal disease control
		Institute teaching program for patient/family, including
		Precipitating factors in crisis—stress, fatigue, infection, constipation
		Avoid infections and exposure, strenuous exercise
		Patient/family's identification of own factors and measures to prevent occurrence
	Patient/family describes activity and dietary regimen	Importance of regular, well-balanced diet
		Planning of daily activities to provide rest periods; prevention of fatigue/overexertion
	Patient/family describes means to achieve maximal independence in ADL, promote safety, and prevent complications	Promotion of maximal independence within capabilities and frustration levels
		Proper use of equipment
		Assistance necessary (type, amount, degree)
		Safety measures
		Prevention of complications
		Importance of 8 hours of sleep or appropriate amount
		Emergency measures that should be implemented for prevention
		Medical alert identification
		Working telephone in home
		Establish ambulance service, police service, fastest local routes to hospital
		Telephone numbers of accessible means to hospital
		If appropriate, home availability/proper use of airway, suctioning equipment, resuscitative equipment and technique
		Signs/symptoms of myasthenic or cholinergic crisis—what to do
		Avoidance of all over-the-counter medications including cold preparations, aspirin; strong cathartics, enemas
	Patient/family describes medication regimen	Medication regimen
		Name and purpose
		Route, dosage, frequency, times
		Side effects and when to notify physician
		Special precautions necessary including drugs, foods, beverages contraindicated or quantity regulated; factors potentiating/decreasing effects/side effects
		If feasible, demand scheduling for medication use to promote optimal management; collaborate with physician in providing necessary information
		Instruct in peak effect times of medications; encourage patient/family planning of ADL at optimal effect times
		Appropriate resources including Myasthenia Gravis Foundation
		Importance of ongoing medical care and regular checkups; that any physician or health facility should be fully informed of disease history, medications
		Proper use of any equipment or therapeutic devices
		If respirator assistance is prescribed for home use, teach utilization, care/maintenance, potential problems/interventions, preventive measures
		Special therapeutic measures prescribed/maintained
		If tracheostomy tube is in place on discharge, teach proper care techniques/maintenance, prevention of complications, signs/symptoms of problems and measures to overcome, when and who to notify for medical intervention

Potential problems	Expected outcomes	Nursing activities
		If vital capacity recordings are indicated, teach method, times, proper equipment use/maintenance, values necessitating notification of physician
		If indicated, teach muscle strength testing, grading, and recording
	Patient/family describes signs/symptoms requiring medical attention	Signs and symptoms of neurological status/medication control requiring medical attention
	Patient/family describes follow-up care regimen	Plan for follow-up care including purpose of appointment, when and where to go, who to see, what to expect, any data recording to bring

THYMECTOMY
Preoperative period

■ Respiratory distress, insufficiency, which may be related to Pulmonary infection Withholding anticholinesterase drugs in hours immediately preceding surgery Thoracic and/or oropharyngeal muscle weakness Excess tracheobronchial secretions	■ Respiratory function sufficient for adequate oxygenation and ventilation in order to achieve Pa_{O_2} and Pa_{CO_2} levels within patient's normal limits Absence of pulmonary infection Effective mobilization of secretions Patent airway	■ Administer systematic, thorough pulmonary toilet, including chest physiotherapy, timed to coincide with peak activity of anticholinesterase medication Administer anticholinesterases as ordered; time activities (e.g., eating, ambulation) to occur at peak activity of medication Administer antibiotics and ultrasonic nebulization treatments as ordered Administer steroid medication preoperatively if ordered Administer long-acting anticholinesterase medication (a time-span capsule) the night before surgery or a few hours preoperatively as ordered Administer atropine for control of secretion production If respiratory insufficiency and production of secretions are marked, nurse or physician should accompany patient to operating room with manual breathing bag and portable suction system
■ Patient/family's anxiety, fears, regarding Hospitalization Disease process Diagnostic procedures Therapeutic regimen Surgery Dependence, altered life-style imposed by myasthenia gravis	■ Reduction in patient/ family's anxiety with provision of information, explanations, and encouragement	■ Assess level of patient/family's anxiety regarding impending diagnostic procedures, surgery Assess level of understanding of anticipated diagnostic procedures and surgery Describe purpose of planned diagnostic procedures and what patient will experience Prepare and support patient before and during procedures Describe purpose of surgery and, in collaboration with physician, the expected outcomes Prepare patient for surgery and provide support and encouragement for patient/family as needed Describe the perioperative experiences, including Preoperative Chest physiotherapy 1. Coughing and deep breathing 2. Incentive spirometry Shave Light dinner, then NPO after midnight Medication for sleep if needed Morning bath/shower Preoperative medications Hospital gown Care of valuables Ride to operating room Scrub suits, masks, and hats worn by operating room staff Anesthesia

Potential problems	Expected outcomes	Nursing activities
		Postoperative
		Waking up in recovery room/intensive care unit
		1. Describe general environment (size of unit, room, etc.)
		2. Nurse always nearby
		3. Dull, continuous noises
		4. Breathing tube may be temporarily in place to ease work of breathing
		Incision with bandage
		IV, arterial lines
		Chest tubes, if anticipated
		ECG monitoring, if anticipated
		Medicine for discomfort, pain
		Policy on family visits
		As patient progresses
		Tubes out
		Deep breathing, coughing, and chest physiotherapy
		Eating again
		Getting stronger, ambulation
		Assess reduction in level of patient/family's anxiety
	Patient/family demonstrates understanding of disease process, therapeutic regimen, and physical limitations imposed by disease	Ongoing assessment of patient/family's level of anxiety, specific fears, and concerns
		Encourage verbalization of fears and concerns; provide information, support as needed
	Patient achieves independence in normal ADL	Assess patient/family's normal life-style, level of activity
		Obtain orders for appropriate referrals such as social service, occupational therapy, physical therapy, Myasthenia Gravis Foundation
	Patient accepts degree of dependence dictated by disease	Encourage and provide for maximal independence in ADL within capabilities, limitations
		Promote patient/family's realistic acceptance of disease, recognizing the therapy available and inherent physical limitations
		See Medical management
Postoperative period		
■ Respiratory insufficiency related to Muscular weakness associated with disease process Phrenic nerve injury	■ Respiratory function adequate for sufficient oxygenation and ventilation; Pa_{O_2} and Pa_{CO_2} levels within patient's normal limits	■ Ongoing assessment of
		Quality of respirations; note presence of respiratory distress
		Respiratory muscle strength; observe diaphragmatic movement, excursion
	Diaphragmatic movements active and within normal limits	Secretions
		Volume
		Nature of
	Effective expectoration of secretions, patent airway	Ability of patient to expectorate
		Breath sounds
		Results of pulmonary function tests, including inspiratory force, vital capacity
	Pulmonary function tests compatible with spontaneous breathing	Arterial blood gas levels; deterioration indicates respiratory insufficiency and may herald respiratory failure
		Results of chest radiograph for
	Patent chest tube drainage system	Infiltrates, atelectasis
		Gross diaphragmatic abnormalities
		Maintain patency of chest tube drainage system
		Monitor amount and nature of chest tube drainage
		Note presence of hemorrhage or air leak; notify physician if either occurs

Potential problems	Expected outcomes	Nursing activities
Pulmonary intersti-tial edema	Absence of pulmonary interstitial edema Weight returns to preoperative baseline level within a few days postoperatively	Keep careful intake and output records Administer fluids and diuretics as ordered, avoiding fluid overload, weight gain, and pulmonary interstitial edema Monitor weight daily for gain or loss Maintain patient on assisted mechanical ventilation; see Standard: *Mechanical ventilation* Provide stiff (tonsillar) suction catheter for patient to aspirate oral secretions as frequently as necessary; patient with myasthenia gravis is usually able to lift hand enough to use these stiff catheters Administer antibiotics as ordered (aminoglycoside medications should not be given) Administer steroids if ordered (as continuation of preoperative therapy)
	Patient successfully weaned from ventilator	Carefully, systematically wean patient from ventilator (usually begins 36 to 48 hours postoperatively) Stay with patient continuously during weaning process; provide for support and encouragement Use intermittent mandatory ventilation system for gradual weaning, if ventilator is so equipped; positive end expiratory pressure (2 to 4 cm H_2O pressure) is usually employed in the system May use T-tube/T-piece system, if ordered, whereby patient is removed from ventilator and allowed to breathe humidified O_2 through wide-bore tubing, using own respiratory muscular effort exclusively Precipitous changes in blood gas values may occur when this method is used Pa_{O_2} values greater than 60 and pH values greater than 7.3 are usually acceptable; Pa_{CO_2} levels may become elevated due to respiratory muscle weakness and hypoventilation; mild elevation is usually acceptable The T-tube/T-piece system is usually applied for 20 to 40 minutes according to the patient's clinical status and arterial blood gas levels
	Vital capacity and inspiratory force measurements steadily increase during weaning process	Monitor serial strength, vital capacity, and inspiratory force measurements during weaning process; if measurements indicate poor patient toleration of weaning effort, notify physician Administer anticholinesterase medication if ordered during period of weaning Monitor effect of medication q15-30min Anticholinesterase medication is often avoided during weaning process because of associated increased secretion production Since patient cannot swallow a pill, the first dose of anticholinesterase medication is given IV or IM; the first dose is usually about one-half the preoperative dose, with increments according to patient's response
Copious secretions Respiratory, oro-pharyngeal muscle weakness	Effective mobilization and expectoration of secretions	Monitor amount and nature of secretions associated with the autonomic (muscarinic) effects of anticholinesterase medication Monitor patient's ability to handle (expectorate) secretions and if marked difficulty is present, notify physician Administer atropine if ordered and closely monitor for decrease in secretion production During and after weaning procedure, administer vigorous chest physiotherapy and aspirate secretions as necessary Closely monitor patient's respiratory status q15-30 min or as patient's condition dictates

Potential problems	Expected outcomes	Nursing activities
		Monitor patient's respiratory status continuously during the first 12 to 24 hours after extubation
		After extubation, monitor patient's ability to phonate, since an inability to phonate properly usually indicates an ineffective cough
		If patient cannot be weaned within 5 to 7 days postoperatively, prepare patient for and assist with tracheotomy according to surgical plan of care, if ordered
■ Hypocalcemia, which can result from inadvertent removal of parathyroid glands lodged within thymus gland	■ Serum Ca^{2+} levels within normal limits	■ Monitor 　For signs and symptoms of hypocalcemia including neuromuscular irritablity, twitching, Chvostek's sign, Trousseau's sign 　Serum Ca^{2+} levels Notify physician of abnormalities Administer Ca^{2+} supplements as ordered
■ Tracheal injury, which may be related to Mechanical stress Infection	■ Proper amount of air maintained in cuff; an air leak around tracheal cuff is apparent on sigh breath An air leak may be permitted with normal tidal volumes Tracheal tube secured in place	■ Prevent by 　Maintaining minimal amount of air in cuff—permitting leak with sigh (and minimal leak with each inspiration) if low pressure cuff used; if high pressure cuff used, regularly deflate (e.g., 5 minutes every hour) 　Recording volume of air in cuff; alert physician if requirements increase, especially if requirements exceed 8 to 10 ml 　Avoiding movement of tracheal tube 　　Note centimeter marking at teeth or nares and record 　　Tape tube securely in place 　　Note placement of tube on radiograph 　　If any change occurs, recheck centimeter marking on tube in relation to mouth and nares 　Using aseptic technique in care of tracheal tube and in suctioning procedures (see Problem, Infection)
■ Infection	■ Absence of or resolution of infection Prompt recognition and intervention if infection occurs	■ Prevent by 　Averting such factors such as urinary retention, pulmonary congestion/aspiration 　Maintaining strict sterile technique for procedures such as catheterization, endotracheal/tracheostomy tube care, suctioning, ventilator maintenance Monitor 　Temperature q4 hr and prn 　IV sites frequently for any signs of redness, tenderness, phlebitis 　For potential infection sources including pulmonary and urinary and exposure to possible sources of infection 　WBC count (may be falsely elevated if patient is receiving steroids) If signs of infection occur, notify physician For other measures, see Medical management
■ Crisis—excessive muscle weakness associated with too much or too little medication, including the following two types Myasthenic—sudden muscular weakness; drug regimen ineffective for unknown reasons	■ Immediate recognition of impending crisis occurrence and intervention Patent airway Adequate ventilation, with Pa_{CO_2} levels within patient's normal limits	■ Careful observations and frequent assessments of neurological/respiratory status Keep emergency equipment and medications readily available—intubation, suctioning equipment; O_2; hand ventilator; airway; mechanical ventilator; cardiopulmonary drugs; etc.—always anticipate potential crisis occurrence Prevent by 　Administering medications and treatments as ordered at precise time and regimen 　Monitoring 　　Effects—maintain flow sheet correlating medication time

Potential problems	Expected outcomes	Nursing activities
Cholinergic—worsening status from overdose of myasthenic drugs		effectiveness on graded muscle strength, cranial nerve functioning, reflexes of swallowing, gag, cough Closely for presence/degree of dysphagia, dyspnea, dysarthria Respiratory status—rate, quality, pattern Vital capacity measurements Averting precipitating factors for crisis such as infection, emotional crisis, constipation Monitor for signs and symptoms of crisis 　Common manifestations of both myasthenic and cholinergic crisis (present in either crisis): skeletal muscular weakness, increased anxiety, restlessness, dyspnea, dysphagia, dysarthria 　Differentiating signs according to crisis type 　　Myasthenic: ocular palsies, ptosis, development/worsening of diplopia 　　Cholinergic: fasciculations/fine twitching; abdominal cramps and diarrhea, nausea/vomiting; increased secretions—salivation, sweating, lacrimation, bronchial; blurred vision; most ominous sign is increased weakness instead of expected improvement 1 hour after medication is administered Notify physician immediately of any signs and symptoms of crisis Administer emergency measures as ordered; see Medical management
▪ Inordinate weakness and fatigue	▪ Optimal muscle strength Early recognition of increased muscle weakness Minimization of fatigue	▪ Establish neurological baseline on admission Monitor ongoing neurological status 　Muscle strength of all groups with repetitive activity 　Ability to raise/lower eyelids completely; if ptosis is present, note location and degree 　Facial muscular strength (cranial nerve VII) bilaterally 　Extraocular movements—presence/degree, location of ocular palsies, nystagmus, diplopia 　Presence/degree of gag and cough reflexes 　Presence/quality of chewing ability 　Speech quality and ability Monitor respiratory parameters (establish baseline on admission) 　Vital signs—respiratory rate, quality, and pattern 　Breath sounds for decreased or absent sounds and presence of rales and/or rhonchi 　Vital capacity measurements 　Muscle strength of diaphragmatic and intercostal muscles 　Presence/quality of cough, gag, and swallowing reflexes 　Presence, amount/quality of secretions/saliva and patient's ability to handle effectively 　Arterial blood gas levels 　Chest radiograph results Patient's history established See Medical management for pertinent historical information that should be collected Ongoing assessment of neurological and respiratory status 　Provide for close observation; place patient close to nurse's station 　Monitor 　　Muscle strengths and vital capacities q2-4 hr and prn 　　　1. Maintain flow sheet of muscle strength; establish specific testing modalities for repetitive muscle strength/fatigue assessments

Potential problems	Expected outcomes	Nursing activities
		2. Maintain flow sheet of vital capacities; use same spirometer and proper position and measurement technique
		Presence/quality of bulbar functioning; facial, hypoglossal, vagal, and glossopharyngeal muscle strength and status
		Presence/quality of gag, swallowing, and cough reflexes
		Presence/quality of extraocular movements and strength of eyelid opening and closure
		For presence/degree of ptosis, diplopia, corneal reflex
		For any signs/symptoms of dysphagia, dyspnea (exertional or at rest), dysarthria—presence, quality, and degree
		Notify physician immediately of any decline in neurological/respiratory status
		Notify physician immediately of any decrease in vital capacity below minimal acceptable level specified for individual patient
		Administer therapy as ordered to improve neurological/respiratory status
		See Problem, Muscle weakness (Medical management)
	Patient demonstrates steady increase in neuromuscular function and strength in postoperative period	Ambulate patient as soon as tolerated; if peripheral weakness is marked, ambulation may have to be delayed until anticholinesterase medication is resumed
		Apply bra for women with large breasts for support and to avoid stretch/stress on incision

Subacute postoperative period

Potential problems	Expected outcomes	Nursing activities
■ Respiratory insufficiency/arrest related to Weakness/paralysis of respiratory muscles due to Pneumonia Atelectasis Dysphagia/aspiration Decreased or absent swallowing, gag, and cough reflexes Dysarthria Dyspnea/respiratory failure	■ Adequate alveolar ventilation Patent airway Respiratory rate and quality within patient's normal limits Arterial blood gas levels within normal limits Swallowing, gag, and cough reflexes at least as good as baseline preoperative level Absence of dysarthria or dysphagia Absence of pulmonary infection/pneumonia	■ Prevention Maintain patent airway Turn and reposition patient q1-2 hr; position to prevent airway obstruction and aspiration of secretions Assist patient with coughing and deep breathing Administer chest physiotherapy q2-4 hr as needed Administer humidified O_2 as ordered to achieve adequate oxygenation and liquefication of secretions Prevent precipitating factors in respiratory failure, especially Severe dysphagia: ongoing monitoring of swallowing reflex and status; keep patient NPO if risk of aspiration is high Respiratory tract infection: protect from potential infection sources; vigorous suctioning and chest physiotherapy to maintain patent airway Prevent aspiration by Assessing foods that patient tolerates best and assisting with diet selection Avoiding fluids that enhance saliva production such as milk Scheduling meals when strength is maximum Staying with patient at mealtimes; monitoring effectiveness of swallowing Prevent pulmonary embolism by Instructing and supervising patient in leg exercises, ROM exercises Applying antithromboembolic stockings or Ace bandages as per physician's order; rewrap or reapply every shift and prn; avoid constriction or looseness Monitor neurological and respiratory status q2 hr and prn, including Muscle strength; cranial nerve functioning; swallowing, cough, gag reflexes For any choking/nasal regurgitation

Potential problems	Expected outcomes	Nursing activities
		Vital signs—respiratory rate, quality, and pattern
		Vital capacities
		Muscle strength of respiratory muscles (diaphragm and intercostal muscles)
		Breath sounds for decrease in or absence of sounds and for signs of obstruction (rales, rhonchi, etc.)
		Patency of upper airway and patient's ability to handle secretions
		Skin color, nail beds, peripheral pulses, and skin warmth
		For signs and symptoms of thrombophlebitis, pulmonary emboli, pulmonary edema, dyspnea/dysphagia
		Arterial blood gas levels and chest radiograph results
		If any impairment in swallowing, gag, or cough reflexes is present, keep patient NPO and notify physician; suction secretions prn; prevent aspiration by positioning, maintaining patent airway
		Have emergency equipment and medications readily available if respiratory problem occurs
		Notify physician immediately of any change in respiratory/neurological status
		Administer medications and treatments as ordered
		Monitor effects and side effects of therapy; notify physician of results
		If respiratory problem occurs, see Medical management
■ Altered communication ability, which may be related to cranial nerve dysfunction, motor paralysis, endotracheal or tracheostomy tube insertion	■ Means for patient to communicate needs are established and in use	■ Monitor communication abilities
		If ability to communicate is altered, establish alternate means of communication based on individual patient needs/status
		Develop alternative communication modes that are the least physically, mentally, and emotionally taxing to patient
		Establish means for patient to get nurse's attention
		Evaluate effectiveness of alternative communication modes with patient/family
		Involve patient/family in planning care
		Involve patient/family in reevaluation/readjustment of modes of communication as necessary
		Anticipate patient's needs
		Encourage staff/family to speak to patient, even if patient cannot respond
■ Bowel or bladder dysfunction	■ Urinary output within normal limits	■ Assess patient's prior elimination patterns
	Absence of bladder distention	Usual voiding pattern
	Pattern of bowel elimination within patient's normal limits	Bowel pattern, problems, dietary/medication measures for elimination
		Monitor
		Intake and output measurements
		Bowel movements—amount, consistency, frequency
		Assess bowel sounds for presence/quality
		Monitor for signs and symptoms of paralytic ileus; notify physician immediately if any signs/symptoms occur
		For any signs and symptoms of urinary retention, overflow voiding, or residual; notify physician if any of these occur
		Administer medications as ordered
		Implement treatments as ordered, such as intermittent catheterization
		Monitor effects and side effects of interventions and notify physician of results
		Continue monitoring urinary output
		Establish and implement individualized bowel/bladder regimen based on patient needs, pattern, previous measures, etc.
		See Medical management

Potential problems	**Expected outcomes**	**Nursing activities**
■ GI bleeding related to CNS factors Stress Steroid administration	■ Absence or control of GI bleeding	■ Prevent by 　Minimizing factors in environment that contribute to patient's stress level 　Helping patient deal with anxiety (see Problem, Patient/family's anxiety) 　Administering antacid as soon as patient is able to take po, if ordered Monitor 　Vital signs, Hgb, Hct 　Stools for Hematest three times a week 　Hematest of aspirate, emesis, urine 　For signs of GI bleeding such as abdominial tenderness, pain, distention 　If patient is receiving steroids, monitor urine glucose and acetone four times a day and prn or as ordered; notify physician of results Report immediately to physician any signs and symptoms of GI bleeding If problem occurs, see Medical management; see Standard: *Acute upper gastrointestinal bleeding*
■ Complications of corticosteroid therapy	■ Prompt recognition of any complications and notification of physician	■ Monitor for any complications of corticosteroid therapy, including 　Signs of GI irritation 　Development or exacerbation of diabetes mellitus 　Increased susceptibility to infection 　Psychosis; behavioral changes 　Hypokalemia 　Hypertension 　Osteoporosis 　Acne For other precautionary measures for the use of steroid therapy in the myasthenic patient, see Medical management
■ Insufficient knowledge to comply with discharge regimen*	■ Sufficient information to comply with discharge regimen Before discharge patient/family accurately 　Describes medication, activity, and dietary regimens 　Describes precautionary measures for the postoperative period 　Is able to demonstrate proper care for suture line 　Verbalizes procedure for follow-up visits	■ Assess patient/family's knowledge regarding disease process, discharge regimen, and follow-up plan of care Consult with physician regarding discharge regimen; ascertain what has been discussed with patient Describe patient's disease process and rationale for discharge regimen Instruct patient/family in medications 　Name and identification of drug 　Purpose 　Indications for use of prn drug 　Dosage/number of pills and schedule 　Precautionary measures 　Potential adverse effects and how to minimize 　Avoidance of over-the-counter medications that can change activity of prescribed medications and to consult physician before using any of these products Describe postdischarge activity progression, precautions Encourage patient to exercise in regular, moderate amounts, with frequent rest periods 　More strenuous activities should be planned for approximately ½ to 2 hours after the anticholinesterase medication is given 　Light activities such as walking, climbing stairs, or cooking are all acceptable in early postoperative period

*If the responsibility of the critical care nurse includes follow-up care.

Potential problems	Expected outcomes	Nursing activities

If sternotomy approach was used, encourage patient to avoid activities requiring strenuous chest muscle activity for several months; examples of activities that should be avoided in the first few weeks at home include
1. Driving a car
2. Vacuuming
3. Lifting a window

More vigorous activities should be avoided for several months, including tennis, swimming, golf and vigorous manual skills such as carpentry work

Explain that a "remission" (or the need for less anticholinesterase medication to accomplish daily activities) may not occur for several months postoperatively; the occurrence and significance of a remission cannot be predicted

Demonstrate and describe care of suture line; provide opportunity for return demonstration

Review plan for follow-up care, including purpose of follow-up visits; when and where to go; who to see; what specimens to bring

Assess potential compliance with discharge regimen

36 □ Guillain Barré syndrome

Guillain Barré syndrome is an inflammatory disease process that involves demyelination and degeneration of the myelin sheath and cylinder of peripheral nerves and the anterior (ventral) and posterior (dorsal) roots at spinal segmental levels. Patients with Guillain Barré syndrome usually present clinically with a rapidly ascending motor and sensory deficit along with cranial nerve involvement. The progression of the disease process is usually complete within 10 to 12 days after symptoms begin. Strangely enough, the progression can stop at any one level without any further deterioration or progression.

Treatment of Guillain Barré syndrome is supportive. Recovery occurs, spontaneously and the patient regains prior motor and sensory function, often in a stepwise fashion. The speed of recovery varies with each individual, but recovery commonly occurs over weeks or months.Complete recovery of normal function occurs in the majority of cases with only a small percentage of patients retaining mild residual defects.

The cause of Guillain Barré syndrome is not known. Two theories of causation are the infective and the immunological. A virus has not been isolated in Guillain Barré syndrome but is considered a strong possibility as the cause of the polyneuritis. The immunological theory involves the autoallergic response of body cells to antibodies formed against infectious agents. The clinical history in 50% of Guillain Barré patients involves the occurrence of a mild respiratory or gastrointestinal infection 1 to 3 weeks before the appearance of neurological symptoms. This high incidence of preceding infection heightens suspicion that a viral agent may be responsible.

SIGNS AND SYMPTOMS

1. Paresthesias: numbness, tingling, and other abnormal sensations frequently beginning in the feet. Pain, temperature, proprioception, vibration, and touch are also diminished in the affected areas due to inflammation and degeneration of the posterior (dorsal) roots of the spinal cord.
2. Paresis/paralysis: the motor involvement is usually a complete lower motor neuron paralysis with flaccidity, decreased or absent deep tendon reflexes, and hypotonia or atonia of muscles. The motor involvement usually corresponds to the areas involved in the sensory deficits and progresses in the same pattern.

Weakness usually appears first bilaterally and then progresses to paralysis of involved areas. The motor deficits are due to inflammation and degeneration of the motor neuron axons that exit from the spinal cord in the anterior (ventral) roots. Commonly, the motor paralysis progresses from legs to trunk, arm, and cranial muscles, attaining peak severity within 10 to 14 days. The motor paralysis of intercostal and phrenic nerves, if it occurs, results in respiratory failure, which is the greatest threat and primary cause of mortality in patients with Guillain Barré syndrome.

3. Cranial nerve dysfunction: the cranial nerves frequently involved in pathology are
   a. Facial (VII)—lower motor neuron weakness or paralysis of facial muscle control unilaterally or bilaterally
   b. Glossopharyngeal (IX), vagus (X), and hypoglossal (XII)—lower motor neuron bulbar palsy causes nasal, dysarthric speech; dysphagia; impaired gag and cough reflexes; and sympathetic dysfunction with postural hypotension, episodes of hypertension, flushing, sweating, and tachycardia
   c. Oculomotor (III) and abducens (VI)—produce diplopia, nonconjugate eye movements, ptosis
   d. Spinal accessory (XI)—produces impaired shoulder shrug and head turning to side abilities

The diagnosis of Guillain Barré syndrome is based on the clinical history, clinical presentation of signs/symptoms, progression, and clinical course. A lumbar puncture is performed to aid in diagnosis. The CSF is under normal pressure, contains a normal leukocyte count with an elevated protein count (this increased protein content and normal leukocyte count is called albuminocytological dissociation). The elevated protein count usually appears several days after the onset of symptoms; the protein level continues to rise, reaching a peak in 4 to 6 weeks. This increased CSF protein content is thought to result from the release of plasma proteins from the inflammation, degeneration, and damage of the nerve roots.

ASSESSMENT

1. Onset, duration, progression, and description of neurological symptoms, especially
   a. Motor system: weakness or paralysis, tone, muscles involved
   b. Sensory system: numbness, tingling; pain, temperature, proprioception, vibratory sensations status
   c. Cranial nerve dysfunctions
   d. Reflex system and status
   e. Respiratory symptoms of muscular weakness such as dyspnea, tachypnea
2. Any previous respiratory or gastrointestinal infection: when, symptoms of, and duration
3. Previous neurological treatment or neurosurgical procedure
4. Presence of any medical problems and therapy employed
5. Any previous vaccination or immunization received: when, specific type, effects, and side effects
6. Patient's perceptions and reaction to diagnosis, disease progression, treatment modalities
7. Presence of any alterations in body image; fears of permanent disability or deficit; altered role in family, normal occupation/performance of ADL
8. Baseline parameters status
   a. Neurological
   b. Respiratory
   c. Cardiac
   d. Circulatory and vascular
   e. Fluid and electrolyte
   f. Hydration/nutritional
   g. Metabolic
   h. Vital capacity
   i. Vital signs
   j. Weight
9. Diagnostic test results, including
   a. Lumbar puncture
   b. Electromyography
10. Results of
    a. CSF determinations
    b. Serum electrolyte levels
    c. Hgb, Hct, platelet count, WBC count/differential
    d. Arterial blood gas levels
    e. Clotting profile
    f. Urinalysis, culture, specific gravity, osmolality
    g. Chest radiograph
    h. ECG

GOALS

1. Optimal neurological functioning
2. Optimal recovery extent and rate; absence of complications
3. Optimal independence in ADL
4. Adequate alveolar ventilation and perfusion
5. Acid-base balance within normal limits
6. Adequate cardiac output

7. Serum electrolyte levels and fluid balance within normal limits
8. Hgb and Hct stable within normal limits
9. Infection free
10. Normal bladder and bowel function
11. Behavior demonstrates reduction of patient/family's anxiety with provision of information, demonstrations, support
12. Before discharge patient/family is able to

a. Describe medication, activity, exercise, and dietary regimens
b. Demonstrate safety measures and techniques; proper use of any equipment, therapeutic devices
c. Describe signs and symptoms requiring medical attention
d. State necessary information regarding follow-up care

Potential problems	Expected outcomes	Nursing activities
■ Increasing severity and level of motor/sensory deficits Progression is usually a rapidly ascending motor and sensory deficit, but cases have occurred in which the progression is descending	■ Maximal neurological functioning Absence or resolution of neurological deficit (after disease course) Absence of complications	■ Establish neurological baseline on admission and continue ongoing assessments of neurological status q1 hr and prn; monitor And specifically record deficit present, degree, level, extremities involved especially motor and sensory functioning; cranial nerve functioning and reflex status (presence and quality) LOC; pupil size, equality, light reactivity; extraocular movements Presence and quality of swallowing, cough, and gag reflexes Vital signs for any abnormalities Notify physician immediately of any decline in neurological status—either worsening severity or progression of level Institute measures and administer supportive treatments and interventions as physician's order and patient's status necessitate
■ Respiratory insufficiency related to weakness/paralysis of intercostal and diaphragmatic muscles	■ Patent airway Adequate alveolar ventilation and perfusion Normal respiratory rate, pattern, and quality Vital capacity within normal limits Arterial blood gas values within patient's normal limits	■ Establish baseline respiratory status and continue ongoing assessments q1 hr and prn Monitor for any abnormality/decline Respiratory rate, quality, and pattern Vital signs Neurological status, particularly muscle strength/functioning of respiratory muscles (intercostal, diaphragmatic) Vital capacity Patency of upper airway and patient's ability to handle secretions Presence/quality of gag, cough, and swallowing reflexes Breath sounds bilaterally for quality of aeration; signs of obstruction Skin color, nail beds, peripheral pulses, and skin warmth Arterial blood gas values Chest radiograph results Signs/symptoms of thrombophlebitis, pulmonary emboli, pulmonary edema Maintain patent airway by Turning and positioning to prevent obstruction or aspiration of secretions q2 hr and prn Deep breathing and coughing q1 hr and prn Suctioning prn Chest physiotherapy and pulmonary toilet q2 hr and prn Intermittent positive pressure breathing as ordered Adequate oxygenation and humidification as ordered Apply antithromboembolic stockings or Ace bandages as ordered; reapply every shift and prn; monitor for constriction/looseness, condition of skin

Potential problems	Expected outcomes	Nursing activities
		Assist patient or perform passive ROM exercises
		Notify physician immediately of any decline in respiratory status, neurological status, vital capacity, vital signs
		If problem occurs
		Assist with emergency measures to maintain patent airway and adequate ventilation
		Administer medications/treatments as ordered; monitor effects and side effects
		Patient will be intubated or tracheotomy will be performed if respiratory muscles are involved in paralysis development/ progression; ensure proper positioning of endotracheal tube q2 hr
		Maintain mechanical ventilator as ordered
		See Standard: *Mechanical ventilation*
		Provide explanations and support to patient/family; explain relationship between neurological status and respiratory insufficiency; necessity for respiratory assistance/interventions; see Problem, Patient/family's anxiety
		Establish alternate means of communication; see Problem, Altered communication ability

■ Flaccid paralysis, paresthesias related to motor and sensory deficits	■ Absence of complications
	Full ROM of all extremities
	Skin intact
	Absence of contractures
		■ Establish and implement care plan based on individual needs and status; ongoing assessments of motor and sensory deficits/ functioning
		Institute measures to prevent complications such as contractures, decubiti, footdrop/wristdrop
		   Turn and position properly q2 hr and prn; maintain alignment and decrease gravity pull
		   Sheepskin or air mattress to decrease pressure factors
		   ROM to all extremities from passive to active exercises as status warrants; maintain exercise regimen within pain limits without stretching or resistance
		   Meticulous skin care and inspection of all skin surfaces q2 hr; massage skin and bony prominences
		   Obtain devices to prevent deformities such as handrolls, footboard, hand/foot splints
		   Obtain order for appropriate referrals such as physiotherapy
		   Monitor sensory deficits and administer medications and treatments as ordered such as analgesics, bed cradle, warm moist packs; turn gently and position comfortably
		   Increase activity level/progression as status improves; see Problem, Long rehabilitative phase, for further specifics

■ Cranial nerve dysfunction
  Oculomotor (III)
  Abducens (VI)
    Diplopia, impaired extraocular movements/nonconjugate eye movements
  Facial (VII)—lower motor neuron
    Facial weakness/ paralysis, impaired mouth/lip movement control, decreased or absent corneal reflex
	■ Absence of complications	■ Ongoing assessments of cranial nerve functioning
		
		Assess pupil size, equality, reactivity; extraocular movements; presence/degree of ptosis
		Apply alternating eye patch if diplopia is present
		Place objects within field of vision according to extraocular movements functioning
		
		Assess facial muscle functioning and strength, chewing ability, presence and quality of corneal reflex, speech ability
		If corneal reflex is decreased or absent, obtain order for administration of protective eyedrops and maintain lid closure on affected side by tape, butterfly patch, etc.
		Ongoing assessments for corneal irritation, abrasions
		Frequent eye care
		If patient is allowed po, help select foods within patient's chewing capabilities

Potential problems	Expected outcomes	Nursing activities
		Frequent oral hygiene and removal of saliva from drooling
		If speech is impaired from facial weakness/paralysis, establish alternate means of communication; see Problem, Altered communication ability
Glossopharyngeal (IX) Vagus (X) Hypoglossal (XII) Lower motor neuron bulbar palsy causing nasal, dysarthric speech; dysphagia; absent/diminished swallowing, gag, and cough reflexes		Assess presence and quality of swallowing, cough, and gag reflexes; speech quality; tongue strength/position If reflexes are absent/diminished, maintain interventions to prevent complications Suction prn; position to prevent obstruction or aspiration of secretions Keep patient NPO Administer IV fluids/NG feedings as ordered; monitor NG tube for proper placement and patency; if endotracheal/tracheostomy tube is in place, inflate cuff for 30 minutes prior to and following feedings When po is allowed, elevate head of bed, and start slowly monitoring quality and effectiveness of swallowing ability Progress diet slowly
Spinal accessory (XI) Impaired/absent shoulder shrug and head turning to side abilities		Assess ability to shrug shoulders, turn head to each side If ability to turn head to side is impaired, place objects within field of vision according to head-turning ability/degree
■ Unstable vasomotor function	■ Absence of complication Resolution of vasomotor instability	■ Maintain absolute bed rest as ordered; change position slowly Apply antithromboembolic stockings/Ace bandages as ordered Monitor ECG recording continually for any abnormality Monitor vital signs q2 hr and prn Monitor for hypotension, hypertension, sweating, flushing; notify physician immediately if any of these occurs Administer medications and treatments as ordered; monitor effects and side effects; notify physician of results When neurological status allows Tilt table if needed Slowly increase head gatch and activity
■ Patient/family's anxiety related to Neurological disease Neurological deficit and progression Fears of permanent disability or deficit	■ Patient/family's behavior demonstrates decreased anxiety with provision of information	■ Ongoing assessment of level of patient/family's anxiety, fears, concerns Collaborate with physician in providing realistic information appropriate to level of understanding Explain the usual signs/symptoms, progression, and clinical course of syndrome Explain that cause is unknown; that shock, fear, frustrations, anger are normal reactions to this insidious, rapid disease onset; accept reactions and help patient/family to deal realistically with reactions Explain the usual prognosis expected; that spontaneous recovery occurs over a period of time with recovery onset and speed of recovery varying with each individual Encourage verbalization of questions, fears, anxieties, and other concerns/reactions Answer questions realistically Provide time and support Reinforce that treatment is supportive, that recovery will occur spontaneously and progress, and that no interventions or "pushing" will promote recovery initiation Continually reassure and reinforce that recovery from disease will occur

Potential problems	Expected outcomes	Nursing activities
		Explain reasons for frequent respiratory/neurological assessments, vital signs and vital capacity monitoring
		Explain reasons why all treatments, measures, interventions are necessary
		Explain tests to patient/family; prepare and support patient during tests such as lumbar punctures, muscle testing
		If possible, provide one nurse to care for patient exclusively; have the same nurses provide care
		Involve patient in planning of care and goals; encourage patient to make decisions regarding care when possible
		Involve family in care planning, decision making, maintaining communication
■ Altered communication ability related to Cranial nerve dysfunction Motor paralysis Endotracheal or tracheostomy tube insertion	■ Alternate means of communication established	■ Monitor communication abilities If ability is altered, set up alternate means of communication based on individual patient needs/status such as writing tablet, word or letter board, eye-blinking system Convey the alternate means of communication utilized to other staff, family; assist in effective use of means Anticipate patient's needs Establish means for patient to get nurse's attention Continue verbal stimulation of patient even if patient is unable to respond; encourage family to talk to patient to maintain stimulation, interests, and contact with reality Evaluate effectiveness of alternative communication means with patient/family Involve patient/family in planning care Involve patient/family in reevaluation/readjustment of alternative communication means as necessary Try to find alternative communication means that are the least physically, mentally, and emotionally taxing to patient Accept the frustrations the patient frequently experiences from altered communication ability and resulting depression; try to minimize frustrations by anticipating needs, constant supervision, having the same nurses provide care, etc.
■ Fluid and electrolyte imbalance	■ Fluid and electrolyte balance within normal limits	■ Monitor and accurately record intake and output, urine specific gravity as ordered Monitor for signs of dehydration or overhydration such as Poor skin turgor Dry mucous membranes Peripheral edema Excessive thirst Change in LOC Monitor for Abnormal vital signs, Hgb/Hct values NOTE: Retention of Na^+ from the effects of increased aldosterone with increased release of ADH may occur as well as K^+ depletion from immobility Weight alterations Temperature elevations Insensible fluid losses including respiratory, diaphoresis, secretions Presence/degree of nausea and vomiting; effectiveness of medications ordered Presence/quality of gag and swallowing reflexes Administer IV fluids, NG feedings as ordered

Potential problems	Expected outcomes	Nursing activities
		■ Administer medications as ordered; monitor effects and side effects; if patient is receiving steroids, monitor urine glucose and acetone levels four times a day Notify physician of any fluid imbalance or electrolyte abnormality

■ Bowel/bladder dysfunction	■ Urinary output adequate
	No bladder distention
	Normal bowel elimination
		■ Assess patient's prior elimination patterns—usual voiding pattern, bowel pattern, problems, dietary/medication measures for elimination
		Monitor
		  Accurate recording of intake and output
		  For any signs/symptoms of urinary retention, overflow voiding, or residual; notify physician if any of these occurs and administer medications/treatments as ordered; monitor effects
		  Bowel movements (amount, consistency, frequency)
		  Bowel sounds, presence/quality; signs/symptoms of paralytic ileus
		Establish and implement individualized bowel regimen based on patient needs, pattern, previous measures, preferences/effectiveness
		  Involve patient in planning
		  Obtain orders for administration of stool softeners, cathartics, enemas as needed
		  Assess effectiveness of regimen; readjust as needed
		  When patient is allowed po, assist in food selection to promote bowel elimination

■ Infection	■ Absence or resolution of infection	■ Prevent precipitating factors such as urinary retention, pulmonary congestion/aspiration
		Maintain strict sterile technique for procedures such as catheterization; endotracheal/tracheostomy tube care, management, suctioning; ventilator maintenance
		Monitor
		  Temperature q4 hr and prn for any elevation
		  IV sites frequently for any signs of redness, tenderness, phlebitis
		  For potential infection sources including pulmonary, urinary, exposure to infection sources
		  WBC count (may be falsely elevated if patient is receiving steroids)
		If temperature elevation or sign of infection occurs, notify physician and culture possible infection sources
		  Monitor sputum/urinary cultures, chest radiograph results
		  Administer medications/treatments as ordered; monitor effects and side effects
		  Continue accurate recording of intake and output; monitor for dehydration/overhydration
		  Monitor for resolution/progression
		  Institute measures to promote resolution of infection souce if possible

■ GI bleeding related to Stress Steroid administration Anticoagulation regimen complication	■ Absence or resolution of GI bleeding	■ Monitor vital signs q2-4 hr, Hgb and Hct; stools for Hematest three times a week; Hematest of aspirate, emesis, and urine for any abnormalities If patient is receiving anticoagulants, monitor for effects and side effects; notify physician of results Monitor clotting profile results and appropriate coagulation values as ordered

Potential problems	Expected outcomes	Nursing activities

Obtain order for antacid adminisration as soon as patient able to take po

Monitor for signs of GI bleeding including abdominal tenderness/distention, hypotension, sudden tachycardia

Notify physician immediately if any abnormality occurs; if problem occurs, see Standard: *Acute upper gastrointestinal bleeding*

- Long rehabilitative phase
  Patient family's anxiety, anger, frustrations, depression related to
  Lengthy rehabilitative phase
  Slow resolution of neurological deficits

- Maximal neurological functioning*
  Maximal level of independence
  Patient/family verbalizes fears, frustrations, and other concerns
  Patient/family copes with lengthy rehabilitative process
  Patient/family demonstrates required care

- Ongoing assessment of neurological status—implementation of individualized plan of care and interventions based on patient's needs and status; plan care in collaboration with physician and department of physical therapy based on disease phase

  Acute phase: rehabilitative aspects include complete bed rest, prevention of complications, passive ROM exercises within pain limits, exercise regimen without stretching or resistance

  Condition stabilization phase but without return of function: exercise regimen progresses to gentle stretching and active exercise with avoidance of overstretching weakened muscles

  Recovery phase: exercise regimen progresses to active-resistant as muscle strength and reflexes return; activity regimen is initiated

  Provide explanations, time, support, reassurance to patient/family of interventions and necessary reasons; ongoing assessment of patient/family's level of anxiety, anger, and other reactions; see Problem, Patient/family's anxiety, for nursing activities

  In addition

  Explain relationship between phases and interventions

  Explain that vigorous exercise during acute phase will not promote function/recovery but may promote damage of muscles; overstretching exercises during phase of stability before recovery phase can cause permanent damage

  Reevaluate and readjust care plan as patient's status/needs necessitate and phase progression occurs

  Implement individualized plan of care to promote maximal neurological functioning, independence in ADL, and patient/family involvement in planning, giving care, and decision making

  Assist patient as needed in performing ADL; promote personal hygiene

  Monitor potential and encourage self-care as patient's rehabilitative phase status allows; encourage return to independence

  Provide rest periods between activities

  Increase activity to tolerance level

  Obtain appropriate referrals such as physical/occupational therapy, social service

  Obtain appropriate equipment/devices to maximize potential for independent functioning and safety

  Try to assist patient/family in coping with illness; channel reactions to positive potentials/interventions to promote maximal independence

*If responsibility of the critical care nurse includes this stage of care.

Potential problems	Expected outcomes	Nursing activities
		Encourage patient/family to maintain prior interests as feasible such as reading, hobbies, social visits
		Reinforce and reassure any progression in rehabilitative/recovery phase
		Reinforce any gains in muscle strength/functioning, independence achieved
		Plan, instruct, demonstrate, and evaluate patient/family's verbalization/performance of needed information/skills for maximal independent functioning such as
		Proper use of therapeutic devices/equipment
		Measures to prevent complications
		Assistance necessary: type, amount, and degree
		Assess patient/family's progress toward maximizing potential and independence in ADL
		Monitor level achieved
		If residual deficit is anticipated; coping means, reactions, knowledge, skills demonstrated by patient/family
		If full recovery is anticipated: level achieved by patient/family toward attainment
		Encourage verbalization of perceptions of possible alterations in life-style whether temporary/permanent
		Assess means to promote as "normal" a life-style as possible and encourage striving for attainment
■ Insufficient knowledge to comply with discharge regimen*	■ Patient/family demonstrates or verbalizes understanding of discharge regimen	■ Assess patient/family's level of understanding of neurological problem and therapy received
		Explain relationship between patient's neurological status and therapies prescribed
		Instruction of patient/family regarding required information and skills so that before discharge patient/family is able to
	Patient/family accurately describes medication, activity, and dietary regimens	Describe medication regimen
		Name and purpose
		Route, dosage, frequency, times
		Side effects
		Special precautions necessary including drugs, foods, beverages contraindicated or quantity regulated; factors potentiating/decreasing effects or side effects; physical restrictions; safety measures
		Describe dietary regimen
		Describe activity regimen, exercise program
		Describe and demonstrate any special therapeutic measures prescribed
	Patient/family describes means to achieve maximal independence in ADL, promote safety, and prevent complications	Describe and demonstrate proper use of equipment or therapeutic devices prescribed
		Reasons for using
		Time, method, and duration of use
		Precautions/safeguards
		Necessary maintenance (type, frequency)
		Measures to promote optimal functioning, upkeep/duration
	Patient/family describes signs/symptoms requiring medical attention	Describe signs/symptoms of neurological status requiring medical care
	Patient/family describes follow-up care regimen	Describe plan for follow-up care including purpose of appointment, when and where to go, who to see, what to expect

*If the responsibility of the critical care nurse includes such follow-up care.

GASTROINTESTINAL

37 □ Peritonitis

Peritonitis is an inflammation of the peritoneum associated with an irritative or infective offending agent.

Primary peritonitis is an infection de novo, resulting from a blood-borne or lymph-borne spread of an infectious organism that "seeds" the peritoneum. It occurs most commonly in patients with a compromised resistance and immunity to infective organisms. Immunological compromise occurs in patients receiving immunosuppressive therapy or chemotherapy. Chronic diseases that reduce host immunity include cancer; kidney disease (e.g., uremia, nephrotic syndrome); liver disease (e.g., postnecrotic cirrhosis); cystic fibrosis; and lupus erythematosus.

Secondary peritonitis results from direct extension of irritative or infective substances from a ruptured organ or infection outside the peritoneum. Etiological factors may include rupture of a viscus (e.g., from trauma, ulcer disease, ulcerative colitis); gangrenous bowel; extension of an extraperitoneal infection (e.g., pyonephrosis); or pancreatitis.

Postoperative peritonitis occurs occasionally after surgery on the biliary tract, stomach, pancreas, and intestine, particularly if difficulties were encountered during surgery.

Nutritional depletion, fluid and electrolyte imbalance, and the aforementioned risk factors for primary and secondary peritonitis increase the likelihood of postoperative peritonitis.

The pathogenesis of peritonitis involves the entry of bacteria and other offending agents* into the peritoneum where they are normally phagocytosed by macrophages, polymorphonuclear leukocytes, and opsonins and cleared from the blood by the reticuloendothelial system and other systemic defense systems. However, the bacteria and their endotoxins may proliferate in the peritoneal cavity, particularly in hosts with impaired immunity and in the presence of the exudation of a large amount of fibrin-containing serous fluid. In the acute phase the systemic defense mechanisms may be exhausted, resulting in septic, endotoxin shock and a high probability of death.

Pain is the predominant symptom, with rebound tenderness and abdominal muscle rigidity. Abdominal pain, nausea, and vomiting often occur together, with systemic symptoms of fever and chills. Bowel sounds are decreased or absent, representing an evolving paralytic ileus.

In making the diagnosis of peritonitis, a leukocyte count may be helpful, although levels are of equivocal value in patients with acquired immunological deficiency. An initial lavage with a peritoneal catheter can be useful in diagnosis. One liter of Ringer's lactate is infused into the peritoneum, allowed to remain for 5 minutes, and then withdrawn. If the WBC count is greater than $500/mm^3$ or the RBC count is greater than $50,000/mm^2$, intraperitoneal disease is considered present. When the lavage is done, the results are correlated with other laboratory test values (e.g., peritoneal, blood, urine amylase levels) and with the patient's clinical picture to permit the development of an appropriate therapeutic regimen.

An abdominal radiograph may reveal free air in the abdomen in the case of a perforated viscus and/or a diffuse ileus. A chest radiograph is done to rule out pneumonia and to detect atelectasis or a sympathetic pleural effusion.

Medical therapy and nursing care are supportive in nature and include restoration of plasma volume, fluid and electrolyte replacement, pain medication (only after a diagnosis and therapeutic regimen have been formulated), systemic and local (peritoneal lavage) antibiotics, control of the fever, gastrointestinal decompression (nasogastric tube), respiratory support, and provision of adequate nutrition, often with hyperalimentation.

Surgery may be indicated to remove foreign material (e.g., after trauma), to drain an abscess, or to repair a ruptured abdominal viscus, which usually involves the

---

*Viral, tuberculous, or fungal organisms occasionally infect the peritoneum.

321

creation of a colostomy. Placement of drains is an effective surgical method of treatment and prevents many types of secondary peritonitis.

ASSESSMENT

1. History of
   a. Abdominal trauma
   b. Abdominal surgery
2. History, presence, and nature of
   a. Chronic disease(s)
   b. Current or chronic infections
3. Dietary habits
4. Medications taken, particularly corticosteroids, antibiotics, analgesics
5. Physical signs/symptoms
   a. Location, severity of discomfort/pain
   b. Radiation, rebound tenderness, and/or rigidity
   c. Nausea and vomiting
   d. Bowel function abnormalities
   e. Decreased or absent bowel sounds
   f. Inability to pass flatus or feces
   g. Fever
   h. Hypotension, tachycardia, tachypnea; signs and symptoms of dehydration
   i. Thirst and oliguria
6. Results of lab and diagnostic tests, including
   a. Serum protein, albumin levels
   b. WBC count
   c. Sedimentation rate
   d. Amylase levels
   e. Chest and abdominal radiographic studies, which may reveal a perforated viscus as the cause of the peritonitis, dilatation of the large and small bowel with edema of the small bowel wall, or some other abnormality associated with peritonitis
   f. Paracentesis
7. Level of patient/family's anxiety concerning disease process, hospitalization, diagnostic procedures, and therapy employed

GOALS

1. Patient/family's behavior indicates reduction in anxiety with provision of information, explanations and encouragement
2. Infection free, afebrile
   a. Absence of or minimal formation of adhesions
   b. Wound intact; no evisceration
   c. Absence of abscess formation or septic shock
3. Normal bowel function; no ileus
4. Fluid and electrolyte balance within normal limits; weight responds in the desired direction
5. Respiratory function sufficient to maintain
   a. Serum Pa_{O_2} and Pa_{CO_2} within normal limits
   b. Absence of atelectasis, pulmonary infection, pneumonia
   c. Absence of pleural effusion, "shock lung" (adult respiratory distress syndrome)
6. Nutritional intake sufficient to maintain body weight, positive nitrogen balance, and adequate wound healing
7. Before discharge patient/family is able to
   a. Describe specific wound, suture line care as ordered with return demonstration as appropriate
   b. Describe dietary regimen
   c. Describe activity regimen
   d. Describe medication regimen
   e. Identify signs and symptoms requiring medical attention
   f. State necessary information regarding follow-up care

Potential problems	Expected outcomes	Nursing activities
■ Patient/family's anxiety related to Hospitalization Disease process Signs and symptoms Diagnostic procedures Therapeutic regimen Altered family roles Dependency	■ Reduction in level of anxiety with provision of information, explanations, and encouragement	■ Ongoing assessment of level of patient/family's anxiety Assess level of knowledge and understanding of disease process, diagnostic procedures, and therapy employed Explain relationship of disease process to signs/symptoms the patient is experiencing Explain in simple terms the disease process and rationale for various therapeutic interventions Describe diagnostic procedures and what the patient will experience; prepare patient for each Provide opportunity for and encourage questions, verbalization of fears and anxieties Provide comfort measures Encourage participation in care as tolerated Assess reduction in level of patient/family's anxiety with provision of information, explanations, and encouragement

Potential problems	Expected outcomes	Nursing activities

■ Infection, which may be associated with
Peritonitis
Abscess formation localized in subphrenic spaces, pelvis, retroperitoneum
Wound evisceration
Sepsis
Septic shock
Failure of resolution or localization of peritonitis
	■ Afebrile
	Infection free
	Bowel function within normal limits (bowel sounds, flatus)
		■ Prevent by
		  Using aseptic technique when indicated
		  Providing oral hygiene q2 hr
		  Administering prophylactic antibiotics after certain procedures and surgeries if ordered
		Monitor for
		  Fever, hypotension, tachycardia in patients at high risk for development of infection, particularly those who are debilitated and/or malnourished
		  Presence, nature, and progression of abdominal discomfort, pain; carefully document and report
		  Nausea and vomiting
		  Decreased or absent bowel sounds, bowel function
		  Altered level of consciousness (LOC)
		  Abnormal results of laboratory and diagnostic tests, including
		    WBC count with differential, sedimentation rate
		    Serum amylase
		    Serial blood, sputum, throat, urine, and if an abdominal suture line/wound is present, wound cultures
		    Chest and abdominal radiograph results
		Notify physician of abnormalities in the aforementioned
		If problem occurs
		  Serially repeat all cultures
		  Administer antibiotics as ordered
		  Monitor progression of fever and other signs/symptoms
		  Administer wound care using aseptic technique
		  Monitor
		    Serial measurements of abdominal girth
		    For progression, alleviation of abdominal discomfort, pain (local or diffuse)
		    Progression/alleviation of tenderness and rigidity of abdomen
		    Intake and output q1 hr
		    Daily weights
		    Hemodynamic measurements q1 hr until stable (e.g., BP, P, central venous pressure [CVP], and pulmonary artery pressure [PAP] if available; urine output, peripheral circulation)
		  Notify physician of abnormalities in the aforementioned measurements
		  Administer fluid replacement as ordered
		  Administer peritoneal dialysis with antibiotics if ordered
		  To prevent continuing unresolved peritonitis, monitor for the presence of ulcer, excess peritoneal exudate; necrotic, infected bowel; appendicitis; localized abscess
		  Prepare patient for additional diagnostic tests as ordered
		  Surgery may be performed to plicate an ulcer, to remove excess peritoneal exudate, for bowel resection, for appendectomy, or to drain localized abscess
		  Prepare patient for surgery according to plan of care

■ Ileus (paralytic)	■ Bowel sounds within normal limits	■ Prevent by administering therapy to treat peritonitis as ordered
		Monitor for
		  Presence of peritonitis
		  Bowel sounds, bowel function, flatus
		  Abdominal girth q4-8 hr for distention
		  Volume of NG aspirates
		  Weight gain or loss

Potential problems	Expected outcomes	Nursing activities

		If ileus occurs
		    Monitor bowel function, abdominal girths, and weights
		    Assist intestinal decompression with long intestinal tube
		    Administer agents such as suppositories, enemas, neostigmine (Prostigmin) to stimulate bowel function as ordered

■ Respiratory insufficiency related to
Discomfort
Abdominal distention
Atelectasis
Pleural effusion
Acute respiratory distress synrome or pulmonary interstitial edema—may be associated with septicemia; large protein losses into peritoneum, which thus decrease serum oncotic pressure; or result from vigorous fluid resuscitation
	■ Adequate oxygenation and ventilation with arterial blood gas levels within normal limits
	Chest radiograph reveals full lung expansion, without atelectasis, interstitial edema
	No dyspnea
		■ Prevent by
		    Placing patient in semi-Fowler's position
		    Administering pain medication sufficient to permit adequate breathing and coughing
		    Administering chest physiotherapy q2-4 hr while patient is on bed rest; thereafter administering as needed
		    Turning at least q2 hr
		Monitor respiratory status
		    Quality of respirations q1 hr; note tachypnea, dyspnea
		    Serial arterial blood gas determinations for hypoxemia, hypercapnia, acidosis q6-12 hr
		    Breath sounds q1-2 hr for decreased or absent sounds and the presence of rales and/or rhonchi
		    Serial chest radiograph results for atelectasis, pleural effusion, and other abnormalities
		    Serial sputum C and S results
		Monitor daily weights for gain or loss
		Notify physician of any of these abnormalities
		If respiratory insufficiency occurs
		    Assess nature, extent of problem
		    Administer humidified O_2 as ordered
		    Provide for vigorous chest physiotherapy to affected areas of lung
		    Assist with aspiration of pleural effusion, if procedure is necessary
		    Assist with intubation if needed (see Standard: *Mechanical ventilation*)
		    Administer antibiotics and/or steroids as ordered
		    Administer diuretics if ordered; closely monitor patient's response

■ Fluid and/or electrolyte imbalance related to
Fluid losses into peritoneum
GI fluid losses related to decompression and, if present, wound losses
May be associated with development of renal failure
	■ Weight within normal limits
	Normovolemia with hemodynamic parameters within normal limits
		■ Prevent by
		    Administering fluid replacement according to serial weights, hemodynamic parameters, as ordered
		    Administering electrolyte replacement according to calculated losses and measured serum levels, as ordered
		Monitor
		    Daily weights for loss or gain
		    Indices of intravascular volume, including serial measurements of BP, P, CVP, PAP, urine output, peripheral circulation, and mentation; correlate with changes in abdominal girth
		    Serum electrolyte levels q6-12 hr
		    For signs/symptoms of electrolyte imbalance including weakness, lethargy, irritability
		Notify physician of abnormalities
		If fluid and electrolyte imbalance occurs administer plasma, fluids, diuretics, and/or electrolytes as ordered; closely monitor patient's response

Potential problems	**Expected outcomes**	**Nursing activities**

■ Malnutrition, metabolic abnormalities related to
Increased catabolism with loss of muscle mass
Glucose intolerance
	■ Weight within normal limits for patient
	Positive nitrogen balance
	Body muscle mass remains stable or increases in size
		■ Assess nutritional status
		  Diet history
		  State of muscle mass, skin turgor, mucous membranes, hair
		Prevent metabolic abnormalities, malnutrition by
		  Monitoring blood and urine glucose levels and notifying physician of abnormalities
		  Administering glucose supplements and insulin as ordered and closely monitoring patient's response
		  If oral intake of nutrients is limited or absent for an extended period of time, administer IV hyperalimentation early in course of therapy as ordered
		Monitor
		  Daily weights for gain or loss
		  Serial blood, urine glucose; urine acetone levels for signs/symptoms of hyperglycemia and hypoglycemia
		If malnutrition or metabolic abnormalities occur, provide nutrients orally by NG tube or intravenously as ordered

■ Renal failure related to decreased perfusion of kidneys	■ Renal function within normal limits	■ Prevent by
		  Administering adequate fluid intake
		  Administering therapy to provide for adequate cardiac output and renal blood flow
		Monitor
		  For hypovolemia by assessing hemodynamic parameters q1-2 hr
		    Note hypotension, tachycardia, low CVP and pulmonary pressure, and signs of peripheral hypoperfusion
		  Serial weights for gain or loss
		  Fluid intake and output q1 hr; note oliguria
		  BUN and serum creatinine levels daily
		  Urine electrolyte levels
		Notify physician of significant abnormalities
		If renal failure occurs, see Standard: *Acute renal failure*

■ Insufficient information for compliance with discharge regimen*	■ Before discharge patient/family accurately describes
	Activity progression
	Dietary management
	Medication regimen
	Plan for follow-up care
		■ Assess patient/family's level of understanding of peritonitis and therapy employed
		Explain relationship between peritonitis and therapy prescribed
		Describe follow-up plan for
		  Activity levels
		  Diet
		  Medications
		    Purpose
		    Identification
		    Route
		    Dosage
		    Frequency, timing
		Describe untoward signs/symptoms requiring medical attention (individualize description according to patient's problem and need to know), including
		  Fever, flushed feeling
		  Abdominal pain, discomfort
		  Tight abdominal muscles
		  Abdominal distention
		  Decreased bowel function and fewer bowel movements
		  Nausea, vomiting
		  Loss of appetite

*If responsibility of critical care nurse includes this type of follow-up care.

Potential problems	Expected outcomes	Nursing activities
		Describe follow-up plan of care, including purpose of follow-up appointments, where and when to go, what specimens to bring, and what activities will be included in the follow-up visit
		Encourage patient/family to ask questions
		Assess potential compliance of patient/famiy with discharge regimen

38 □ Liver failure/decompressive portovenous shunting procedures

Liver failure is the derangement of one or all of the functioning units of the liver. The extent of derangement depends on how much each unit has been affected, including (1) parenchymal cells, (2) reticuloendothelial cells, and (3) biliary ducts.

The liver aids in initial digestion and emulsification by secreting bile. It controls carbohydrate, protein, and fat metabolism (both anabolism and catabolism) to supply energy to meet the body's needs, build up muscle tissue, and supply proteins and enzymes to perform many important bodily functions. The liver acts as a warehouse by storing glycogen, iron, minerals and metals, and some vitamins (A, B_{12}, D, E, K). The liver metabolizes nitrogenous waste products into ammonia, urea, and bilirubin. Hormones are conjugated in the liver and secreted in bile. The liver protects the body by removing bacteria and by detoxifying endotoxins and drugs.

The liver has a remarkable regenerative power that allows it to recover from such major insults as hepatitis and to regenerate tissue after a major resection. Approximately 70% of the hepatic parenchymal tissue must be damaged before the liver function tests become consistently abnormal. The associated liver dysfunction involves a disturbance in all the normal hepatic functions described before.

Liver failure may result from indirect or direct hepatotoxins or as part of a disease process. Indirect hepatotoxins interfere with a specific metabolic pathway, with a variable latent period followed by hepatitis. Excessive alcohol intake produces an indirect toxic effect by accelerating triglyceride synthesis, which produces an increase in smooth endoplasmic reticulum and intracellular fat deposits, resulting in alcoholic hepatitis with hepatocellular necrosis. Some drugs act as indirect hepatotoxins and, in persons with a hypersensitivity response, produce a similar picture.

Diseases that can produce hepatic dysfunction and failure include hepatitis, Wilson's disease, Budd-Chiari syndrome, metastatic cancer, schistosomiasis, venooclusive disease, extrahepatic vein thrombosis, postanesthesia hepatic failure, glycogen storage diseases, homozygous-familial hypercholia, tularemia, and cryptogenic hepatic failure.

Advanced liver failure is manifested by ascites, hypersplenism, gastric and esophageal varices, hypoproteinemia, and abnormal coagulation studies. Severe portal hypertension may result in variceal bleeding and increase circulatory levels of nitrogenous products.

Prognosis varies according to the severity of liver dysfunction and other body variables. Mortality is high in patients with encephalopathy, ascites, renal failure, and certain lab abnormalities, (i.e., prolonged prothrombin time, hyperbilirubinemia, high BUN levels, and leukocytosis).

DECOMPRESSIVE PORTOVENOUS SHUNTING PROCEDURES

The objective of surgery is to reduce the risk of esophageal and gastric bleeding by lowering the portal esophageal, and gastric venous pressures. Venous blood that would normally traverse the portal vein is diverted into another vein that eventually empties directly into the vena cava. The systemic load of nitrogenous waste products is thereby increased, usually producing some degree of encephalopathy.

Shunts that provide the greatest reduction in the risk of bleeding also divert a greater proportion of blood away from the esophagogastric veins and from the liver and are associated with the greatest incidence of encephalopathy (e.g., portacaval shunts). Other decompressive shunts provide less diversion of blood away from varices and less reduction in the risk of bleeding, but are also associated with a less severe encephalopathy (e.g., mesocaval, splenorenal, coronary/left gastric–caval, splenocaval).

Potential candidates for surgery are rated on the presence of certain prognostic parameters. Parameters that reflect a good surgical risk include albumin levels greater than 3 g/100 ml, bilirubin level less than 2 mg/100 ml, normal or only slightly prolonged prothrombin time, transaminases less than 80 units, alkaline phosphatase normal or only slightly elevated, absence of ascites and advanced encephalopathy, and good nutritional status.

ASSESSMENT

1. History of
   a. Any disease affecting the liver
   b. Amount of alcohol intake on a daily/weekly basis
   c. Exposure to toxins such as carbon tetrachloride
   d. Any injections in the past 6 months, including blood tests, dental treatments, tattooing
   e. Signs and symptoms that suggest cholelithiasis or choledocholithiasis
   f. Dark urine and light stools; jaundice and pruritis; icteric sclera
   g. Anemia; splenectomy, cholecystectomy; congenital or familial hyperbilirubinemia; tremors or neurological abnormalities
   h. Medications taken recently—note those known to affect liver function
   i. Adverse reactions to any drugs taken
2. Presence and extent of
   a. Jaundice—hues
      (1) Muddy yellow: may indicate hemolysis of RBC
      (2) Orange: may indicate parenchymal disease
      (3) Deep greenish: may indicate prolonged biliary obstruction
   b. Icteric sclera

   c. Cachexia, wasting of extremities
   d. Dilated veins in flank, anteroabdominal region; hemorrhoids
   e. Enlarged, nodular, firm liver; or atrophied, small liver
   f. Tender hepatic margins
   g. Enlarged gallbladder (Courvoisier's sign)
   h. Splenomegaly
   i. Asterixis, any neurological abnormalities
   j. Mental, personality changes
   k. Stigmata of cirrhosis
   l. Parotid gland enlargement
   m. Dupuytren's contracture
   n. Gynecomastia
   o. Diminished axillary or pubic hair
   p. Skin ecchymosis
   q. Palmar erythema, spider angiomas; scratch marks, pruritis
   r. Clubbing of nails
   s. Xanthomas
3. Lab data
   a. Serum proteins, including total protein, albumin levels; albumin-globulin ratio
   b. Immunoglobulins; gamma globulin
   c. Coagulation studies, including clotting factors and platelets
   d. Hct, Hgb
   e. WBC count
   f. Bilirubin (total, indirect, direct)
   g. Ammonia
   h. Lipids; esterified cholesterol
   i. Flocculation and turbidity tests
4. If indicated
   a. Bromsulphalein excretion (BSP) study
   b. Ceruloplasmin and copper levels
   c. Schistosomal levels
   d. Antigen for hepatitis B
   e. Urine levels of
      (1) Conjugated bilirubin—glucuronide (note levels above 0.4 mg/100 ml)
      (2) Urobilinogen
      (3) Electrolytes
5. Results of diagnostic tests
   a. Abdominal roentgenography
   b. Liver-spleen scan (scintiscan)
   c. Angiography, venography
   d. Splenoportography
   e. Barium studies of the gastrointestinal tract

f. Emergency celiac angiography and endoscopy for emergency bleeding
g. Endoscopy
h. Laparoscopy
i. Liver biopsy
j. Cholecystography and cholangiography
k. Portal and hepatic vein manometry
6. Anxiety about and understanding of disease process, diagnostic procedures, purpose of hospitalization, therapy planned; if appropriate, surgery and the expected outcome and what the patient will experience in the perioperative period
7. Patient's perception of and reaction to the diagnosis and therapy

GOALS

1. Reduction in patient/family's anxiety with provision of information, explanations, and encouragement
2. Liver dysfunction does not further deteriorate; absence or resolution of coagulation abnormalities
3. Absence or resolution of gastrointestinal bleeding
4. Hemodynamic stability
5. Absence or no exacerbation of encephalopathy
6. Absence or resolution of ascites
7. Electrolyte levels within normal limits
8. Renal function within normal limits; absence of hepatorenal syndrome
9. Respiratory function sufficient to maintain adequate oxygenation, ventilation
10. Absence of emboli
11. Adequate nutritional intake, positive nitrogen balance
12. Patent decompressive shunt
13. Before discharge patient/family is able to describe discharge regimen, including
    a. Medication, dietary, and activity regimens
    b. Identify untoward signs and symptoms requiring medical attention
    c. Describe plan for follow-up care

Potential problems	Expected outcomes	Nursing activities
Medical management		
■ Patient/family's anxiety related to Hospitalization Disease process Therapy prescribed Diagnostic procedures	■ Reduction in patient/family's anxiety with provision of information, explanations, and encouragement	■ Ongoing assessment of anxiety Assess patient/family's knowledge of disease process, therapy prescribed, and diagnostic procedures Explain the disease process and its relationship to the therapy employed Describe rationale for planned diagnostic tests; prepare patient for and, if appropriate, assist with diagnostic tests Provide opportunity for and encourage patient/family's questions, verbalization of fears and anxieties Assess reduction in level of patient/family's anxiety
■ Ascites related to Increased portal hydrostatic pressure Decreased plasma colloid osmotic pressure associated with decreased albumin synthesis Hypovolemia, which may stimulate increased aldosterone production and retention of Na^+ and H_2O by the kidney Increased lymph formation in cirrhosis and in hepatic venous obstruction Loss of newly formed albumin into the free peritoneal space	■ Absence of or resolution of ascites; abdominal girth remains stable or decreases in size Weight remains stable Serum protein, albumin levels within normal limits	■ Administer plasma, colloids as ordered to maintain oncotic pressure, serum protein and albumin levels within normal limits Promote/support liver function (see Problem, Unresolved progressive liver failure: nursing activities, for prevention of liver failure) Salt and/or H_2O restriction if ordered Monitor for Anasarca; presence and extent of edema in various body areas Daily weight changes Serial abdominal girths; note progression of ascites Abnormal serum protein and albumin levels Abnormal serum electrolytes, particularly Na^+ levels Notify physician if the aforementioned abnormalities occur Employ the following measures as ordered Salt restriction, which may be limited to 500 mg Na^+/day (occasionally is limited to 250 mg Na^+/day); because salt restriction limits protein intake to some degree, administer protein supplements in the form of powdered milk low in Na^+ if ordered H_2O restriction is employed for some patients with an impaired free H_2O clearance to help prevent dilutional hyponatremia; may be limited to 1500 ml/day in adults as ordered

Potential problems	Expected outcomes	Nursing activities
		Administer diuretics as ordered; diuretics should be given cautiously so that depletion of extracellular fluid volume does not occur; since capacity to absorb ascitic fluid is limited to about 800 ml/day, depletion of the extracellular fluid volume should not proceed at a rate greater than this
		Monitor for electrolyte loss and imbalance associated with diuretic administration q12-24 hr
		Bed rest may be ordered for patients with ascites; after diuresis has begun, a gradual increase in activity is usually permitted
		Assist with paracentesis, which may be done if abdominal distention is severe; not more than 1000 to 1500 ml of fluid should be withdrawn at a time or hypotension, shock, and encephalopathy may ensue
		Monitor vital signs q1-2 hr
		Monitor for potential complications of paracentesis—hemorrhage, protein depletion, shock
		Protein supplementation
		Administer salt-poor albumin—25 g/day IV for 3 to 4 days, if ordered, to augment intravascular osmotic pull and to enhance movement of ascitic fluid into the intravascular space, thus promoting diuresis
		Corticosteroids
		In addition to diuretics, administer corticosteroids, if ordered, to augment free H_2O clearance in patients in whom the extracellular fluid volume is markedly expanded and hyponatremia is severe; corticosteroids are usually administered for 7 to 10 days in moderate to large doses, then discontinued

■ Encephalopathy precipitated by
  Medications that require liver metabolism
  GI bleeding with an increased protein load
  Hypotension, shock
  Diuretic therapy with associated hypokalemic alkalosis, which increases ammonia production
  Abnormal cerebral metabolism of glucose associated with high ammonia levels
	■ Absence and/or resolution of encephalopathy
	BUN levels remain stable or decrease
	State of consciousness, mentation, behavior, gait, speech, and neuromuscular function remain the same or improve
		■ Avoid the following abnormalities and therapies that can increase ammonia production
		  Administration of ammonium chloride
		  Diuresis of more than 1 to 2 kg/day
		  Dehydration, shock
		  Sedatives, narcotics, tranquilizers
		  Anesthesia, decompressive shunting procedures
		  Infection
		  Acid-base, electrolyte imbalance (avoid hypokalemic alkalosis); if acidification is needed, lactulose may be ordered to acidify the bowel
		Prevent by
		  Administering lactulose, if ordered, to induce movement of ammonia from blood to colon; lactulose also has a laxative action that promotes excretion of the ammonium ion
		  Administering poorly absorbed antibiotics, if ordered (orally, by enema), to reduce nitrogen-forming intestinal bacteria
		  Administering antacids and/or an anti–H_2 medication, if ordered, to reduce the risk of GI bleeding
		  NOTE: If GI bleeding is present, institute therapy to control it; see Standard: *Acute upper gastrointestinal bleeding*
		  Administering fluid volume repletion as ordered, usually including salt-poor albumin
		Monitor
		  Blood ammonia and BUN levels; assist in titrating the patient's protein intake to a level that does not raise circulating ammonia and BUN to unacceptable levels
		  The patient's state of consciousness, mentation, speech, behavior, gait, and neuromuscular function
		  Results of EEG, which may reflect diffuse slowing

Potential problems	Expected outcomes	Nursing activities

		If encephalopathy occurs
		  Maintain safe environment
		  Reorient patient frequently to time, place, and person
		  Explain procedures simply and clearly
		  Avoid medications that depend heavily on liver metabolism: ammonia-containing drugs, amino compounds
		    If sedation is needed, phenobarbital and chloral hydrate are preferred; occasionally diazepam is given in very small quantities
		  Administer a cathartic such as sorbitol in H_2O or magnesium citrate, as ordered, to reduce intestinal flora
		  Reduce dietary intake of protein while providing adequate calories as ordered
		    Low-protein tube feedings are available such as Lipomul-Oral*
		    When protein intake is resumed, start with 20 to 40 g protein/day or as ordered and increase by 10 to 20 g q2 to 4 days as tolerated in adults
		  Administer lactulose (adults: 35 to 70 g/day), if ordered, to produce an acidic colonic pH, which favors movement of ammonia into stool
		    Arginine or glutamic monochloride is sometimes ordered in an effort to inactivate excess ammonia

■ Unresolved, progressive liver failure related to Viral hepatitis—patient may follow a fulminant course
Drug sensitivity
Phosphorous poisoning
Reye's syndrome
	■ Liver dysfunction does not further deteriorate
	Absence of clotting abnormalities, encephalopathy
		■ Monitor
		  For signs/symptoms of liver failure, including progressive jaundice, encephalopathy
		  Serial liver function tests, including serum bilirubin and transaminases (usually 2 times a week in the acute phase), prothrombin levels
		  For abnormal coagulation studies
		  For signs/symptoms of bleeding, including petechiae and ecchymoses
		Assist with liver biopsy (done if diagnosis unclear or patient in prolonged or relapsing hepatitis)
		If bleeding occurs, notify physician; administer therapy as ordered, which may include fresh whole blood, fresh frozen plasma, or products containing only clotting factors, platelets; monitor for transfusion reaction
		Administer corticosteroids if ordered; they may be given to patients with chronic, active hepatitis and hepatic necrosis, and/or in the presence of anorexia, encephalopathy, and clotting abnormalities
		  The effect of steroids on healing and on the progression of the necrotic process has not been conclusively determined
		Institute bed rest until acute liver failure episode subsides (if it does) or until fever abates, abnormal liver function tests begin to show return to normal, and clinical improvement occurs, as ordered
		Monitor results of liver function tests

*Lipomul-Oral, The Upjohn Co., Kalamazoo, Mich.

Potential problems	Expected outcomes	Nursing activities
		Administer or assist with unusual supportive measures as ordered, including exchange blood transfusions, plasma exchanges, hemodialysis or peritoneal dialysis, saline washout, extracorporeal pig liver perfusion, or cross-circulation with human volunteers or primates

■ Malnutrition related to fulminant liver failure and associated with
  Insufficient intake of protein
  Impaired absorption of fat-soluble vitamins
  Macrocytic anemia, vitamin B_{12} deficiency related to
  Hepatitis
  Chronic, active hepatic necrosis
  Acute alcoholic hepatitis
  Anorexia, encephalopathy
  Clotting abnormalities
	■ Sufficient intake of protein for liver regeneration, but not so much that blood nitrogenous waste product levels significantly increase
	Liver function within normal limits
	With medications tailored to specific liver dysfunction, liver function tests return toward normal and clotting abnormalities and/or encephalopathy, if present, subside
		■ The patient's dietary intake of protein should be titrated to toleration for the nitrogen load; if tolerated, the intake may be as much as 100 to 125 g protein/day and 3000 calories/day, with approximately one half of the total calories supplied as carbohydrates; if encephalopathy develops, notify the physician; the protein load should be reduced accordingly
		If patient is in fulminant liver failure, the protein intake may be as little as 20 to 40 g/day, with increments of 10 g every 2 to 3 days if the liver failure is resolving; remainder of diet is moderate in fat, high in carbohydrates; salt restriction is usually needed to limit fluid retention
		  If anorexia impairs food intake, tube feedings may be administered as ordered
		  If adequate intake of nutrients is impossible using these methods, IV hyperalimentation may be employed; see Standard: *Total parenteral nutrition through central venous catheter*
		Administer vitamins, particularly A, D, and K as ordered; B vitamins are often ordered, particularly if a macrocytic anemia is present

■ Hepatorenal syndrome
  Acute renal failure in advanced liver disease may be related to
    Circulating pressor substance that cannot be detoxified by an impaired liver
    The production of vasoactive substances by a dysfunctional liver
    Decreased effective plasma volume associated with ascites
  AV shunts (which may be surgically created)
	■ Absence and/or resolution of hepatorenal syndrome
	Renal function within normal limits
	BUN and creatinine levels are within normal limits
	Absence of hypotension and oliguria
	Serum Na^+ levels within normal limits
	Urinary creatinine and creatinine clearance within normal limits
	Absence of proteinuria
		■ Observe measures to prevent decreased renal blood flow including
		  Slow removal of ascitic fluid during abdominal paracentesis with careful fluid, albumin repletion as needed
		  Avoidance of vigorous diuretic therapy
		  Preparing patient for a Levine shunt, which may be placed to connect the peritoneal space, where much of the ascitic fluid lies, with the vena cava, thus permitting recirculation of ascitic fluid
		Administer therapy as ordered to improve liver function
		Monitor for signs of portal hypertension: ascites, encephalopathy, jaundice, and oliguria; notify physician if any of these occurs; conditions such as urinary obstruction or prerenal failure should be ruled out as causes of oliguria, and treatment should be altered accordingly
		Monitor
		  Serum electrolyte levels for hyponatremia
		  Serum creatinine concentrations (0.7 to 1.5 mg/100 ml is normal)
		  Urine creatinine excretion (25 mg/kg/24 hours is normal)
		  Creatinine clearance (ml/minute), which is the urine concentration × urine volume ÷ the plasma concentration (normal creatinine clearance is 90 to 140 ml/minute)
		  For proteinuria
		Administer dopamine in low doses, if ordered, to augment renal blood flow and to produce natriuresis and diuresis
		Administer antibiotics, if ordered, to reduce circulating ammonia levels
		  In the presence of renal dysfunction, antibiotic doses should be appropriately reduced

Potential problems	Expected outcomes	Nursing activities

■ Bleeding resulting from Esophageal and gastric varices, esophageal laceration, peptic ulcer, gastritis, and, occasionally, carcinoma of the esophagus
 	
Hepatic disease
  Deficient production of clotting factors; coagulopathy
	■ Absence or resolution of bleeding (e.g., GI)
	Hct, Hgb remain stable or, with supplementation of blood products, return to normal limits
		■ Prevent by administering therapy to support/promote liver function and to limit portal hypertension (see Problem, Unresolved progressive liver failure)
		Monitor for
		  Hematemesis
		  Hematest-positive stools and vomitus/NG aspirate
		  Dropping Hct
		  Hypotension, tachycardia
		Notify physician of any abnormality
		If bleeding occurs
		  Administer fluids and blood products to maintain hemodynamic parameters and Hct within normal limits
		  Control bleeding as ordered with iced saline NG lavages and, if necessary, esophagogastric pressure balloons—maintain air pressure in balloons at a predetermined level; see Standard: *Acute upper gastrointestinal bleeding.*
		Prepare patient for and assist with endoscopy and other diagnostic tests or therapeutic procedures as ordered
		Prepare patient for surgery if planned

■ Emboli
  Pulmonary
  Mesenteric
  Renal
  Cerebrovascular
  Coronary
	■ Absence of emboli
	Absence of signs, symptoms of ischemia or infarction of pulmonary, intestinal, renal, cerebral, or myocardial tissue
		■ Administer fluids and blood products as ordered to prevent low, sluggish blood flow and associated ischemia
		Administer low-dose heparinization, if ordered, in high-risk surgical patients
		Provide for early mobilization and ambulation as ordered
		Monitor for
		  Signs of thrombophlebitis, including Homans' sign (calf pain on dorsiflexion)
		  Signs of peripheral arterial emboli
		  Signs and symptoms of various types of emboli (e.g., coronary, pulmonary, mesenteric, renal, and cerebrovascular)
		If embolus occurs, administer therapy as ordered
		For other preventive, monitoring activities and the therapeutic interventions, see Standard: *Embolic phenomena*

■ Insufficient information to comply with discharge regimen*	■ Sufficient information to comply with discharge regimen
	Before discharge patient/family is able to
	  Verbalize knowledge of discharge regimen, including medications, dietary regimen, and activity progression and is able to perform specific therapeutic interventions
	  Identify untoward signs/symptoms requiring medical attention
	  Describe plan for follow-up care, including purpose of visits, when and where to go, who to see, what specimens to bring
		■ Assess patient/family's knowledge and understanding of discharge regimen
		Instruct patient/family as needed in
		  Medications, including identification, dosage, frequency, timing, and precautionary measures
		  Dietary regimen
		  Activity progression
		  Specific therapeutic measures, such as dressings, if appropriate; provide opportunity for practice and return demonstration
		Describe signs and symptoms that require attention
		Describe plan for follow-up care, including purpose of visits, when and where to go, who to see, and what specimens to bring
		Provide opportunity for and encourage patient/family to ask questions
		Assess patient's potential compliance with discharge regimen

*If this type of follow-up care is the responsibility of the critical care unit nurse.

Potential problems	**Expected outcomes**	**Nursing activities**

SURGICAL MANAGEMENT: DECOMPRESSIVE PORTOVENOUS SHUNTING PROCEDURES

Preoperative

■ Patient/family's anxiety related to
  Diagnostic, preparatory tests before surgery
  The surgery, its expected outcomes, and potential problems
	■ Reduction in patient/family's anxiety with provision of information, explanations, and encouragement
	Patient/family verbalizes anxiety and asks questions
	Absence of nonverbal responses suggestive of anxiety
		■ Ongoing assessment of patient/family's level of anxiety
		Assess patient/family's knowledge and understanding of certain diagnostic tests, the rationale for these tests, and what patient will experience
		Explain, in simple terms, disease process, need for surgery, expected outcomes (and associated benefits), and potential problems
		Explain purpose of diagnostic tests and what the patient will experience
		Encourage patient/family to verbalize fears and to ask questions
		Assess reduction in level of anxiety with provision of information, explanations, and encouragement

Postoperative

■ Hemodynamic instability related to
  Hemorrhage
  Fluid depletion from
    Loss of ascitic fluid when the abdomen is surgically opened and/or during paracentesis
    Loss of lymphatic fluid during surgery
    Prolonged NG suctioning
	■ Hemodynamic stability; BP, P, CVP, PAP, urine output, peripheral circulation, and mentation within normal limits	■ Monitor for (q½-1 hr)
		  Hypotension
		  Tachycardia
		  Low CVP and PAP
		  Reduced peripheral circulation
		  Restlessness
		  Signs and symptoms of hemorrhage including
		    Bloody aspirate from NG tube or other drains
		    Increasing tenseness of abdomen and size of abdominal girth
		    Hct, Hgb, platelet, and albumin levels q6-12 hr until stable
		    Daily weights
		    Excessive amounts of NG drainage
		Notify physician of any abnormality
		If hemodynamic instability occurs
		  Administer fluids, fresh whole blood, fresh frozen plasma, platelets, clotting factors, and/or vitamin K as ordered
		  Closely monitor patient's response

■ Shunt closure related to
  Small caliber of shunt
  Low blood flow through shunt (hypotension)
	■ Patent decompressive shunt
	Severe portal hypertension does not recur
		Administer fluids, blood products as ordered
		Monitor for hypotension, increasing abdominal girth, recurring ascites, increasing weight, progressive encephalopathy, signs of increased pressure in esophageal varices, esophageal bleeding
		Monitor indices of liver function for the following
		  Decreasing protein, albumin, and fibrinogen levels
		  Abnormal coagulation studies
		  Elevated bilirubin, ammonia levels
		  Elevated liver enzymes (alkaline phosphatase, transaminases)
		Notify physician of significant abnormalities in any of the aforementioned measurements

■ Abnormal electrolyte levels
  Hyponatremia
  Hypokalemia—often associated with diuretic therapy
	■ Electrolyte levels within normal limits
	Absence of signs/symptoms of electrolyte imbalance
		■ Monitor for
		  Signs and symptoms of electrolyte imbalance
		  Serum and urine electrolyte levels q12-24 hr
		Notify physician of any abnormality
		Administer electrolyte replacement as ordered

Potential problems	Expected outcomes	Nursing activities
■ Progressive liver dysfunction related to Decreased circulation to the liver, which can produce central lobular necrosis with marked deterioration in liver function within 36 hours after surgery A slow progressive deterioration in liver function that may result from deficient hepatic blood supply associated with a bypass operation	■ Liver function tests reveal no postoperative deterioration Absence of encephalopathy, ascites, and bleeding (coagulation disorders)	■ If possible, a decompressive shunt is chosen that does not significantly impair hepatic blood flow, such as the renal-splenic shunt Progressive liver dysfunction is prevented with careful postoperative maintenance of blood flow to the liver by administering fluids and blood products as ordered Monitor for parameters indicating liver dysfunction (encephalopathy, jaundice, bleeding, ascites) Notify physician of any abnormality If liver failure occurs, see Medical management
■ Coagulation abnormalities related to Liver dysfunction with reduction of prothrombin, clotting factors Administration of stored blood in the perioperative period, particularly in the presence of low circulating levels of clotting factors, prothrombin	■ Hgb, Hct levels remain stable without exogenous blood administration Coagulation studies within normal limits Absence of bleeding from mucous membranes or petechiae, ecchymoses	■ Prevent bleeding by using small-gauge needles for injections; maintain indwelling catheters for regular collection of blood specimens Provide for a safe environment Padded siderails can be employed to prevent trauma, hematoma formation Administer vitamin K as ordered to assist in the synthesis of prothrombin Assess extent of coagulation abnormality: presence of ecchymoses, petechiae, any spontaneous bleeding from mucous membranes or puncture sites Monitor (q6-12 hr until stable) Prothrombin, partial thromboplastin times Hct, Hgb, and platelet levels Hematest results on all drainages or specimens including NG aspirates, urine, and stool Notify physician of any abnormality If coagulation abnormalities occur, administer replacement in the form of fresh blood, fresh frozen plasma, and/or platelets as ordered
■ Encephalopathy related to Venous blood, carrying nitrogenous waste products, is shunted away from the liver Protein (nitrogen) load from surgical blood loss and blood remaining in the GI tract from preoperative bleeding Anesthetics	■ Minimal or no encehalopathy after decompressive liver shunt Patient oriented to place and person	■ See Medical management

Potential problems	Expected outcomes	Nursing activities
■ Respiratory insufficiency related to Cerebral depression from anesthesia Encephalopathy Splinting from incisional pain Diaphragmatic elevation from ascites	■ Absence of respiratory insufficiency Full diaphragmatic excursion and lung expansion sufficient to maintain Pa_{O_2} and Pa_{CO_2} levels within normal limits	■ Prevent by Encouraging patient to cough and deep breathe q1 hr Repositioning patient q1-2 hr Administering chest physiotherapy q3-4 hr or as needed Administering incentive spirometry and/or intermittent positive pressure breathing as ordered Administering supplemental humidified O_2 as ordered Administering analgesics as ordered for pain relief and to permit effective pulmonary physiotherapy Administering analgesics that require little liver metabolism, with decreased dosages to prevent mental or respiratory depression Monitor patient's ongoing respiratory status, particularly noting presence of Dyspnea, tachypnea, shallow breathing Difficulty in effective deep breathing, coughing, and/or turning Signs/symptoms of hypoxia Arterial blood gas results indicating hypoxemia, hypercapnia Notify physician of any abnormality If respiratory insufficiency occurs, see Standard: *Acute respiratory failure*
■ Malnutrition	■ Positive nitrogen balance Weight stability or weight gain in the form of muscle mass, not ascites	■ See Medical management Maintain NG aspiration, as ordered, for the first few postoperative days until bowel sounds return Administer antacids to neutralize gastric hyperacidity associated with hypersecretion if ordered Administer nutrients as ordered after surgery (to prevent a sustained negative nitrogen balance)
■ Insufficient information to comply with discharge regimen*	■ Sufficient information to comply with discharge regimen Before discharge patient/family is able to Verbalize knowledge of discharge regimen, including schedule for medications, dietary regimen, activity levels; and perform specific therapeutic interventions Identify untoward signs/symptoms requiring medical attention Describe plan for follow-up care, including purpose for visits, when and where to go, who to see, and what specimens to bring	■ Assess patient/family's knowledge and understanding of discharge regimen Instruct patient/family as needed in Medications, including identification, dosage, frequency, timing, and precautionary measures Dietary regimen Activity progression Specific therapeutic measures (e.g., dressings); provide opportunity to practice and for a return demonstration Describe signs and symptoms that require medical attention Describe plan for follow-up care, including the purpose for the visits, when and where to go, who to see, and what specimens to bring Provide opportunity for and encourage patient/family's questions Assess patient's potential compliance with discharge regimen

*If critical care nurse is responsible for this type of follow-up care.

39 ☐ Pancreatitis

Pancreatitis is a sterile inflammation of the pancreas, which may occur with a mild or fulminant course. It can be classified as either an *acute edematous* or *hemorrhagic (necrotic)* type of inflammation.

Acute edematous pancreatitis includes interstitial pancreatic edema with escape of enzymes into nearby tissues and peritoneal entry. Peritoneal fluid accumulates and is accompanied by tenderness across the upper abdomen, abdominal and back pain, and nausea and vomiting. Lipase causes fatty necrosis of the omentum; blood lipase and amylase levels are elevated.

Acute interstitial pancreatitis may become hemorrhagic where enzymatic digestion of the pancreas is more widespread. Blood escapes into the pancreatic tissue and into the retroperitoneum, resulting in more severe abdominal and back pain, often with clinical signs and symptoms of peritonitis. The peripancreatic tissue becomes necrotic.

The normal function of the pancreas is to produce digestive enzymes for protein, carbohydrate, and fat metabolism and to produce insulin and glucagon for glucose metabolism. This function is altered in patients with pancreatitis, resulting in digestive and metabolic abnormalities.

Pancreatitis can also be induced by alcohol abuse. Alcohol increases gastric and pancreatic secretions, induces duodenal wall inflammation, and stimulates edema and spasm of the ampulla of Vater, thereby producing partial obstruction. Alcohol intake also causes a decreased gastric pH, which stimulates constant secretion of pancreatic juices in the face of a partially obstructed ampulla, resulting in acute edematous pancreatitis and eventually in hemorrhagic pancreatitis and/or in fibrosis.

Other abnormalities that are associated and can precipitate pancreatitis include

Vasculitis of the different vessels in systemic erythematosis
Steroid and/or thiazide therapy
Infectious organisms from the bloodstream, that is, mumps, scarlet fever
Staphylococci food poisoning
Hyperlipemia, hyperparathyroidism
Dietary indiscretion with higher fat intake
Biliary tract stones

Trauma (blunt or penetrating injury in upper abdominal trauma)
Complications of pregnancy
Genetic disorders, that is, defects in renal tubular reabsorption of lysine and cystine

ASSESSMENT

1. History that includes
   a. Alcohol intake—type and amount
   b. Biliary tract disease (''gallstone'')
   c. Duodenal ulcer
   d. Recent abdominal surgery
   e. Recent trauma to abdomen
   f. Hereditary pancreatitis
   g. Hyperlipemia
   h. Any other diseases present
   i. Medications, particularly steroids, diuretics
2. Presence, nature, and severity of
   a. Nausea and vomiting
   b. Abdominal distention, adynamic ileus, constipation
   c. Peritonitis
   d. Fever
   e. Severe intense abdominal pain; determine the location of pain to assist in localizing the lesion in the head, body, or the tail of the pancreas; lesions in the tail are associated with left upper quadrant (LUQ) pain, those in the body are associated with epigastric pain, those in head are associated with epigastric or right upper quadrant pain
   f. Weakness
   g. Distress, restlessness, anxiety
   h. Dyspnea (diaphragmatic instability)
   i. Hypotension, tachycardia, diaphoresis, even shock, with an associated oliguria
   j. Mottled skin, cold extremities
   k. Weight gain or loss
   l. Nutritional status, including dietary history, appearance of mucous membranes, general strength, degree of muscle atrophy
3. Presence of the following signs (most often seen in hemorrhagic pancreatitis and related to extravasation of sloughing tissue)
   a. Grey Turner's sign: bluish green, brown discolo-

ration in the flank (blood in retroperitoneal routes)

 b. Cullen's sign: bluish discoloration around umbilicus (blood dissecting beneath anterior abdominal muscles)

 c. Tetany: tonic spasm of any muscle with occasional generalized convulsions (calcium binds with free lipids)

4. Results of lab and diagnostic tests

 a. Blood amylase, lipase levels

 b. Complete blood count: Hgb, Hct, WBC levels (neutrophils elevated in 90% of patients with pancreatitis)

 c. Electrolyte levels; hyperglycemia or hypoglycemia, abnormal protein, albumin, globulin, bilirubin, and calcium levels

 d. Urine amylase levels—note diagnostic elevation of more than 500 μm/hour in patients with acute interstitial pancreatitis; no elevation in amylase output may be present in patients with hemorrhagic pancreatitis

 e. Urine glucose and fat levels

 f. Fecal fat and trypsin levels, particularly if steatorrhea is present

 g. Chest radiograph for elevation of the left side of diaphragm and left pleural effusion

 h. Abdominal radiograph for presence of distended, gas-filled loops of intestine, signs of paralytic ileus

 i. Arteriography

 j. Biliary tract studies, intravenous cholangiography

 k. Sonogram studies

 l. ECG for presence of transient S-T segment depression, T wave changes

5. Level of patient/family's anxiety related to the disease process, accompanying signs and symptoms, diagnostic and lab tests, therapeutic regimen, and prognosis

GOALS

1. Reduction in patient/family's anxiety with provision of information and explanations
2. Hemodynamic stability
3. Pancreatic stress minimized; function adequate for digestion of nutrients, maintenance of blood glucose within normal limits
4. Adequate intake of nutrients, vitamins to meet calculated daily requirements, weight stabilization or weight gain
5. Respiratory sufficiency, with Pa_{O_2} and Pa_{CO_2} within normal limits
6. Absence of pleural effusions, pulmonary interstitial edema, or pulmonary microemboli
7. Infection free—absence of peritonitis
8. Electrolyte levels and acid-base balance within normal limits
9. Absence or resolution of potential problems, including pseudocyst, cyst, or abscess formation
10. Before discharge patient/family correctly verbalizes postdischarge regimen, including

 a. Medications

 b. Dietary management

 c. Activity progression

 d. Plan for follow-up visits

Potential problems	Expected outcomes	Nursing activities
■ Patient/family's anxiety related to insufficient knowledge of disease process, planned therapeutic intervention, and/or diagnostic procedures	■ Reduction in patient/family's anxiety with provision of information regarding disease process, therapy, and/or diagnostic procedures	■ Assess patient/family's level of anxiety Assess patient/family's understanding of disease process and therapy employed Explain in simple terms the disease process and its relationship to therapy employed Assess patient/family's understanding of diagnostic procedures and results Explain purpose of planned diagnostic procedures and what the patient will experience Evaluate reduction in anxiety
■ Hemodynamic instability, which may be associated with Fluid loss into the peritoneum, retroperitoneal space	■ Hemodynamic stability BP, P, CVP, PAP, peripheral circulation, urine output within normal limits Stable Hct and Hgb	■ Monitor for Extent of hemodynamic instability: BP, P, CVP, and PAP if available (q2-4 hr); daily weight; urine output; peripheral circulation; and mentation Signs of internal bleeding (hemorrhagic pancreatitis) Low Hgb, Hct levels q6-12 hr

Potential problems	Expected outcomes	Nursing activities

Serum, plasma, albumin, blood loss into peritoneum, peritoneal space
Fever
Dehydration from nausea and vomiting
Coagulation defects, with blood loss associated with disseminated intravascular coagulation (DIC)
	Absence of bleeding
	Afebrile
		Measure for increasing abdominal girth q4-8 hr, depending on rate of progression
		Notify physician of any abnormality
		If problem occurs
		  Administer fluid, blood, or blood products as ordered
		  Administer vitamin K as ordered
		  Administer antipyretic agents as ordered
		  See Standard: *Disseminated intravascular coagulation*

■ Pancreatic dysfunction with altered production of digestive enzymes, insulin, and glucagon	■ Minimal pancreatic stress; function adequate for digestion of nutrients and maintenance of blood glucose within normal limits	■ Monitor for (q6-12 hr)
		  Serial serum amylase, lipase levels
		  Urine amylase levels
		  Serial blood glucose levels
		  Signs of hyperglycemia: polydipsia, polyuria, polyphagia, weakness
		  Urine for elevated glucose, acetone levels
		  Digestive disturbances
		  Steatorrhea
		  Nature, severity of clinical signs/symptoms of pancreatitis, i.e., nausea, and vomiting, pain, fever
		Notify physician of any abnormality
		Administer therapy to include
		  NPO in acute phase
		  NG tube to continuous low suction; note character and amount of drainage q2-4 hr
		  Frequent mouth care; apply lubricant around NG tube and nares
		  Evaluate for presence of earaches and parotitis if use of NG tube is prolonged
		  Nonabsorbable antacids q1-2 hr
		  Cimetidine or another H_2 antagonist as ordered
		  Anticholinergics as ordered
		  Antipyretics if needed, as ordered; alcohol sponges, cooling blanket as needed
		  Calm and quiet environment
		Reduce metabolic requirements to a minimum
		  Keep patient resting; bed rest in acute phase
		  Administer sedation if needed, as ordered
		  O_2 therapy if hypoxia develops (reduces respiratory effort)
		Provide adequate nutritional intake with minimal stimulation of pancreas; may be done with IV hyperalimentation
		Administer supplemental insulin and/or enzyme preparations if needed, as ordered
		Administer other medications/agents as ordered
		  Steroids
		  5-Fluorouracil: decreases metabolism of pancreatic cells and production of enzymes
		  Propylthiouracil: decreases metabolism of pancreatic cells and production of enzymes
		  Bile salts to prevent loss of fat in stool and to facilitate digestion and absorption of vitamins A, D, E, and K

Potential problems	Expected outcomes	Nursing activities
■ Malnutrition related to Alcoholism Low vitamin and nutrient intake Abnormal, inefficient metabolism	■ Absence or resolution of malnutrition Weight gain or maintenance Positive nitrogen balance	■ Assess nutritional status and general appearance for presence of Dry, flaky, and cracked skin Tongue—dry and discolored Sunken eyeballs Loss of appetite Lethargy Poor skin turgor; flaccidity Decreased muscle control; tremors and twitching Provide adequate nutritional intake as ordered IV hyperalimentation may be employed in the acute phase, followed by a bland, low-fat, high caloric diet Avoidance of coffee, tea, alcohol, and spicy, hot, or rich foods Supplementary pancreatic enzyme preparations (pancreatin [Viokase], pancrelipase [Cotazym]) and/or insulin may be ordered Vitamin supplements, including vitamin K, may be ordered Ongoing assessment of nutritional status and therapy, including Weight loss or gain Muscle atrophy, weakness Changes in skin turgor Altered mental status—restlessness, irritability, confusion
■ Respiratory failure related to Pain, producing splinting and hypoventilation Atelectasis Respiratory distress syndrome (pulmonary interstitial edema) related to inflammatory process and vigorous fluid administration Pleural effusion with exudation of serous fluid from pancreatic area Microemboli	■ Respiratory sufficiency with adequate oxygenation and ventilation (Pa_{O_2} and Pa_{CO_2} within normal limits) Absence and/or resolution of pleural effusion, pulmonary interstitial edema, or pulmonary microemboli	■ Administer analgesics (usually meperidine and dihydromorphinone [Dilaudid]) as ordered for pain to prevent splinting and hypoventilation Administer vigorous chest physiotherapy q2-4 hr Reposition q1-2 hr Monitor chest radiograph results for presence of atelectasis, pleural effusion, pulmonary interstitial edema, and microemboli every day Provide cool, oxygenated vapor therapy as ordered for adequate oxygenation and humidification of secretions If microemboli are suspected, monitor results of coagulation studies Monitor For pain and associated splinting Respirations for rate and quality q1-2 hr; note tachypnea, dyspnea, wheezing Breath sounds q1-2 hr; note decreased or absent breath sounds or the presence of adventitious breath sounds Secretions for amount, consistency, and color Chest radiograph results for atelectasis, interstitial edema Arterial blood gas results for hypoxemia, hypercapnia, or acidosis If problem occurs, see Standard: *Acute respiratory failure* and, if appropriate, *Mechanical ventilation* and *Positive end expiratory pressure*
■ Peritonitis related to leakage of pancreatic enzymes into peritoneum causing inflammation and infection	■ Absence and/or resolution of peritonitis Afebrile	■ Monitor for signs and symptoms of peritonitis, including abdominal pain, rigidity; fever, elevated WBC count daily If problem occurs, see Standard: *Peritonitis*

Potential problems	Expected outcomes	Nursing activities
■ Electrolyte imbalance related to Hypocalcemia—fatty acids combine with Ca^{2+} Hyperkalemia/hypokalemia from diuretics, vomiting and NG suctioning	■ Electrolyte levels within normal limits Absence of signs, symptoms of electrolyte imbalance	■ Monitor serial serum electrolyte levels Monitor for signs/symptoms of electrolyte imbalance: weakness; altered mental status (e.g., lethargy, irritability); arrhythmias; tetany, particularly from the second or third day in an episode of acute pancreatitis Notify physician of any abnormality If problem occurs, administer electrolyte replacement as ordered
■ Ketoacidosis, which may be related to low insulin levels and diabetes, with incomplete fat metabolism and ketosis	■ Absence and/or resolution of ketoacidosis	■ Monitor (q 6-12 hr) Blood and urine pH levels Abnormal electrolyte levels For glucose and acetone in urine Notify physician of any abnormality If ketoacidosis occurs, see Standard: *Diabetic ketoacidosis*
■ Pseudocyst—a capsule of cellular debris and irritating substances that may lead to Cysts in the pancreas (collection of fluid usually rich in pancreatic enzymes and necrotic tissue, which is enclosed by a fibrous wall) Abscess Bleeding	■ Absence of pseudocyst, cyst, abscess formation	■ Administer antibiotics as ordered to prevent or combat secondary infection and secondary abscess formation Monitor for Pattern (location and intensity), progression of pain and abdominal discomfort Fever q1-2 hr Leukocytosis q6-12 hr Signs/symptoms of large cyst pressing against stomach or colon Notify physician of any abnormality If pseudocyst, cyst, or abscess occurs, surgery may be employed for drainage Prepare patient for procedure
■ Insufficient information to comply with discharge regimen*	■ Sufficient information to comply with discharge regimen Patient/family correctly verbalizes postdischarge medication, dietary, and activity progression regimen Patient/family describes signs and symptoms that require medical follow-up Patient/family correctly describes plan for follow-up visits	■ Assess patient/family's level of understanding regarding discharge regimen Explain in simple terms what pancreatitis is and the purpose of the therapy employed If appropriate, teach about hazards of continued alcohol intake; Alcoholics Anonymous may be recommended If diabetes is present, teach patient how to control this disease (see Standard: *Diabetic ketoacidosis*) Describe signs and symptoms of a recurrent attack of pancreatitis and indicate how and where patient should get help Discuss dietary modifications, including the avoidance of spicy, hot foods; heavy meals (eat smaller, more frequent meals); alcohol, tea, and coffee Discuss the medication regimen, including Identification, dosage, frequency, timing Pancreatic supplement Antibiotics, if being continued Analgesic, if needed and ordered Insulin, if needed Describe progression in level of activity in the postdischarge period Discuss plan for follow-up care, including purpose of visits, when and where to go, who to see, and what specimens to bring Provide opportunity for and encourage questions and verbalization of anxiety regarding discharge regimen Assess potential compliance with discharge regimen

*If critical care nurse is responsible for this type of follow-up care.

40 □ Pancreatic surgery

Pancreatic surgery involves partial or total removal of the pancreas and resection/repair of contiguous organs. It may be performed for several pathophysiological problems, including tumors (e.g., carcinomas), hemorrhagic pancreatitis unresponsive to medical therapy, recurrent relapsing pancreatitis, and complications of acute pancreatitis such as abscess, pseudocyst, and pancreatic ascites.

A *whipple* is a surgical procedure in which a tumor of the head of the pancreas, the adjacent stomach, and the distal portion of the common bile duct are removed. The remaining portion of the common bile duct is sutured to the end of the jejunal segment, and the remaining pancreas and gastric remnant are anastomosed to the side of the jejunal loop. This procedure is performed for tumors invading contiguous organs including adenocarcinomas, beta or alpha cell tumors, and cystoadenocarcinomas. If a whipple procedure is not possible, obstruction and jaundice may be relieved by a cholecystojejunostomy, choledochojejunostomy or in order to divert bile from the gallbladder into the jejunum.

Radiotherapy and chemotherapy may be employed to shrink the tumor and achieve pain relief. Low cure rates associated with partial pancreatectomy have resulted in increasing employment of total pancreatectomy to achieve removal of all cancer cells. This surgery results in less frequent anastomotic disruption but often produces a brittle type of diabetes.

Surgical intervention for hemorrhagic pancreatitis not responding to medical therapy may include debridement of necrotic pancreatic tissues, a choledochotomy, insertion of a T tube for any common bile duct obstruction, and placement of large drains near the pancreas. Surgery may be considered for chronic relapsing pancreatitis to establish a free flow of bile into the duodenum and to eliminate obstruction of the pancreatic duct. This is accomplished by sphincterotomy, or dilatation of the sphincter of Oddi, or reimplantation of the distal end of the duct into a limb of the jejunum.

A vagotomy may be performed to reduce the volume of gastric acid, which can ulcerate a fresh anastomosis.

Trauma may result in a persistent pancreatic fistula formation or delayed formation of a pseudocyst. Fistulas can be surgically treated by implantation of the duct or tract into the duodenum or jejunum; a pseudocyst can be simply drained externally or internally with a cystogastrostomy or cystojejunostomy.

Whenever pancreatic surgery is performed, a gastrostomy attached to suction/gravity drainage may be employed to decrease gastric contents in the duodenum and reduce stimulation of pancreatic secretion. A jejunostomy may be placed for feedings to prevent duodenal stimulation of pancreatic function and/or to bypass duodenal obstruction.

ASSESSMENT

1. Presence, nature, and extent of
   a. Abscess: episodic temperature elevations; elevated WBC count, erythrocyte sedimentation rate (ESR); chest and abdominal radiographs may indicate subdiaphragmatic collection
   b. Pseudocyst: LUQ mass; chest and abdominal radiographs may indicate subdiaphragmatic mass
   c. Pancreatic ascites: abdominal ascites and distention
2. Result of lab and diagnostic data
   a. Elevated alkaline phosphatase, bilirubin levels if common duct obstruction or hepatic metastasis is present; neoplastic obstruction produces higher bilirubin levels than are seen with benign biliary obstruction
   b. Diagnostic secretin stimulation of pancreatic secretions may induce release of malignant cells, collected in the duodenum
   c. Upper gastrointestinal series may reveal invasion (filling defect) by tumor
   d. Angiography of the pancreas often reveals distortion of pancreatic vessels by the tumor and increased vascularization within the tumor
   e. Transhepatic cholangiogram or retrograde cannulation of biliary system may reveal common bile duct obstruction
3. Patient/family's knowledge regarding operative therapy—what they have been told, their expectations, fears regarding surgery and the outcomes, previous experiences with surgery, if any
4. Information and detail surgeon has provided about the need for surgery, the actual surgery to be done, and the expected outcome
5. Patient/family's level of anxiety related to the surgery and prognosis

341

GOALS

1. Reduction in patient/family's anxiety with provision of information and explanations
2. Pancreatic secretory function kept at a minimum, yet adequate for digestion of nutrients and maintenance of blood glucose levels within normal limits
3. Hemodynamic stability
   a. Absence of intraoperative, postoperative hemorrhage
   b. Anastomosis intact
4. Respiratory function sufficient to maintain adequate oxygenation and ventilation
5. Adequate intake of nutrients; weight gain or weight stabilization
6. Infection free—absence of wound infection, peritonitis, or sepsis
7. Prevention of or resolution of potential problems, including pseudocyst, cyst, or abscess formation
8. Before discharge patient/family is able to verbalize
   a. Medication regimen, dietary management, and activity progression
   b. Signs and symptoms necessitating medical attention
   c. Plan for follow-up visits

Potential problems	Expected outcomes	Nursing activities
Preoperative		
■ Patient/family's anxiety related to insufficient information regarding Disease process Medical therapy employed Anticipated diagnostic procedures Surgical intervention	■ Reduction in patient/family's anxiety with provision of information, explanations	■ Assess patient/family's level of anxiety Assess patient/family's understanding of disease process and ongoing medical therapy Explain in simple terms the disease process and its relationship to medical therapy employed Assess patient/family's understanding of diagnostic procedures and results Explain purpose of diagnostic procedures and what the patient will experience Describe the preoperative experiences and therapeutic regimen, including Preoperative Orient patient to chest physiotherapy (call therapist if available) 1. Coughing and deep breathing 2. Incentive spirometry 3. Postural drainage Shave Light dinner, then NPO after midnight Morning bath/shower Preoperative medications Hospital gown Care of valuables Ride to operating room Scrub suits, masks, and hats worn by operating room staff Anesthesia Postoperative Waking up in recovery room/intensive care unit Describe general environment (size of unit, room, etc.) Dull, continuous noises If anticipated, breathing tube that may be temporarily in place Incision with bandage IV, arterial lines ECG monitoring Medicine for discomfort, pain Policy on family visits As patient progresses Tubes out Ambulation Coughing and deep breathing, chest physiotherapy

Potential problems	Expected outcomes	Nursing activities
		Describe responsibility of patient in achieving a speedy recovery by taking an active role in coughing and deep breathing to keep lungs clear and so on Encourage patient/family's questions Encourage verbalization of anxiety, fears related to hospitalization, diagnostic procedures, therapeutic regimen, surgery, and anticipated surgical outcomes Evaluate reduction in patient/family's level of anxiety
■ Malnutrition	■ Weight gain, at least back to preoperative baseline level Positive nitrogen balance Absence or resolution of any signs of malnutrition	■ Assess nutritional status including 　Dietary history 　History of weight loss 　Appearance of mucous membranes 　Skin turgor; dry, flaky skin; spongy gums that bleed easily 　Swollen joints, muscle atrophy Notify physician of presence of these abnormalities Administer nutrients and IV hyperalimentation as ordered SEE STANDARD: *Total parenteral nutrition through central venous catheter*
■ Dehydration	■ Absence and/or resolution of dehydration Patient's appearance including eyes, skin, mucous membranes indicates good level of hydration	■ Assess state of hydration, including 　History of nausea and vomiting 　History of acute weight loss (over hours to 2 to 3 days) 　Appearance of mucous membranes 　Poor skin turgor 　Dull sunken eyes Monitor 　Intake and output q1 hr 　BP, P, CVP, PAP, urine output, and peripheral circulation q½-1 hr until stable 　Daily weights 　LOC q2-3 hr Notify physician of any abnormalities If dehydration occurs, administer fluids as ordered

Postoperative

Potential problems	Expected outcomes	Nursing activities
■ Hemorrhage related to Leakage of pancreatic enzymes, digestive acids during and after surgery, causing a breakdown of vascular (capillary) membranes	■ Absence of hemorrhage Hct and Hgb within normal limits Adequate cardiac output Hemodynamic stability with BP, P within normal limits	■ Monitor 　Vital signs q1-2 hr and prn until stable 　Note hypotension, tachycardia 　CVP and PAP q1-2 hr; note low values 　Intake and output q1 hr; note oliguria 　Hct and Hgb levels q6 hr and more frequently if signs of bleeding occur Notify physician of abnormalities If hemorrhage occurs 　Administer blood and blood products as ordered; carefully monitor patient's response 　Monitor for continued bleeding
■ Pancreatic insufficiency secondary to Initial excessive production/release of enzymes, insulin, glucagon Deficient production of enzymes, insulin, glucagon	■ Blood glucose, urine glucose and acetone levels within normal limits	■ Monitor 　Serum amylase levels daily 　Serial blood glucose levels q6-12 hr and prn 　Urine glucose and acetone levels q1 hr Notify physician of abnormalities in the aforementioned If problem occurs 　Administer glucose and/or insulin as ordered; carefully monitor patient's response SEE STANDARD: *Pancreatitis*

Potential problems	Expected outcomes	Nursing activities
■ Peritonitis 　Occurs in approximately 30% of pancreatectomy patients 　May result from 　　Preoperative peritonitis 　　Leakage of irritating pancreatic enzymes and exudate into the peritoneum during surgery	■ Absence of or resolution of peritonitis 　Abdomen undistended, supple/soft, and pain free 　Afebrile 　Absence of pancreatic enzymes leakage 　Intact anastomosis	■ Prevention 　Administer prophylactic antibiotics if ordered 　Surgery may be planned before preoperative peritonitis ensues 　Monitor 　　For signs and symptoms of peritonitis q1 hr, particularly fever, general abdominal discomfort, nausea and vomiting 　Notify physician of any abnormalities 　If signs and symptoms of peritonitis occur 　　Assist in careful insertion of drains into the operative area, which may reveal exudate indicative of anastomotic rupture, formation of fistulas 　　Assist in dye studies to document further anastomotic defect 　If problem occurs, administer appropriate antibiotics if ordered and assist with local drainage if instituted 　SEE STANDARD: *Peritonitis*
■ Peritonitis associated with ileus and/or abscess formation	■ Bowel function within normal limits 　Absence of or resolution of abscess formation	■ Prevention 　Encourage and assist in early ambulation 　Provide for patent NG tube and maintain on low suction 　Monitor for 　　Presence and nature of bowel sounds q6-12 hr 　　Serial measurements of abdominal girth daily and more often if signs of peritonitis occur 　　Presence/absence of flatus and stool q12 hr 　　Pain pattern q2 hr indicative of peritonitis, ileus, and/or abscess 　　Complete blood count q6 hr for leukocytosis and increased sedimentation rate (during acute phase) 　　Chest and abdominal radiograph daily for detection of subdiaphragmatic and peritoneal abscesses 　Notify physician of any abnormality 　If peritonitis occurs, see Standard: *Peritonitis*
■ Metabolic/digestive abnormality	■ Absence of and/or resolution of metabolic/digestive abnormality	■ Prevention 　Provide for preoperative nutritional supplementation, which may include IV hyperalimentation as ordered 　Administer pancreatic enzyme supplements, if ordered, just before meals 　Administer insulin as ordered 　Monitor for digestive disturbances q12-24 hr 　　Indigestion 　　Steatorrhea (persistent fatty diarrhea) 　　Weight loss 　Notify physician of presence of any of these, and implement changes in therapy as ordered 　If problem occurs, see Standard: *Pancreatitis*
■ Fluid and electrolyte imbalance (see Standards: *Gastrointestinal surgery* and *Pancreatitis)*	■ Fluid and electrolyte levels within normal limits	■ Prevention 　Provide proper hydration and electrolyte replacement if needed, as ordered 　Monitor 　　For signs and symptoms of electrolyte imbalance q1-2 hr 　　Serial serum electrolyte levels q6 hr 　　Accurate intake and output q1-2 hr; daily weights 　Notify physician of any abnormality 　If problem occurs, administer therapy as ordered 　SEE STANDARDS: *Gastrointestinal surgery* and *Pancreatitis*

Potential problems	Expected outcomes	Nursing activities
■ Liver dysfunction related to Obstruction of splenic vein by tumor, causing splenomegaly and segmental portal hypertension with bleeding esophageal varices Obstruction of hepatic veins may cause the Budd-Chiari syndrome (thrombosis of the hepatic veins)	■ Liver function tests within normal limits Coagulation studies, transaminase levels within normal limits Absence of hepatomegaly, icteric sclera	■ Prevention by early detection of precipitating cause and implementation of therapy as indicated Monitor Liver function tests, including total protein, serum albumin levels; fibrinogen, prothrombin levels, coagulation studies; transaminase levels q6-12 hr during acute phase For hepatomegaly, jaundice, icteric sclera q6-12 hr Notify physician of any abnormality If problem occurs, see Standard: *Liver failure*
■ Wound and skin irritation, breakdown, which may result from Contact with irritating pancreatic drainage Malnutrition with poor healing	■ Wound intact, without erythema, pain, and drainage Skin intact, without signs of irritation (redness, swelling) Adequate intake of nutrients, sufficient to maintain weight, considering age and pathophysiological abnormalities	■ Prevention and management Monitor for reddened excoriated skin Administer alimentation for adequate nutritional requirement as ordered Keep skin around wound dry Protect skin by applying A protective agent on skin that repels drainage Peristomal (Stomahesive) pad to form an occlusive protective covering Ostomy bag if drainage is leaking around as well as through a sump drain
■ Pancreatic and duodenal fistulas including biliary fistulas related to Partial anastomotic disruption Distal obstruction Total disruption of anastomosis due to inadequate blood supply to jejunal limb Pancreatic fistula	■ Pancreatic and duodenal membrane intact Absence of or resolution of fistula formation	■ Maintain continuous patent suction system Monitor for Continued large volume drainage (400 to 600 ml) for more than 5 to 8 days Skin breakdown (due to activation of bile and pancreatic enzymes present) Presence of obstruction as evidenced by plain abdominal radiography and upper GI series with contrast media results Signs of subhepatic abscess and/or obstructive jaundice indicating anastomotic disruption Notify physician of any of these abnormalities If problem occurs Administer alimentation as ordered, often including IV hyperalimentation; see Standard: *Total parenteral nutrition through central venous catheter* Administer skin care around fistula, including application of protein powder or agents to protect skin Prepare patient for reconstructive surgery if planned
■ Intra-abdominal abscess related to inadequate drainage and collection of fluid in subphrenic or subhepatic space	■ Absence of or resolution of intra-abdominal abscess	■ Maintain continuous patent suction system Monitor for Spiking fevers; check vital signs, and temperature q1-2 hr Ileus; note quality of bowel sounds q2 hr Abdominal pain and tenderness q6-12 hr Presence of pleural effusion, elevated diaphragm and collection of fluid in abdomen, and distended bowel as evidenced in the daily chest and abdominal radiograph results; note sonogram results if procedure done Elevation in bilirubin and alkaline phosphatase daily Notify physician of any abnormality

Potential problems	Expected outcomes	Nursing activities
		If intra-abdominal abscess occurs Administer antibiotics and fluids as ordered Administer sufficient nutrients, often in the form of hyper-alimentation, as ordered; see Standard: *Total parenteral nutrition through central venous catheter* Prepare patient for surgery if planned
■ Malnutrition related to prolonged absence of adequate nutritional intake Abnormal metabolism of nutrients due to pancreatic dysfunction	■ Weight stable or gain Appearance and character of skin indicates good hydration, sufficient nutrient intake Moist, pink mucous membranes Muscle mass remains stable or increases in size and is firm	■ Determine presence of recent weight loss or gain Assess patient's dietary, beverage intake history Note adequacy of nutritional intake and the intake of foods, beverages that may be related to the present pathophysiology requiring surgery (e.g., amount of alcohol intake and amount of sugar-glucose in diet) Assess present nutritional status, including weight and appearance and character of skin, mucous membranes, muscle mass Monitor daily weights; intake of nutrients as ordered Provide for intake of required/needed nutrients If malnutrition occurs, administer nutrients as ordered, which may include hyperalimentation in the presence of (or anticipation of) extended periods of NPO See Standard: *Pancreatitis* or *Total parenteral nutrition through central venous catheter* as appropriate
■ Insufficient information to comply with discharge regimen*	■ Sufficient information for compliance with discharge regimen Patient/family correctly verbalizes postdischarge regimen regarding medications, diet, fluid intake, and progression in activity levels Patient/family describes signs and symptoms that require medical follow-up Patient/family correctly describes plan for follow-up visits	■ Assess level of patient/family's understanding of discharge regimen Explain in simple terms the patient's pathophysiological problem and rationale for the postdischarge regimen If appropriate, explain hazards of continued alcohol intake; Alcoholics Anonymous may be recommended Discuss importance of dietary modifications, including avoidance of spicy, hot foods, heavy meals, alcohol, tea, and coffee If diabetes is present, teach patient how to control this disease (see Standard: *Diabetic ketoacidosis*) Instruct patient/family about prescribed medications, including identification, dosage, frequency, timing Pancreatic supplement Antibiotic, if being continued Analgesic, if needed Insulin, if needed Discuss signs and symptoms of recurrence and indicate how/where patient should seek medical attention Explain plan for follow-up care, including purpose of the visits, when and where to go, who to see, and what specimens to bring Assess patient/family's potential compliance with the discharge regimen

*If responsibility of critical care nurse includes discharge teaching.

41 □ Acute upper gastrointestinal bleeding

Patients bleeding from the upper gastrointestinal tract are always at risk of death from exsanguination and shock.

The clinical manifestation of upper gastrointestinal bleeding varies with the underlying disease and extent of bleeding. Overt clinical manifestations are usually present including hematemesis, melena, and hematochezia (which is the passage of bright red blood from the rectum).

Hematemesis of bright red or dark red blood indicates that the origin of bleeding is above the ligament of Treitz, usually in the stomach and esophagus. Hematemesis indicates a rapidly bleeding lesion, and generally surgery is required in a high percentage of patients. Coffee ground vomitus is blood that has been in the stomach long enough for the gastric acid to convert hemoglobin to methemoglobin. This does not indicate origin or time of bleeding.

Melena (which is the passage of tarry black stools) is indicative of bleeding from the upper gastrointestinal tract. The appearance of melena, however, is not an accurate gauge of the time in which bleeding has occurred. It is thought that melena is the product of oxidation of heme by intestinal and bacterial enzymes.

Hematochezia may occur as a result of rapid intestinal transit of blood from the gastrointestinal tract. The presence of blood in the stomach often produces increased gastric motility with gastric retention, vomiting, and hematochezia.

Orthostatic changes in blood pressure, pulse, and a low-value hematocrit are reliable indices of hemodynamic compromise in acute bleeding but may indicate a fluid loss that is underestimated. Renewed or major loss of circulating blood volume is evidenced by tachycardia; restlessness; pallor; diaphoresis; cool, clammy skin; and thirst.

The most common causes of upper gastrointestinal hemorrhage include

Esophagus—esophageal varices; Mallory-Weiss syndrome

Stomach—gastritis secondary to alcohol and drug intake; gastric ulcers; gastric varices

Duodenum—duodenal ulcer

Esophageal or gastric varices are frequently related to the portal hypertension associated with liver cirrhosis.

Although bleeding tends to be massive and abrupt, minor bleeding can occur for days before detection.

The Mallory-Weiss syndrome is a longitudinal laceration of the mucosa near the esophagogastric junction associated with nonbloody vomiting followed by hematemesis after episodes of forceful retching.

Gastritis can include either generalized or localized erosions or ulcerations of the gastric mucosa associated with hyperacidity related to alcohol intake, drug ingestion, or stressful situations.

Ulcers are the most common cause of upper gastrointestinal bleeding. The majority of these ulcers are found in the duodenum. About 25% of patients with ulcers will have at least one episode of gastrointestinal bleeding.

Therapy is directed toward maintaining intravascular volume, stopping the hemorrhage, and defining the source of bleeding within a reasonable period of time.

ASSESSMENT

1. Baseline data regarding clinical history of
   a. Ulcer disease or epigastric pain relieved by food, milk, or antacid
   b. Previous bleeding episodes, vomiting, diarrhea, cramps, weight loss, fever, bleeding from other sites, that is, skin, mucous membrane, etc.
   c. Family history of intestinal disease or hemorrhagic diathesis
   d. Recent ingestion of drugs known to irritate gastric mucosa
   e. Alcoholism; recent alcoholic binge
   f. Jaundice
   g. Forceful retching before hematemesis
   h. Frequent stressful and anxiety-provoking situations
   i. Smoking; number of packs per day
   j. Dietary habits
   k. Seasonal occurrence
   l. Associated diseases including hyperparathyroidism, polycythemia vera, chronic liver disease, chronic respiratory disease, uremia, and any malignancy, that is, presence of rectal shelf, etc.
2. Presence, extent, and/or nature of
   a. Nonintestinal source of bleeding, that is, rule out hemoptysis, epistaxis, and any pharyngeal lesions
   b. Associated conditions including signs of liver dis-

ease: jaundice, telangiectasia, spider angiomas, hepatomegaly, ascites, edema, and unusual skin pigmentation

   c. Abdominal masses, nodes, and hepatospleno-megaly

   d. Dilated veins in flank, anteroabdominal region, hemorrhoids

   e. Any obvious neurological or personality abnormalities

   f. Frequency and character of vomitus and bowel sounds

   g. Cachexia, especially of extremities

3. Baseline lab and diagnostic data for

   a. Abnormal serial blood counts particularly leukocytosis; low Hct and Hgb; and red cell morphological abnormalities

   b. Abnormal serum electrolytes

   c. Serial BUN measurements for elevation

   d. Abnormalities in clotting studies

   e. Extent of positive Hematest of gastric aspirate, vomitus, and stool

   f. Results of endoscopic procedures

   g. Angiography and upper gastrointestinal studies if done

   h. Abdominal radiograph for any visible free air

4. Patient/family's perception of and reaction to disease process, symptoms, diagnostic procedures, and therapy planned

5. Patient/family's understanding of disease process,

purpose of hospitalization, therapy planned, expected prognosis, and, if appropriate, the surgery, expected outcome, and what the patient will experience in the perioperative period; if patient is an alcoholic, assess psychosocial effect on patient/family

GOALS

1. Reduction of patient/family's anxiety with provision of information and explanations

2. Absence and/or resolution of gastrointestinal bleeding

3. Absence and/or resolution of any complications including pulmonary edema, renal failure, and coagulopathy

4. Hemodynamic stability

5. Complete blood count, acid-base balance, and electrolyte levels within normal limits

6. Absence of any further deterioration of associated diseases related to upper gastrointestinal bleeding

7. Nutritional intake sufficient to maintain body weight and positive nitrogen balance

8. Before discharge patient/family is able to

   a. Describe medication regimen

   b. Describe dietary regimen

   c. Describe activity regimen

   d. List signs and symptoms requiring medical attention

   e. State necessary information regarding follow-up care

Potential problems	Expected outcomes	Nursing activities

■ Anxiety related to hemorrhage	■ Patient demonstrates decreased level of anxiety with provision of emotional support and information	■ Assess level of anxiety
		Demonstrate interest and concern
		  Reassure and stay with the patient
		  Explain all procedures before administering them
		  Perform procedures in an unhurried manner
		  Maintain calm and pleasant manner whenever ministering to patient
		Encourage verbalization of any anxiety or fears related to hemorrhage
		Prepare patient for and assist in diagnostic procedures
		Provide an environment conducive to mental, physical, and emotional rest
		  Keep patient dry, warm, and comfortable
		  Allow for rest periods between treatments
		  Limit visitors according to patient's needs; inform visitors to avoid upsetting conversations

■ Anxiety related to insufficient knowledge of Disease process Diagnostic procedures Therapy employed	■ Patient/family's behavior demonstrates decreased level of anxiety with provision of information and explanations	■ Ongoing assessment of anxiety Describe nature of disease process and rationale for various therapeutic interventions Explain anticipated procedures involved in diagnostic process/plan of care and what patient will experience Assure that proper preparation is made before any diagnostic procedures

Potential problems	Expected outcomes	Nursing activities
	Patient/family verbalizes understanding of disease process and its relationship to therapy employed Patient/family participates actively in planning and implementing care	Encourage patient/family's questions, verbalization of fears and anxieties Involve patient/family in planning for care

■ Hemorrhage	■ Control or resolution of hemorrhage
	Absence of blood volume deficit
	Normal circulating blood volume
		■ Monitor for
		  Any transfusion reactions
		  Hypoperfusion or hemodynamic instability including
		    Orthostatic vital signs and temperature q30 min until stable or as frequently as indicated by condition
		    Measurement of CVP, cardiac output, pulmonary pressures if available until stable q1 hr
		    Presence of tachycardia, diaphoresis, cold, clammy extremities, daily weights below what is expected
		    Oliguria, hourly intake and output until stable
		    Frequency, amount, nature of hematemesis and melena
		  Signs and symptoms of respiratory distress
		  Giddiness, restlessness, syncope, and any alterations in LOC
		  Arrhythmias, especially atrial arrhythmias
		  Serial blood count; Hct, and Hgb
		  Serial electrolytes; elevated BUN, ESR, etc.
		  Presence or absence and nature of bowel sounds
		  Clinical manifestations of perforation, including
		    Severe persistent abdominal pain, increasing in intensity
		    Pain radiating to shoulder
		    Boardlike rigidity, extremely tender abdomen
		    Abdominal radiographs showing presence of free air under diaphragm
		  Notify physician of any abnormalities
		Administer continuous, chilled saline lavage until clear with continuous suction
		Maintain parenteral fluids, blood expanders, and blood as ordered
		Administer medications, i.e., vitamins K and B_{12}, sedatives, antacids, and H_2 inhibitors if ordered
		Maintain patent airway, position to sides, aseptic suctioning if necessary; administer O_2 if ordered; frequent oral hygiene
		Reassure and stay with patient
		Endoscopy and angiography may be done to determine etiology of hemorrhage and to tailor therapy
		  Explain procedure
		  Assist with procedure
		If surgery is indicated, see Standard: *Gastrointestinal surgery*

■ GI distress related to
 	
Gastritis secondary to alcohol and drug abuse
Ulcers—gastric and duodenal
	■ Absence or remission of
	Gastritis
	
	Ulcers
		■ Refer to Problem, Hemorrhage, for parameters permitting detection of hemorrhage and activities for control
		Intra-arterial or IV infusion of vasopressin (Pitressin) may be ordered specifically for patients with gastritis
		Monitor for vasopressin (Pitressin) side effects, including
		  Facial pallor, discomfort, abdominal colic, hypertension, abnormal ECG, chest pain, abdominal tenderness and distention, oliguria, and hyponatremia
		  Catheter insertion site for infection, thrombosis, and embolism

Potential problems	Expected outcomes	Nursing activities
		Administer cimetidine and H$_2$ inhibitor if ordered
		Administer an antacid (that does not contain aluminum hydroxide and/or calcium carbonate) q1 hr as directed
		Administer anticholinergic drugs and sedatives if ordered specifically for patients with ulcers
		If surgery is indicated, see Standard: *Gastrointestinal surgery*
		Institute dietary regimen appropriate for gastric problem
		Provide an environment conducive to physical and mental rest
		Allow for rest periods between treatments
		Limit visitors; inform them of need to avoid upsetting conversations
		Monitor effectiveness of therapy/intervention
		Evaluate for health teaching regarding control of excessive drug and/or alcohol intake
Mallory-Weiss syndrome	Complete occlusion of tear either by embolization or surgical repair	Refer to Problem, Hemorrhage, for parameters permitting detection of hemorrhage and activities for control
		If embolization therapy is required
		Explain procedure to patient
		Prepare and shave area as ordered
		Postembolization monitoring activity same as in Problem, Hemorrhage, with decreasing frequency as condition stabilizes
		If surgery is required, see Standard: *Gastrointestinal surgery*
Varices—esophageal and/or gastric	Absence or resolution of bleeding from varices	Refer to Problem, Hemorrhage, for control of hemorrhage
		Monitoring activity same as in Problem, Hemorrhage, decreasing in frequency as condition stabilizes
		Administer arterial or IV infusion of vasopressin (Pitressin) if ordered
		Monitor for side effects of vasopressin (Pitressin) therapy (see Problem, GI distress: Nursing activity—monitor for vasopressin (Pitressin) side effects
		Sengstaken-Blakemore (SB) tube may be employed
		Assist in insertion of SB tube
		Check patency of each lumen
		Check gastric and esophageal balloon for weak spots and leaks under H$_2$O after air inflation
		Explain procedure to patient
		Stay and reassure patient while tube is being inserted
		Once in place ensure proper inflation of balloon
		Gastric balloon is usually inflated with 200 to 500 cc of air; esophageal balloon is inflated with air to level of 30 to 40 mm Hg pressure—attached to a sphygmomanometer
		Secure tube in place and connect to intermittent suction
		Keep a pair of scissors taped at bedside for emergency deflation of SB tube in case of acute respiratory distress secondary to occlusion of airway by balloon
		Assist with radiograph for proper placement of SB tube
		Assist in insertion of NG tube to remove secretions coming from mouth if patient is unable to cough oropharyngeal secretions; connect NG tube to low suction
		Monitor for respiratory distress
		Ongoing care
		Maintain traction on SB tube if ordered
		Irrigate SB tube q1 hr and prn for patency with cold sterile H$_2$O or saline; note color, amount, and nature of aspirate; continuous gastric lavage may be ordered
		Check patency of NG tube q1 hr; irrigate with saline solution if necessary

Potential problems	Expected outcomes	Nursing activities
		Check for prescribed pressure readings q½-1 hr and that lumens of SB tube are secured properly
		Deflate and inflate esophageal balloon if ordered
		Monitor for
		Gross bleeding q1 hr
		Abnormal vital signs q15-30 min
		Lethargy, drowsiness, confusion, and unconsciousness
		Chest pain, any respiratory distress
		Serial Hct, Hgb, and electrolyte levels
		Keep head of bed elevated to 30 degrees unless patient is in shock
		Mouth and nares care q1 hr and prn
		Position to sides q1-2 hr and provide skin care
		Instruct patient not to gag, cough, or strain
		Reassure patient/family
		Encourage deep breathing exercise q1 hr
		Assist in removal of SB tube, usually 24 hours after bleeding has been controlled
		Notify physician of any abnormality
		If surgery is indicated, see Standard: *Gastrointestinal surgery*
■ Pulmonary edema due to fluid overload	■ Absence or resolution of pulmonary edema Normal respiration pattern No obvious sign of chest congestion	■ Prevent by cautious administration of colloid and crystalloid solution with careful monitoring of hemodynamic response
		Monitor for
		Sudden coughing, restlessness, and anxiety
		Marked dyspnea and orthopnea, tachycardia
		Cyanosis, audible wheezing, and rales throughout lung fields
		White or pink-tinged frothy sputum
		Abnormal arterial blood gas levels
		Any tachyarrhythmias
		Hypotension and/or hypertension
		Accurate intake and output, daily weights
		Abnormal CVP, cardiac output, and pulmonary pressures if available
		Notify physician of any abnormalities
		If problem occurs, see Standard: *Acute respiratory failure*
■ Coagulopathy and/or continued bleeding as a result of massive transfusion reaction	■ Absence of and/or control of coagulopathy No continued bleeding Bleeding stops and does not recur	■ Prevent by administration of platelets and fresh frozen plasma (about 1 unit per 3 to 4 units of banked blood) to replace the factors necessary for coagulation
		Monitor for
		Serial blood counts for leukocytosis, low Hgb and Hct; abnormal prothrombin and thrombin time, fibrinogen levels, bleeding tests, and immunoassay tests
		Continuous gross bleeding: hematemesis and hematochezia
		Any spontaneous skin discoloration including petechiae, bruises
		Prolonged bleeding or oozing of injection sites, hematoma
		Presence of hematuria
		Notify physician of any abnormality
		If problem occurs, see Standard: *Disseminated intravascular coagulation*

Potential problems	Expected outcomes	Nursing activities
■ Renal failure related to decreased renal perfusion	■ Absence and/or resolution of renal failure	■ Prevent by 　Careful administration of colloid and crystalloid solution 　Monitoring for adequate urine output Monitor for 　Hypotension, BP q1 hr until stable 　Oliguria and/or polyuria; accurate hourly intake and output 　Abnormal CVP, cardiac output, and PAP if available 　Serial blood and urinary electrolyte levels 　Serial increase in BUN and creatinine levels 　Any alterations in LOC 　Presence of albumin in urine, high specific gravity, and urine-to-plasma creatinine concentration (ratio is usually greater than 20) 　Notify physician of any abnormality If problem occurs, see Standard: *Acute renal failure*
■ Insufficient information to comply with discharge regimen*	■ Sufficient information to comply with discharge regimen Patient/family verbalizes dietary, medication, and activity regimens	■ Assess patient/family's level of understanding and ability to comprehend; determine any physical limitations regarding follow-up plan of care or discharge regimen Describe discharge regimen, including 　Dietary regimen—antacids may be ordered to prevent mucosal irritation between meals 　Explain therapeutic diet and need for good eating habits, including 　　Nutritionally adequate diet 　　Meals to be eaten in a quiet, relaxed environment 　　Frequent small feedings; do not miss a meal 　　Foods to be chewed well 　　Avoidance of irritating and hard-to-digest foods including fried foods, coffee, highly seasoned foods, and alcohol 　　Need for bland diet and foods high in fat to neutralize acid 　　Assist patient/family in planning diet 　　Adjust diet to cultural and socioeconomic needs 　　Vitamins may be ordered 　Medication regimen 　　Names of drugs and purpose 　　Specific dosage schedule in hours, considering patient's eating habits 　　Expected adverse side effects, how to deal with them, and when to report to physician 　　Avoidance of medications that will irritate the esophageal and gastric mucosa, including aspirin, etc.; if necessary take them with meals, milk, or crackers 　　Avoidance of over-the-counter medications 　Activity regimen 　　Planned and regular exercise and rest activities; avoidance of fatigue 　　Avoidance of certain activities such as eating a heavy meal, 　　Avoidance of straining at stool due to constipation, heavy lifting, severe coughing, and vomiting 　　Avoidance of smoking to prevent increase of gastric acid 　　Encourage family involvement with activity progression
	Patient/family describes signs and symptoms that will require medical intervention	Identify signs and symptoms of 　Early bleeding 　　Dizziness and blurred vision 　　Coffee ground vomitus

*If critical care nurse is responsible for this type of follow-up care.

Potential problems	**Expected outcomes**	**Nursing activities**
	Patient/family verbalizes information on Alcoholics Anonymous association	Sudden or gradual weakness
		Dark stool, heme positive on testing
		Common colds and/or respiratory distress requiring medical attention
	Patient/family accurately describes plans for follow-up care	Provide information and referral services for available community resources to patient/family (e.g., Alcoholics Anonymous)
		Describe follow-up visits including reason for, when and where to go, who to see, and what specimens to bring
		Provide opportunity for and encourage patient/family's questions and verbalization of anxiety regarding discharge regimen
		Assess patient/family's potential compliance with discharge regimen

42 □ Gastrointestinal surgery

Gastrointestinal surgery is performed when medical management is inadequate to control the adverse signs and symptoms of certain gastrointestinal abnormalities. Surgery may also resolve or at least halt the progress of gastrointestinal problems.

Operative therapy may be used to treat gastric or duodenal ulcers* in patients with the following conditions: intractable ulcers (recurrent despite therapy) and in the presence of perforation, hemorrhage, and gastric outlet obstruction. A duodenal ulcer may be treated with pyloroplasty and vagotomy or antrectomy with vagotomy. A gastric ulcer is treated by plication or by a partial or total gastrectomy with either a gastroduodenostomy (Billroth I) or gastrojejunostomy (Billroth II).

Tumors are removed if they are malignant or if they are benign but are causing bleeding, obstruction, and intussusception. Gastric neoplasms are removed by partial or total gastrectomy. Small adenomas and mucosal excrescences may be removed by surgical excision using cold forceps and diathermy.

Surgery is frequently required to resolve obstructive conditions of the gastrointestinal tract, including simple mechanical obstruction and strangulation obstruction. Lesions that can produce bowel necrosis may also require surgery, such as a hernia, volvulus, intussusception, obturation, and complete obstruction caused by

*For medical management of ulcers, see Standard: *Acute upper gastrointestinal bleeding.*

chronic adhesions. Surgery may also be necessary for a partial obstruction that does not adequately respond to medical decompressive efforts.

A superior mesenteric artery embolus can cause a "vascular obstruction" and necrosis of the bowel in that region. Early surgical intervention may permit adequate resolution with a mesenteric embolectomy, although a resection of the severely ischemic or necrotic bowel is usually required.

Regional enteritis, including regional ileitis, regional enterocolitis, and Crohn's disease are inflammatory diseases that commonly occur in the terminal ileum, although they may occur anywhere along the gastrointestinal tract. Surgery is indicated when medical management fails to control symptoms or when complications, including obstruction, bleeding, colonic perforation, or fistula formation, occur. If surgery becomes necessary in a period of acute exacerbation, a temporary ileostomy may be created.

Diverticulosis and diverticulitis are treated with surgery if any of the following occur: perforation, obstruction, fistula formation to surrounding tissue, massive hemorrhage, and chronic or recurrent symptoms. In general, surgery is avoided during an acute attack. Rather, antibiotics are administered and the inflammatory process is given time to subside. (If surgery appears to be necessary, it is postponed for 3 to 6 months whenever possible.) *If* acute symptoms persist for 1 week or more, surgery is usually indicated and may include the establishment of a transverse colostomy and drainage of any collections or abscesses present.

Essential components of the postoperative regimen include gastrointestinal decompression of the bowel (until function resumes) and careful fluid and electrolyte replacement. Much of the nursing care is focused on prevention of and monitoring for potential postoperative problems, with appropriate revision of the plan of care should any occur.

ASSESSMENT

1. History, presence, and nature of
   a. Factors that predispose to intestinal obstruction
      (1) Previous abdominal surgery
      (2) Presence of marked adhesions
      (3) Abdominal injuries or wounds
      (4) Peritonitis
      (5) Volvulus, intussusception, diverticulitis, adenoma, or carcinoma of colon or rectum
   b. Factors that predispose to paralytic ileus
      (1) Recent abdominal surgery
      (2) Blunt trauma to abdomen
   c. Factors that predispose to vascular obstruction
      (1) Aneurysm of aorta
      (2) Severe atherosclerosis of aorta
      (3) Low cardiac output, atrial fibrillation, congestive heart failure
   d. Inflammatory diseases that can produce an obstruction or require primary resection
      (1) Ulcerative colitis
      (2) Regional enteritis
      (3) Diverticulitis and diverticulosis
   e. Abnormalities that require primary resection or surgical revision
      (1) Upper gastrointestinal hemorrhage
      (2) Peptic ulcer disease
      (3) Appendicitis
      (4) Diverticula
      (5) Familial intestinal polyposis
      (6) Small bowel fistulas
      (7) Hemorrhoids
2. Signs and symptoms, including
   a. Abdominal pain—manner of onset, location, radiation and intensity; note pain that is
      (1) Continuous—may indicate strangulation, peritonitis
      (2) Crampy
   b. Abdominal tenderness, rebound tenderness
   c. Abdominal rigidity (muscles over area of inflammation become spastic)
   d. Abdominal distention
   e. Bowel sounds—hyperactive, borborygmus, diminished, or absent
   f. Anorexia, nausea and/or vomiting
   g. Gastrointestinal bleeding
      (1) Hematemesis
      (2) Bloody mucus in rectum (may indicate intussusception—more common in children)
      (3) Bloody diarrhea (mesenteric infarction)
   h. Signs of recent abdominal trauma—wounds, contusions, lacerations
   i. Signs of rupture of hollow viscus (bladder, peritoneum)
   j. Signs of rupture of solid viscus ([spleen, liver, kidney] see Standard: *Multiple trauma*)
   k. Fever
   l. Tachycardia
3. Lab and diagnostic data, including
   a. WBC count with differential—note presence of leukocytosis
   b. Electrolyte imbalance
   c. Stool test positive for occult blood
   d. Chest radiograph (upright, posterior, anterior) and abdominal radiograph (upright and supine)—note results indicating free air or intestinal obstruction
   e. Peritoneal tap after abdominal trauma; note presence of blood and results of gram stain, amylase determination, and culture
   f. Urinalysis for WBC and RBC counts
   g. Liver function tests (particularly in the presence of gastrointestinal bleeding)
      (1) Coagulation study results
      (2) Transaminase levels
      (3) Alkaline phosphatase levels
      (4) Serum total protein, albumin levels
      (5) Albumin-globulin ratio
      (6) Blood ammonia levels
   h. Esophagogastroscopy
   i. Gastroduodenoscopy
   j. Fiberoptic endoscopy (if patient is not bleeding massively)
   k. Abdominal scans
   l. Arteriograms (trauma, vascular obstruction)
   m. Dye studies (ulcer disease, occasionally in obstruction)
4. Patient/family's understanding and level of anxiety regarding disease process, purpose of hospitalization, and therapy planned, including potential surgery and expected outcome

5. Patient/family's knowledge regarding operative therapy
   a. What they have been told
   b. Their expectations
   c. Previous experiences with surgery

GOALS

1. Reduction in patient/family's anxiety with provision of information, explanations, and encouragement
2. Gastrointestinal function within normal limits
   a. Anastomosis intact
   b. Normal peristalsis—absence of ileus
   c. Absence of intestinal obstruction, marginal ulceration, dumping syndrome, or "nine-day" syndrome
3. Hemodynamic stability
   a. BP, P within patient's normal limits
   b. Absence of intraoperative or postoperative hemorrhage
4. Respiratory function sufficient to maintain Pa_{O_2} and Pa_{CO_2} within patient's normal limits
5. Infection free; patient afebrile; no wound infection, peritonitis, or sepsis
6. Patient/family verbalizes understanding of disease condition, signs and symptoms, and specific therapy
7. Before discharge patient/family is able to describe accurately
   a. Medication regimen
   b. Dietary alterations and activity progression
   c. Signs and symptoms requiring medical attention
   d. Plan for follow-up visits

Potential problems	Expected outcomes	Nursing activities
■ Patient/family's anxiety related to Disease process Medical therapy Need/purpose for surgery Expected surgical outcomes Diagnostic procedures	■ Patient/family demonstrates decreased anxiety with provision of emotional support, encouragement, and explanations Patient/family verbalizes understanding of disease process and its relationship to therapy employed Patient/family participates actively in planning and implementing care	■ Ongoing assessment of patient/family's level of anxiety Assess patient/family's level of understanding of disease process and therapeutic regimen Explain in simple terms disease process, medical management, need/purpose for surgery, and expected outcomes Describe in simple terms the purpose of diagnostic procedures and what the patient will experience Encourage verbalization of questions, anxieties, and fears Provide emotional support, appropriate encouragement Encourage patient/family's participation, including decision making, in care Evaluate for reduction in level of patient/family's anxiety
■ Obstruction Small bowel obstruction related to Adhesions (account for 30% to 40% of small bowel obstruction) Volvulus Intussusception Internal hernia Large bowel obstruction related to Neoplasm Volvulus of sigmoid colon Strangulated hernia	■ Absence and/or resolution of small bowel obstruction Absence and/or resolution of large bowel obstruction	■ Prevention Evaluate the progression of signs and symptoms of the patient with "an acute abdomen" Correlate signs and symptoms to assist in diagnostic process and for appropriate therapeutic intervention Monitor for Signs and symptoms indicating bowel obstruction q1 hr and prn, including Persistent and crampy abdominal pain Continuous pain, which suggests strangulation or peritonitis Tenderness, which may be diffuse or localized Bowel sounds, hyperactive borborygmus (may decrease after a prolonged course), tympany Abdominal distention Nausea and vomiting Absence of and inability to pass gas or stool Fever (particularly if strangulation or peritonitis is present) Dehydration q1-2 hr; note hypotension, tachycardia, low CVP, oliguria, high urine specific gravities, and ketonuria

Potential problems	Expected outcomes	Nursing activities

		Abnormal results of lab and diagnostic data, including
		   Metabolic acidosis; check arterial blood gas results q1-2 hr
		   Hemoconcentration—increased Hct, Hgb
		   WBC count for leukocytosis (suggests strangulation) q4-8 hr or as ordered
		   Electrolyte imbalance (Na^+, K^+, Cl^-, CO_2, and BUN abnormalities); check electrolyte levels q4-8 hr or as ordered
		   Abdominal radiographs daily or as ordered (upright or lateral decubitus) for presence of free air in abdomen, dilated bowel, fluid levels in bowel
		Notify physician of any abnormality
		Administer therapy for patient stabilization until surgery can be performed
		Keep NPO
		NG tube to low suction
		Monitoring activities as given previously

■ Strangulation of bowel related to
   Paralytic ileus—often associated with
     Surgery
     Acute peritonitis
     Local trauma
   Acute peritonitis—often associated with
     Acute pancreatitis
     Gastroduodenal perforation
   Perforation and/or necrosis of GI tract
	■ Bowel function within normal limits
	   Absence of strangulation, paralytic ileus, or acute peritonitis
		■ Monitor (q1-2 hr) for signs and symptoms of
		   Strangulation
		     Constant, severe abdominal pain
		     Signs of peritonitis
		     Fever
		     Tachycardia
		     Increasing leukocytosis
		     Blood in rectum
		     Associated abdominal, pelvic, rectal mass
		   If strangulation occurs, administer therapy as ordered
		   Paralytic ileus
		     Silent abdomen, absent bowel sounds
		     Absence of cramping
		     Radiographic evidence of gas throughout small and large intestines
		   If paralytic ileus occurs, administer therapy as ordered
		   Acute peritonitis
		     Malaise
		     Abdominal discomfort, pain
		     Rebound tenderness, with muscular rigidity over primary area of inflammation
		     Leukocytosis
		     Fever
		     Nausea, vomiting
		     Fluid and electrolyte imbalance
		   If problem occurs, see Standard: *Peritonitis*

■ Vascular obstruction related to
   Mesenteric arterial thrombosis associated with aortic aneurysms, severe aortic atherosclerosis
   Mesenteric vasoconstriction, hypoxia, and vasospasm of bowel associated with low cardiac output
	■ Vascular sufficiency
	   Bowel sounds within normal limits
		■ Monitor for
		   Signs and symptoms of arterial mesenteric occlusion q1 hr
		     Occult blood in stools
		     Do Hematest on all stools
		     Vital signs, including temperature; note hypotension, tachycardia
		   Signs and symptoms of mesenteric venous occlusion q1 hr
		     Tender abdomen
		     Diminished or absent peristalsis
		     Gradually developing distention
		     Vital signs, including temperature; note hypotension, fever
		   Lab reports for leukocytosis; check complete blood count results for WBC count q12-24 hr
		Note results of abdominal tap, if done, indicating presence of blood in peritoneum (may indicate infarcted bowel)

Potential problems	**Expected outcomes**	**Nursing activities**
Mesenteric venous thrombosis, which may be associated with appendicitis, strangulation hernia, or an abdominal hernia		Notify physician of any of these abnormalities If vascular obstruction occurs, administer therapy as ordered, which may include Fluid, electrolyte, and blood replacement Antibiotics Preparation of patient for surgery to resect infarcted bowel or to perform an embolectomy or thrombectomy of artery, vein involved
■ Diverticulitis	■ Resolution of diverticulitis and associated problems	■ Monitor for Progression of characteristic signs and symptoms of *chronic* diverticulitis q1 hr Altered bowel habits, e.g., constipation, diarrhea, flatulence Recurrent left lower quadrant pain and tenderness Rectal bleeding (occasional) Signs and symptoms of *acute* sigmoid diverticulitis q1 hr Rapid onset of marked lower left quadrant pain Lower abdominal tenderness, peritoneal irritation Fever—check vital signs including temperature Leukocytosis; note complete blood count results q6 hr Mass in the area of acute pain Notify physician of any abnormality Prepare patient for barium enema, sigmoidoscopy as ordered Administer low-residue diet if ordered Administer anticholinergic drugs and laxatives if needed, as ordered For patients with *acute* diverticulitis Administer antibiotics as ordered Prepare patient for surgery if procedure is necessary (if medical measures do not sufficiently arrest the inflammatory process or if an abscess is documented)
■ Ulcerative colitis	■ Resolution and/or early remission	■ Monitor for Severe bloody diarrhea; determine frequency and amount Fever; check vital signs, including temperature q1 hr and prn Weight loss Accurate intake and output q1 hr BP, CVP, PAP readings q1 hr, if available Specific signs and symptoms of acute fulminating ulcerative colitis, including Abdominal pain and distention Leukocytosis, complete blood count q6 hr or as ordered Toxemia Peritoneal sepsis Toxic dilatation of the colon Notify physician of any abnormality Prepare for and assist with sigmoidoscopy, barium enema as ordered For patients with *fulminating ulcerative* colitis Administer fluids, antibiotics, blood transfusions as ordered Administer analgesics and sedatives if needed, as ordered For persisting acute symptoms, administer steroids as ordered For patients with *chronic debilitating* colitis Administer bland diet as ordered Administer anticholinergic, antidiarrheal agents and sedatives if needed, as ordered

Potential problems	Expected outcomes	Nursing activities

■ Diaphragmatic hernia, which may be one of two types
Esophageal hiatal hernia
	■ Resolution of diaphragmatic hernia	■ Monitor for progression of signs and symptoms of an esophageal hiatal hernia, including
		  Esophagitis
		  Substernal or epigastric distress and heartburn, made worse by patient being in reclining position after eating
		  Nausea, vomiting, dysphagia (occur occasionally)
		  Bleeding; check vital signs q1 hr and prn
		  Hematest on all stools and vomitus
		  Notify physician of any abnormality
		  Prepare patient for barium study, esophagoscopy as ordered
		  Administer bland diet, antacids, anticholinergic drugs if ordered
		  Place head of bed in a semiupright position, particularly after patient eats
		  Prepare patient for surgery if ordered

Traumatic diaphragmatic hernia		Monitor for signs and symptoms of traumatic diaphragmatic hernia, particularly respiratory distress Notify physician of any abnormality Prepare patient for radiograph, barium study, and/or esophagoscopy as ordered Prepare patient for surgery if procedure is necessary

Postoperative

Potential problems	Expected outcomes	Nursing activities

■ Hemodynamic instability
Hemorrhage related to
  Bleeding arteriole
  DIC
Hypotension related to
  Insufficient fluid administration
  Inadequate myocardial function
	■ Hemodynamic stability	■ Intraoperatively, administer blood products and fluids to replace blood losses as ordered; observe for transfusion reaction
		Monitor
		  BP, P q1-2 hr; note hypotension, tachycardia
		  CVP, PAP, cardiac output, urine output with specific gravity q1 hr
		  Peripheral circulation, mentation
		  Hct and Hgb, coagulation studies
		  Drainage (e.g., NG, wound) for presence of blood and amount; weigh dressing if wound drainage is copious
		  Abdomen for tenseness q1 hr and girth q4-8 hr and prn
		Notify physician of any abnormality
		Maintain accurate fluid intake with accurate intake and output records including specific gravity; daily weights
		If hemodynamic instability occurs, administer fluids and blood products as ordered; closely monitor patient's hemodynamic response and urine output

■ Respiratory insufficiency—atelectasis related to
Anesthesia and prolonged immobility during surgery
Pain, splinting, and decreased diaphragmatic movement
NG tube producing sore throat and difficulty with effective cough
	■ Patient breathes without distress; respiratory rate within normal limits
	Adequate oxygenation, ventilation, with Pa_{O_2} and Pa_{CO_2} within normal limits
	Clear lungs determined by auscultation, radiograph
		■ Monitor for
		  Fever, tachypnea, tachycardia, and hypertension; check vital signs including temperature q1 hr
		  Decreased chest wall movement on affected side
		  Amount, color, consistency of secretions
		  Presence of rales, rhonchi, and other adventitious breath sounds
		  Elevated diaphragm on one or both sides
		  Presence of atelectasis, local or diffuse infiltrates, pleural effusion; check chest radiograph results daily
		  Infection; note C and S of sputum results
		  Acidosis; note arterial blood gas results q12 hr and prn
		  Decreasing LOC
		Notify physician of any abnormality
		Postural drainage and chest physiotherapy q2-4 hr and prn; nasotracheal suction if patient is unable to cough up secretions
		Administer pain medication, as needed, for effective coughing and breathing exercises

Potential problems	Expected outcomes	Nursing activities
		Assist patient with use of spirometer
		Administer intermittent positive pressure breathing treatment if ordered
		Ambulate as soon as possible according to plan of care
		If aforementioned measures fail, prepare for and assist with intubation; see Standard: *Mechanical ventilation*

■ Pulmonary emboli, thrombophlebitis related to
  Venous stasis associated with immobility
  Hypercoagulability associated with stress of surgery
	■ Absence of pulmonary emboli, thrombophlebitis	■ Prevention
		  Apply antithromboembolic stockings
		  Assist patient with ROM exercises, isometric exercises, ambulation
		  Administer low-dose anticoagulation therapy, if ordered, for high-risk surgical patients
		  Monitor for
		  Signs and symptoms of thrombophlebitis of lower extremities q4-8 hr
		    Calf tenderness
		    Homans' sign
		    Swelling, redness along vein
		  Signs and symptoms of pulmonary embolism
		    Chest pain
		    Tachypnea, dyspnea (q1 hr)
		    Elevated BP, tachycardia; determine vital signs, including temperature, q1 hr and prn
		  Notify physician if these signs and symptoms occur
		  If pulmonary emboli, thrombophlebitis occur, see Standard: *Embolic phenomena*

■ Fluid and electrolyte imbalance related to
  Large GI, wound, ostomy losses
  Hypovolemia due to inadequate fluid replacement in the preoperative and intraoperative periods
  Hypervolemia due to vigorous fluid replacement
  Inordinate electrolyte losses and/or inadequate electrolyte replacement
	■ Fluid intake and output in balance
	  Weight approximates preoperative baseline level
		■ Monitor
		  Fluid intake and output records q1-2 hr (including GI, wound, ostomy losses)
		  Daily weights for significant gain or loss
		  For signs and symptoms of electrolyte imbalance q4-8 hr: lassitude, irritability, weakness, nausea, vomiting, neuromuscular abnormalities, twitching
		  Serum electrolyte levels q6-12 hr
		  Notify physician of any abnormalities
		  If fluid and electrolyte imbalance occurs
		  Administer fluid and electrolyte replacement as ordered; closely monitor patient's response
		  Administer special therapy according to the causal factors, e.g., low-residual diet; antidiarrheal/H_2 antagonist medication in patients with ileostomy

■ Infection: wound	■ Infection free, afebrile
	  Wound clean and dry, intact (healing well)
		■ Prevention
		  Aseptic dressing change
		  Provide for adequate intake of nutrients to facilitate wound healing
		  Monitor for
		  Appearance of incision line and surrounding tissues; note any irritation—redness, warmth, and swelling; any complaints of localized tenderness, pain
		  Wound drainage—amount, color, and odor
		  Results of wound C and S if infection is suspected
		  Leukocytosis; check complete blood count results every day
		  Fever; note vital signs including temperature q2 hr and prn
		  Notify physician of any abnormalities
		  If wound infection occurs
		  Administer antibiotics as ordered
		  Wound care as ordered

Potential problems	Expected outcomes	Nursing activities
■ Infection: peritonitis related to Duodenal stump leakage Leakage of bile during surgery Necrotic bowel resulting from deficient blood supply Intussusception of jejunum, often related to decreased blood supply that causes necrosis of a segment of bowel with herniation of one part of bowel into another	■ Absence and/or resolution of peritonitis Intact anastomosis GI, bowel function within normal limits including Bowel sounds Bowel movements begin soon after patient resumes dietary intake	■ Prevention Careful wound care Adequate intake of nutrients to facilitate healing as ordered Monitor for signs and symptoms of peritonitis q1-2 hr, including Continuing large NG drainage Fecal or bilious contents in wound drainage Distended, rigid, tender, abdomen with rebound tenderness Increasing size of abdominal girth Presence and characteristics of pain; note constant increasingly intense discomfort Fever, tachycardia; check vital signs including temperature Elevated WBC count and ESR Nausea and vomiting Notify physician of any abnormality If peritonitis occurs Monitor accurate intake and output q1-2 hr Monitor daily weights Administer fluids as ordered Send cultures of wound drainage, blood as ordered Administer antibiotics as ordered Assist in peritoneal dialysis if ordered See Standards: *Peritonitis; Peritoneal dialysis*
■ Infection: localized abdominal abscess, subphrenic abscess	■ Infection free; afebrile Absence of signs of localized abdominal infection	■ Monitor for Elevation of diaphragm, obliteration of the costophrenic angle in chest radiograph results Discomfort and pain q2 hr; note localization of pain Fever, often occurring in the late afternoon or evening q2 hr Leukocytosis, elevated ESR Scans and ultrasonography results, if tests done Notify physician of any abnormality If localized abdominal or subphrenic abscess occurs Administer antibiotics Prepare for surgery if ordered
■ Infection: sepsis	■ Infection free; afebrile	■ Monitor (q1-2 hr) for signs and symptoms of Sepsis Shock Diaphoresis, hyperthermia, hypothermia Altered mentation and malaise Fever Notify physician of any abnormality If sepsis is suspected, obtain cultures as ordered If sepsis occurs, administer antibiotics as ordered, and monitor for resolution
■ Paralyic ileus related to operative stress and manipulation	■ Normal GI function Bowel sounds present 1 to 2 days after surgery	■ Monitor for signs and symptoms of paralytic ileus q2 hr Increasing gastric output per NG tube Absent or diminished bowel sounds Absent or diminished passage of flatus Increasing abdominal girth; measure q4-8 hr and prn Notify physician of any of these abnormalities If paralytic ileus occurs Administer suppository, enema, or neostigmine (Prostigmin) if ordered (to stimulate peristalsis) Administer oral/IV nutrients as ordered

Potential problems	Expected outcomes	Nursing activities
■ Marginal ulceration related to Damage of the tissue along the anastomosis from acidic gastric secretions or alkaline pancreatic secretions Inadequate vagotomy	■ Intact surgical anastomosis	■ Monitor for signs and symptoms of Bleeding; Hematest all stool and NG aspirates Hypotension; take vital signs including temperature q1-2 hr Notify physician of any abnormality If marginal ulceration occurs, administer antacid or an H₂ antagonist as ordered; prepare patient for surgery if procedure is necessary
■ Obstruction, retention in GI tract, which may include	■ Absence or resolution of obstruction	■ Prevent by Ensuring continuous function of NG tube; irrigate as necessary Avoiding removal of NG tube
Dilatation of gastric remnant after a partial gastrectomy Gastric retention following a Billroth I or II operation associated with A constricting anastomosis Edema and subsequent scarring and stricture of proximal loop	Intact anastomosis without signs and symptoms of gastric dilatation	Monitor q1-2 hr for Nausea, vomiting Hiccups Continued large NG aspirate Distended upper abdomen Signs and symptoms of shock and pulmonary embolus if dilatation is severe Notify physician of presence of any of these abnormalities If obstruction/retention occurs Administer fluid and electrolyte replacement as ordered Check for patency of NG tube q1/2-1 hr to ensure continuous gastric decompression
Dumping syndrome consists of nausea and vomiting caused by intake of high carbohydrate food, which pulls large amount of fluids into intestinal tract, resulting in dehydration, nausea, and vomiting	GI function within normal limits No nausea and/or vomiting Nutrient intake consists of low-medium carbohydrate concentration and is isotonic	Prevent by Administering nutrients with low-medium carbohydrate content and isotonic osmolality Administering frequent small meals Monitor for Any complaints of nausea, vomiting Accurate intake and output q1-2 hr Serial serum electrolyte levels q12 hr Notify physician of any abnormality If dumping syndrome occurs Administer fluid, electrolyte replacement as ordered Reevaluate content of patient's nutritional intake and alter as indicated and ordered
Adhesion formation promoted by extensive surgical manipulation, infection, and peritonitis	Absence and/or resolution of adhesions	Monitor for Adequacy of bowel function Presence, nature of bowel sounds Presence of flatus Suppleness/rigidity of abdomen Patient's complaints of specific area of tenderness, signs/symptoms of peritonitis Changes in abdominal girth Weight loss/gain Amount, character of NG aspirates
Intussusception of bowel related to Decreased blood supply, causing necrosis and herniation of one part of bowel into another	Absence and/or resolution of intussusception	Monitor for signs and symptoms of complete intestinal obstruction Nausea and vomiting Pain, tenderness Distended abdomen Increased, then decreased bowel sounds Air and fluid levels (by radiograph) proximal to the point of obstruction

Potential problems	Expected outcomes	Nursing activities

Adhesion formation resulting in "nine-day syndrome," which begins to occur 6 to 7 days postoperatively		Notify physician of any abnormality
		If intussusception of bowel occurs
		  Monitor progress of signs and symptoms
		  Maintain decompression of GI tract with nasogastric (NG) tube or a long intestinal tube (Miller-Abbott, Cantor)
		  Serial measurements of abdominal girth q4-8 hr and prn
		  Maintain scrupulous fluid intake, output records q1 hr
		  Monitor serum electrolyte levels
		  Administer fluid, electrolyte replacement as ordered
		  Monitor for signs of systemic infection: note temperature, vital signs, mentation, lab values—WBC count, sedimentation rate
		  Provide optimal chest physiotherapy
		  Maintain patient in semi-Fowler's position
		  Reposition at least q2 hr
		  Ensure effective deep breathing and coughing; administer pain medication as ordered, if needed
		  Monitor arterial blood gas values q6-12 hr
		  Prepare patient for surgery for lysis of adhesions and/or resection of a portion of gangrenous bowel if necessary

■ Jaundice related to Intravascular hemolysis of RBC
Edema of the duodenal stump in Billroth I and II surgeries, causing occlusion of the common bile duct
Surgical occlusion of common bile duct
	■ Absence or resolution of jaundice	■ Monitor for
		  Jaundice
		  Presence of upper abdominal pain (every shift)
		  Bilious drainage (q2 hr)
		  Results of liver function tests (every day)
		Notify physician of any abnormality
		If jaundice occurs, administer therapy as ordered

■ Wound dehiscence, evisceration related to obesity, malnutrition, debilitation
Dehiscence involves disruption of several layers of the wound (e.g., peritoneum, outer fascia)
Evisceration is the escape of abdominal viscera through the wound and is associated with inadequate support from all fascial layers
	■ Suture line intact, healing well, and without signs of dehiscence, evisceration	■ Perioperative use of abdominal binders for the obese may be useful for some patients
		Monitor for a sudden discharge of serosanguineous fluid, which may indicate dehiscence
		The patient may complain of a "popping" sensation during coughing
		If dehiscence is suspected
		  Notify physician
		  Cover wound with sterile dressing or towels
		  Instruct patient to avoid further straining
		  Prepare patient for surgery as ordered
		Monitor for appearance of abdominal contents in wounds subsequent to dehiscence, indicating that evisceration is occurring
		Notify physician
		If dehiscence/evisceration occurs, cover with sterile towels
		Prepare patient for surgery as ordered

■ Malnutrition, negative nitrogen balance	■ Weight maintenance or weight gain (unless patient is obese)
	Positive nitrogen balance
		■ Monitor for
		  Return of bowel sounds after surgery q4-8 hr
		  Daily weight (without adequate nutrition, 0.5 pound [0.23 kg] of muscle mass can be lost per day)
		  Nitrogen balance results if done
		Administer alimentation as ordered
		  Through oral feeding, gastrostomy, or jejunostomy tube
		  For parenteral alimentation, see Standard: *Total parenteral nutrition through central venous catheter*

Potential problems	**Expected outcomes**	**Nursing activities**

■ Prolapse
  Rectal—related to in-adequate abdominal support
  Of an ileostomy—related to weak abdominal ring or to inadequate internal fixation of the ileum
	■ Absence or resolution of intestinal prolapse	■ Prevent by instructing patients not to strain excessively at school; if difficulty with defecation is present, stool softeners and small enemas may be useful
		Monitor for rectal prolapse
		  A mass felt by patient, particularly when walking or during defecation
		  Soiling of clothing from discharge, bleeding, fecal incontinence
		Notify physician of these abnormalities
		Prepare patient for diagnostic modalities to document the problem
		Monitor for prolapse of an ileostomy
		  Appearance of additional intestinal mucosa/lining through the ileostomy opening, which often appears superficially infected, edematous and ulcerated
		Notify physician if the aforementioned signs occur
		Prepare patient for surgery if ordered

■ In the hiatal hernia or esophagogastrectomy patient reflux from incompetent cardiac sphincter, which may result in aspiration of gastric contents into the lungs	■ Minimal to no reflux of gastric contents into esophagus
	Absence of aspiration of gastric contents into lungs
		■ Prevention
		  Place patient in semi-Fowler's position unless contraindicated
		  When oral intake resumes, administer small, frequent meals that are low in bulk and are easily digested
		Monitor for
		  Patient's complaints of gastric acidity, discomfort, and heartburn and reflux of acidic gastric contents into upper esophagus/throat
		  Aspiration of gastric contents into lungs
		Notify physician of these abnormalities
		If reflux of gastric contents occurs
		  Reevaluate patient's position and dietary intake and revise appropriately
		If aspiration of gastric contents into lung occurs
		  Notify physician immediately
		  Immediately suction patient's airway
		  Administer humidified O_2
		See Problem, Respiratory insufficiency (postoperative)

■ Undue gastric fullness occurring with surgery including vagotomy, in which the stomach becomes atonic and empties more slowly, permitting food fermentation	■ Absence of undue gastric fullness after meals	■ Prevent by providing for small, frequent meals
		Monitor for
		  Patient's complaints of fullness, discomfort after eating
		  Gastric distention
		  Inordinate flatus, diarrhea
		If problem occurs reevaluate patient's dietary intake and alter accordingly

■ Nausea and vomiting after eating (the dumping syndrome) related to
  High carbohydrate intake
  Occurs a few minutes after eating and really represents a jejunal hyperosmolar syndrome, in which carbohydrates, high in osmolarity, pull H_2O
	■ Absence of nausea and vomiting after eating	■ Provide diet that includes
		  Frequent, small amounts
		  A moderate to high fat content helps to retard passage of food and to maintain weight
		  Relatively low carbohydrate content
		  Avoidance of milk, sweets, alcohol, or carbonated beverages
		  A high protein content to help rebuild tissue and maintain weight
		Monitor for the following signs/symptoms after meals
		  Patient's complaints of fullness, nausea
		  Vomiting
		  Tachycardia
		  Weakness, dizziness
		  Diarrhea

Potential problems	Expected outcomes	Nursing activities

into the intestine, causing intravascular volume depletion		Notify physician of these signs/symptoms
		If nausea and vomiting occur
		  Assist in the reevaluation of dietary intake and revise the fat, carbohydrate content as ordered
		  Omit beverages that induce the syndrome

■ Skin irritation
  Occurs most frequently in patients with diversion of fecal material to the skin (e.g., ileostomies)
	■ Skin intact and dry	■ Prevent by protecting skin with a properly fitted ileostomy appliance and meticulous skin care
		Monitor for reddened, irritated skin around ileostomy site
		If problem occurs
		  Alter skin care to provide additional protection and permit healing to occur
		  If skin irritation is severe, notify physician and administer therapy as ordered

■ Insufficient information for compliance with discharge regimen*	■ Sufficient information for compliance with discharge regimen
	Before discharge patient/family
	  Verbalizes knowledge of discharge program, including medication regimen, dietary management, activity progression
	  Is able to perform specific therapeutic interventions
		■ Assess patient/family's knowledge and understanding of discharge regimen
		Instruct patient/family as needed in
		  Therapeutic interventions such as dressings; provide opportunity for practice
		  Medication regimen, including
		    Purpose
		    Identification
		    Dosage
		    Frequency and timing
		    Potential adverse effects
		    Precautions
		  Dietary management
		    For all patients after GI surgery a slow progression in diet with small frequent meals is recommended
		    Avoid foods high in roughage, residue in the early postoperative period
		    Dietary alterations are made according to the specific GI surgery done and individual tolerance
		    For gastrectomy and hiatal hernia repair patients
		      1. Resumption of oral intake should occur gradually with small frequent meals consisting of food that is easily digested, mild, and low in bulk and residue (an ulcer-type diet works well)
		      2. Advise patient not to eat for several hours before bedtime
		    For hiatal hernia patients with dysphagia from residual postoperative esophageal edema, encourage patient to eat slowly and chew food well; encourage patient to avoid certain meats that are hard to swallow, eggs, fresh bread, spicy or hot foods, salads, and carbonated beverages until the dysphagia subsides
		    If patient has signs/symptoms of dumping syndrome
		      1. A low carbohydrate, high protein (meat, eggs, cheese), moderately high fat diet is recommended
		      2. Foods to avoid include those high in sugar (e.g., sweets), alcohol, sweet carbonated beverages
		      3. Fluids are taken between meals, at least 1 hour before and 1 hour after meals
		  Activity progression
		    Avoid lifting heavy objects (over 15 pounds) in first few postoperative months

*If responsibility of critical care nurse includes this type of follow-up care.

Potential problems	Expected outcomes	Nursing activities
		Activities that require vigorous abdominal muscular effort should be avoided (e.g., opening stuck windows, tennis) Straining at stool should be avoided
	Identifies untoward signs and symptoms requiring medical attention	Describe untoward signs and symptoms that require medical attention
	Describes plan for follow-up care	Discuss plan for follow-up care, including purpose of the visits, when and where to go, who to see, and what specimens to bring Provide opportunity for and encourage patient/family's questions Assess patient's potential compliance with discharge regimen

43 □ Jejunal-ileal bypass surgery

A jejunal-ileal bypass operation involves resection of 14 inches of jejunum and 4 inches of ileum (or 12 and 6 inches, respectively) to reduce the intestinal absorption of nutrients consumed, resulting in weight loss.

Relative indications for surgery include the presence of morbid obesity for most of the patient's lifetime (at least for 5 years), the absence of endocrine imbalances such as hypothyroidism and Cushing's disease, and the failure of medical measures for modification of the obesity, including psychosocial counseling, behavior modification programs, weight reduction groups, and various dietary and medication regimens.

The incidence of medical problems related to obesity is high and includes cardiac and cardiovascular disease, diabetes, osteoarthritis, and the pickwickian syndrome (somnolence, hypoventilation, and hypoxia). The hazards of the continued presence of these medical problems if surgery is not performed should be weighed against the disadvantages of surgery. Possible hazards associated with the surgery include the psychosocial adjustment to weight loss, diarrhea, easy fatigability, progressive hepatic dysfunction due to fatty necrosis, renal stone formation, hyperuricemia, arthritic symptoms (probably related to circulating cryoproteins formed by colonic bacteria), and a small incidence of operative mortality.

The psychosocial evaluation should reveal sufficient stability and motivation to comply with the discharge regimen for jejunal-ileal bypass surgery and indication of the patient's ability to tolerate the psychosocial changes associated with significant weight loss and the potential problems associated with the surgery. A psychosocial evaluation often reveals a negative body image, a feeling of helplessness in dealing with an obsessive eating habit, depression, and a dependent type of personality. These individuals often describe feelings of isolation and psychosocial, employment, and financial difficulties.

Postoperative care is focused on achieving adequate oxygenation and ventilation and on management of problems that are frequently associated with the procedure (e.g., diarrhea, psychological adjustment difficulties). To assist the patient to successfully adjust to the many postoperative changes that take place, the patient and family are encouraged to verbalize their fears and anxieties. Encouragement and support from the staff and a plan of care that provides for patient and family participation in its planning and delivery can enhance the surgical outcome.

ASSESSMENT

1. History, presence, nature, and severity of medical problems frequently associated with sustained obesity, including
   a. Cardiac and cardiovascular abnormalities
      (1) Heart failure
      (2) Angina
      (3) Hypertension
      (4) Symptoms of pulmonary edema
      (5) Shortness of breath, dyspnea on exertion
   b. Pulmonary abnormalities
      (1) Pulmonary disease

(2) Respiratory distress

(3) History of smoking

2. Nature of weight gain
   a. Actual weight
   b. Amount of recent weight loss or gain
   c. Length of time and pattern of weight gain
   d. Pertinent circumstances related to weight gain
   e. Weight loss programs employed
   f. Typical food and alcohol intake
   g. Medications taken; note those that may impair liver function

3. Previous and current medical therapy; past surgical procedures

4. Psychosocial factors that are pertinent to patient's sustained obesity and that are also important factors in the postoperative period
   a. Feelings about weight gain
   b. Factors that precipitate eating
   c. Previous counseling in weight reduction, including formal weight reduction programs
   d. Pertinent psychosocial factors in family background, support systems
   e. Employment history
   f. Educational and comprehension level

5. Results of lab tests that affect surgical outcome, including
   a. Liver function tests—alkaline phosphatase and transaminases, bilirubin levels
   b. Protein and albumin levels
   c. Coagulation studies
   d. Indices of kidney function, particularly BUN, creatinine
   e. Pulmonary function tests
   f. Arterial blood gas values
   g. Chest radiograph results

6. Patient/family's anxiety regarding hospitalization and altered family roles

7. Patient/family's knowledge regarding operative therapy

   a. What they have been told
   b. Their expectations, fears regarding surgery and the outcomes
   c. Previous experiences with surgery, if any

8. Information and detail surgeon has provided about the need for surgery, the actual surgery to be done, and the expected outcomes

9. Patient/family's level of anxiety related to the surgery and prognosis

GOALS

1. Reduction of patient/family's anxiety with provision of information, explanations, and encouragement
2. Hemodynamic stability
3. Respiratory function sufficient to maintain arterial blood gas levels within normal limits
4. Fluid balance adequate to maintain hemodynamic stability and adequate urine output; electrolyte levels within normal limits
5. Liver function tests within normal limits, including serum proteins, enzyme levels, bilirubin and coagulation studies
6. Blood glucose levels within normal limits
7. Infection free
   a. Wound heals without infection, dehiscence, wound evisceration
   b. Absence of pulmonary infection
8. Bowel function within normal limits; diarrhea controlled
9. Absence of thrombophlebitis, pulmonary emboli, cerebral emboli, or other types of emboli
10. Urinary function within normal limits; absence of urinary calculi
11. Absence of arthralgia
12. Hair thickness at approximately baseline levels
13. Patient/family accurately verbalizes discharge regimen, including dietary management, medication regimen, and plan for follow-up visits

Potential problems	Expected outcomes	Nursing activities
■ Patient/family's anxiety related to Obesity and associated complications Hospitalization Diagnostic procedures Therapeutic regimen Anticipated surgery and expected outcomes	■ Reduction in patient/family's anxiety with provision of information, explanations, and encouragement	■ Ongoing assessment of the level of patient/family's anxiety Assess patient/family's knowledge and understanding of the surgery, expected outcomes, potential problems, postoperative medical regimen Assess patient/family's response to hospitalization Arrange for psychiatric consult and follow-up as ordered Encourage participation in care as tolerated Perform treatments in unhurried manner Provide comfort measures Explain anticipated diagnostic procedures and what patient will experience

Potential problems	**Expected outcomes**	**Nursing activities**

Assist in preparing patient for diagnostic procedures

Explain the rationale for the intestinal bypass procedure

Teach patient about medical regimen to enhance success of surgery
  No alcohol intake
  Dietary modifications
  Demonstrate respiratory exercises; teach and encourage patient until he/she is able to exercise properly

Describe the perioperative experience including
  Preoperative
    Orient patient to chest physiotherapy (call therapist for assistance if available)
      1. Coughing and deep breathing
      2. Incentive spirometry
      3. Postural drainage
    Shave and prep
    Light dinner, then NPO after midnight
    Medication for sleep if needed
    Morning bath/shower
    Preoperative medications
    Hospital gown
    Care of valuables
    Ride to operating room
    Scrub suits, masks, and hats worn by operating room staff
    Anesthesia
  Postoperative
    Waking up in the recovery room/intensive care unit
    Describe the general environment (size of unit, room, equipment)
    Nurse always nearby
    Dull, continuous noises
    Breathing tube temporarily in place to ease patient's work of breathing and the load on the heart
    NPO until "breathing tube" removed
    Incision with bandage
    IV, arterial lines
    ECG monitoring
    Medicine for discomfort, pain
    Policy on family visits
  As patient progresses
    Tubes out
    Eating again
    Getting stronger, ambulation
    Postural drainage, coughing, and deep breathing
    Diarrhea expected with therapy to control

Describe responsibility of patient in achieving a speedy recovery by taking an active role in coughing and deep breathing to keep lungs clear

Encourage patient/family's questions

Encourage verbalization of anxiety, fears related to hospitalization, diagnostic procedures, therapeutic regimen, surgery, and anticipated surgical outcomes

Potential problems	**Expected outcomes**	**Nursing activities**
■ Hemodynamic instability, which may be related to Low cardiac output Heart failure Increased metabolic requirements of obesity with increased O_2 needs Angina, myocardial ischemia, and infarction Arrhythmias	■ Hemodynamic stability Absence of Low cardiac output/ heart failure Angina Myocardial ischemia and infarction Arrhythmias ECG within normal limits Absence of signs of myocardial ischemia, infarction	■ Prevent hemodynamic instability by Carefully monitoring hemodynamic parameters, fluid intake and output measurements, and weight Administering fluids and diuretics to keep these parameters within normal limits Administering humidified supplemental O_2 as ordered to prevent tachycardia associated with hypoxemia Administering measures to prevent emboli formation, which contributes to hemodynamic instability (see Problem, Embolus formation) Early, gradual ambulation as ordered Monitor BP, P q½-1 hr until stable; CVP and PAP if available q½-1 hr until stable Urine output with specific gravity q1 hr; note oliguria with high specific gravities Indices of peripheral circulation and mentation; note signs of reduced peripheral circulation and altered mentation Daily weights for gain or loss For chest pain ECG and/or apical and radial pulse for arrhythmias, signs of myocardial ischemia, infarction Notify physician of abnormalities in the aforementioned If problem occurs Administer fluids, blood, and blood products as ordered; carefully monitor patient's response in terms of hemodynamic parameters and fluid intake and output measurements Administer cardiotonic/vasopressor medications if necessary, as ordered If arrhythmias, heart failure, angina, or myocardial infarction occur, see Standards: *Arrhythmias; Heart failure; Angina pectoris; Acute myocardial infarction* as appropriate
■ Respiratory insufficiency related to Atelectasis Pneumonia Pulmonary interstitial edema Emboli	■ Full lung expansion Arterial blood gas levels within patient's normal limits No abnormal or adventitious breath sounds Clear chest radiograph	■ Prevention Place patient in semi-Fowler's position Careful fluid intake and output records Notify physician of imbalance, and adjust fluid intake or administer diuretic agent as ordered Turn, reposition q1-2 hr Administer chest physiotherapy q2 hr Administer humidified O_2 supplementation as ordered Monitor Respirations for sudden dyspnea or tachypnea and for restlessness and tachycardia; the composite of these symptoms may indicate a pulmonary embolus Serial arterial blood gas levels for hypoxemia, hypercapnia Breath sounds q1-2 hr for decreased or absent sounds or the presence of rales, rhonchi, and wheezes Chest radiograph results for atelectasis, pneumonia Quality and amount of secretions Obtain serial sputum cultures as ordered, particularly when the character of the sputum suggests infection Temperature for elevation (q2 hr) Notify physician of abnormalities in the aforementioned If respiratory insufficiency occurs Administer antibiotics as ordered Continue monitoring as described before

Potential problems	Expected outcomes	Nursing activities
		If signs of acute respiratory insufficiency occur, monitor arterial blood gas results for hypoxemia, hypercapnia, and acidemia
		Monitor and document patient's pattern of respiratory insufficiency; note progression of respiratory parameters
■ Fluid imbalance	■ Fluid administration adequate to maintain BP, P, CVP, PAP, urine output, peripheral circulation, and mentation within normal limits Steady loss of weight after the first few postoperative days	■ Prevention Careful administration of fluids, as ordered, according to patient's intake and output record, BP, P, CVP, PAP, and daily weight changes Monitor Fluid intake and output q1 hr; correlate with hemodynamic parameters and weight changes Daily weights Hemodynamic parameters: BP, P, CVP, and PAP q1 hr and prn until stable Notify physician of abnormalities in any of these parameters If fluid imbalance occurs Restrict fluid intake or administer additional fluids as ordered; closely monitor patient's response Administer diuretics as ordered; closely monitor urine output and hemodynamic indices
■ Electrolyte imbalance related to NG suction in the early postoperative period Diarrhea	■ Blood electrolyte levels within normal limits	■ Prevent by administering electrolytes as ordered to replace electrolytes lost in NG drainage, diarrhea Monitor Serum electrolyte levels q6-12 hr For signs and symptoms of electrolyte imbalance: neuromuscular irritability, weakness, lassitude Notify physician of these abnormalities If electrolyte imbalance occurs Administer electrolyte supplements as ordered Administer therapy for cause of electrolyte loss as ordered, e.g., antidiarrheal agents
■ Liver dysfunction related to Malabsorption due to creation of shunt Fatty degeneration Toxic substances may be produced by shunted remnant of intestine	■ Liver function tests within normal limits Coagulation studies and serum protein levels within normal limits	■ Prevent by Administration of a special diet as ordered, which is usually low fat and low oxalate; protein levels are titrated to the toleration of patient's liver for protein load, monitored by ammonia and BUN levels Administering an amino acid preparation if ordered Monitor daily Liver function tests, including alkaline phosphatase, transaminase levels Bilirubin, ammonia, and BUN levels Serum protein levels Coagulation studies Notify physician of abnormalities in the aforementioned If problem occurs, see Standard: *Liver failure*
■ Abnormal glucose metabolism, diabetes	■ Blood glucose levels within normal limits	■ Monitor daily Urine glucose and acetone levels For signs and symptoms of hyperglycemia and hypoglycemia Serial blood glucose levels Notify physician of any abnormality If hyperglycemia occurs, administer insulin and institute dietary alterations as ordered If hypoglycemia occurs, administer glucose as ordered; institute dietary changes as appropriate

Potential problems	Expected outcomes	Nursing activities
■ Wound infection, which is related to Delayed, poor healing of suture line due to inadequate blood flow through thick layers of abdominal fat Wound dehiscence Hypoalbuminemia associated with liver failure	■ Infection free Wound heals without infection, dehiscence	■ Prevent by Application of abdominal binder for support as needed and as ordered Employing careful aseptic technique with dressing changes, wound care as indicated Carefully cleaning and assisting patient to clean skin folds Monitor Nature of wound drainage; note presence of any purulent drainage and notify physician; obtain wound culture as ordered on such drainage For fever q2 hr; signs of local wound infection daily WBC levels daily for leukocytosis Notify physician of any abnormality If wound infection occurs Continue monitoring as before Assist with or administer as ordered local irrigation; change dressing frequently, as needed Administer antibiotics as ordered
■ Diarrhea, which occurs in nearly every patient with a jejunal-ileal bypass	■ Absence or resolution of diarrhea	■ Monitor Stool for consistency, frequency, color Note frequent loose stools For presence of occult blood and chart results If diarrhea occurs Notify physician regarding nature of diarrhea Administer antidiarrheal agent as ordered Note presence of associated rectal excoriation; cleanse and apply lubricant Support patient/family psychologically; assure them that diarrhea is common, can be treated, and will decrease as the intestine adjusts to its new length Keep careful intake and output records, including diarrheal losses Monitor serial electrolyte determinations, since electrolyte losses can be significant with diarrhea
■ Embolus formation, which may be related to Thrombophlebitis Obesity Immobility	■ Absence or resolution of emboli	■ Prevent by Early mobilization, ambulation Applying antithromboembolic stockings Administering prophylactic anticoagulation if ordered Monitor for signs and symptoms of Thrombophlebitis Positive Homans' sign with dorsiflexion Pain in calf muscles Redness, warmth along vein Swelling distal to suspected site of embolus Pulmonary emboli Sharp chest pain Dyspnea, tachypnea Restlessness Signs and symptoms of hypoxemia, including tachycardia, restlessness If suspected, an arterial blood gas sample should be drawn immediately to determine the presence of hypoxemia and a significant drop in Pa_{O_2} Cerebral emboli Altered consciousness, restlessness, aphasia, dysphasia Unilateral weakness, ptosis Other types of emboli including renal, mesenteric, splenic; see Standard: *Embolic phenomena*

Potential problems	Expected outcomes	Nursing activities

■ Metabolic imbalance and associated problems
Urinary calculi, oxalate renal stones
	■ Urine function within normal limits
	Urinary tract remains patent
		■ Assess metabolic status
		  Diet history, weight
		  Physical appearance including skin, mucous membranes
		Prevent by
		  Administering and teaching patient/family about low oxalate diet
		  Administering cholestyramine therapy and increased Ca^{2+} intake if ordered
		  Administering fluids as ordered to provide adequate fluid intake and urine output
		Monitor for signs and symptoms of urinary calculi
		  Flank pain
		  Nausea and vomiting (in some cases)
		  Fever, if secondary infection is present
		  Dysuria, if stone is present in neck or outlet area of bladder
		If problem occurs
		  Determine any deviations from prescribed diet, and notify physician and dietitian
		  Instruct patient in revised diet

Arthralgia related to
Increased circulating levels of cryoproteins
Altered activity of colonic bacteria
	Musculoskeletal function within normal limits
	Absence of arthralgia
		Prevent by administering an antianaerobic antibiotic, if ordered, which is prophylaxis against the intestinal syndrome that often precedes arthralgia
		Monitor for
		  Signs and symptoms of arthralgia: achiness, pain in one or more joints, bones; these may be preceded by watery diarrhea, fever, lower abdominal discomfort, pain, diffusely tender abdomen, distended lower abdomen followed by symptoms of arthritis
		Notify physician if any of these occur
		If problem occurs
		  Apply soaks if needed, as ordered
		  Administer analgesic and/or anti-inflammatory agent as ordered
		  Administer an antianaerobic antibiotic, if ordered, for relief of the intestinal syndrome and arthritic symptoms

Hair loss related to
Altered carbohydrate metabolism
Decreased blood proteins
	Hair thickness at baseline, preoperative level	Prevention
		  Minimize metabolic abnormality by providing sufficient intake of nutrients for building of body proteins, including hair
		Monitor for hair thickness, hair loss
		If problem occurs
		  Assure patient/family that with resumption of more normal metabolism, hair usually grows back to its original thickness
		  Provide for high protein, moderate carbohydrate diet, as ordered, if liver can handle the protein load
		  If the nitrogenous metabolite levels increase, the protein intake may need to be decreased

Potential problems	Expected outcomes	Nursing activities
■ Psychological dependence, depression	■ Patient progresses from a dependent role to a more independent one	■ Ongoing assessment of patient's psychological status and stress level Arrange for psychiatric consult and follow-up as ordered Determine nature of current stresses and patient's ability to cope with them; assist patient in mobilization of resources to deal with these problems; enlist support of family/significant others Carefully encourage and provide opportunity for patient progression from a dependent role to a more independent one by the time of discharge from the critical care area Encourage patient's decision making and participation in his/her care Include family in care; encourage their support of patient Provide emotional support and encouragement; acknowledge patient's progress Encourage verbalization of anxieties, fears, and feelings of depression

■ Insufficient knowledge to comply with discharge regimen*	■ Before discharge patient/family is able to
	Accurately verbalize discharge regimen regarding dietary management and the medication regimen
	Describe signs and symptoms requiring medical attention
	Accurately describe plan for follow-up care
		■ Assess patient/family's understanding of discharge regimen
		Arrange for a dietary consult
		Instruct patient/family in
		  Diet
		    Foods to avoid
		    Vitamin B supplements, other vitamins
		    Fluid: avoid alcohol—describe hazard regarding increased risk of liver dysfunction
		  Weight
		    Explain that weight loss does not occur for several days postoperatively; that steady weight loss will occur during the first year; thereafter that weight may plateau because the bowel progressively dilates and thereby increases in absorption capacity
		  Medication
		    Identification of dosage, timing/frequency; potential adverse effects
		    Medications may include antidiarrheal agent, vitamins
		    Oral contraceptives are usually not recommended because absorption is unreliable
		Encourage patient/family's communication of feelings regarding weight loss
		Review signs and symptoms requiring medical attention
		Review plan for follow-up visits, including when and where to go, who to see, and what specimens to bring
		Briefly review purpose and importance of follow-up visits
		Provide opportunity for and encourage patient/family's questions

*If responsibility of critical care nurse includes this type of follow-up care.

RENAL

44 □ Acute renal failure

Acute renal failure is a sudden onset of kidney dysfunction caused by impaired renal blood flow or glomerular/tubular damage. The function of the kidney in excreting nitrogenous waste products is impaired, resulting in azotemia with high serum ammonia, uric acid, and creatinine levels.

Acute renal failure is characterized by the onset of a variable period of oliguria or anuria, acidosis, and electrolyte abnormalities. In some cases of acute renal failure, it is possible to have normal or large amounts of urine in the early period, although this is rare. The period of oliguria is followed by polyuria and, finally, recovery of renal function. Usually acute renal damage is reversible.

The etiology of renal failure can be categorized into prerenal, renal, and postrenal events. The *prerenal* event includes physiological abnormalities that cause diminished renal perfusion such as decreased cardiac output, dehydration, and bilateral renal vascular obstruction. These conditions may result in oliguria, anuria, and azotemia.

The *renal* event is caused by two major types of conditions—namely, ischemic insult, which is secondary to severe prolonged volume depletion as in hypotension, disseminated intravascular coagulation (DIC), severe dehydration, and "third spacing" as in third-degree burns, sepsis and following major vascular surgery; and direct, chemical damage by toxins taken by ingestion, injection, or inhalants such as chemotherapeutic agents, exogenous toxins, drugs, organic solvents, or heavy metals.

The *postrenal* event is caused by lower urinary tract obstruction, such as renal calculi and prostatic hypertrophy.

Both the prerenal and the postrenal causes, if uncorrected, may lead to acute renal failure. However, if therapy is immediate, renal perfusion and urine output usually will be restored, thus ensuring continued kidney function.

The diagnosis of acute renal failure is based on clinical findings, lack of increased urine output in response to a fluid or a diuretic challenge, and characteristic abnormalities in the urinalysis. The tubular dysfunction accompanying acute renal failure results in inefficient concentrating ability. Other common findings are urinary sodium greater than 20 mEq/liter and specific gravity less than 1.015.

The patient in acute renal failure appears critically ill, very lethargic, and sometimes confused. Anorexia, nausea, vomiting, and diarrhea are often present. Skin and mucous membranes are dry from dehydration/uremia, and urinary output is scanty, bloody, and has a low specific gravity.

The three clinical phases of acute renal failure include the oliguric, diuretic, and convalescent phases. The oliguric phase, when the urine output is less than 400 to 600 ml/24 hours, is accompanied by an increase of serum concentration of elements usually excreted by the kidney (urea, creatinine, uric acids, and the intracellular cations potassium and magnesium).

The oliguric phase is usually followed by a phase of high urine output called the diuretic phase of renal failure. In "high output failure" nitrogenous waste products are retained even though 2 to 3 liters of urine are excreted daily. In some patients the oliguric phase is transient, and the high output phase is the primary clinical sign of renal dysfunction. The third phase, or period of convalescence, is marked by restoration of renal function, a process that occasionally takes 6 to 12 months.

ASSESSMENT

1. History, presence, and nature of
   a. Chronic renal disease
   b. Previous radiation therapy
   c. Infection involving kidneys
   d. Diseases/conditions that are associated with low kidney perfusion, causing renal ischemia
   e. Ingestion/injection/inhalation of various nephrotoxins; any drugs patient has recently taken
   f. Recent hypersensitivity response
   g. Disease of glomeruli and small blood vessels

    h. Major blood vessel disease

    i. Lower urinary tract obstruction; presence of wide fluctuations of urine output; enlarged prostate; distended bladder

    j. Massive hemorrhage, trauma

    k. Cardiac disease

    l. Pulmonary insufficiency

    m. Hypertension

    n. Hepatomegaly, jaundice, ascites

2. Signs/symptoms (if any) of chronic renal failure complications

    a. General appearance

      (1) Anemia, pallor

      (2) Swelling of eyelids

      (3) Pruritus

      (4) Poor skin turgor

      (5) Dry mucous membranes

    b. Cardiovascular

      (1) Pericarditis

      (2) Hypertension

      (3) Retinopathy

    c. Respiratory

      (1) Deep sighing, Kussmaul's respirations

      (2) Urine smell on breath

      (3) Chest radiograph signs of hilar pneumonitis

    d. Urinary—urine produced may reflect proteinuria, hematuria, pyuria, casts

    e. Gastrointestinal—hiccups, anorexia, nausea and vomiting, coated tongue, patient's complaints of taste of ammonia

    f. Central nervous system (CNS)—headache, lassitude, confusion, disorientation, drowsiness, insomnia, muscle twitching, weakness

3. Parameters to include

    a. BP, P, noting orthostatic changes

    b. Pallor

    c. Level of consciousness (LOC)

    d. Pattern of urine output, urine volumes, specific gravity, state of hydration

    e. Weight

4. Results of lab and diagnostic tests

    a. Urinalysis; urinary sediment, osmolality, creatinine, electrolytes

    b. Serum creatinine, uric acid, ammonia, bilirubin, BUN, electrolyte, and magnesium levels

    c. Coagulation studies

    d. Hct, Hgb, platelets, WBC with differential

    e. Liver function studies particularly serum albumin and protein levels, liver enzymes

    f. Blood type and crossmatching

    g. Abdominal flat plate roentgenogram

    h. Tomography

    i. Renal scan

    j. Intravenous pyelogram

    k. Cystoscopy

    l. Arteriogram

    m. Renal biopsy

    n. Echogram (for kidney size)

5. Patient's perception of and reaction to the diagnosis and therapy

GOALS

1. Normovolemia, removal of excess body fluids

2. Hct, Hgb, and coagulation studies within normal limits

3. Blood levels of nitrogenous waste substances within normal limits

4. Serum electrolyte levels and acid-base balance within normal limits

5. Infection free

6. Nutrition adequate to prevent protein catabolism; positive nitrogen balance

7. Normal cardiovascular, gastrointestinal, neuromuscular, and integumentary function

8. Patient's behavior demonstrates decreased anxiety with provision of information

9. Patient oriented to time, place, and person; clear sensorium

10. Before discharge,* patient is able to

    a. Explain relationship between process and therapy prescribed

    b. Successfully identify all medications and take the proper dosage on the proper schedule

    c. Briefly describe signs/symptoms of chronic renal dysfunction

    d. Describe and follow prescribed diet

    e. Describe follow-up regimen

    f. Ask pertinent questions

---

*Applies when chronic management and/or prevention is required.

Potential problems	Expected outcomes	Nursing activities
■ Patient's anxiety related to limited understanding of renal dysfunction, its effects on the body, and diagnostic procedures	■ Patient's behavior demonstrates decreased anxiety with provision of information Patient asks questions and demonstrates understanding of disease	■ Ongoing assessment of level of anxiety Describe in simple terms the nature of the patient's renal disease and its relationship to the signs/symptoms the patient is experiencing Explain the relationship of the renal failure to the plan of care Explain briefly the diagnostic procedures involved in the plan of care Encourage patient/family's questions, verbalization of fears

■ Hypervolemia	■ Normovolemia	■ Careful administration of fluid replacement
		Maintain diet with sodium restriction
		Strict intake and output q1-2 hr; daily weights
		Monitor for presence of
		  Moist rales
		  Dyspnea, tachycardia
		  Pulmonary congestion
		  Edema, distended neck veins
		  Increased central venous pressure (CVP), cardiac output, pulmonary artery pressure (PAP), and pulmonary capillary wedge pressure (PCWP)
		  Hypertension
		  Abnormal skin turgor
		Notify physician of any abnormality
		If hypervolemia occurs
		  Administer diuretics as ordered
		  Monitor pressures (CVP, cardiac output, PCWP, and BP) q½-1 hr
		  Head gatch at 45-degree angle
		  Dialysis may be ordered; see Standards: *Peritoneal dialysis; Hemodialysis*

■ Electrolyte imbalance
  Hyperkalemia
  Hypernatremia
  Other ions, including
    Low serum Ca^{2+} levels
    Elevated serum Mg^{2+} levels
    Elevated serum phosphate levels
	■ Electrolyte levels within normal limits	■ Monitor for presence of
		  Acidosis—check arterial blood gas levels q4-8 hr
		  Skin turgor, flaccid paralysis, and anxiety
		  Arrhythmias
		    Ventricular tachycardia
		    Conduction defect
		    Presence of peaked T wave
		  Abnormal electrolyte levels q4-6 hr
		  Hypertension
		  Congestive heart failure
		  Tetany
		Notify physician of any abnormality
		If electrolyte imbalance occurs
		  Administer therapy as ordered
		  Antacid-phosphate binders
		  Vitamin D
		  Kayexalate to bind K^+
		  Infusion of sodium bicarbonate, calcium solutions, glucose and insulin, cation-exchange resins
		  Restriction of potassium and sodium intake
		  Continuous cardiac monitoring may be ordered
		  Monitor electrolyte levels q1-2 hr
		  Assess effect of therapy
		  Assist in dialysis if ordered; see Standards: *Peritoneal dialysis; Hemodialysis*

Potential problems	Expected outcomes	Nursing activities
■ Infection	■ Infection free	■ Prevention 　Administer good hygiene 　Observe aseptic technique when ministering to the patient 　Administer Foley catheter care every shift and prn 　Aseptically change and dress IV sites 　Pulmonary physiotherapy q2-4 hr Monitor for presence of 　General malaise 　Hypothermia/hyperthermia; check TPR q2-4 hr 　Abnormal WBC counts q6-12 hr 　Signs of local infection 　Positive C and S results of blood or secretions Notify physician of any abnormality If infection occurs 　Appropriate cultures redone as ordered 　Protective isolation may be ordered (neutropenia) 　Administer antibiotic therapy as ordered
■ Cardiovascular disorders: hypertension related to Fluid retention Renin angiotensin system disturbance	■ Resolution of hypertension BP within normal limits	■ Monitor for 　Diastolic pressure greater than 100 mg Hg 　Possible seizures 　Headache and restlessness Notify physician of any abnormality If hypertension occurs 　Monitor vital signs q½ hr and prn 　Maintain low sodium diet as ordered 　Strict intake and output q1 hr; daily weights 　Administer antihypertensive medications as ordered 　Administer diuretics and sedatives as ordered 　Assist in dialysis if ordered; see Standards: *Peritoneal dialysis; Hemodialysis*
■ Cardiovascular disorders: pericarditis	■ Adequate cardiac output Normal pericardium	■ Monitor for presence of 　Chest pain, pain on deep inspiration and change of position 　Paradoxical pulse 　Pericardial friction rub 　Arrhythmia Notify physician of any abnormality If pericarditis occurs 　Monitor arterial pressure and cardiac activity continuously 　Position for comfort 　Administer medication for chest pain 　Assist in dialysis or pericardiocentesis as ordered, if needed; see Standards: *Pericarditis; Peritoneal dialysis; Hemodialysis*
■ Uremia: central and peripheral nervous disorders Disorientation Confusion Neuropathy	■ Patient is oriented to time, place, and persons Clear sensorium Normal neuromuscular function	■ Prevention 　Orient patient to time, place, date, and persons 　Placement of a clock and calendar in room 　Planning and participation in own care if able 　Passive and active range of motion (ROM) exercises Monitor for 　Inability to concentrate for long periods of time 　Periods of agitation, excitation, and depression 　Changes in LOC 　Peripheral neuropathy progressing to numbness, difficulty in position sense with eventual loss of muscle power Notify physician of any abnormality

Potential problems	Expected outcomes	Nursing activities
		If central and peripheral nervous disorders occur 　Administer therapy as ordered 　Position for comfort 　Provision for protection against injury, i.e., padded siderails, 　　restraints if needed, as ordered 　Physiotherapy if needed, as ordered
■ Uremia: GI manifestation 　Nausea 　Ulcers	■ Normal GI function 　Absence of nausea, 　vomiting, ulcers	■ Test vomitus or NG aspirate and stool for Hematest Monitor for Hct and Hgb daily Observe for nausea, vomiting, and anorexia Notify physician of any abnormality If GI manifestation of uremia occurs 　Alterations in diet therapy may be ordered 　Administer antiemetic drugs if needed, as ordered 　Provide frequent mouth care 　Administer iron supplement as ordered 　If blood transfusion is administered, observe for transfusion 　　reaction
■ Uremia: hematopoietic 　system disturbances 　Normochromic 　Normocytic anemia 　Coagulation abnormalities	■ Hct, Hgb, and coagulation studies within normal limits 　Increased reticulocyte count	■ Monitor: 　Hgb and Hct daily; Hct may fall to 11% to 12% if untreated 　Platelet count daily; quality may be defective 　For subcutaneous hemorrhage 　For pale skin, mucosa, and nail beds 　Weakness and fatigability Notify physician of any abnormality If hematopoietic system disturbances occur 　Blood transfusion may be ordered; observe for transfusion 　　reaction 　Protect patient from injury with padded siderails
■ Uremia: integumentary 　system disturbances 　Skin thickened, rough, 　and dry	■ Skin reflects good turgor and hydration 　Absence of pruritus	■ Provide frequent mouth care and good skin care; apply lotion Reposition frequently Administer calamine lotion for pruritus Administer antihistaminic if needed, as ordered
■ Progressive renal dysfunction related to renal osteodystrophy in hyperparathyroidism	■ BP, P within normal limits 　Normal renal function 　Normovolemia 　Normal blood levels of nitrogenous waste substances 　Electrolyte levels within normal limits	■ Administer therapy as ordered to preserve kidney function, including 　Antibiotics that are not nephrotoxic 　Compatible blood products Administer therapy to maintain cardiac output and renal blood flow Administer phosphate binders as ordered Careful administration of vitamin D as ordered Subtotal parathyroidectomy is sometimes necessary followed by vitamin D and calcium supplements Monitor 　TPR, BP, CVP q2-4 hr 　Peripheral circulation, color 　LOC 　Urine output q2 hr 　Phosphate and Ca^{2+} levels daily Notify physician of any abnormality, and alter the aforementioned activities as ordered

Potential problems	Expected outcomes	Nursing activities
■ Malnutrition	■ Nutrition adequate to prevent protein catabolism Positive nitrogen balance Weight maintained or weight gain if appropriate	■ Assess baseline nutritional status Set required therapeutic diet and fluids with physician and dietitian Monitor for signs and symptoms of malnutrition; increased BUN daily Monitor strict intake and output every shift, daily weights Provide frequent oral care Ensure intake of therapeutic diet and fluid required Provide for small frequent feedings if necessary Mobilize, ambulate as soon as possible to decrease tissue catabolism Provide good hygiene Administer anabolic steroids if ordered Administer hyperalimentation if ordered; see Standard: *Total parenteral nutrition through central venous catheter*

■ Insufficient knowledge to comply with discharge regimen*	■ Sufficient knowledge to comply with discharge regimen
	Patient/family accurately describes dietary, medication, and activity regimens
	
	Patient/family identifies signs and symptoms of acute and chronic renal dysfunction requiring immediate medical attention
	Patient/family accurately describes plans for follow-up care
		■ Assess patient/family's level of understanding, ability to comprehend follow-up plan of care or discharge regimen
		
		Discuss
		  Prescribed therapeutic diet and fluids
		  Medications including purposes, side effects, route, dose, schedules/times, and precautions
		  Activity progression: avoid overfatigue; allow for rest and relaxation
		Describe signs and symptoms of acute and chronic renal dysfunction
		
		Describe follow-up plan of care, clinic visits, when and where to go, who to see, and what specimens to bring
		Provide opportunity for and encourage questions and verbalization of anxiety regarding discharge regimen
		Arrange follow-up care with community health organization if necessary

*If this type of follow-up care is the responsibility of the critical care unit nurse.

45 □ Peritoneal dialysis

Dialysis is a method of removing metabolic waste products, electrolytes, and excess body fluid during renal failure. Certain toxic substances may be similarly removed when the kidney is inadequate to perform the task. Dialysis is based on the principle that a substance present in different concentrations on two sides of a semipermeable membrane moves from the side of greater concentration to that of lesser concentration (diffusion).

Peritoneal dialysis uses the patient's peritoneum as the semipermeable membrane, permitting transfer of nitrogenous waste products and other substances from the blood through the peritoneum into the dialysate, a solution composed of dextrose and electrolytes in concentrations that facilitate this transfer. The glucose in the dialysate creates an osmotic gradient such that the solvent (water) moves from an area of greater water concentration to one of lesser water concentration.

The equipment needed for the procedure includes the peritoneal dialysis catheter, administration tubing, cutdown tray, sterile towels, surgical gloves, and dialysis fluid (dialysate) of a specified osmolarity, either a 1.5% or 4.25% glucose solution. Both are hypertonic to normal plasma and will provide an osmotic gradient for the passage of fluid through the peritoneal membrane into the dialysate, with the 4.25% solution providing the great osmotic gradient. Generally, 1.5% is used initially; if a greater or faster body fluid loss is required, 1.5% and 4.25% solutions may be used alternately, or 4.25% may be used continuously (in adults).

Potassium may be added to the dialysate, even in the presence of hyperkalemia, to allow a more gradual rate of potassium ion diffusion and loss.

Heparin may be added to the dialysis fluid to prevent coagulation at the catheter tip and to ensure free flow of the solution.

Peritoneal dialysis is superior to hemodialysis in that it uses a simpler technique and produces a more gradual physiological change. Peritoneal dialysis, however, is less useful when rapid removal of toxic substances, metabolites, body fluid, and/or electrolytes is necessary. The technique is also less useful when the peritoneal membrane surface is not intact and cannot retain the dialysate, such as occurs in the early postoperative period after abdominal surgery. Peritoneal dialysis is associated with an increased risk of infection, particularly pulmonary and peritoneal; significant protein (albumin) loss; and patient discomfort.

Careful observation of the patient while receiving and immediately following peritoneal dialysis is an important aspect of this procedure. Various changes in the regimen may be based on these observations according to metabolic, fluid, and electrolyte changes that occur. Problems that arise may also require alterations in the therapeutic regimen, including difficulties with the peritoneal dialysis system, respiratory embarrassment, hemodynamic instability, and infection.

ASSESSMENT

1. History of ingestion/injection of drugs or other toxic substances
2. History, presence, and nature of the following
   a. Cardiac decompensation and other abnormalities that decrease renal blood flow
   b. Coronary heart disease; "cardiac" medications

taken, such as digitalis, antianginal agents, beta-blocking agents
   c. Hypertension—antihypertensive medications taken
   d. Lower urinary tract obstruction
   e. Kidney disease
   f. Previous peritoneal dialysis
   g. Previous surgery, particularly abdominal surgery
   h. Related medical problems
   i. Malnutrition
   j. Uremia and related problems
      (1) Anemia
      (2) Metabolic bone disease
      (3) Gout
      (4) Coronary artery disease
      (5) Cardiovascular complications
      (6) Infections
      (7) Neuromuscular complications
      (8) Gastrointestinal complications—ulcers
   k. Other health problems
3. Signs and symptoms of kidney/bladder dysfunction—costovertebral pain (flank pain, lower back discomfort); hematuria; dysuria
4. Lab and diagnostic tests, including indices of renal function
   a. Urine specific gravity
   b. Urine osmolality
   c. Urine sediment
   d. Urine electrolytes
   e. Urine creatinine
   f. Serum electrolytes
   g. Serum creatinine, uric acid, BUN
   h. Blood levels of certain toxic substances based on patient's history
   i. WBC count
   j. Liver function studies including transaminase levels and coagulation studies; serum protein levels
   k. Chest radiograph results
   l. Abdominal flat plate roentgenogram results
   m. Kidney, ureter, and bladder radiograph results
   n. Cystoscopy
   o. Arteriogram
   p. Ultrasonography
5. Hemodynamic/respiratory status
   a. BP, P, peripheral circulation, temperature, respirations for rate and quality
   b. Urine volume
6. Weight
7. Level of patient/family's anxiety regarding patient's

renal dysfunction, the need for peritoneal dialysis, the procedure itself, and other related concerns

GOALS

1. Reduction of patient/family's anxiety with provision of information, explanations, and encouragement
2. Minimal discomfort associated with peritoneal dialysis
3. Infection free; absence of peritonitis
4. Respiratory function adequate to maintain blood gas levels within patient's normal limits, without pulmonary infection
5. Cardiovascular stability—BP and P within patient's normal limits; no ectopic beats
6. Normovolemia—desired alteration in body fluid volume achieved
7. Efficient dialysis, adequate to achieve levels of nitrogenous waste products (BUN, creatinine, uric acid) within normal limits, serum electrolyte values within normal limits and adequate to remove toxic substances (drugs, etc.); normoglycemia; and adequate blood protein/albumin levels are maintained
8. Acid-base parameters in balance
9. Nutrition adequate to prevent protein catabolism and to maintain positive nitrogen balance
10. Before discharge patient/family is able to
    a. Properly care for catheter insertion site
    b. Identify each medication and describe the administration regimen
    c. Keep accurate fluid intake and output records
    d. Accurately record daily weight
    e. Consume proper diet and describe dietary guidelines
    f. Maintain progressive activity level in the hospital and describe expected daily schedule after discharge
    g. Describe plan for follow-up visits

Potential problems	Expected outcomes	Nursing activities
■ Patient/family's anxiety related to Hospitalization Disease process Diagnostic procedures Therapy employed	■ Patient/family's behavior demonstrates decreased anxiety with provision of explanations and encouragement	■ Assess level of patient/family's anxiety Evaluate psychosocial dynamics of family If complex problems are present, mobilize other resources, which may include a social worker, a clergyman, and a psychiatrist for consults and follow-up Explain in simple terms patient's disease process and need for dialysis Explain procedure to patient/family Encourage and provide opportunity for patient/family to ask questions and verbalize fears and anxieties Encourage and comfort patient/family during procedure; reassure them that certain responses during dialysis are normal (e.g., feeling of fullness) Assess reduction in level of patient/family's anxiety with provision of information, explanations, and encouragement
■ Improper choice and preparation of dialysate	■ Dialysis solution properly prepared with dialysate able to efficiently dialyze patient to achieve Normovolemia and desired weight changes Acid-base balance and electrolyte levels within normal limits	■ Ongoing assessment of BP CVP if available Weight Acid-base balance P Temperature Parameters of kidney function Urine output Specific gravity Urine sediment Osmolality—serum, urine Electrolytes—serum, urine Creatinine—serum, urine Serum uric acid, BUN Serum levels of certain toxic substances based on patient's history Hgb, Hct

Potential problems	Expected outcomes	Nursing activities
		Liver function studies, including transaminases, coagulation studies, and serum protein levels
		Prevent by
		Properly preparing patient for dialysis
		Ensure empty bladder by having the patient void or by placing a bladder catheter
		Place patient in supine position with slight head elevation
		Assist physician during catheter insertion
		Properly preparing dialysate and equipment
		Add medications ordered to dialysate bottle and label it with the additives, the number of the exchange, date, and time
		Warm dialysate to 37° C (98.6° F)
		Connect administration set to dialysate bottle and prime tubing with dialysate
		Connect primed administration tubing to peritoneal catheter
		Ascertaining and implementing the prescribed regimen for dialysis; guidelines should include
		Type of dialysate to be used
		Times for inflow/equilibration/outflow (usually 10 minutes/20 to 30 minutes/20 to 30 minutes)
		Total number of exchanges (usually 48 to 72), medications to be added (usually potassium, heparin)
		Frequency of weights; specimens to be sent, i.e., blood electrolyte levels and culture of dialysate

■ Traumatic insertion of catheter
  Bleeding
	■ Atraumatic insertion
	
	  Blood-tinged returns subside after the first few runs
		■ Monitor for frank bloody drainage that continues past the first few runs (blood-tinged drainage normally subsides after the first few runs)
		Notify physician immediately of significant bleeding
		If bleeding occurs
		  A pressure dressing, sandbags, ice packs may be applied
		  The area where a bleeding arteriole is suspected may be infiltrated with solution containing epinephrine
		  Monitor BP, P closely

Bowel perforation	Absence or resolution of bowel perforation	Monitor for
		  Fecal contents in the dialysate returns
		  Urge for defecation, eventually producing a stool mixed with large amounts of fluid
		  Hypotension, tachycardia
		If bowel perforation occurs
		  Notify physician immediately; stop dialysis
		  An antibiotic is usually added to dialysate with the antibiotic lavage continuing for several days
		  Monitor BP, P, q15-30 min
		  A surgical repair of the tear may be done immediately, then lavage started; prepare patient for procedure
		  Notify physician if pronounced hypotension, tachycardia occur

Bladder perforation	Absence/resolution of bladder perforation	Monitor for
		  Intense urge to urinate with large urine outputs
		  Production of large amounts of urine through a bladder catheter; if this occurs, test for high glucose concentration
		If bladder perforation occurs
		  Notify physician of signs/symptoms
		  Stop dialysis as ordered
		  Assist with removal of catheter as needed

Potential problems	Expected outcomes	Nursing activities

■ Leakage of dialysate from the insertion site of peritoneal catheter, resulting in Excoriation of skin	■ Absence of or minimal leakage of dialysate around catheter insertion site
	Absence of excoriation of skin around catheter insertion site
		■ Monitor for frequent need to change dressing and for dialysate leakage around insertion site
		If dialysate leakage occurs
		  Weigh dressing and include in record of fluid loss
		  Assist physician to tighten and/or place a suture in the skin around the catheter insertion site
		  Change dressing at the catheter insertion site as frequently as needed
		  Protect the skin at the insertion site by applying a spray that forms a barrier to the irritating dialysate returns

Inaccurate intake and output records	Accurate dialysate inflow/outflow records	

■ Ileus, usually related to irritation/inflammation from dialysis procedure	■ Normal bowel function	■ Monitor for any of the following that persist after the day of catheter insertion
		  Absence of bowel sounds
		  No bowel movements
		  Malaise, loss of appetite
		  Abdominal distention
		  Large NG aspirates if NG tube in place
		Notify physician if aforementioned abnormalities occur
		If ileus occurs
		  Apply warm packs to help stimulate peristalsis
		  Administer medications to increase bowel activity as ordered
		  Provide for adequate nutritional intake as ordered either by oral or intravenous/central venous route

■ Pain, irritation, discomfort occurring during and/or immediately after catheter placement related to
Catheter too long; catheter irritation of bladder, vagina, root of penis
	■ Absence of/or minimal discomfort during dialysis treatment
	
	Absence and/or resolution of irritation
		■ Assess presence, nature, and severity of pain, discomfort
		Monitor for
		  Pain occurring at point of catheter insertion into abdomen
		  Localized pain in region of catheter tip
		  Complaints of pain in lower abdomen, perineal region or discomfort localized in the bladder, vagina, or at the root of the penis
		Notify physician of these abnormalities
		If pain, irritation, discomfort occur
		  Administer analgesics if needed, as ordered
		  If pain occurs at time of insertion, the catheter will be repositioned by the physician
		    A short length of the catheter is usually pulled out to alleviate discomfort
		    With repositioning, discomfort should subside within a short period of time
		Note alleviation of mild discomfort

Cold dialysate	Absence of or minimal discomfort during dialysis treatment	Prevent by warming dialysate to 37° C (98.6° F) If inadequate warming is suspected Monitor for presence and nature of pain that begins when inflow is initiated and continues through much of equilibration phase
Acidic dialysate		Monitor for pain that starts during inflow and continues during equilibration phase If this type of pain occurs, add bicarbonate to the dialysate or into the administration tubing before the run; procaine may also be added to the tubing as ordered

Distention of peritoneum, abdomen with dialysate		Monitor for discomfort most pronounced toward the end of inflow and the beginning of the outflow phases
		If distention of peritoneum, abdomen with dialysate occurs
		  Assure patient that discomfort usually lessens after the first few runs
		  Place patient in semi-Fowler's position
		  Administer analgesics if needed, as ordered
		  For significant continuing discomfort, notify physician; smaller infusion volumes may be ordered

Potential problems	Expected outcomes	Nursing activities
Air infusion through administration tubing		Prevent by allowing no air entry during connections and by using an administration set with a drip chamber and rubber diaphragm (that closes over the tubing when the chamber is empty) Monitor for symptoms that include pain in the shoulder blade area If air infusion occurs, air can sometimes be removed from the peritoneum through the catheter with the patient in a knee-chest or Trendelenburg position
Intraperitoneal infection		Monitor for severe continuing pain, which may indicate infection in the peritoneum (peritonitis); see Problem, Peritonitis

■ Peritonitis
NOTE: Sterile peritonitis is an inflammatory process and may occur in response to the composition of the dialysate
	■ Absence of peritonitis
	Afebrile
		■ Prevent infection by
		  Changing administration tubing according to hospital protocol
		  Changing dressing frequently, since small amounts of dialysate inevitably leak around the insertion site
		  Cleansing insertion site and surrounding skin with an antiseptic solution; a protective skin barrier spray or cream may be applied to protect the skin
		  Between dialysis treatments, assisting physician in the removal of dialysis catheter and aseptic replacement with a peritoneal button to keep the tract open *or* disconnecting administration tubing from peritoneal catheter and placing cap on hub of catheter; placing a sterile dressing over the catheter
		  After catheter or peritoneal ''button'' is removed, ensuring that the wound is completely closed with Steri-strips or butterfly bandages and a sterile dressing
		Monitor
		  Temperature q2 hr and prn for elevation
		  For persistent cloudy dialysate returns
		  For persistent unexplained localized or diffused tenderness, particularly if in association with elevated WBC count in dialysate returns
		  Results of serial cultures of dialysate returns
		  For unexplained fever and malaise
		  For elevated WBC count in the dialysate returns (300 cells/mm^3 or more)
		  Elevated serum WBC levels
		  Catheter tract or insertion site for infection
		  For late catheter obstruction that cannot be corrected by irrigation
		If peritonitis occurs
		  Send a stat sample of the dialysate returns for C and S determination, as ordered
		  Monitor results of stat blood cultures, if done
		  Add antibiotics to the dialysate if ordered
		  Administer systemic antibiotics if ordered (often given if septicemia is documented)
		  Administer a local antibiotic with a short half-life in the dialysate if ordered

Potential problems	Expected outcomes	Nursing activities

- Pulmonary insufficiency
Pulmonary infection, pneumonia
Dialysate elevates diaphragm, which decreases diaphragmatic excursion and tidal volumes, producing respiratory embarrassment
Uremic patient is particularly susceptible as a result of
Depressed cough reflex and respiratory effort due to CNS depression
Increased viscosity of pulmonary secretions due to dehydration and mouth breathing
Pulmonary congestion and "shock lung" syndrome

- Breathing without respiratory distress
Adequate exchange of blood gases, with Pa_{O_2} and Pa_{CO_2} within normal limits
No atelectasis, respiratory infection

- Prevention
Place patient in semi-Fowler's position
Provide respiratory support to maintain adequate oxygenation and ventilation, which may include humidified O_2 through a mask or artificial ventilation if necessary
Turn side to side q1-2 hr
Administer chest physiotherapy as indicated
Assist extubated patient with deep breathing and coughing, breathing exercises, incentive spirometry

Monitor
Quality of respirations q½ hr until stable; note tachypnea, dyspnea, shortness of breath, shallow breathing
Breath sounds q1 hr and prn
Note decreased, absent, or adventitious breath sounds
Amount, color, and consistency of secretions
Arterial blood gas results; note hypoxemia, hypercapnia
Chest radiograph results
Serial body weights
Temperature q1-2 hr for fever
Notify physician of clinical abnormalities
If pulmonary insufficiency occurs
Augment activities to keep lungs clear (see prevention activities)
Administer humidified O_2 support as ordered
Assist with intubation if procedure is necessary (see Standard: *Mechanical ventilation*)
If pneumonia occurs
Administer antibiotic therapy as ordered
Monitor sputum C and S results
Monitor temperature q1 hr until stable
Administer antipyretics if needed, as ordered
Provide for a quiet, restful environment
Reassure patient that nurse is always nearby

- Hemodynamic instability related to hypotension, resulting from
Rapid removal of intravascular fluid
Vena caval compression (children more susceptible to this)

- Hemodynamic stability with BP, P within normal limits

- Prevent by
Holding or decreasing the dosage of cardiac drugs and antihypertensive medications in the presence of renal failure; adjust dosages at time of dialysis as ordered
Avoiding rapid fluid shifts and loss by administering 1.5% dialysate, at least for the first few runs
Monitor
Weight every 6 to 10 runs; weigh patient when peritoneum is empty
BP and P q15 min during the first complete cycle (run) of dialysis; thereafter monitor BP and P q1-2 hr
Monitor ECG continuously if monitor is available
CVP and PAP if available
Urine output with specific gravity q1 hr
Notify physician of significant abnormalities in these parameters
If *mild* hypotension occurs
Open drainage tubing and begin the outflow phase to reduce pressure exerted by the fluid on the vena cava
Turn patient to side in an effort to reduce direct vena caval pressure and enhance the outflow phase
If a *marked* hypotension occurs
Notify physician
Alter dialysate regimen as ordered, which may include changing from exclusive use of 4.25% dialysate to a regimen of alternating 4.25% and 1.5% (in adults)
Reduce the volume of each run (infusion) as ordered

Potential problems	Expected outcomes	Nursing activities

■ Hemodynamic instability related to hypertension	■ Hemodynamic stablity with BP, P within normal limits	■ Monitor BP q½-1 hr during dialysis; note hypertension
		If significant hypertension occurs, notify physician
		    Evaluate level of discomfort; alleviate any cause of pain (see Problem, Traumatic insertion of catheter)
		    Evaluate for fluid overload, particularly if 1.5% concentration has been used and the overall dialysis fluid balance is positive
		Notify physician of these abnormalities

■ Arrhythmias
Premature beats associated with cold dialysate, respiratory distress
Bradyarrhythmias related to overdistention with dialysate (may be a reflex response)
	■ Absence or resolution of arrhythmias, bradyarrhythmia
	Adequate cardiac output
	Hemodynamic stability
		■ Prevent by
		    Minimizing discomfort associated with peritoneal dialysis by
		      Positioning
		      Implementing measures to prevent respiratory distress
		      Warming the dialysate
		    Administering humidified O_2 supplements to provide for adequate oxygenation if needed, as ordered
		    Administering therapy to achieve acid-base parameters and electrolyte levels within normal limits
		Monitor
		    ECG continuously via bedside oscilloscope and meter if possible
		    For arrhythmias
		      Ectopic beats
		      Premature beats
		    P q1 hr and prn for bradycardia
		    Arterial blood gas results for hypoxemia, acidosis
		    Serum electrolyte levels for imbalance
		Notify physician of any significant incidence of ectopic beats (more than 4 to 6/minute) or a significant drop in pulse rate
		If arrhythmias and/or bradycardia occur
		    Administer antiarrhythmic agent as ordered; closely monitor patient's response
		    Decrease size of dialysate infusion volume if ordered
		    Administer therapy to correct predisposing factors such as hypoxia, acid-base imbalance, or electrolyte abnormalities as ordered

■ Hypervolemia, fluid overload related to
The sole use of the 1.5% dialysate, particularly in adults
Hyponatremia (dilutional) occurring just before dialysis treatment
	■ Normovolemia
	Desired alteration in body fluid volume and weight is achieved
		■ Prevent by
		    Keeping an accurate record of intake and output, providing for an even or negative balance, as the patient's plan of care requires
		    Administering salt-poor albumin as ordered
		Monitor
		    Serial body weights (q8 hr) during dialysis therapy
		    For positive fluid balance (patient retaining fluid)
		    For elevated BP, P, CVP, and PAP
		    For elevated urine output
		    For confusion or disorientation
		    Serum electrolyte results
		    For hyponatremia
		Notify physician of abnormalities
		If hypervolemia occurs
		    Alter dialysate regimen as ordered; the proportion of runs using dialysate of 4.25% glucose concentration may be increased
		    If electrolyte imbalance is present, administer therapy to correct as ordered

Potential problems	Expected outcomes	Nursing activities
■ Inefficient dialysis related to difficulties in drainage of dialysate (outflow phase)	■ Efficient dialysis sufficient to achieve Normovolemia—desired alteration in body fluid volume (desired weight change achieved) Acid-base balance within normal limits Blood levels of nitrogenous waste products within normal limits, including BUN, creatinine, uric acid	■ Monitor for signs of difficulty in drainage or a protracted outflow phase If difficulty in drainage occurs, enhance drainage of dialysate By turning patient from side to side By pressing hands against patient's retroperitoneal spaces (use this method particularly if turning is not well tolerated) By sitting patient up in bed (if patient's physiological status permits)
■ Inefficient dialysis related to difficulties in inflow caused by Obstructed catheter Clots Fibrin Fat deposits Malpositioned catheter The catheter may be nestled in an area of dense adhesions from previous surgery or peritonitis	■ Peritoneal dialysis system patent and optimal inflow/outflow phases of dialysis achieved	■ Prevent catheter obstruction by adding heparin to the dialysate, if ordered, in an effort to prevent occlusion of the catheter with fatty, fibrin aggregates Monitor for slow or absent progress in infusion of dialysate If catheter is obstructed, assist physician with irrigation of catheter If catheter malposition is apparent, notify physician Assist with repositioning catheter if needed
Kinks in catheter, tubing	Patent catheter	Prevent kinks in administration tubing, catheter; anchor catheter such that good inflows/outflows are achieved Monitor for difficulty in both inflow and outflow phases If kinks in catheter and/or tubing occur Note external position of catheter; change the angle at which it enters the skin, if necessary, to achieve better catheter alignment, obviate kinking If the aforementioned maneuvers do not work, notify physician and assist with catheter replacement, if procedure is necessary
Dialysate bottle not high enough Air in administration tubing		The drip chamber of the dialysate administration tubing should be 4 feet above the patient Prevent air entry into the administration tubing during connections If the outflow tubing becomes partly or completely filled with air, it may need to be reprimed with dialysate from the inflow tubing
Peritonitis (see Problem, Peritonitis)	Peritoneum free of infection	Prevent peritonitis (see Problem, Peritonitis) Observe for signs and symptoms of peritonitis If peritonitis develops Add antibiotics to the dialysate if ordered Administer systemic antibiotics if ordered

Potential problems	Expected outcomes	Nursing activities
Adhesions may develop subsequent to repeated intraperitoneal instillation of dialysate	Peritoneum free of adhesions	Observe for difficulties in both inflow/outflow phases; adhesions should be suspected if patient has had previous abdominal surgery, peritonitis, peritoneal dialysis or if the catheter has been in place for several days If problem occurs Notify physician Assist with catheter replacement if procedure is necessary Prepare patient for hemodialysis if ordered
■ Hyperglycemia related to infusion of 4.25% glucose dialysate solution, which can lead to cellular dehydration, confusion, and eventually coma	■ Blood glucose level within normal limits	■ Monitor Blood glucose levels by Labstix* (at the bedside) Serial glucose determinations q6 hr when dialysis is initiated Urine sugar levels for glycosuria For clinical signs of hyperglycemia Notify physician of abnormalities If hyperglycemia occurs Alternate dialysate concentrations—4.25% and 1.5% if ordered Add insulin to dialysate bottle or give subcutaneously as ordered Monitor serial K^+ levels closely (hypokalemia should be avoided, particularly if the patient is receiving digoxin)
■ Protein loss	■ Serum protein/albumin levels within normal limits	■ Monitor Serum albumin/protein levels as ordered Dialysate returns for protein levels If significant protein loss occurs Administer salt-poor albumin to replace albumin lost through peritoneum, as ordered Administer nutritional replacement of protein/albumin as ordered; if po diet is possible, an 80 g protein diet is often instituted in adults
■ Malnutrition, protein catabolism, which may be related to Anorexia Nausea and vomiting Altered mentation, malaise Decreased absorption of Ca^{2+} and iron Stomatitis	■ Adequate nutritional intake Positive nitrogen balance Weight maintenance or weight gain	■ Prevent by Controlling nausea and vomiting with medication as ordered, if necessary Providing for adequate calories, essential amino acids Administering low sodium, high protein, high carbohydrate diet as ordered, with potassium and sodium restriction depending on BP and serum Na^+ levels (if patient can take po diet) Administering small, frequent meals Administering vitamins (particularly vitamin D), calcium, and iron supplements as ordered Administering phosphate binders, folic acid, and nandrolone decanoate (Deca-Durabolin) if ordered Monitor for signs/symptoms of malnutrition If malnutrition occurs, reevaluate and alter aforementioned preventive activities as ordered; if needed, administer sufficient calories via a peripheral or central venous catheter as ordered (see Standard: *Total parenteral nutrition through central venous catheter*)
■ Insufficient knowledge to comply with discharge regimen†	■ Sufficient knowledge to comply with discharge regimen	■ Discuss extended plan of care with physician and ascertain what has already been discussed with the patient Assess patient's understanding of need for dialysis and what his/her responsibilities in care are

*Labstix, Ames Co., Elkhart, Ind.
†If intensive care unit nurse is responsible for this type of follow-up care.

Potential problems	Expected outcomes	Nursing activities
		For patients undergoing long-term dialysis*
		Discuss psychological, social, financial, and physical implications of long-term dialysis with patient; refer patient to a special training program for patients undergoing dialysis at home for further discussion of these aspects
	Before discharge patient/family is able to	Instruct the patient in the following (the patient may be able to assume many of these self-care activities while in the hospital)
	Do proper dressing of catheter insertion site if appropriate	Protection of peritoneal catheter and prosthesis, insertion site, and catheter tract
	Identify each medication and describe the regimen for administration	Aseptic technique and prevention of infection
		Control of (and recording of) fluid intake and output
	Keep accurate fluid intake and output records	Daily weights to be done at same time of day using the same scale
	Describe proper diet	Prescribed diet—adequate in calories and essential amino acids
	Describe activity progression	Medication regimen and precautions
		Reasonable activity level
		Describe preventive measures to avoid exacerbation of renal failure
		If peritoneal dialysis is to be continued at home, refer patient to a special teaching program designed to prepare patient/family to do the dialysis safely and effectively at home
		Provide opportunity for patient/family to ask questions
		Assess patient/family's potential compliance with discharge regimen
		Describe the plan for follow-up visits, including when and where to go, who to see, and what specimens to bring
	Patient successfully, accurately records daily weight on a log form	On follow-up visits the patient will be evaluated for signs/symptoms of protein and calorie malnutrition (weakness, apathy, weight loss, decreased serum albumin levels, and edema)
	Weight is maintained without significant incidence of edema	Fluid balance, including signs/symptoms of under or over hydration and weight, will also be assessed

---

*If intensive care unit nurse is responsible for preparing the patient for long-term dialysis.

46 □ Hemodialysis

Dialysis is a method of removing metabolic waste products, electrolytes, and excess body fluid during renal failure or of removing toxic substances. Dialysis is based on the principle that a substance present in different concentrations on two sides of a semipermeable membrane moves from the side of greater concentration to that of lesser concentration.

The patient's blood is drawn out from the body through tubing into the dialysis machine where it comes into contact with a semipermeable cellophane membrane. The dialysate is made of essential electrolytes in ideal concentrations, including sodium, potassium, calcium, and magnesium, and the anions chloride and acetate. Through the process of diffusion, electrolytes move from the area of greater concentration to that of lesser concentration. Diffusion is also responsible for removal of creatinine, urea, uric acid, potassium, magnesium, and phosphate. Similarly, calcium and acetate may be added to the blood by the same diffusion process. Gradients in osmolality and hydrostatic pressure are created so that excess body fluid can be removed (by a process called ultrafiltration).

Various methods of vascular access are available. The external arteriovenous (AV) shunt was the first device available and is still used. It consists of Teflon cannulas inserted into the radial artery and an adjacent vein. There have been many problems and restrictions regarding the preservation of these shunts and their life span has been short (6 to 12 months).

Internal AV fistulas avoid many of the problems with external Teflon shunts and may last for several years. An artery, either radial or femoral, is connected by a side-to-side anastomosis to an adjacent vein. Internal fistulas can also be created from autogenous saphenous vein grafts, bovine grafts, and Dacron prostheses. After insertion of a graft or prosthesis, the vein into which it is inserted gradually dilates and is able to accommodate blood returning from the dialyzer.

If hemodialysis is necessary and neither a mature internal nor an external fistula or shunt is available, catheters may be inserted into a large artery and/or vein for the treatment.

Heparin is added to the blood to prevent coagulation, using systemic or regional heparinization. Regional heparinization is often preferred in patients who have coagulation deficiencies or who have pericarditis.

Careful observation of the patient while receiving and immediately following hemodialysis is an important aspect of this procedure. Various changes in the regimen may be based on these observations according to metabolic, fluid, and electrolyte changes that occur. Problems that arise may also require alterations in the therapeutic regimen, such as malfunction of the shunt or fistula, hemodynamic instability, and infection.

ASSESSMENT

1. Etiology and/or history of
   a. Renal dysfunction
   b. Lower urinary tract obstruction
   c. Ingestion/injection of drugs or other toxic substances
2. History, presence, nature, and severity of
   a. Malnutrition
   b. Uremia and associated anemia, metabolic bone disease, gout, cardiovascular complications (peri-

carditis), neuromuscular complications, gastrointestinal complications (particularly ulcers)
   c. Infections, hepatitis
   d. Signs/symptoms of kidney/bladder dysfunction—costovertebral pain, hematuria, dysuria, pyuria
   e. Signs and symptoms of chronic renal dysfunction
      (1) Costovertebral pain (flank pain, lower back discomfort)
      (2) Anemia, pallor
      (3) Eyelid swelling
      (4) Pruritus
      (5) Poor skin turgor
      (6) Dry mucous membranes
      (7) Gout
      (8) Malnutrition
   f. Cardiac and cardiovascular abnormalities
      (1) Coronary artery disease; use of medications such as nitroglycerin, digitalis preparations, propranolol (Inderal)
      (2) Hypertension—antihypertensive medications taken
      (3) Pericarditis
      (4) Heart failure
   g. Respiratory abnormalities
      (1) Deep sighing, Kussmaul's respirations
      (2) Urine smell on breath
      (3) Chest radiograph for hilar pneumonitis
   h. Renal abnormalities—if urine is produced, may reflect proteinuria, hematuria, pyuria, casts
   i. Gastrointestinal abnormalities—hiccups, anorexia, nausea and vomiting, coated tongue, patient's complaints of taste of ammonia, ulcers
   j. CNS abnormalities
      (1) Headaches, lassitude
      (2) Confusion, disorientation
      (3) Drowsiness, insomnia
      (4) Muscle twitching, weakness
   k. Retinopathy
3. Results of lab and diagnostic tests, including
   a. Parameters of kidney function
      (1) Urine volume
      (2) Specific gravity
      (3) Sedimentation
      (4) Osmolality
      (5) Electrolytes
      (6) Creatinine
      (7) Serum electrolytes, creatinine, and uric acid; BUN, levels of certain toxic substances based on patient's history

b. Liver function tests, particularly coagulation studies, serum protein, albumin levels

c. Hgb, Hct, and platelets levels; WBC count

GOALS

1. Patient/family's behavior demonstrates reduction in anxiety with provision of information, explanations, encouragement, and psychosocial/spiritual support
2. Hemodynamic stability, absence of arrhythmias or angina, absence of disequilibrium syndrome
3. Dialysis effectively achieves physiological levels of
   a. Metabolic waste products
      (1) BUN
      (2) Creatinine
      (3) Uric acid
      (4) Ammonia
   b. Toxic substances (drugs, etc.)
   c. Electrolytes
   d. Blood volume (normovolemia); excess body fluids removed; weight gain of approximately 0.5 kg/day in adults between treatments
4. Hct, Hgb, platelet levels within normal limits
5. Coagulation studies mildly prolonged during hemodialysis
6. Fistula or shunt patent—fistula walls intact; tissue around shunt or fistula viable and intact
7. Infection free; without hepatitis
8. Nutrition adequate to prevent protein catabolism, to maintain/build body muscle mass, and to preserve protein/fat stores with reasonable blood levels of nitrogenous waste products and minimal uremic symptoms
9. Before discharge the patient is able to
   a. Comply with dietary/fluid restrictions
   b. Keep daily log of weight, fluid intake, and a record of dietary intake if asked
   c. For adults, keep daily weight gain between dialysis treatments at about 0.5 kg/day
   d. Identify foods high in sodium and potassium that will be avoided altogether
   e. Accurately take the proper dose of medications at the correct time and record it accurately on a chart (if hospital permits self-administration)
   f. Properly care for shunt or fistula, using aseptic technique and providing for proper shunt alignment and prevention of injury to shunt or fistula
   g. Properly ascertain shunt/fistula patency
   h. Accurately describe precautionary measures that help to ensure longevity of shunt/fistula
   i. Accurately describe sign/symptoms of complications of chronic renal failure and ways these complications can be prevented
   j. Accurately describe plan for follow-up visits

Potential problems	Expected outcomes	Nursing activities
■ Patient/family's anxiety related to limited understanding of disease and its relationship to need for dialysis and related therapy	■ Patient/family's behavior demonstrates decreased anxiety with provision of information, explanations, and encouragement	■ Ongoing assessment of level of anxiety Assess patient/family's understanding of disease process and its relationship to need for dialysis; explain in simple terms this information as needed Explain procedure for hemodialysis Reassure patient during procedure that certain responses are normal Encourage questions from patient/family
■ Dialysis procedure inadequate for patient's needs related to Improperly prepared hemodialysis system Inappropriate dialysis regimen Excessive ultrafiltration rate (or the rapidity with which body fluid is removed)	■ Effective dialysis sufficient to achieve Blood levels of metabolic waste products within normal limits Removal of desired amount of excess body fluid; desired weight loss during dialysis achieved; normovolemia	■ Prevention Before dialysis is started, perform observations or tests to ensure Accuracy of the dialysate concentrate Dialysate compatibility with blood Patency of blood tubing and membrane Secure connections Intact electrical system Absence of air in tubing Sterile blood circuit (ensure that aseptic technique is used to make all connections) Before hemodialysis is started, ascertain the following guidelines for the treatment as ordered Type of equipment for and frequency and length of dialysis Composition of dialysate

Potential problems	Expected outcomes	Nursing activities
		Fluid administration and/or replacement
		Transfusions to be administered if ordered
		Weight adjustment
		Acceptable flow rates
		Degree of ultrafiltration
		Anticoagulation regimen; other medications to be administered
		Dietary management
		Lab requests, specimens to send
		Other special therapies during dialysis
		Ascertain guidelines for the following emergency situations
		Hypotension
		Hypertensive crisis
		Massive blood loss
		Convulsion
		Equipment failure that is life threatening
		Monitor
		Serial weights for desired amount of weight loss with the hemodialysis treatment
		Lab tests indicating levels of metabolic waste products: BUN, creatinine, uric acid, ammonia
		Serum electrolyte levels
		Arterial blood gas results for acid-base balance
		Notify physician of any abnormality
		If problem occurs
		Examine dialysis system for leaks, air
		Change composition of dialysate as ordered
		Alter hemodialysis regimen if ordered (e.g., adjust flow rates; alter degree of ultrafiltration by decreasing positive pressure in the blood chamber or by decreasing negative pressure in the dialyzing bath, as ordered)
■ Inadequate dialysis with poor blood flow related to	■ Desired degree of dialysis achieved	■ Prevention
Vessel that goes into spasm easily	Blood levels of metabolic waste products within normal limits (BUN, creatinine, uric acid, ammonia)	Allow freshly placed arterial venous fistula to heal and "mature" before using it for dialysis (2 to 4 weeks)
Immature vessel or immature vessels around shunt		Maintain cuff pressure at 300 mm Hg
		For the first few dialysis treatments, smaller needle sizes (fistulas) and slower blood flows may be employed; maintain flows sufficient to keep arterial side of tubing filled
Mature but small vessels	Blood levels of electrolytes within normal limits	In large adults a fistula can usually accommodate a large 14-gauge needle; the fistula in smaller adults and children may not accept such a large needle
Needle, cannula improperly positioned	Removal of excess body fluid; desired weight loss achieved	Initiate dialysis by slowly increasing blood flows
Flow rates set too high (in the presence of a satisfactorily functioning vessel, cannula)	Normovolemia	Monitor for indices of poor blood flow
		Note low flowmeter readings
	Acid-base balance within normal limits	Collapsed tubing on arterial and/or venous side of dialysis tubing, indicating vessel spasm, improper positioning of one or both needles on sides of the cannula, or too high a pump speed
Incorrect needle gauge		Abnormalities at vessel cannulation sites, particularly during the first few minutes of operation
		For significant patient discomfort associated with poor blood flows, which may indicate placement of needle tip against vessel wall
		Notify physician of any of these abnormalities
		If vessel spasm occurs, the patient may be instructed to immerse limb in warm/hot water prior to fistula venipuncture
		Warm compresses may be continued during dialysis
		Correct needle position or pump speed as needed

Potential problems	Expected outcomes	Nursing activities

■ Hypotension related to Diversion of approximately 300 ml of patient's blood into dialysis machine Hypovolemia	■ Hemodynamic stability	■ Prevent by
		  Priming dialysis machine with saline solution, albumin, or blood as ordered
		  Avoiding weight loss of more than 3 to 4 kg during dialysis
		Monitor
		  Weight before, during, and after hemodialysis for excessive weight loss
		  BP, P, urine output, and peripheral circulation q15-30 min before, during, and after dialysis until stable; note hypotension, tachycardia, oliguria
		  CVP and PAP, if available, continuously during dialysis via monitor (or measure q15-30 min)
		Notify physician of abnormalities in the aforementioned
		If hypovolemia occurs
		  Place patient in a more horizontal position
		  Administer Albumisol, blood, or blood products as ordered
		  Administer vasopressor medication if ordered
		  Adjust blood flows and ultrafiltration pressures according to protocol or as ordered

■ Hypotension caused by antihypertensive medication When relative hypovolemia occurs during dialysis, an antihypertensive medication may not permit sympathetic vasoconstriction to maintain BP within normal limits	■ Hemodynamic stability BP within normal limits	■ Physician may order omission of antihypertensive medication several hours before dialysis is begun Closely monitor BP, P, and peripheral circulation in patients receiving antihypertensive medication Notify physician if marked hypotension occurs during dialysis procedure Administer therapy as ordered, including fluids and adjustment of the dosage of antihypertensive medication If dramatic hypotension occurs, administer vasopressor medication if ordered

■ Hypotension caused by kinked tubing, vessel spasm, blood leaks in dialyzer	■ Efficient dialysis Patent, unobstructed, intact dialysis system	■ Prevent by ensuring that all connections are tight before dialysis begins and that tubing is intact
		Monitor
		  For kinked tubing, vessel spasm, blood leaks in machine
		  Blood leak detector, if the machine is so equipped, and the dialysate for evidence of a blood leak
		  Serial Hct results
		If tubing is kinked, straighten it and position so that kinking is not likely to recur
		If leak occurs, immediately clamp off cannula tubing and shut machine off; replace the dialysate bath, replace the extracorporeal tubing, ensure the absence of leaks, and resume dialysis
		If vessel spasm occurs, reduce flow rate; if the fistula/shunt is newly placed, reduced flow rates may be necessary for the first few dialysis treatments

■ Hemorrhage related to technical problems in fistula cannulation	■ Hemodynamic stability Hemodialysis needles remain properly placed in fistula Hgb, Hct, and coagulation studies within normal limits or mildly prolonged during dialysis	■ Prevent by
		  Preventing needle dislodgement by securely taping needle in place; observe needle placement frequently
		  Positioning patient's extremity to prevent abrupt movements and needle dislodgement
		Monitor
		  Needle position and security throughout dialysis procedure
		  BP, P, peripheral circulation, urine output, and other available hemodynamic parameters; notify physician of significant abnormalities
		  For bleeding from needle puncture sites (fistula)
		  Serial Hct levels

Potential problems	Expected outcomes	Nursing activities
		If needle becomes dislodged, immediately clamp both the arterial and venous lines; monitor BP, P closely; notify physician; apply pressure for 10 to 15 minutes or until bleeding stops; then apply pressure dressing and leave in place for 3 to 4 hours; another needle may be inserted and dialysis resumed
		If hematoma occurs, apply cool compress or ice bag until effects of heparin have worn off; then apply warm compress to relieve soreness and aid in resolution of hematoma
		If needle is improperly positioned
		Slow blood flow (pump speed) temporarily and check needle/cannulas
		Pull needle back slightly and retape
		Needle/cannula may need to be lifted up by placing a gauze square under the hub of needle or cannula; decrease blood pump speed while doing this maneuver
■ Hemorrhage related to accidental disconnection of shunt between treatments	■ Shunt remains in situ without dislodgement Shunt cannulas remain connected and intact between treatments	■ Prevent by carefully dressing external shunts to protect them from accidental dislodgement Monitor for shunt disconnection If disconnection occurs, clamp both sides of the cannula; notify physician immediately; follow protocol for aseptic reconnection If one cannula comes out of its insertion site, apply pressure to the bleeding side and clamp the cannula that is still in place; notify physician immediately

■ Hemorrhage related to
Systemic heparinization with inadvertent hemorrhage related to altered coagulation times
Repeated punctures of fistula through thin, dry skin
Puncture of external shunt
Tissue breakdown around cannula/fistula insertion sites
Aneurysm formation around insertion site
Cannula tip erosion through subcutaneous tissues or erosion of fistula vessel walls after repeated punctures
	■ BP, P remain within normal limits
	Hgb, Hct remain within patient's normal limits, and no clinical signs of bleeding are evident
	Clotting times, prothrombin time (PT), and activated partial thromboplastin time (APTT) are moderately prolonged during dialysis
	No bleeding from puncture sites occurs
	External shunt intact
	Vessels around cannula tip are viable and intact without aneurysm formation
	Tissue around cannula tips is viable and intact
		■ Prevent extraordinary pressure stress on the extremity used for dialysis by preventing cuff BP measurements on the extremity, both during dialysis and between treatments
		Apply pressure dressing after needle is removed; remove dressing after 3 to 4 hours; if bleeding/oozing continues, reapply pressure dressing for another 2 to 4 hours
		Apply shunt dressing so as to minimize stress on the cannula insertion sites
		Instruct patient to avoid tight clothing on affected extremity
		Rotate fistula vessel puncture sites
		Permit no punctures of external shunt
		Monitor
		  Serial clotting times, PT, and APTT during dialysis
		  For signs/symptoms of external/internal bleeding during and after the dialysis procedure
		  Tissue around cannula insertion site and over the place where an internal fistula joins the patient's artery and vein for redness, swelling, discomfort, and dilatation
		Notify physician of any of these abnormalities
		If bleeding occurs in the presence of systemic heparinization, notify physician; protamine sulfate, the antidote for heparin, is administered as ordered

■ Hypertension related to
Body fluid overload
Disequilibrium syndrome or disorientation caused by
Cerebral edema
Rapid dialysis or removal of serum solutes or fluid
	■ Hemodynamic stability
	BP within patient's normal limits
	Weight gain not more than 0.5 kg/day in adults between dialysis treatments
	Absence of signs and symptoms of disequilibrium syndrome
		■ Prevent by instituting the following as ordered
		  Restrict fluid and sodium intake
		  Individualize the dialysate composition, blood flow rate, and dialysate bath flow rate
		  Correct fluid and electrolyte imbalance slowly and cautiously
		  Administer renin-releasing inhibitors such as propranolol
		Monitor
		  BP, P q15-30 min during treatment
		  For signs of disequilibrium syndrome (hypertension, headache, confusion, nausea and vomiting; in severe cases convulsions have occurred)

Potential problems	Expected outcomes	Nursing activities

		If body fluid overload occurs
		    Alter dialysis treatment to remove excess fluid
		    Review with patient the necessary fluid and sodium restrictions
		If disequilibrium syndrome occurs, administer therapy as ordered, which may include
		    Reducing rate of solute/fluid movement during dialysis
		    Altering dialysate to be more compatible with patient's serum solute or fluid load

■ Angina pectoris, which may be related to
Hypotension
Excessive ultrafiltration
Anxiety
	■ Absence of anginal pain	■ Prevent by slowly increasing blood flow rate (through dialysis machine)
		Monitor
		    BP, P q15-30 min during dialysis
		    For patient's complaints of chest pain
		If problem occurs, notify physician
		Alter the regimen as ordered, including
		    Decreasing the blood flow rate
		    Administering antianginal medication
		    Administering additional crystalloid or colloid fluids if needed, as ordered
		Reassure patient
		A sedative that requires little renal excretion may be ordered
		SEE STANDARD: *Angina pectoris*

■ Arrhythmias related to
Rapid K$^+$ shifts
Hypokalemia or other electrolyte imbalance
Hypotension
	■ Absence of arrhythmias during dialysis
	Serum electrolyte levels within normal limits
		■ Prevent by
		    Maintaining K$^+$ concentration of dialysate bath at a level that will minimize rapid K$^+$ shifts
		    Correcting cause of hypotension (an increase in the rate of fluid administration and/or a decrease in the ultrafiltration rate may increase BP)
		Monitor bedside ECG and apical and radial pulse for the presence and incidence of serious, unperfused arrhythmias
		Notify physician of abnormalities
		If problem occurs
		    Administer antiarrhythmic medication as ordered
		    See Standard: *Arrhythmias*

■ Air embolus related to air entering tubing
Large amounts of air in right ventricle interfere with pulmonary blood flow and oxygenation
Can occur if IV bottle runs dry and blood pump continues to run, pulling air into tubing
	■ Intact hemodialysis system without air in system	■ Prevent by
		    Avoiding kinks in system; pay careful attention to alignment of tubing
		    Carefully taping all connections
		    Avoiding negative pressure between patient and pump; pay careful attention to blood flows
		    Hanging fresh IV bottle/bag before the previous one is completely empty
		Monitor for
		    Air in dialysate tubing
		    Hemodynamic instability
		    Signs and symptoms of pulmonary air embolus
		        Chest pain
		        Cyanosis
		        Cough
		        "Mill wheel murmur" over precordium (sounds like whipping bubbles in motion)
		If a significant amount of air is delivered to patient, turn patient on left side and notify physician; turn off machine immediately

Potential problems	Expected outcomes	Nursing activities

■ Electrolyte imbalance	■ Blood electrolyte levels within normal limits	■ Prevent by using dialysate bath tailored to patient's serum electrolyte values
		Monitor
		    Serum electrolyte levels
		    For signs/symptoms of electrolyte imbalance
		Notify physician of abnormalities
		If problem occurs
		    Alter dialysate bath as ordered
		    Reduce ultrafiltration pressure as ordered

■ Infection
    Of shunt or fistula
    Systemic
	■ Absence or early resolution of local or systemic infection
	    Afebrile
		■ Prevent by
		    Using aseptic technique in preparing dialysis machine, in making all connections
		    Using scrupulous care to ensure uncontaminated dialysis machine tubing
		    Using aseptic technique for daily shunt dressing
		    Aseptically inserting needles into fistula
		Monitor for signs of local infection
		    Swelling, redness, or warmth in skin temperature around shunt or fistula site
		    Drainage of exudate around insertion sites of shunt
		    Decreased circulation to extremity
		    Fever
		Monitor for systemic sepsis
		    Fever
		    Shaking chills
		    Hypotension, signs of peripheral vasoconstriction
		Notify physician of these clinical abnormalities
		If *local or systemic* infection occurs
		    Monitor temperature q1-2 hr until stable
		    Administer antipyretics if needed, as ordered
		If *systemic sepsis* occurs
		    Administer antibiotics IV as ordered
		If *local* infection occurs
		    Administer systemic and/or local antibiotic as ordered
		    Monitor results of C and S of exudate around shunt/fistula insertion sites
		    Apply warm soaks to affected arm if ordered
		    Prepare patient for and assist with drainage of infected local collection or shunt/fistula removal if either procedure is necessary

■ Shunt or fistula closure related to clotting	■ Patent shunt/fistula	■ Prevent shunt/fistula closure by
		    Permitting no cuff BP readings or venipunctures in extremity with shunt or fistula
		    Instructing patient not to sleep on affected extremity
		    For shunts in the leg, avoiding weight bearing for 3 weeks or until edema subsides and healing is in progress
		    Elevating legs to relieve edema
		Monitor for patency frequently after shunt or fistula placement
		    Listen for bruit
		    Palpate for thrill by lightly depressing fistula or lightly pressing shunt; note presence of weak pulsation
		For shunts, frequently monitor color of blood in shunt, observing for
		    Uniform medium red color
		    Dark purplish red color, which may indicate sluggish blood flow and the beginning of a clot

Potential problems	Expected outcomes	Nursing activities
		Dark reddish black color adjacent to a clear yellow fluid, indicating full clot formation with separation of red cells from serum Feel the shunt for warmth, indicating blood flow at body temperature
■ Secondary failure of fistula or shunt related to Repeated cannulation, inflammation, and/or clotting with sclerosis of the vessels Vessels around the fistula/shunt do not dilate Aneurysmal dilatation of vessels around the fistula/shunt Infection at puncture sites (fistula)	■ Patent fistula/shunt Absence of aneurysmal dilatation of vessels around shunt insertion site or of fistula and the surrounding vessels	■ Prevent by Maintaining flows within limits that will provide for efficient dialysis without complications Using aseptic technique during cannulation and applying sterile pressure dressing after completion of hemodialysis treatment Monitor for Inflammation of shunt or fistula site Signs of local infection Dilatation of fistula or of vessels around shunt insertion site Patency of fistula/shunt Note signs of fistula/shunt occlusion by a clot Notify physician of clinical abnormalities If local infection occurs Administer local and/or systemic antibiotics as ordered Administer antipyretic agent if needed, as ordered Apply warm soaks If fistula/shunt clots Prepare patient for and assist with clot removal Prepare patient for surgery for fistula/shunt removal and for insertion of a new fistula/shunt if procedure is necessary
■ Secondary failure of shunt related to Kinking, bending, indentations, or roughening of the shunt tip, thereby enhancing clot formation Irritation at shunt insertion site	■ Patent shunt	■ Prevention Silicone rubber cannulas and Teflon parts help to prevent clot formation Discard bent, indented, roughened tip of connector and replace it Handle shunt carefully; avoid malrotation, bending of shunt back or up Apply dressings to achieve minimal tension on cannula sites Monitor Results of radiograph revealing injury to Teflon tips inside the vessel For clotted shunt; see Problem, Shunt or fistula closure For irritation at shunt insertion site If problem occurs, reevaluate and alter preventive activities; prepare patient for surgical removal of shunt if procedure is necessary
■ Psychosocial difficulties related to Depression Dependency on machine for survival Presence of ''terminal'' illness Alteration of body image Alteration of role in family	■ Patient's behavior demonstrates decreased anxiety with psychosocial support and counseling, occupational counseling, and other support or counseling as indicated	■ Ongoing assessment of patient's level of anxiety Assess psychosocial adjustment in relation to Renal failure Dependence on hemodialysis machine Altered family roles Constant feelings of lethargy, fatigue Assess presence of Impotence Loss of job Marital problems Financial strain Depression

Potential problems	Expected outcomes	Nursing activities

In some cases
  Breakdown of marital, family relationship(s)
  Job loss
		Allow patient to make decisions regarding the scheduling and the process of care as much as possible
		Provide for the following as needed
		  Psychosocial support from staff, physicians, social worker, clergy
		  Arrange for financial or marital counseling if needed; if signs of sexual problems are apparent, assess their nature and provide for counseling as necessary; support family and mobilize their psychosocial resources

■ Anemia with hemolysis of RBCs related to
Dialysate that is too warm or too cold
Inadequate heparinization
Dialysate of wrong concentration, composition
Increased RBC fragility; turbulent blood flows in dialysis machine
Decreased erythropoietin production by diseased kidneys
Splenomegaly with shortened RBC survival
Uremia
Transfusion reaction
	■ Hct, Hgb, platelet levels within normal limits
	Absence of bleeding during hemodialysis
		■ Prevent by
		  Warming dialysate bath to body temperature before dialysis treatment
		  Providing for adequate heparinization by monitoring serial clotting times, APTT during dialysis
		  Mixing small amount of dialysate with patient's blood to check for coagulation before initiating dialysis
		  Carefully regulating blood flows during dialysis treatment; replace frayed, bent parts of shunt; transfuse patient with blood as necessary
		  Avoiding situations that increase RBC hemolysis, consumption of platelets
		  Minimizing uremia with dietary control of protein intake and regulating the frequency of dialysis procedures
		Monitor
		  Slips and tags of all blood and blood products administered for compatibility with patient's blood
		  For transfusion reactions
		  Serial Hct, Hgb, and platelet levels before, during, and after dialysis
		  For enlarged spleen; a splenectomy is occasionally necessary
		Notify physician of abnormalities
		If problem occurs, administer blood products as ordered

■ Hepatitis acquired by
Transfusion with blood-borne hepatitis virus
	■ Patient remains infection free, without hepatitis	■ Monitor serial liver function test results
		Periodically test patient for hepatitis B antigen as ordered
		Periodically test staff for asymptomatic carriers of the hepatitis virus
		If hepatitis occurs
		  Isolate patient
		  Administer supportive care as ordered
		  Monitor patient's liver function tests

■ Congestive heart failure related to repeated hypervolemia between dialysis treatments	■ Patient's cardiac output remains within normal limits
	Patient gains approximately 0.5 kg/day between treatments
		■ Prevent by
		  Restricting patient's fluid intake to the amount prescribed during dialysis
		  Reviewing with patient the proper amount of fluids to be taken between treatments
		Monitor for signs/symptoms of heart failure, particularly low cardiac output and venous congestion
		If problem occurs, see Standard: *Heart failure*

Potential problems	Expected outcomes	Nursing activities

■ Malnutrition related to Protein catabolism (negative nitrogen balance) Loss of protein, fat stores Loss of body muscle mass, weight	■ Nutrition adequate to prevent protein catabolism, maintain/build body muscle mass, preserve protein, fat stores with reasonable BUN and creatinine levels and a reduction in uremic symptoms	■ Assist in evaluation of patient's degree of impairment in renal function and uremic symptoms, which, together with age and physical activity, will determine prescription for protein intake
		Take a diet history
		Assess home situation regarding food preparation
		Ascertain dietary, fluid restrictions
		Arrange with dietitian for dietary consult
		Apply dietary restrictions to patient's dietary habits
		Instruct patient/family in a dietary regimen based on the following guidelines
		  Proteins
		    Usual prescription for adult is 0.5 to 1 g protein/kg/day (40 to 60 g); at least two thirds of the protein should be of high quality, that is, consist primarily of foods high in essential amino acids (eggs, milk, meat, fish, fowl); foods with protein that are low in these essential amino acids are vegetables and cereals
		    The usual proportion of dietary calories composed of protein is about 15%
		    Adequate protein intake reflected by a BUN to serum creatinine ratio of 10 to 1
		  Carbohydrates
		    Sufficient calories in the form of carbohydrates should be ingested to maintain body weight
		    Recommended ratio of nonprotein (carbohydrates and fat) to protein calories is usually 5 to 1
		    Total recommended calorie intake is 40 to 50 calories/kg ideal body weight for an average adult
		    Carbohydrates should be ingested within 4 hours of protein intake for a protein-sparing effect on the body
		    Carbohydrate intolerance may be present, requiring curtailment of concentrated glucose preparations
		  Fats
		    It is usually recommended that less than 35% of the diet consist of fats with an emphasis on the intake of polyunsaturated fats to avoid hyperlipoproteinemia, hypertension, and vascular disease, which occur with a higher incidence in patients with renal disease
		    The prescribed proportion/amount of fat intake is reviewed with the patient/family, with an emphasis on polyunsaturated fats
		    A list of foods high in saturated and unsaturated fats may be shared with the patient

■ High total body Na^+ levels associated with Fluid overload Edema Hypertension Cardiac complications	■ Serum Na^+ levels within normal limits with no signs/symptoms of fluid overload, edema, and hypertension	■ Instruct patient/family according to the following guidelines regarding sodium
		Provide a list of foods/fluid with moderate sodium content; discuss those to be consumed in limited amounts
		  The exact sodium content may be included in the list provided
		
		    1 g NaCl = 40 mg Na
		    1 mEq Na = 23 mg Na
		
		No salt should be added to foods during cooking or at the table
		Salt substitutes should also be limited to some extent, since they contain potassium, which is also restricted
		Water softeners often add sodium to tap water and should be considered
		Many medications contain sodium and should be considered in the daily intake

Potential problems	Expected outcomes	Nursing activities
		Tips for improving palatability of food in light of a salt restriction are shared (by the dietitian if possible) including the use of spices, herbs, and other seasonings
■ Fluid overload occurring between hemodialysis treatments	■ Normovolemia BP, P within normal limits Weight gain between treatments about 0.5 kg/day	■ Instruct patient/family according to the following guidelines regarding fluids Discuss prescribed fluid intake with patient/family Intake of fluids may vary according to patient's residual kidney function, body weight, physical activity, type of food intake (some foods such as ice cream are 90% fluid), ambient temperature, and tolerance to excess fluid accumulation between dialysis treatments An acceptable daily weight gain is 0.5 kg/24 hours (adults) Excess fluid gain may produce hypertension and edema Usual fluid intake for adults is 500 to 800 ml plus the urine volume for previous 24 hours in addition to the fluids in foods; liquids low in both sodium and potassium are emphasized (e.g., H_2O; cranberry, grape, and apple juices) Fluids should be carefully spaced and refreshingly cool to quench thirst Frequent oral hygiene Patient/family should be allowed and encouraged to tally intake of fluids and urine output while still in hospital
■ Hyperkalemia	■ Serum K^+ levels within normal limits	■ Instruct patient/family according to the following guidelines regarding potassium Potassium restriction depends on residual kidney function and the 24-hour loss of potassium Review food that should be avoided altogether Protein restriction automatically restricts potassium intake The dietary potassium restriction is usually 40 to 70 mEq/day for adults (or 1 mEq/kg of ideal weight/day) 30 mg K = 1 mEq K 1200 mg K = 40 mEqK Patient/family may be encouraged to tally sodium and potassium intake while still in the hospital A suggested meal plan may be shared and reviewed with patient/family
■ Insufficient knowledge to comply with discharge regimen*	■ Before discharge Patient accurately takes medications, maintains careful intake and output restrictions and records, and sodium-restricted diet Patient describes potential problems related to long-term dialysis, how they will be prevented, and signs/symptoms by which they are recognized	■ Discuss extended plan of care with physician and ascertain what has already been discussed with patient Discuss psychological, social, financial, and physical implications of long-term dialysis with patient Arrange for assistance from social worker, vocational rehabilitation therapists, and clergy to counsel patient as appropriate Instruct patient in Careful recording of intake and output and daily weights Fluid and sodium restrictions Dietary restrictions in protein, cholesterol, and saturated fats Activities, which, in combination with diet, are designed to build muscle mass, maintain/build strength, ameliorate headaches, and improve psychological well-being Medications If home dialysis to be done 1. Instruct patient in procedure with emphasis on aseptic technique, prevention of infection, and careful preservation of vascular access

*If critical care unit nurse is responsible for such follow-up care.

Potential problems	Expected outcomes	Nursing activities

2. Instruct patient that if unexplained bleeding occurs from around shunt/fistula site, apply pressure dressing and perhaps a BP cuff or other tourniquet to the arm; patient should notify physician immediately and arrange transportation to the appointed health facility for assessment/treatment of the problem

■ Patient has limited understanding of how to safely care for shunt/fistula*
Patency

■ Shunt/fistula remain patent, in situ, and infection free

■ Patency
Shunt and fistula
Instruct patient/family in how to monitor for shunt/fistula patency
Palpate for thrill (pulsation) or a "buzzing" sensation
If it is difficult to palpate thrill, a stethoscope can be used to hear *bruit*
Monitor for indices of circulation to extremity (warmth, color)
Shunt
Monitor for warmth of shunt, for uniform red, not dark color; for pain, tingling sensation under dressing
If blood flow in *shunt/fistula* has decreased but is not completely occluded, instruct patient according to physician's order; guidelines may include
Injection of heparin into the shunt every few hours
Opening the shunt, squeezing out a few drops of blood, followed by reconnection of arterial and venous ends of cannula
For *total shunt/fistula occlusion*
Notify physician; a declotting procedure is performed and may be followed by intermittent injection with heparin
For *partial shunt occlusion*
If one side of a cannula is occluded, the other side may be kept open by continuous or intermittent infusion until the clotted side of the cannula can be revised/replaced
Instruct patient/family
To avoid constricting clothing
To avoid sleeping on arm with shunt or acutely flexing extremity for long periods; a cast or brace is sometimes helpful in developing the habit of not sleeping on shunted extremity
To avoid exposing extremity to extremes of heat and cold
To avoid situations in which the shunt or fistula could be traumatized
To avoid fast movements with the affected extremity; to avoid lifting heavy objects and doing strenuous activities with the affected extremity

Infection

Instruct patient/family in proper shunt dressing, using aseptic technique
Describe and demonstrate proper alignment of the shunt; dressing must be kept dry
Describe untoward signs
Irritation, with a skin rash around the shunt resulting from sensitivity to iodine or Betadine; if this occurs, notify physician; solutions will be changed
Signs/symptoms of local infection—redness, swelling, warmth, purulent drainage
If these signs occur, encourage patient to notify physician so that cultures can be taken and the infection treated

---

*If intensive care unit nurse is responsible for preparing patient for long-term dialysis.

Potential problems	Expected outcomes	Nursing activities
Shunt dislodgement		Demonstrate application of dressing such that tubing is not easily disconnected; two clamps should be carried on dressing at all times to be used to clamp the shunt tubings should a disconnection occur
		Should a tubing come out of the vessel, instruct patient/family to clamp the cannula side that is still in place and to apply direct pressure to the bleeding site
		A tourniquet (a necktie or something like it will do) may be tightly tied above the site; if a BP cuff is available, it should be inflated to a pressure just above the patient's own systolic BP
		Instruct patient with an *external shunt* in related self-care activities
		Whether bathing the shunted extremity is permitted and, if so, whether a protective waterproof covering is to be used
		If dressing becomes damp, the patient is usually told to change it
		Prescribe physical activities on an individual basis
		Encourage patient to wear medical alert bracelet
■ Patient/family has insufficient knowledge of complications of long-term renal failure including anemia, malnutrition, polyneuropathy, hyperparathyroidism, bony abnormalities	■ Patient identifies and, when appropriate, performs activities necessary to prevent potential long-term complications of hemodialysis Patient accurately records daily weight on a log form Weight maintained without significant incidence of edema	■ Review potential problems of long-term renal failure and the care that will minimize associated problems Anemia, unusual weakness, loss of energy, apathy, headache Malnutrition, weight loss, nausea and vomiting Polyneuropathy Hyperparathyroidism Bony abnormalities Signs of fluid and electrolyte imbalance and acidosis—muscular irritability, twitching, weakness, lethargy Provide opportunity for patient/family to ask questions Describe plan for follow-up visits with the patient/family, including when and where to go, who to see, and what specimens to bring Explain that follow-up visits will include evaluation for Signs/symptoms of protein and calorie malnutrition (weakness, apathy, weight loss, decreased albumin levels, and edema) Weight changes; the patient's daily weight log is reviewed Fluid balance; signs of underhydration or overhydration

47 □ **Renal transplantation**

In renal transplantation a functioning kidney is removed from one individual and used to replace a nonfunctioning kidney in another individual.

Renal transplantation is performed for a variety of reasons. Hemodialysis may be inadequate for control of renal failure. Medication and dietary management in the hemodialysis patient may not adequately control the signs/symptoms of renal failure. Psychosocial factors such as the realization of life-threatening aspects of renal failure, its "terminal" nature, and the concurrent dependency on the hemodialysis machine have an adverse effect on self-image and interpersonal relationships. Physiological effects of renal failure and hemodialysis, including constant fatigue, possible impotence, and job loss, further strain intimate relationships.

Renal transplantation can offer these persons a more

normal life-style, an improved sense of well-being, and a more liberalized medication and dietary regimen than is possible with a hemodialysis regimen. Renal transplantation provides for a greater feeling of independence than is usually possible during hemodialysis therapy. Psychosocial difficulties that occur with long-term hemodialysis may also be ameliorated or avoided altogether. Potency may return in males, and libido may increase in women. Moreover, renal transplantation may result in decreased long-term financial cost.

Appropriate candidates for kidney transplantation include patients who anticipate long-term dialysis, are within a predetermined age range, and have had no cancer within a predetermined length of time.

In the early postoperative period, these patients are usually cared for in a surgical intensive care unit or in a special transplant-dialysis unit.

Postoperatively, the goal of therapy is to prevent irreversible rejection of the donor kidney with the use of immunosuppressive agents. These medications depress the patient's immunological reaction against the donor tissue. Unfortunately, this therapy decreases the patient's ability to engulf and destroy unwanted bacteria, fungi, and viruses. The bacteria can multiply at an accelerated rate, producing a fulminant infection. Measures to prevent infection are thus an essential component of the postoperative regimen.

The nurse must monitor for infection and rejection on an ongoing basis. Should signs of either occur, the physician should be notified and the therapeutic regimen appropriately revised.

ASSESSMENT

1. History that includes
   a. Etiology, natural history of renal dysfunction
   b. Results of biopsies done
   c. Start and length of therapy with peritoneal dialysis and/or hemodialysis, including complications
   d. Presence and date of insertion of shunt and/or fistula
   e. Previous operations, particularly
      (1) Nephrectomy—left and/or right
      (2) Parathyroidectomy
      (3) Pericardiectomy
   f. Presence of chronic systemic disease or any disorders compromising life expectancy (e.g., cancer)
2. Signs and symptoms of chronic renal failure; see Standard: *Acute renal failure*
3. Hemodynamic status

   a. BP
   b. P
   c. Peripheral circulation
4. Results of lab and diagnostic tests, including
   a. Parameters of kidney function
      (1) Urine (if present) volume, specific gravity
      (2) Sedimentation
      (3) Osmolality
      (4) Electrolytes
      (5) Blood—electrolyte levels particularly potassium, calcium, phosphorus levels; creatinine, uric acid, BUN; drug levels, if appropriate
   b. Liver function tests
      (1) Transaminase levels (SGOT, SGPT)
      (2) Serum protein, albumin levels
   c. Complement levels
   d. WBC count with differential
   e. Hct, Hgb, platelets, coagulation profile
   f. Australian antigen (serum hepatitis antigen)
   g. Viral studies (especially herpes, cytomegalovirus)
   h. Blood type
   i. Tissue type
   j. Histocompatibility studies
      (1) Mixed lymphocyte cytotoxicity inhibition
      (2) Panel cross-match
      (3) Final cross-match with donor leukocytes
   k. Immunological determinations
      (1) Blast cell count
      (2) Antibody titers
      (3) E-rosette levels
   l. Baseline radiographs of major bone areas—shoulder, hips, joints
   m. Tests performed to assure the absence of cancer and ulcers
   n. Cultures
      (1) Blood
      (2) Throat
      (3) Sputum
      (4) Urine
      (5) Stool or rectal
5. Level of patient/family's anxiety regarding hospitalization, transplant surgery, expected outcomes, and related therapy employed (e.g., immunosuppression)
6. Patient/family's knowledge regarding operative therapy
   a. What have they been told
   b. Their expectations
   c. Previous experience with surgery

7. Information and detail surgeon has provided patient/family about need for surgery, actual surgery to be performed, and expected outcome

GOALS

1. Reduction of patient/family's anxiety with provision of information, explanations, and encouragement
2. Physiological serum levels of
   a. Metabolic waste products (BUN, ammonia, uric acid, creatinine)
   b. Electrolytes
   c. Toxic substances (drugs, etc.)
3. Hct, Hgb, and coagulation studies within normal limits
4. Normovolemia
5. Acid-base balance within normal limits
6. Infection free
7. Nutrition adequate to prevent protein catabolism
8. Positive nitrogen balance
9. Absence or alleviation of signs and symptoms of chronic renal failure
10. Normal cardiovascular, gastrointestinal, neuromuscular, and integumentary function
11. Before discharge patient/family is able to describe
    a. Dietary and fluid management
    b. Activity progression
    c. Medication regimen
    d. Special procedures required (e.g., wound care)
    e. Untoward signs and symptoms
    f. Plan for follow-up care
12. Absence of long-term complications of immunosuppression

Potential problems	Expected outcomes	Nursing activities
Preoperative and Postoperative		
■ Patient/family's anxiety related to Disease process Hospitalization Diagnostic procedures Therapeutic regimen Anticipated surgery and expected outcomes	■ Patient/family's behavior indicates reduction in anxiety with provision of information, explanations, and encouragement	■ Ongoing assessment of level of patient/family's anxiety Assess patient/family's knowledge and understanding of disease process and rationale for surgery Assess patient/family's understanding of diagnostic procedures, therapeutic regimen, anticipated surgery, expected outcomes Explain the aforementioned as needed; individualize instruction in terms of approach, timing, and sequence Arrange for psychiatric consult and follow-up if needed, as ordered Encourage patient to participate in decisions regarding his/her care Encourage participation in care as tolerated Perform treatments in unhurried manner Provide comfort measures Describe the perioperative experiences, including Preoperative Chest physiotherapy Coughing and deep breathing Incentive spirometry Shave Light dinner, then NPO after midnight Morning bath/shower Preoperative medications Skin tests for immune status if appropriate Hospital gown Care of valuables Ride to operating room Scrub suits, masks, and hats worn by operating room staff Anesthesia Postoperative Waking up in the recovery room/intensive care unit 1. Describe the general environment (size of unit, room, etc.) 2. Nurse always nearby 3. Dull, continuous noises

Potential problems	Expected outcomes	Nursing activities
		Incision with bandage
		IV, arterial lines
		ECG monitoring
		Medicine for discomfort, pain
		Policy on family visits
		Measures to prevent postoperative infection
		Protective isolation if planned
		Measures to keep lungs clear of secretions
		Use of immunosuppressive medications
		As patient progresses
		Tubes out
		Eating again
		Getting stronger, ambulation
		Postural drainage, coughing, deep breathing
		Discuss the long-term therapy of a kidney transplantation, including
		Immunosuppression and possibility of rejection
		Prevention of infection
		Describe responsibility of patient in achieving a speedy recovery by taking an active role in coughing, deep breathing, and so on
		Encourage patient/family's questions
		Encourage verbalization of anxiety and fears related to hospitalization, diagnostic procedures, therapeutic regimen, surgery, and surgical outcomes
■ Inadequate stabilization of preoperative medical problems	■ Preoperative medical problems under control	■ Monitor
		Results of lab studies
		Hepatitis B antigen
		Viral titers (e.g., herpes, cytomegalovirus)
		Hct, Hgb, platelet levels
		Coagulation profile
		WBC count with differential
		Electrolyte levels
		Temperature
		BP; note hypertension
		Notify physician of any of these abnormalities
		Administer therapy as ordered to correct acid-base imbalance, electrolyte abnormalities, and low Hgb/Hct and platelet levels

Postoperative

Potential problems	Expected outcomes	Nursing activities
■ Hemodynamic instability	■ Hemodynamic stability Cardiac output, BP, P within normal limits	■ Note baseline preoperative BP, P, and CVP (if available)
		Monitor vital signs q15 min until stable, then q30 min four times; if stable, decrease frequency to q1 hr for duration of first postoperative day
		Monitor for other signs: adequate cardiac output, CVP, peripheral circulation, mentation, urine output
		Urine output of the transplanted kidney may be very low in the early postoperative period
		Monitor for arrhythmias
		Administer fluids and medications as ordered by physician to maintain BP and fluid balance within normal limits
■ Fluid overload related to dysfunction of transplanted kidney	■ Normovolemia BP, P, CVP, weight, and urine output within normal limits	■ Prevent by administering fluids as ordered; closely monitor urine output and other parameters of fluid balance (weight, BP, P, CVP, skin turgor)
		Monitor
		BP, P, CVP, and PAP, if available, q½-1 hr until stable
		Urine output q1 hr until stable
		Daily weights
		Skin turgor

Potential problems	Expected outcomes	Nursing activities
		Notify physician of a significantly decreased urine output or of an increase in BP, CVP, and change of skin turgor
		If fluid overload occurs
		Administer diuretics as ordered; closely monitor patient's response
		Institute fluid restrictions as ordered
		Prepare patient for and, if appropriate, assist with hemodialysis if procedure is necessary
■ Hypertension related to Hypervolemia Hypernatremia	■ BP within normal limits Serum Na$^+$ levels within normal limits	■ Prevent by
		Preparing patient for bilateral nephrectomies, if procedure is necessary, to reduce circulating levels of renin; this is done several weeks before transplantation
		Administering fluids as ordered to keep patient's weight, intake and output records, and hemodynamic parameters within prescribed limits
		Administering sodium as ordered to keep serum Na$^+$ levels within normal limits
		Monitor
		BP, P, CVP, and PAP, if available, q½-1 hr until stable
		Urine output and specific gravity q1 hr
		Daily weight
		Serum and urine Na$^+$ levels
		If hypertension occurs
		Administer diuretics, if ordered
		Alter levels of sodium administration as ordered
		Administer antihypertensive medications if ordered; closely monitor patient's response
■ Pulmonary insufficiency, which may consist of Inadequate oxygenation Hypercapnia Atelectasis Infection (see Problem, Infection)	■ Adequate exchange of blood gases Adequate oxygenation (arterial Pa$_{O_2}$ within normal limits) Adequate ventilation (arterial Pa$_{CO_2}$ within normal limits)	■ Prevent by
		Administering vigorous chest physiotherapy, including
		Turning at least q2 hr; early ambulation
		Deep breathing and coughing
		Chest physiotherapy in the early postoperative period and later as indicated
		Administration of humidified oxygenated air in the early postoperative period and later as indicated
		An incentive inspirometer or intermittent positive pressure breathing device may be ordered; assist patient to use and follow with encouragement to cough up mobilized secretions
		Monitor
		Quality of respirations, secretions
		Breath sounds serially for diminished or absent breath sounds or the presence of rales, rhonchi, and other adventitious breath sounds
		Serial arterial blood gas measurements
		For signs/symptoms of hypoxia and/or hypercapnia including restlessness, altered mentation, tachypnea, tachycardia, and dusky color
		Notify physician of any abnormality, and alter therapy as ordered
■ Renal dysfunction related to Obstructed urinary drainage system	■ Indices of renal function within normal limits Patent urinary drainage system	■ Prevent by
		Maintaining patent urinary drainage system: bladder catheters are connected to a bag and maintained as a closed, intact drainage system
		Note presence of clots or other particles
		If present, milk or irrigate the tubing and catheter as needed

Potential problems	Expected outcomes	Nursing activities

		Monitor
		  Urine output; note volume, color, odor, presence of particles (hematuria, casts)
		  Lower abdomen for distention
		  Serially palpate bladder for distention

■ Acute renal failure, which may be related to
  Ischemic damage before surgery
  Kinking of ureter
  Kinking of renal artery
  Rupture of anastomosis (urine enters peritoneum)
  Renal vein thrombosis
	■ Absence of acute renal failure
	
	  Absence and/or resolution of ischemic damage before and during surgery
		■ Prevent by administering fluids and, if needed, cardiotonic/vasopressor drugs such as dopamine or dobutamine to maintain adequate renal blood flow and urine output
		Monitor
		  Urine output q1 hr in the early postoperative period
		  Daily weights
		  Kidney function tests
		  Urine creatinine; BUN and urine Na^+ levels
		  Spot urines as ordered for analysis of
		    RBC casts
		    Epithelial cells
		    WBC
		  Urine C and S results
		  For abdominal distention, which may result from kinking of the renal artery or anastomotic rupture
		  Results of renograms

■ Rejection due to incompatibility of recipient and donor tissue	■ Blood types A, B, and O (ABO) compatibility
	  Absence of signs of cytotoxicity
	  Immunological studies indicate optimal immunosuppression
		■ Prevent rejection by assisting in verifying patient/donor tissue compatibility
		Monitor results of histocompatibility studies, which may include
		  ABO compatibility studies
		  Result of tissue typing and comparison of human leukocyte antigen (HLA) constellations
		    Parents share one chromosome, and siblings share two, one, or no chromosomes; siblings sharing both chromosomes are preferred donors
		    Cadaver donors are similarly tissue typed; the recipient who is most closely matched from a pool of potential recipients is chosen
		    Histocompatibility studies
		      Mixed lymphocyte cytotoxicity inhibition—donor lymphocytes are put in contact with recipient lymphocytes in tissue culture to test for preformed cytotoxic antibodies; if marked aggregation occurs (antigen-antibody response), the donor is incompatible
		  Panel cross-match
		  Final cross-match with donor leukocytes
		  Immunological studies
		    Antibody titers, blast cell count, E-rosette levels
		Prevent by administering immunosuppressive agents, as ordered, to suppress rejection of donor kidney
		Monitor lab indices of adequate immunosuppression, including
		  Blast cell counts
		  E-rosette levels
		  Panel cross-match
		  Mixed lymphocyte cytotoxicity inhibition
		  Antibody titers
		Monitor tolerance of immunosuppression and for adverse effects
		  Hct, Hgb, platelet, and reticulocyte levels; WBC count with differential; bleeding time, stool specimens for blood; liver function
		  Note the occurrence of the following
		    Depression, anxiety, psychosis, other behavioral changes
		    Increased BP
		    Edema
		    Visual changes

Potential problems	Expected outcomes	Nursing activities
		Monitor for signs and symptoms of *hyperacute rejection,* which usually occurs within minutes of surgery due to reformed cytotoxic antibodies to donor tissue; preoperative testing for such antibodies should prevent this type of rejection
		Monitor for *accelerated rejection* within 5 days of surgery (etiology not clear); treatment may be unsuccessful
		Monitor for signs and symptoms of *acute cell-mediated rejection,* which appears from 1 week to 3 months after transplantation: fever, malaise, tenderness over graft site, deterioration in indices of renal function, Na⁺ retention, and reduction in creatinine clearance
		Treatment with high steroid doses and antithymocyte globulin may be successful in reversing such rejection
		Monitor for signs and symptoms of *chronic humoral antibody-mediated rejection:* progressive deterioration in indices of renal function, proteinuria, and hypertension; treatment is often unsuccessful
		Monitor for signs/symptoms of rejection, including
		Results of periodic renal scans, which may show blood vessel compromise
		Deteriorating parameters of renal function
		Malaise and temperature elevation, concurrent with parameters that reflect impaired renal function
		Decreased urine output, increased BP, and significant temperature elevation
		Pain over graft site
		Elevated blood levels of Na⁺, BUN, creatinine
		Arthralgias
		If any of these signs/symptoms occur, notify physician
		Assist with plasmapheresis, which may be done to minimize the patient's rejection of the donor kidney tissue
		If rejection occurs
		Administer increasing dosages of immunosuppressive agents; gradually taper dosage as renal function improves
		Prepare patient for radiotherapy, if ordered
		Prepare patient for hemodialysis, if procedure is necessary
		If therapy for rejection is unsuccessful, removal of the kidney may be necessary; prepare patient for procedure
		Keep patient informed of progress
		Give the patient/family simple explanations
		Provide opportunity for expression of fears, anxieties
		Provide for kind, supportive care
■ Electrolyte imbalance, which may include	■ Serum electrolyte values within normal limits	■ Monitor serial blood and urine samples for electrolyte levels
Hypernatremia in oliguric phase of renal failure with concurrent administration of sodium		Notify physician of significant abnormalities
		Administer electrolyte replacement, which is ordered with consideration for urinary losses and concurrent therapeutic measures
Hyponatremia related to diuretic phase of renal failure or dilutional hyponatremia		Monitor for signs/symptoms of electrolyte imbalance
		Neuromuscular changes: weakness, irritability, twitching, and/or seizures
Hyperkalemia in oliguric phase of renal failure		Abnormal neurological signs: headaches, confusion, disorientation, restlessness, lethargy
Hypokalemia		Skin
In diuretic phase of renal failure		Temperature: warm or cold, clammy or dry
With vigorous diuretic therapy		Turgor: taut, firm, or loose
		Mucous membranes: moist, dry, cracked, or coated
		Daily weight for loss or gain

Potential problems	Expected outcomes	Nursing activities

■ Metabolic abnormalities: acidosis associated with renal dysfunction/ failure	■ Acid/base balance within normal limits	■ Monitor serial arterial blood gas samples for adequate oxygenation and acid-base balance
		  Provide for adequate oxygenation with supplemental humidified O_2 and vigorous chest physiotherapy
		  Institute therapy to correct primary abnormalities
		  Allow patient's body to compensate for metabolic imbalances with respiratory compensation
		  Administer bicarbonate and electrolyte replacement, as ordered to correct metabolic disturbances

■ Infection	■ Infection free	■ Prevent by
		  Implementing protective isolation during period of maximum immunosuppressive therapy if ordered
		  Limiting contact of patient with personnel and extended family members
		    Keep infected patients, visitors, and personnel away from patient
		  Providing for scrupulous hygiene of mouth, perineum, and skin
		  Providing for early ambulation
		  Providing for adequate nutrition to promote healing, prevent infection
		  Keeping vascular access for hemodialysis clean; change shunt dressing q24-48 hr using aseptic technique
		  Monitor temperature; reculture patient for any significant temperature elevation as ordered

■ Infection of
  Kidney
  Urinary tract
	■ Kidney and urinary tract infection free	■ Prevent by discontinuing bladder catheter as soon as possible
		Monitor for
		  Patient's complaints of
		    Frequency
		    Dysuria or burning on urination
		    Lower back pain
		    Malaise
		    Cloudy urine
		Notify physician of the presence of any of these symptoms, and send stat specimens for urinalysis and C and S determinations
		Monitor
		  Urine WBC and bacterial levels (specimens usually sent every 1 to 2 days while catheter is in place, then three times a week or as ordered)
		  Urine C and S results (specimens usually sent every 1 to 2 days while catheter in place, then 2 to 3 times a week)
		If kidney, urinary tract infection occurs
		  Administer bladder catheter irrigation if ordered
		  Administer antibiotic therapy if ordered

■ Pulmonary infection	■ Absence or resolution of pulmonary infection	■ Prevent pulmonary infection by
		  Providing for vigorous chest physiotherapy (see Problem, Pulmonary insufficiency)
		  Administering humidified O_2 supplements as ordered based on arterial blood gas measurements
		  Administering additional humidity and/or medications to liquefy secretions if ordered
		  Repositioning patient q1-2 hr
		    Bed rest, with a 30-degree head elevation, is usually ordered for the first 2 to 3 days
		Monitor for
		  Fever
		  Increased tenacity, amount, and abnormal color of secretions
		  Breath sounds q1-2 hr for decreased or absent breath sounds or rales, rhonchi

Potential problems	Expected outcomes	Nursing activities

		Signs of respiratory distress: tachypnea, dyspnea, shallow breathing
		 Chest radiograph results for areas of consolidation or collapse
		 Notify physician of any of these abnormalities
		 If pulmonary infection occurs
		     Send additional sputum specimens for C and S as ordered
		     Administer antibiotics as ordered
		     Administer vigorous chest physiotherapy to affected areas of lung

■ Wound infection	■ Infection-free wound	■ Prevention
		     Administer aseptic care of wounds, puncture sites, and in-dwelling catheters
		     Monitor wound, puncture sites for erythema, discomfort or pain, and signs of infected drainage (odor, color, amount)
		     Notify physician of any signs of wound infection
		     Reculture wound/drainage when status changes as ordered

■ Oral infection	■ Infection-free mouth	■ Prevent by providing for scrupulous mouth care
		     Monitor for white coating in mouth, oral lesions
		     Notify physician if either of these occurs
		     If oral infection occurs, administer antifungal mouthwash or lozenges according to the plan of care

■ Hyperglycemia related to
   Endogenous production of cortisone in response to stress of surgery
   Large doses of exogenous steroids in the early postoperative period
	■ Blood glucose levels within normal limits	■ Monitor
		     Serial blood glucose levels
		     Urine glucose and acetone levels
		     For signs and symptoms of hyperglycemia, including confusion, disorientation, dry mucous membranes
		     Notify physician of any of these abnormalities
		     If hyperglycemia occurs, administer insulin if ordered

■ Malnutrition	■ Nutrition adequate to prevent protein catabolism
	 Positive nitrogen balance
		■ Arrange for dietary consult
		     Administer postoperative diet according to kidney function (see Standard: *Acute renal failure*) as ordered
		     After the early postoperative renal dysfunction has subsided, diet progression as ordered
		     If the patient continues on high doses of steroids and/or is hypertensive, institute sodium restriction as ordered

■ Insufficient knowledge to comply with discharge regimen*	■ Before discharge patient/family accurately verbalizes discharge regimen regarding
	 Prevention of infection
	 Activity progression
	 Dietary management
	 Fluid intake and output measurements
	 Weights, BP measurements
	 Medications
		■ Assess patient/family's understanding of discharge regimen
		 Instruct patient/family regarding
		     Prevention of infection
		         Avoid contact with persons with respiratory infections and so on
		         Demonstrate proper wound care
		         Describe signs of symptoms of infection
		     Activity progression
		     Dietary management
		         Fluid intake and output measurements (may be recorded daily in chart form)
		     Daily weights, BP measurement
		     Medications: purpose, dosage, timing, precautionary measures, and potential adverse effects

*If responsibility of the critical care nurse includes follow-up care.

Potential problems	Expected outcomes	Nursing activities

	Untoward signs and symptoms requiring medical attention	Describe signs and symptoms requiring medical attention, including
		Fever
		Tenderness of implanted site
		Anorexia
		Malaise
		Acute depression, anxiety
		Yellow-bronze color of skin
		Yellowish tint in white of eyes (sclera)
		Drug reaction
		Decreased urine output
		Significant changes in BP
		Significant changes in weight
		According to medications patient is receiving, instruct in the potential adverse effects of
		Immunosuppression, including signs of cancer, infection
		Long-term steroid therapy
		    Diabetes
		    Aseptic necrosis of bones
		    GI hemorrhage
		    Pancreatitis
		    Others
		Cyclophosphamide therapy: hemorrhagic cystitis
		Azathioprine therapy
		    Hepatitis
		    Pancreatitis

	Patient accurately describes follow-up plan of care	Describe plan for follow-up care Location, date, times of appointments Specimens to bring Activities during visits Provide patient/family opportunity to discuss Family relationships Sexual adjustments Emotional problems Employ assistance of auxiliary services as needed Social service Vocational rehabilitation Others Assess potential compliance with discharge regimen

METABOLIC

48 □ Diabetic ketoacidosis

Diabetic ketoacidosis is an acute metabolic disorder, which results primarily from a sustained lack of insulin that produces a condition called *hyperglycemia.*

Insulin is required to transport blood glucose for cell metabolism. Without insulin the glucose remains outside the cell and, despite the rising blood glucose levels, the cells "starve." Dehydration and metabolic abnormalities then ensue.

Both intracellular and extracellular dehydration occur in the presence of hyperglycemia. Intracellular dehydration is the result of high extracellular osmolarity that causes a shift of intracellular water into the extracellular space. Extracellular dehydration is caused by an osmotic diuresis, and as glucose passes into the urine it obligates the loss of hypotonic fluid and electrolytes, particularly potassium and sodium.

Metabolic abnormalities include ketoacidosis and abnormal potassium and sodium levels.

Increased utilization of fats and proteins in place of glucose produces accumulation of free fatty acids. Free fatty acids are metabolized in the liver to ketone bodies (acetone, acetoacetic acid, and beta-hydroxybutyric acid), which can then be oxidized for energy. Production of ketone bodies in excess of their utilization and elimination results in ketosis and ketoacidosis.

The osmotic diuresis caused by glycosuria results in loss of potassium and a decrease in intravascular volume. The decrease in intravascular volume activates the renin-angiotensin system, releasing aldosterone and causing further loss of potassium. However, with acidosis intracellular buffer proteins release potassium ions into the serum, and serum potassium may be low, apparently normal, or high. Total body potassium is almost always low.

Total body sodium is usually low as a result of increased urinary losses. The serum sodium measurements in the pesence of hyperglycemia are usually low. However, if dehydration is severe as a result of vomiting and excessive urinary loss of hypotonic fluid, the serum sodium may be normal or even high. Therefore, a high or normal serum sodium in the presence of hyperglycemia is a clue to severe dehydration.

Other causes of ketoacidosis include salicylate intoxication and excessive alcohol intake. Salicylate intoxication alters normal metabolism and leads to production of organic acids including ketone bodies. Patients with salicylate intoxication may have ketones in serum and urine. Alcohol in the absence of starvation has been shown to cause increased serum ketones unrelated to diabetes. Unlike patients with diabetes, these patients have adequate endogenous insulin, but its release and action have been temporarily inhibited by alcohol and the humoral response to hypoglycemia. These patients will respond to glucose infusion, hydration, and small amounts of supplemental insulin.

Factors that can precipitate diabetic ketoacidosis include

1. An undiagnosed diabetes
2. A known diabetic who has
   a. Failed to take prescribed insulin according to specified needs
   b. Not followed prescribed dietary requirement
   c. Severe infection
   d. Prolonged nausea and vomiting
   e. Physiological stresses, that is, trauma, surgery; emotional and mental stresses; and pregnancy
   f. Untreated renal insufficiency

These factors increase glucose utilization, impair glucose metabolism, and/or are associated with insufficient insulin availability.

Therapy in diabetic ketoacidosis is directed toward administration of insulin and treatment of dehydration, metabolic and electrolyte abnormalities, and correction of any underlying conditions that may have precipitated the ketoacidosis.

ASSESSMENT

1. Baseline information regarding history of
   a. Polydipsia, polyuria, and polyphagia related to dramatic weight fluctuations

411

b. Number of years as diagnosed diabetic

c. Inability to follow prescribed diabetic regimen and degree of adherence, that is
   (1) Omission of insulin intake
   (2) Failure to adhere to prescribed dietary and fluid requirements

d. Recent conditions necessitating increased insulin intake including overeating, trauma, etc.

e. Family members with diabetes

f. Any associated illnesses including renal disease, pancreatitis, hepatitis, and endocrine disorders related to pregnancy, infection, obesity, cardiac disease

g. Alcoholism

h. Recent drug ingestion including salicylates, etc.

2. Physical signs and symptoms of
   a. Anorexia, nausea, vomiting, and general malaise
   b. Abdominal pain and tenderness, which may be severe and can mimic surgical emergencies
   c. Abdominal distention, absence of bowel sounds
   d. Hepatomegaly
   e. Headache and visual disturbances
   f. Drowsiness leading to coma
   g. Skin appearance
      (1) Flushed—due to local vasodilatation caused by ketone bodies
      (2) Dry—due to dehydration; may note "tenting" when skin is pinched and soft or sunken eyeballs
   h. Tachycardia
   i. Hypothermia—may accompany coma and hypotension; suggestive of gram-negative sepsis
   j. Hyperthermia—may suggest sepsis
   k. Air hunger with deep heavy respirations called *Kussmaul's respirations*
   l. Acetone breath or fruity odor on breath
   m. Polyuria or oliguria
   n. Decrease or absence of reflexes

3. Lab and diagnostic data results, including
   a. Urine sugar and acetone, specific gravity, and osmolality
   b. Blood for electrolytes, ketones, BUN, and lipid levels; elevation and/or depletion of sodium, potassium, chloride, and bicarbonate
   c. Fasting blood glucose tolerance test
   d. Complete blood count for leukocytosis and elevated Hct
   e. Arterial blood gas results for acidosis
   f. ECG for any S-T segment and T wave abnormalities

g. Results of throat, blood, sputum, urine, and stool cultures

4. Patient/family's knowledge and understanding of disease process, purpose of hospitalization, and therapy planned
   a. Assess patient/family's level of anxiety related to disease process, diagnostic procedures, and therapy planned
   b. Determine diabetic control regimen patient has been on at home, if any, and the degree of patient/family compliance

GOALS

1. Patient/family's behavior indicates reduction in level of anxiety with provision of information and explanations

2. Patient adheres to prescribed therapeutic diet, maintaining blood glucose and weight at desired levels

3. Respiratory function within normal limits
   a. Respiratory assessment and arterial blood gas levels within patient's normal limits
   b. Absence of pulmonary edema

4. Hemodynamic stability
   a. Absence of arrhythmias
   b. Adequate cardiac output

5. Fluids, electrolytes, and complete blood count levels are within normal limits; weight gain or loss in desired direction

6. Absence of and/or resolution of any complications including paralytic ileus secondary to hypokalemia, hypoglycemia, congestive heart failure

7. Prevention and/or resolution of associated medical problems precipitating diabetic ketoacidosis including infection, renal insufficiency, physiological stress, etc.

8. Before discharge patient/family is able to
   a. Describe cause, pathophysiology, diagnosis, therapy, and prognosis of diabetes
   b. Discuss early signs and symptoms of hypoglycemia and ketoacidosis, and what to do about them, including when to report them to physician
   c. Discuss signs and symptoms of infections that will require medical attention
   d. Verbalize and demonstrate, if appropriate, good health practices to prevent infections
   e. Describe and demonstrate, if appropriate, activity, dietary, medication, and follow-up regimens

Potential problems	Expected outcomes	Nursing activities
■ Patient/family's anxiety related to insufficient knowledge of Disease process Diagnostic procedures Therapy employed	■ Patient/family's behavior demonstrates decreased level of anxiety with provision of information and explanations Patient/family verbalizes understanding of disease process and its relationship to therapy employed Patient/family participates actively in planning and implementing care	■ Ongoing assessment of level of anxiety Describe nature of the disease process and its relation to signs and symptoms the patient is experiencing Explain the relationship of the disease process to the rationale for various therapeutic interventions Explain the anticipated procedures involved in the diagnostic process/plan of care and what the patient will experience Assist in preparing patient for diagnostic procedures Encourage patient/family's questions, verbalization of fears and anxieties Involve patient/family in planning for care Demonstrate concern and warmth in providing care to the patient Evaluate for decrease in level of anxiety with provision of information, explanations
■ Metabolic and electrolyte abnormalities Metabolic abnormalities Ketoacidosis as a result of increased ketone bodies, causing a decrease in bicarbonate	■ Absence or resolution of metabolic and electrolyte abnormalities Absence or resolution of ketoacidosis	■ Monitor and notify physician of abnormalities Vital signs including temperature q1 hr until stable; note presence of fever and hypotension Intake and output with glucose and acetone determination, specific gravity q1 hr until stable; daily weight Central venous pressure (CVP) readings if available q1 hr Serum electrolytes and anions/cations such as ketones, phosphate q1 hr For presence of signs and symptoms of hyperkalemia, hypokalemia, hyponatremia, and hypophosphatemia BUN and creatinine levels q6-12 hr Serial serum acetone dilutions q1 hr Serial arterial blood gas results for acidosis q1 hr until stable Serial complete blood count for leukocytosis and elevated erythrocyte sedimentation rate (ESR) Chest radiograph to rule out infection Serial ECG for any T wave and/or S-T segment abnormalities Presence or absence of Kussmaul's respirations and acetone breath Alterations in level of consciousness (LOC), seizure activity, reflex status Skin color for cyanosis Absence or presence of bowel sounds and gastric dilatation
Compensatory respiratory alkalosis (Kussmaul's) Hyperglycemia	Arterial blood gas levels within normal limits Regular and even respirations Absence or resolution of hyperglycemia Blood sugar within normal limits	If patient is comatose, other lab and diagnostic tests may be ordered and results monitored, including C and S of blood, sputum, urine, throat, stool, and cerebrospinal fluid Ca^{2+}, amylase, lactic acid, serum and urine osmolalities Lumbar puncture for spinal fluid pressure and electrolyte determinations Appropriate samples for drug detection Type and cross-match Place patient on continuous cardiac monitor Maintain parenteral infusion and plasma expanders as ordered
Electrolyte abnormalities, particularly imbalance in K^+, Na^+, and abnormal phosphate levels	Serum electrolyte levels within normal limits, particularly K^+, Na^+, and phosphate	Administer electrolyte replacements, i.e., K^+, Na^+, Cl^-, and the anion phosphate if ordered Administer insulin as ordered Check that blood specimens drawn at specified time Insert Foley catheter and connect to closed gravity drainage as ordered Administer O_2 therapy if ordered Maintain a diabetic flow sheet, including glucose and acetone determinations, specific gravity, electrolytes (anion gap), arterial blood gas results, intake and output, and CVP results

Potential problems	Expected outcomes	Nursing activities
		Keep patient NPO until nausea and ileus have cleared; then administer diet according to tolerance as ordered
		Assist in NG tube insertion and connect to low continuous suction if ordered
		Seizure precautions may be necessary; see Standard: *Seizures*
		Maintain low Fowler's position unless contraindicated
		Administer skin care with position change q2 hr; check bony prominences and other areas for any skin breakdown
		Encourage deep breathing exercises q1 hr
		Oral hygiene q2 hr and prn
		Provide an environment conducive to physical, mental, and emotional rest
		Keep patient warm, dry, and comfortable
		Allow for rest periods between treatments
		Limit visitors according to patient's needs
■ Dehydration related to hyperglycemia and increased serum levels of ketone bodies	■ Fluid balance, CVP readings, urine output within normal limits for patient's age and size Weight remains within 5% of patient's normal baseline weight	■ Refer to Problem, Metabolic and electrolyte abnormalities, for parameters permitting detection of hyperglycemia and increased ketone bodies, and activities for control

■ Hypoglycemia related to therapy	■ Absence and/or resolution of hypoglycemia
	Resolution of ketoacidosis with proper therapy
		■ Prevent by careful monitoring of parameters in Problem, Metabolic and electrolyte abnormalities, and activities for control of hyperglycemia
		Monitor or observe for signs and symptoms of hypoglycemia q1 hr, including
		  Sudden lowering of blood sugar level (usually below 60 mg/ 100 ml of blood)
		  Signs and symptoms of
		    Tachycardia
		    Slight increase in systolic BP
		    Sweating
		    Numbness
		    Dilated pupils
		    Pallor
		    General weakness
		    Faintness
		  Cerebral manifestations
		    Nervousness
		    Apprehension
		    Visual disturbances
		    Headache
		    Thick speech
		    Muscle twitching
		    Tonic and clonic spasm
		    Urinary incontinence
		    Unconsciousness
		    Convulsions
		    Babinski's reflex often present
		  Unexpected behavioral reaction
		    Restlessness, negativism, personality changes, catatonia, and maniacal behavior
		If problem occurs
		  Administer glucose IV as ordered
		  If patient is able to swallow, orange juice with sugar or other sources of glucose can be given orally

Potential problems	Expected outcomes	Nursing activities
		Administer glucagon if ordered and start IV 5% dextrose in water (D5W)
		Reevaluate and restandardize therapy to control and/or prevent hypoglycemia
		Monitor lab and diagnostic studies for control
■ Coma or altered mental status related to Metabolic and electrolyte abnormalities Sepsis, meningitis Embolic phenomenon due to myocardial infarction	■ Patient is alert and oriented to time, place, and person Absence and/or resolution of etiologic factors	■ Refer to Problems, Metabolic and electrolyte abnormalities and Dehydration, for parameters permitting detection of metabolic and electrolyte abnormalities and activities for control See Standards: *Meningitis/encephalitis; Embolic phenomena* If problem occurs Identify etiological factors and treat accordingly (see aforementioned problems) Provide for adequate airway patency, including Place in semi-Fowler's position; turn patient side to side q2 hr; suction q1 hr and/or prn; connect NG tube to suction to prevent aspiration Administer O_2 with humidification as ordered Pulmonary toilet q2 hr and prn Auscultate for any abnormal breath sounds q2 hr Vital signs, including temperature, q2 hr until stable Serial arterial blood gas results q1-2 hr or as indicated If mechanical ventilation is indicated, see Standard: *Mechanical ventilation* Neurological assessment q2 hr Monitor LOC q2 hr Provide eye, ear, nose, mouth, and skin care q2 hr or as necessary Maintain proper body alignment and perform passive range-of-motion (ROM) exercises to all extremities q2 hr and prn Maintain seizure precautions Provide for elimination, i.e., perineal care, external catheter; check for bowel movement Maintain quiet environment Provide nursing support as indicated by patient's changing condition, i.e., restlessness Notify physician for any changes or abnormalities Provide emotional support to patient/family
■ Presence of precipitating factors, including Cardiac ischemia, i.e., myocardial infarction	■ Absence or resolution of Myocardial ischemia	■ Monitor ECG for abnormalities—S-T segment and T wave changes and arrhythmias; notify physician if present If cardiac ischemia occurs, see Standards: *Angina pectoris; Acute myocardial infarction* or *Arrhythmias*
Pancreatitis	Pancreatitis	For moderate to severe left upper quadrant pain; notify physician if present If pancreatitis occurs, see Standard: *Pancreatitis*
Significant trauma or CNS catastrophe	Trauma or CNS dysfunction	For altered LOC (restlessness, agitation); pupils for inequality and unreactivity; notify physician if present If trauma or CNS catastrophe occurs, see Standard: *Head trauma*
Sepsis, i.e. Meningitis Pneumonia Cellulitis Pyelonephritis	Sepsis	For hypotension, hypothermia, hyperthermia, tachycardia, altered LOC; if present notify physician If sepsis occurs, see Standard: *Shock*

Potential problems	Expected outcomes	Nursing activities

Potential problems

- Insufficient information to comply with discharge regimen*

Expected outcomes

- Sufficient information to comply with discharge regimen

Patient/family verbalizes understanding of patient teaching and discharge regimen, including
Knowledge of diabetes
Signs and symptoms, causes and treatment of hypoglycemia and hyperglycemia
Importance of reporting early signs and symptoms to physician

Dietary and exercise regimen

Patient/family is able to
Test urine for sugar and acetone
Administer insulin and oral hypoglycemics

Nursing activities

- Assess patient/family's level of understanding, ability to comprehend, and any physical limitations regarding follow-up plan of care or discharge regimen

Develop patient teaching and discharge regimen at patient/family's level of understanding

Involve patient/family in planning for discharge regimen

Describe patient teaching and discharge regimen
Discuss the disease process and fears, and correct misconceptions of diabetes
Provide booklets and pamphlets from the American Diabetes Association, Inc.† and pharmaceutical companies
Describe early signs and symptoms of hyperglycemia and hypoglycemia, including causes of and actions to take

	Hyperglycemia	Hypoglycemia
Onset	Gradual	Sudden
Behavior	Drowsy	Excited
Breath	Fruity odor	Normal
Breathing	Deep and labored	Normal to rapid, shallow
Hunger	Absent	Present
Skin	Dry and flushed	Pale and moist
Sugar in urine	Large amount	Absence or slight
Thirst	Present	Absent
Tongue	Dry	Moist
Vomiting	Present	Absent

If signs of hypoglycemia occur, instruct patient to drink a glass of orange juice or suck on hard candies
If signs of hyperglycemia occur, instruct patient to notify physician immediately

Discuss the importance of
Regularity of diet and exercise
Plan prescribed diet and substitutes with dietitian and patient/family, allowing for cultural and religious preference and economic status
Same amount of exercise daily
Importance of weight control

Demonstrate how to test urine for sugar and acetone
Need to be consistent with type of testing equipment (tablets, reagent strip [dipstick], or test tape)

Discuss the dosage, frequency of administration, time effect begins, maximum action, duration, and side effects, i.e., skin reaction and hypoglycemia

Discuss factors requiring adjustment of insulin dosage, and notify physician before adjusting dose

Demonstrate the proper technique of insulin administration with return demonstration from patient/family

Discuss the importance of
1. Never missing a dose
2. Preventing dosage error
3. Recording dosage or pills taken
4. Insulin storage
5. Consulting physician before taking any other medications

*If responsibility of critical care nurse includes such follow-up care.
†American Diabetes Association, Inc., 18 East 48th St., New York, N.Y. 10017.

Potential problems	Expected outcomes	Nursing activities
	Patient/family's behavior indicates understanding of	Discuss importance of and demonstrate
	Importance of recognition and maintenance of proper health care	Good hygiene
		Careful foot care
		Avoid crowds or people with infections
		Regular routine activities of daily living
		Regular physical check-up
		Use of medical alert identification tag/bracelet
	Signs and symptoms of infections that may require medical intervention	Identify signs and symptoms of infection, including
		Fever
		Colds
		Flu
	Patient/family accurately describes plans for follow-up care	Nausea and vomiting
		Any reddened, swollen, and painful areas; wounds or cuts that do not heal
		Difficulty or burning sensation with urination
		Discuss why diabetics are prone to infection and ways to prevent it
		Describe follow-up visits including purpose of, when and where to go, who to see, and what specimens to bring
		Provide opportunity for and encourage questions and verbalization of anxiety regarding discharge regimen
		Assess potential compliance with discharge regimen

49 □ Total parenteral nutrition through central venous catheter

Total parenteral nutrition (TPN) is the method of delivering carbohydrates, proteins, minerals, vitamins, trace minerals, and/or fat through the intravenous route. Parenteral infusions administered via a central venous catheter can meet the total nutritional needs of patients who cannot ingest the needed nutrients or who cannot or should not absorb them from the gastrointestinal system.

Pathological conditions that necessitate the use of TPN may include (1) conditions that include gastrointestinal abnormalities, such as the malabsorption component of ulcerative colitis, regional enteritis, granulomatous colitis, fistulas, and surgical "short-gut" syndromes; (2) states in which the alimentary tract cannot be used, as in patients with central nervous system (CNS) dysfunction for whom oral feedings are not possible and nasogastric feedings are associated with a high incidence of aspiration; (3) situations in which bowel rest with resulting decreased gastrointestinal secretions is desired, such as in pancreatitis and in some biliary problems; (4)

pediatric patients with congenital gastrointestinal anomalies, chronic diarrhea, surgical short-gut syndromes, and perhaps prematurity; and (5) conditions in which the demand for nutrients is dramatically increased, as in trauma, burns, infection, and other hypermetabolic states.

Electrolytes and minerals that are added to the solution usually include sodium, potassium, chloride, phosphate, magnesium, and calcium. If the patient has a base-losing condition, acetate may be added instead of chloride. In children, 3 mEq/kg body weight/day of sodium and 2 mEq/kg body weight/day of potassium are the usual requirements. In adults the requirements are variable.

A commonly formulated TPN solution is made by mixing a 50% dextrose solution and an amino acid solution. Electrolytes, vitamins, minerals, and trace elements are added as required by the patient. The typical solution used for adults contains 1000 calories/liter of a 25% dextrose solution and 6 g of nitrogen.

Recently, fat emulsions have been approved for parenteral use in the United States. These preparations provide concentrated calories in a small fluid volume (1.1 calories/milliliter) as well as providing a source of essential fatty acids. Essential fatty acids are particularly important to the long-term TPN patient with depleted stores of these nutrients.

Adequate monitoring of the patient is mandatory. This is accomplished by closely monitoring serum glucose, electrolytes, minerals, proteins, liver and kidney function tests, triglycerides, and cholesterol.

Regular, meticulous care of the venous catheter is imperative. It is generally recommended that the dressing over the catheter be inspected and changed at least three times a week.

The presence of a team of nutrition experts, including a physician, nurse, pharmacist, and dietitian has been shown to minimize complications in parenteral nutrition therapy. The functions that this group can serve include patient selection, nutritional assessment, catheter insertion, TPN fluid preparation, metabolic monitoring, TPN dressing changing, and staff education. A coordinated effort on the part of this team can maximize the success of total parenteral nutrition therapy.

PARENTERAL NUTRITION VIA PERIPHERAL VENOUS ROUTE

Peripheral parenteral nutrition (PPN) is the technique in which the administration of carbohydrates, protein, fat, and electrolytes through a peripheral vein provides nutrients to persons who cannot ingest or absorb the needed food from the gastrointestinal system. Feeding a patient by the peripheral venous route is different from TPN in that the blood flow through a peripheral vein is lower and the infusate osmotic density is less; thus the glucose concentration of the solutions should not exceed 10%. The total caloric needs of patients cannot be met within physiologically acceptable fluid volumes. Lipid emulsions, however, can be used in combination with the glucose and protein regimen to provide the additional caloric need. These calorically dense fluids are isotonic and also provide essential fatty acids.

PPN is indicated in a number of disease conditions. These are (1) surgical disorders of the gastrointestinal tract, (2) malabsorption, (3) CNS dysfunction, and (4) hypermetabolic conditions such as burns and trauma. The peripheral venous route is generally recommended for those patients who will require parenteral nutrition for no more than 7 to 10 days or who do not have accessible peripheral veins for infusion of fluids for 7 to 10 days. However, the final choice of either the peripheral

or central route should be based on the physiological condition of the patient. A severely depleted patient may need the advantages of central vein access to replace body stores of nutrients.

The protein and electrolyte infusions are similar to those for patients receiving central venous TPN. The metabolic complications, with the exception of hyperglycemia, are also similar. The insertion and care of the peripheral catheter is different in that insertion and removal are obviously simpler procedures and the major potential problem is the risk of local tissue damage from infiltration of the fluid. The risk of sepsis is reduced by the fact that the needle or peripheral catheter is changed more often than the central catheter. Care in preparation and delivery of the infusates, however, remains a major consideration.

ASSESSMENT

1. History and presence of medical or surgical problem that would require total parenteral alimentation
   a. Gastrointestinal abnormalities
      (1) Major gastrointestinal surgery
      (2) Impaired absorption of nutrients: ulcerative colitis, regional enteritis, granulomatous colitis, Crohn's disease, intractable diarrhea in infancy
   b. Increased demand for nutrients as occurs in burn and trauma patients
   c. CNS dysfunction
   d. Pediatric patients with congenital gastrointestinal abnormalities, chronic diarrhea, surgical short-gut syndrome, or, in some cases, prematurity
2. Results of lab and diagnostic tests
   a. Blood glucose
   b. Serum proteins
   c. Kidney function tests
   d. Liver function tests; cholesterol levels
   e. Blood ammonia levels
   f. Serum electrolytes
   g. Acid-base determination
   h. Serum osmolalities
   i. Urine osmolality
   j. Urine glucose
   k. Chest radiograph
3. Patient/family's level of anxiety related to disease condition and therapy prescribed

GOALS

1. Reduction of level of anxiety with provision of information, comfort, support

2. Absence of catheter-related sepsis
3. Absence of sensitivity to the amino acid solution administered
4. Blood glucose levels within normal limits
5. Blood levels of ammonia, BUN, and creatinine within normal limits
6. Serum electrolyte levels within normal limits
7. Absence of vitamin, mineral, fatty acid deficiency
8. Positive nitrogen balance; weight maintenance or weight gain without fluid retention; preservation of body's muscle mass, protein, and fat stores
9. Acid-base balance and blood gas values within normal limits

10. BP, P, and urine output within normal limits
11. Liver function tests within normal limits
12. Intact infusion system, without air; no catheter dislodgement
13. Absence of signs/symptoms of emboli formation
14. Absence of psychological disturbances from change of feeding modality
15. Before discharge, if patient is going home on TPN, referrals are made to regional center where facilities and personnel are available for home services

Potential problems	Expected outcomes	Nursing activities
■ Patient/family's anxiety related to Insufficient knowledge and understanding of TPN IV mode of nutrient intake Disease process requiring IV alimentation Limited oral intake (if necessary)	■ Reduction in patient/family's anxiety with provision of information, explanations, and encouragement	■ Assess patient/family's level of anxiety Explain rationale for IV alimentation Explain method of TPN delivery and monitoring Discuss with physician the recommended oral intake of nutrients and permissible foods; provide for oral intake, considering patient's food preferences Provide opportunity for and encourage patient/family's questions, verbalization of anxieties, fears Support and encourage patient/family Provide for comfort measures Provide for diversional activities (e.g., reading, television) Particular attention should be paid to providing *the infant* with adequate psychosocial stimulation
■ Inadequate preparation of patient/family for insertion of catheter	■ Patient/family properly prepared for catheter insertion	■ *Central* Explain what the patient will experience during the insertion Assess need for sedation Shave and prep skin of neck as well as scalp in the infant receiving a jugular vein catheter Prepare infant/child/adult for insertion of catheter as needed (usually is done in operating room) Position patient supine in bed Procure all necessary equipment Maintain sterile technique throughout the procedure Monitor for Complaints of tingling, numbness of fingers, which may indicate brachial plexus injury Brisk bleeding during the insertion procedure may indicate puncture of subclavian artery; if occurs, apply direct pressure for at least 10 to 15 minutes Presence of respiratory distress or change in vital signs, which may indicate potential pneumothorax, hydrothorax, or hemothorax Infuse hypertonic infusate only after proper position of central venous catheter is verified by radiograph *Peripheral* Explain that the insertion of the peripheral catheter will be similar to a regular IV infusion needle placement Remind patient/family to notify staff of any pain or swelling at insertion site Check needle of peripheral catheter site regularly for evidence of infiltration

Potential problems	Expected outcomes	Nursing activities

■ Infusion of improperly prepared solution	■ Infusion of properly prepared solution, free of precipitate, with proper formulation for patient's caloric and physiological needs	■ Check each new solution for clarity, proper constituents, and date mixed
		Change solution and administration tubing at least q24 hr
		Review caloric intake daily for the first week and at least weekly thereafter
		For lipid administration
		  Check tubing during infusion for evidence of a precipitate
		  Inspect bottles for separation of emulsion and any change from milky white color
		  Do not shake bottle as it may cause fat particles to aggregate
		  Follow instructions on bottle concerning need for refrigeration
		  Do not use filter on lipid line
		  Connect lipid line to primary line by a Y connector at junction closest to insertion site, as it is not stable for long periods of time if mixed with other infusates
		  Hang lipid bottle (if gravity flow is used) higher than bottles of amino acid/dextrose solution to prevent backflow into amino acid/dextrose line due to low specific gravity of lipids
		Keep amino acid/dextrose solutions refrigerated and out of light until needed
		Store bottles out of light to prevent light-sensitive vitamin degradation

■ Sepsis related to TPN solution	■ Absence/resolution of infection	■ *Central*
		  Maintain aseptic system
		  Restrict use of line to nutritional infusates
		  If sepsis is suspected
		    Send, if appropriate, and monitor results of urine, peripheral blood, and infusates for bacteria and fungi
		    Assist with lumbar puncture for spinal fluid specimen
		  If TPN related sepsis occurs
		    Assist with catheter removal, if catheter is the probable source
		    Administer antibiotics as ordered
		    Administer a solution of moderate dextrose concentration (e.g., D10W) through a peripheral vein as ordered
		    Monitor patient's response to therapy

■ Complications related to presence of catheter
Vessel thrombosis/emboli
Vessel injury
	■ Absence/resolution of thrombosis/emboli	■ Use microbial (22 μm) filter in glucose/amino acid line
		Central
		  Monitor patient for swelling of head and chest above nipple line, which is indicative of superior vena cava syndrome
		  Monitor patient for edema along catheter route
		  Monitor patient for widened mediastinum on chest radiograph, which may indicate thoracic duct injury
		Peripheral
		  Observe peripheral needle or catheter site for local phlebitis and peripheral thrombosis/emboli
		  SEE STANDARD: *Embolic phenomena*

Catheter displacement and infiltration	Catheter in place
	Absence of infiltration
		Central
		  Ensure that skin sutures are intact
		  Secure tubing from central line to skin with tape to minimize possibility of accidental dislodgement
		  Observe track of catheter for evidence of swelling or bleeding
		  Assess need for restraints for infants, toddlers, and delirious patients
		  Obtain radiograph of catheter track if displacement is suspected; use radiopaque solution to visualize catheter if necessary

Potential problems	Expected outcomes	Nursing activities
	Absence of infiltration	*Peripheral* Observe site and limb for local infiltration of infusate
Air embolism (an air embolism is a life-threatening problem)	Absence of air embolism	*Central or peripheral* Use air elimination filter Secure connections of tubing well, and remove all air from tubing Have patient perform Valsalva's maneuver during tubing changes If air enters tubing Using aseptic technique, remove air from tubing while maintaining patency of line by slow sterile flush with appropriate dextrose solution If air is suspected in right ventricle Turn patient to left side and place in Trendelenburg position to keep air out of pulmonary artery; monitor vital signs frequently Assist physician with aspiration of air through central line while patient performs Valsalva's maneuver If procedure is necessary, monitor for cardiopulmonary instability
■ Allergic response to amino acids/peptides	■ Absence of allergic response to amino acids/peptides	■ Monitor for signs and symptoms of allergic response, including Headache Fever Chills Nausea Vomiting Rash Vasodilation Abdominal pain If problem occurs, notify physician and slow or stop infusion as ordered
■ Metabolic imbalance	■ Glucose, electrolyte, and BUN levels within normal limits Absence of signs/symptoms of fatty acid deficiency, trace element deficiency, acid-base imbalance, or fluid imbalance	■ Monitor established biochemical schedule closely and review results Establish nursing monitoring system Decrease the infusion system rate gradually Control rate of infusion by use of graduated infusion chambers and infusion pump Check rate of infusion at least q1 hr to avoid any variance greater than 10% of the rate ordered Monitor urine glucose and specific gravity during glucose infusion
Hypoglycemia	Serum glucose levels within normal limits	Monitor blood glucose levels when infusion rates are decreased If infusion must be discontinued, administer a glucose solution of moderate concentration as ordered Monitor for signs of hypoglycemia including pallor, listlessness, dizziness, staring, muscular weakness, tremors, sweating If any of these occur, notify physician and alter therapy as ordered
Electrolyte imbalance	Serum electrolyte levels within normal limits	Monitor for signs of electrolyte imbalance, including Tremors Muscular cramping Irritability Restlessness Serum electrolyte levels If these signs/symptoms occur, notify physician and alter therapy as ordered

Potential problems	Expected outcomes	Nursing activities

Elevated BUN	BUN within normal limits	Monitor for signs of increased BUN, including
		  Vomiting
		  Lethargy, stupor
		  Headaches
		  BUN levels
		Administer lipid solution 1 to 2 times a week if ordered

Fatty acid deficiency	Absence of signs/symptoms of fatty acid deficiency	Monitor for signs of fatty acid deficiency
		  Dry, scaly skin
		  Weight loss
		  Increase in heart rate
		Notify physician if occurs; administer therapy as ordered
		Monitor for immediate adverse reaction to lipid solution, including
		  Flushing
		  Dyspnea
		  Chest and back pain
		  Nausea
		  Dizziness
		  Headache
		Monitor vital signs q10 min for first 30 minutes of infusion
		Monitor for delayed lipid intolerance reaction
		  Headache
		  Irritability
		  Low-grade fever
		  Abdominal pain
		  Nausea
		  Anemia
		  Coagulopathy
		  Turbid serum
		Monitor baseline and serial triglyceride levels
		Notify physician of abnormalities, and alter therapy as ordered

Trace element deficiency	Absence of signs/symptoms of trace element deficiency	Prevent by adding trace elements to TPN solution if ordered Monitor for trace element deficiency after long-term TPN therapy

Zinc deficiency		Monitor for zinc deficiency
		  Poor wound healing
		  Loss of hair
		  Hypogeusia

Copper deficiency		Monitor for copper deficiency
		  Anemia
		  Neutropenia
		  Hypogeusia
		Notify physician of these signs and symptoms and alter therapy as ordered

Acid-base imbalance	Absence of signs/symptoms of acid-base imbalance
	Arterial blood gas levels within normal limits
		Monitor for acid-base imbalance
		  Tachypnea
		  Headache
		  Mentation alterations (fatigue, drowsiness, restlessness, apathy, inattentiveness)
		Monitor arterial blood gas results for pH, bicarbonate, base excess, and CO_2 levels
		Note increased blood lactate levels
		Notify physician of abnormalities and alter therapy as ordered

Fluid overload; dehydration	Absence of fluid imbalance
	Normovolemia
	Weight stable or weight gain consisting of increased muscle mass
		Weigh patient daily
		Note presence of edema
		Observe for
		  Respiratory distress
		  Signs of congestive heart failure
		Notify physician if either of the aforementioned occurs; see Standard: *Heart failure*

Potential problems	Expected outcomes	Nursing activities
		Administer diuretics, as ordered: closely monitor patient's response
■ Hepatomegaly	■ Absence of hepatomegaly Liver function tests within normal limits	■ Monitor results of liver function tests for abnormalities, including Serum glutamic oxaloacetic transaminase (SGOT), serum glutamic pyruvic transaminase (SGPT), alkaline phosphatase, gamma glytamyl transpeptidase (GGTP), lactic dehydrogenase (LDH), and bilirubin levels Coagulation studies (prothrombin time [PT], activated partial thromboplastin time [APTT]) Protein albumin/globulin levels Monitor for right upper quadrant fullness, elevated diaphragm on right side Notify physician of abnormalities and alter therapy as ordered
■ Insufficient knowledge to comply with discharge regimen*†‡	■ Sufficient knowledge to comply with discharge regimen	■ Refer patient to regional center where facilities and personnel are available for home hyperalimentation services

*If responsibility of critical care nurse includes follow-up care.
†Note that a small number of children and adults are receiving hyperalimentation at home via implanted central venous catheters.
‡Note that extensive teaching and follow-up care of these patients are essential to success.

GENERAL

50 ☐ Multiple trauma

Multiple trauma refers to injury of two or more systems of the body. When an accident involves significant force, the body may sustain multiple injuries. Assessment is based on the principle of *triage*. Assessment for detection of life-threatening injuries should be employed first, followed by administration of appropriate life-sustaining therapy.

A triage system for evaluation of the trauma patient has been developed* with life-threatening injuries given first priority in the following order:
1. Life-threatening injuries
   a. Cardiovascular
      (1) Cardiac arrest
      (2) Cardiopericardial injuries
      (3) Hypovolemia (e.g., hemorrhage or severe burn)
   b. Respiratory
      (1) Obstructed airway
      (2) Injured chest wall—flail chest
      (3) Decreased thoracic air space
         (a) Pneumothorax
         (b) Hemothorax
         (c) Diaphragmatic rupture
   c. Central nervous system (CNS)
      (1) Coma—closed head injury
      (2) Spinal cord injury
2. Urgent injuries
   a. Visceral
      (1) Spleen and liver—intraperitoneal bleeding
      (2) Bowel and pancreas
         (a) Bowel and pancreas—intraperitoneal bleeding
         (b) Bowel—bacterial contamination
         (c) Pancreas—liberation of pancreatic enzymes

      (3) Kidney and bladder
         (a) Kidney trauma
         (b) Ruptured bladder, urethra
   b. Cardiovascular
      (1) Traumatic aortic injury—impending rupture
      (2) Continued bleeding from intra-abdominal and vascular injuries
      (3) Laceration of arterial or venous supply to an extremity—viability of extremity threatened
3. Delayed injuries
   a. Fractures of extremities
   b. Soft tissue
   c. Spine and pelvic trauma, fractures
   d. Maxillofacial

Immediate management of the trauma patient includes provision of a patent airway with adequate oxygenation, blood volume replacement as needed, control of hemorrhage, and emergency relief measures (e.g., pericardiocentesis, chest tube, intubation) for life-threatening injuries.

These initial resuscitation activities continue while efforts for repair of specific injuries are begun, with priority attention given to the most life-threatening cardiac and respiratory injuries.

Trauma patients that are most likely to be cared for in the critical care unit include those with
1. Multisystem injury
2. Blunt thoracic trauma with cardiac and/or pulmonary injury
3. Pulmonary aspiration of gastric contents
4. Posttraumatic pulmonary insufficiency
5. Multiple transfusions
6. Prolonged hypotension
7. Sepsis and/or grossly contaminated wounds
8. Preexisting cardiovascular, respiratory, or renal disease

Hemodynamic monitoring in the critical care unit usually includes measurement of arterial pressure, central venous pressure (CVP), pulmonary artery pressure (PAP), cardiac output, and other hemodynamic param-

---

*Civetta, J. M.: Assessment of the patient following multisystemic trauma, Summary proceedings, Seventeenth Annual Symposium on Critical Care Medicine, Las Vegas, Nev., 1979, University of Southern California School of Medicine, Postgraduate Division, and Institute of Critical Care Medicine.

eters. Pulmonary artery catheters are particularly useful in assessing the response of an impaired left ventricle to fluids and blood products. PAP and pulmonary capillary wedge pressure (PCWP) can also assist in differentiating pulmonary and cardiac abnormalities.

ASSESSMENT

1. History and nature of trauma sustained, including time, events, and weapons, if any
   a. Known foreign objects that remain in wound
   b. Wound, contusions, or abrasions to any body parts
   c. Apparent bleeding sites
   d. Suspected presence of abdominal crisis
   e. Neurological abnormalities; progression/regression of level of consciousness (LOC) from pre-admission status
2. Stabilization treatment in progress
   a. Means to establish and maintain a patent airway, oxygenation
   b. Means for control of hemorrhage (e.g., pressure dressings, volume replacement)
   c. Treatment for hypotension, shock
   d. Treatment for fractures, including splints, backboards
   e. Prophylactic antibiotic therapy may be given to clear bacteria from circulation
   f. Means to maintain adequate urinary output
3. Hemodynamic stability; adequacy of cardiac output and tissue perfusion
   a. Signs and symptoms indicating specific cardiac abnormalities
      (1) Pericardial friction rub
      (2) Evidence of progressing tamponade
      (3) Radiographic evidence of enlarged heart; widened mediastinum indicative of aortic injury
      (4) ECG evidence of myocardial injury
      (5) Recurrent arrhythmias
      (6) New conduction defects
      (7) Distention of neck veins
      (8) Sinus tachycardia with small, diminishing pulse pressure
   b. Results of lab studies, including
      (1) Chest radiograph
      (2) ECG
      (3) Ultrasound study
      (4) Intravenous contrast study
      (5) Pericardiocentesis
      (6) Cardiac enzymes
      (7) Radioisotope scanning
      (8) Cardiac catheterization
      (9) Aortography
4. Adequacy of respiratory function
   a. Patent airway
   b. Respiratory rate and quality
   c. Respiratory distress—note presence of dyspnea, gasping, stridorous breathing, wheezing, cyanosis, retractions
   d. Subcutaneous emphysema
   e. Chest movements—note presence of asymmetrical movements
   f. Diaphragmatic movements
   g. Intact chest wall
   h. Midline trachea
   i. Breath sounds—note decreased, distant, and/or dull breath sounds
   j. Hyperresonant chest on percussion
   k. Signs/symptoms of pulmonary edema
   l. Signs/symptoms of hypoxia including agitation, tachypnea, dyspnea, and labored respirations
   m. Signs and symptoms revealed by roentgenographic studies consistent with
      (1) Pneumothorax
      (2) Hemothorax
      (3) Intrapulmonary hematoma
      (4) Pulmonary contusion
      (5) Foreign object (e.g., bullet) within pulmonary parenchyma
      (6) Mediastinal widening
      (7) Pneumomediastinum
      (8) Apical or another area of increased density (may suggest injury to a major vessel or contusion of the lung)
      (9) Laceration of the lung
5. Adequacy of CNS function
   a. Peripheral motor activity—note presence of purposeful movements or spontaneous responses
   b. LOC—note presence of confused, disoriented, lethargic, stuporous, or even unresponsive behavior and dulled mentation; if stuporous or unresponsive, assess reaction to verbal, noxious stimuli
   c. Vision
      (1) Pupils—note size, inequality of pupils and their response to light
      (2) Visual disturbances
      (3) Concurrent vertigo, dizziness, headache
   d. Signs and symptoms of increased intracranial pressure

e. Presence and nature of drainage from ears, nose, mouth, and head; test for presence of glucose

f. Presence of seizure activity
   (1) Note body source and progression
   (2) Duration
   (3) Type of tremor/seizure

g. Results of lumbar tap
   (1) Increased intracranial pressure
   (2) Bloody or cloudy cerebrospinal fluid

h. Signs and symptoms of fractures
   (1) Skull radiograph results indicating a large separation of fractured bone fragments
   (2) Depression of any area on the scalp
   (3) Leakage of cerebrospinal fluid from nose or ear
   (4) Severe ecchymosis of eyelids or over mastoid process

6. Signs and symptoms of injury or rupture of an intra-abdominal organ
   a. Localized or generalized peritonitis
      (1) Increasing abdominal discomfort/pain/distention
      (2) Tenderness, rebound tenderness
      (3) Muscle rigidity, spasm
      (4) Decreased bowel sounds
      (5) Tachycardia, fever
      (6) Shoulder pain (may be from diaphragmatic irritation)
   b. Injury of solid viscera (liver, spleen, pancreas) including hemorrhage, enlargement of organ, abdominal distention, reflex ileus, rectal bleeding
   c. Results of lab and diagnostic tests
      (1) Radiographs—note presence of pneumoperitoneum: retroperitoneal air, elevation of diaphragm
      (2) Abdominal tap
      (3) Intraluminal studies and selective celiac and superior mesenteric angiography
      (4) Complete blood count; note presence of leukocytosis
      (5) Elevated serum and urine amylase levels

7. Signs and symptoms of genitourinary system injury
   a. Tenderness in the suprapubic area, perineum, scrotum, and pubic rami on pelvic compression
   b. Expanding masses or masses in the flank and suprapubic area, perineum, and scrotum
   c. Laceration, contusions, avulsion, or amputation of the penis
   d. Hemorrhage

e. Hematuria

f. Pelvic examination revealing pelvic hematoma, lesions of the urethra, and blood at urethral meatus

g. Results of abdominal radiographs indicating lower rib fracture, presence of foreign body near the genitourinary system

8. Musculoskeletal system for injuries, function
   a. Sensation, motor function of extremities
   b. Pain—location, nature of
   c. Bruises, lacerations
   d. Swelling, deformity
   e. Pulses, pallor

9. Results of lab and diagnostic tests, including
   a. Complete blood count
   b. Coagulation studies: prothrombin time (PT), activated partial thromboplastin time (APTT)
   c. ECG
   d. Pertinent radiographs—chest, abdomen, or fracture site(s)
   e. Electrolytes
   f. Liver function tests, cardiac enzymes
   g. Indices of renal function
   h. Urinalysis
   i. Arterial blood gas levels
   j. Specific scans, echograms, angiograms, endoscopies (depending on the injury sustained)

10. Assess level of patient/family's anxiety regarding the traumatic injury sustained, immobility and disabilities, diagnostic procedures, and therapeutic regimen

GOALS

1. a. Respiratory function sufficient for adequate oxygenation and ventilation
   b. Patent airway
   c. Full lung expansion

2. a. Hemodynamic stability
   b. Adequate cardiac output

3. a. Patient alert and oriented to time, place, and person
   b. Sensations and spontaneous movements of extremities and torso within normal limits
   c. Absence or resolution of head injury; stabilization of spinal cord injury

4. a. Function of abdominal organs within normal limits
   b. Absence and/or resolution of signs of abdominal trauma, catastrophe, including injury to
      (1) Liver

(2) Spleen

(3) Pancreas

(4) Kidney, bladder, urethra

(5) Bowel, peritoneum

5. a. Stabilization of fractures present

 b. No apparent bleeding from fracture site

6. a. Infection free

 b. Absence of atelectasis

 c. Absence of infection associated with open traumatic injuries

7. Resolution and/or prevention of complications, including renal insufficiency, stress ulcer, embolic phenomena, coagulopathy

8. Absence and/or minimal deformity or contractures

9. Restoration to optimal physical, emotional, and psychological functioning

10. Reduction in patient/family's anxiety with provision of information, explanations, and comfort

11. Before discharge, patient/family is able to

 a. Verbalize knowledge of

 (1) Activity progression and precautions

 (2) Dietary management and modifications

 (3) Medications—identification, dosage, schedules for administration, possible adverse effects, and precautionary measures

 (4) Untoward signs and symptoms requiring medical follow-up

 b. Perform specific therapeutic measures such as dressing changes

 c. Describe plan for follow-up care

Potential problems	Expected outcomes	Nursing activities
■ Respiratory insufficiency related to *obstructed airway,* which may result from Mandibular fracture(s) Massive bleeding from intraoral injuries Disordered sensorium Aspiration of blood, gastric contents Edema of larynx (frequent in auto crash trauma)	■ Respiratory sufficiency with patent, unobstructed airway Absence of respiratory distress Alveolar ventilation adequate with Pa_{CO_2} within patient's normal limits	■ Monitor for Absence of respirations Respiratory distress—note presence of deep, gasping, rapid, shallow, labored, dyspneic, or stridorous breathing; wheezing Adequacy of ventilation Hold hand above patient's nose and mouth and feel force of expired air Observe chest movements Observe Pa_{CO_2} levels Occlusion of airway by tongue, secretions, or blood Arterial blood gas results for hypoxemia, hypercapnia If partial/total obstructed airway is apparent Hyperextend head (except in patients with suspected cervical or spinal cord injury) If airway obstruction is still present, remove clotted blood, loose teeth, dentures, vomitus, foreign objects from patient's mouth with fingers Apply humidified O_2 mask as ordered Prepare patient for and assist with intubation for mechanical ventilation, which is often required for patients with Fractures of two or more ribs Severe mandibular fractures Massive oropharyngeal tissue injury Obtundation from a head injury SEE STANDARD: *Mechanical ventilation*
■ Respiratory insufficiency related to *flail chest,* which may result from Fracture of four or more ribs Fracture of sternum at junction of ribs (separation of costochondral cartilages producing a free-floating sternum)	■ Flail chest stabilized with adequate alveolar ventilation, without undue splinting, and without further lung contusion due to fractured ribs Cardiac output and arterial O_2 saturation, Pa_{O_2} within normal limits	■ Monitor for Splinting Swelling and/or crepitation over rib cage Light palpation revealing fractured rib Paradoxical movement of chest with breathing Arterial blood gas results for decrease in arterial O_2 saturation Pain Chest radiograph results indicating fracture Notify physician of these abnormalities If flail chest occurs Administer analgesics as ordered

Potential problems	Expected outcomes	Nursing activities
		Assist physician with local infiltration of anesthetic Maintain sandbag traction, light hand pressure, or a pillow splint for stabilization if intubation is not immediately possible Prepare patient for and assist with intubation; see Standard: *Mechanical ventilation*
■ Respiratory insufficiency related to *pulmonary vessel injury* with *hemothorax,* which may be associated with bleeding from the following arteries Pulmonary Main hilar Pleurocutaneous	■ Hemodynamic stability with adequate cardiac output, normovolemia Pulmonary vessels intact	■ Monitor for Signs and symptoms of shock, hypovolemia, blood loss, hypoxemia, and hypercapnia Signs and symptoms of pulmonary contusion Atelectasis Decreased breath sounds Bloody secretions Hazy chest radiograph in area of suspected contusion Chest radiograph results revealing Pneumothorax Hemothorax Prepare patient for and assist with chest tube insertion if procedure is necessary Monitor chest tube drainage; note amount, nature of blood loss If dark and pulsatile, a pulmonary artery tear may be the source If bright red and pulsatile, a pulmonary vein or surrounding artery may be torn If chest entrance wound is present, monitor for tear of aorta and other major arterial vessels and for cardiac tamponade; see Problem, Hemodynamic instability, if chest entrance wound is present If pulmonary vessel injury occurs, assist with needle aspiration or tube thoracotomy Prepare patient for surgery, if planned (often required for major, ongoing blood losses, a large retained clot after chest tube insertion, a major bronchial tear)
■ Respiratory insufficiency related to *sucking wound* Destroys pressure gradient between atmosphere and pleural space Leads to atelectasis, pneumothorax, mediastinal shift, impaired venous return to heart	■ Adequate alveolar ventilation Absence or resolution of sucking chest wound Absence of air leak	■ Monitor for Sound of sucking wound of chest; note open wound Signs/symptoms of pneumothorax, mediastinal shift, impaired venous return to heart, atelectasis If sucking wound occurs Maintain airtight dressing (gauze with petroleum jelly coating); should be applied at the end of expiration when the diaphragm has expelled residual air and fluid from the pleural space through the wound opening Prepare for and assist with insertion of chest tube Maintain patient in semi-Fowler's position
■ Respiratory insufficiency related to *pulmonary contusion* with hemorrhage and edema Signs of pulmonary contusion become more obvious hours after trauma due to the natural inflammatory process and because the low pressure pulmonary system is	■ Absence or resolution of pulmonary contusion	■ Monitor for Dropping Pa_{O_2} levels Requirements for greater inspired O_2 concentrations to achieve adequate oxygenation (Pa_{O_2}) Higher inspiratory pressures required for delivery of desired tidal volume (decreased compliance) Chest radiograph results revealing a diffusely hazy picture throughout the lung fields; localized pattern of haziness and atelectasis consistent with pulmonary contusion Notify physician of these abnormalities If pulmonary contusion occurs Administer respiratory support if needed, as ordered

Potential problems	Expected outcomes	Nursing activities

prone to accumulation of fluid used during resuscitation		Supplemental humidified O_2
		Intubation and mechanical ventilation
		See Standard: *Mechanical ventilation*
		Administer fluids cautiously
		  Accurate intake and output
		  Administer diuretics as ordered
		  Weigh daily; note weight gain, which is to be avoided

■ Posttraumatic respiratory insufficiency related to Sepsis (systemic and pulmonary) Long bone fracture (fat emboli) Direct pulmonary injury Massive transfusion of whole blood Aspiration of gastric contents Fluid overload Ischemic pulmonary injury (i.e., hemorrhagic shock)	■ Adequate oxygenation and ventilation Arterial blood gas levels within normal limits Clear lungs as evidenced by chest radiograph and auscultation	■ Monitor for syndrome, particularly in patients at high risk, including Hypoxemia Decreased pulmonary compliance Measurements of lung volumes reveal a fall in resting volume or functional residual capacity (FRC) in lung Diffuse infiltrates, which may progress to consolidation, indicating worsening of syndrome If posttraumatic respiratory insufficiency occurs, administer therapy as ordered directed at recruiting collapsed and partially occluded alveoli, which will directly increase the FRC of the lung and improve oxygenation/ventilation If artificial mechanical ventilation is instituted, see Standard; *Mechanical ventilation* If mechanical ventilation with positive end expiratory pressure (PEEP) is instituted, see Standard: *Positive end expiratory pressure* Administer fluids carefully to avoid hypervolemia and pulmonary interstitial edema (which is directly associated with fluid overload) Administer diuretics as ordered—monitor patient's response carefully Monitor weight daily; improvement in respiratory function is often associated with a loss of some of the extra body fluid used for resuscitation
■ Respiratory insufficiency related to reduced air space that results from Pneumothorax Bronchial tear Hemothorax Diaphragmatic tear Phrenic nerve injury and diaphragmatic paralysis	■ Adequate alveolar ventilation with full lung expansion Absence of respiratory distress	■ Monitor for signs and symptoms of a pneumothorax and/or hemothorax Tachypnea Respiratory distress Asymmetrical chest movements Signs that are indicative of pneumothorax Shift of trachea to unaffected side Distended neck veins Altered LOC due to hypoxia Swelling and palpable crepitations around neck (particularly injuries to apex of lung) Distant breath sounds Hyperresonance on percussion Signs that are indicative of hemothorax Dullness with percussion Chest radiograph results revealing fluid level in pleural space area Drop in Hct if blood loss is significant Sudden drop in BP, CVP, and cardiac output If pneumothorax and/or hemothorax occur, prepare patient for and assist with Thoracentesis Chest tube insertion If hemothorax occurs (in addition) Monitor vital signs q15-30 min and serial Hct levels Administer fluids, blood, and blood products as ordered; closely monitor patient's response

Potential problems	Expected outcomes	Nursing activities

		Monitor for signs of bronchial tear
		  Signs/symptoms of a pneumothorax
		  Massive air leak
		  Persistent atelectasis
		  Inability to sufficiently expand the injured lung
		Monitor for signs of diaphragmatic tear, particularly in patient's with history of blunt chest and abdominal trauma
		  Elevated diaphragm by radiograph and clinical examination
		  Persistent lower lobe atelectasis
		Assist with upright chest radiograph, fluoroscopy, and other tests to rule out injury to phrenic nerve and paralysis of diaphragm, revealed in part by reduced diaphragmatic movement

■ Hemodynamic instability related to *hemorrhage* resulting from
  Torn or ruptured aorta
  Tear of coronary artery
  Cardiac rupture
  Tear of subclavian or innominate artery
	■ Hemodynamic stability
	  Adequate cardiac output, blood volume
	  Hemodynamic parameters and vital signs within patient's normal limits
	  Urine output 0.5 ml/kg/hour in adults; 1 to 2 ml/kg/hour in children/infants
		■ Monitor
		  Vital signs q¼-1 hr until stable
		  For presence of signs/symptoms of shock
		    Marked hypotension, tachycardia
		    Weak, thready pulses
		    Peripheral vasoconstriction (coolness, clamminess)
		    Pallor
		    Restlessness
		  For external blood loss (through wounds, body orifices, tubes inserted for drainage)
		  For presence of expanding chest wall hematoma
		  Results of serial Hct and Hgb (q6-12 hr until stable)
		  Fluid intake and output, scrupulously
		  For signs/symptoms of cardiac tamponade due to accumulation of blood in pericardium, mediastinum
		  For presence of chest or upper abdominal wound; monitor for chest radiograph results revealing widened mediastinum; contused myocardium; hematoma at apex of heart; foreign body (e.g., bullet) near major vessels; rib fractures; flail chest and/or fractured sternum; hemothorax; and for injury to a major artery
		Note diminished or absent pulses on the affected upper extremity; monitor for
		  Neurological deficits associated with ischemia, thrombosis, or cerebral embolism; ischemic brachial plexus injury, which is revealed by neurological deficits of the arm
		  Presence of a bruit over a major vessel (may indicate traumatic arteriovenous fistula formation)
		  Substernal pain
		Notify physician of any abnormality
		If hemorrhage occurs
		  Administer fluids, blood, and blood products as ordered into a catheterized vessel proximal to a suspected arterial/venous tear
		  Carefully monitor patient's hemodynamic response
		  Keep patient supine until resuscitation effort improves hemodynamic—circulatory parameters; avoid Trendelenburg position if head, neck, and chest injuries have not been ruled out
		  Prepare patient for arteriography and/or surgery as planned
		  Assist with insertion of central venous, pulmonary artery lines
		  Monitor CVP and PAP q½-1 hr and prn during resuscitation efforts
		  Measure circumference of all body systems parts that may be bleeding, particularly abdomen and lower extremities

Potential problems	**Expected outcomes**	**Nursing activities**
■ Hemodynamic instability related to *myocardial contusion*	■ Hemodynamic stability Resolution of signs/ symptoms of myocardial contusion	■ Monitor for ECG evidence of myocardial ischemia, injury New conduction defect Recurrent arrhythmias, particularly sinus tachycardia, atrial arrhythmias, bundle branch block, and ventricular arrhythmias Elevated serum cardiac enzyme levels Concurrent hemodynamic compromise—low cardiac output not produced by obvious valvular or septal rupture Signs of heart failure Pericardial rub, other signs of pericarditis Cardiac tamponade Exsanguinating intrathoracic hemorrhage (e.g., in pericardial laceration) Ventricular aneurysm Notify physician of any of these abnormalities If myocardial contusion occurs Administer supportive therapy as ordered Mild inotropic agents Beta–adrenergic-blocking agents Diuretics Fluids O_2 See standards appropriate for problems associated with myocardial contusion: *Arrhythmias; Heart failure; Acute myocardial infarction* Prepare patient for diagnostic studies, as planned, which may include Ultrasound study Radioisotope scan Intravenous contrast study of right heart
■ Hemodynamic instability related to *cardiac tamponade*	■ Absence or resolution of cardiac tamponade	■ Monitor for signs/symptoms of cardiac tamponade, including Rapidly advancing signs of shock—hypotension, decreasing pulse pressure, rising venous pressure, tachycardia, cold clammy skin Progressive venous distention in neck and arms Kussmaul's sign (neck veins paradoxically expand with inhalation) Pulsus paradoxus (pulse stronger with exhalation, weaker with inhalation) Distant heart sounds Decreasing voltage of QRS complex on ECG Characteristic pericardial friction rub and ECG S-T segment and T wave abnormalities Widening mediastinum, cardiac silhouette as evidenced by chest radiograph results Notify physician of these abnormalities If cardiac tamponade occurs Prepare patient for pericardial aspiration, if planned, and assist with procedure; after procedure, monitor for recurrent cardiac tamponade, which may indicate a bleeding artery and need for a pericardial window Administer IV fluid, blood products as ordered; carefully monitor patient's response Administer cardiotonic, diuretic agents as ordered for cardiac failure and pulmonary edema See Standard; *Pericarditis* for nursing activities regarding pericardial effusion/cardiac tamponade

Potential problems	Expected outcomes	Nursing activities
■ Hemodynamic instability related to traumatic *pericardial rupture,* resulting from Herniation of heart Torsion of great vessels Rupture of heart itself	■ Resolution of traumatic pericardial rupture	■ Monitor for signs of traumatic pericardial rupture, primarily signs of cardiac decompensation and low cardiac output Notify physician of signs of cardiac decompensation Prepare patient for emergency surgery if planned
■ Hemodynamic instability related to *valvular injuries* Mitral regurgitation resulting from Laceration of a leaflet Rupture of chordae tendineae Hemorrhage into and avulsion of a papillary muscle (necrosis, then rupture) Aortic regurgitation associated with Tear of aortic leaflet Avulsion of a commissural attachment Aortic intimal tear with prolapse of the leaflet into the ventricular outflow tract Tricuspid regurgitation	■ Valvular function adequate for sufficient forward blood flows Absence and/or resolution of valvular injuries	■ Monitor for Holosystolic murmur, heard best at apex of axilla and not transmitted to neck—S_1 soft; S_3 present Chest radiograph results revealing enlarged left atrium ECG revealing Left ventricular hypertrophy Left atrial hypertrophy Left axis deviation Cardiac catheterization revealing Little or no pressure gradient at mitral valve Mitral regurgitation on cineangiography Elevated left atrial pressure—big V waves Notify physician of any of these abnormalities Monitor for Basal decrescendo diastolic murmur Early systolic murmur Midsystolic murmur at apex Wide pulse pressure Quick-rising pulses Chest radiograph results revealing dilated aorta ECG revealing signs of left ventricular hypertrophy Cardiac catheterization results revealing Little or no pressure gradient at aortic valve Aortic regurgitation with cineangiocardiography Notify physician of any abnormality Monitor for Holosystolic murmur—maximum point near sternum; increased with inspiration; not transmitted to axilla V waves in jugular venous hypertension and congestive heart failure Pulsating liver Chest radiograph revealing enlarged right atrium, vena cava ECG revealing right axis deviation Cardiac catheterization revealing Elevated right atrial pressure V waves in and proximal to right atrium If valvular insufficiency occurs, administer therapy to support cardiac function as ordered, which may include Cautious fluid administration so as not to overload the heart Diuretics Inotropic agents If signs of heart failure occur, see Standard: *Heart failure* Prepare patient for cardiac catheterization if planned Prepare patient for surgery if planned

Potential problems	**Expected outcomes**	**Nursing activities**
■ Hemodynamic instability related to *rupture of cardiac septa, chamber walls,* which may include Ventricular wall rupture Interatrial septal defect Ventricular septal defect Left ventricular–right atrial communication Aortic–right ventricular communication Process may include acute laceration or less acute contusion and hemorrhage, followed by necrosis, sloughing, and perforation	■ Hemodynamic stability Cardiac chambers, septum intact	■ Monitor for signs of septal, chamber rupture (in patients with history of chest compression) Cardiovascular collapse Low cardiac output Profound heart failure Pulmonary congestion, interstitial edema Notify physician of these abnormalities If rupture occurs Administer fluid, blood, blood products as ordered Monitor patient's vital signs continuously via oscilloscope; note q5 min Prepare patient for surgery according to the plan of care
■ Altered LOC related to Closed head injury Concussion Skull fracture (brain damage) Trauma associated with acute exacerbation/onset of a medical problem (e.g., diabetes) Cerebrovascular accident Drug overdose, poisoning Hysteria	■ Patient oriented to person, place, and time Neurological examination within normal limits Absence or resolution of increased intracranial pressure	■ Assess LOC and note in particular Decreased alertness, orientation to surroundings Restlessness, confusion, stupor Monitor for Hemodynamic changes associated with increased intracranial pressure Widening pulse pressure Slow bounding pulse, bradycardia Slowed, slurred speech Neck stiffness Abnormal respiratory pattern Inequality of pupil size and reaction to light Mild fever Nausea and/or vomiting Fluid intake and output imbalance; particularly note polyuria associated with increased intracranial pressure Patient's movement and sensation of all extremities; note differences and notify physician Presence of ecchymoses around eyes, chin, and/or ears If these signs and symptoms are present Evaluate for skull fracture (frontal and basal), and palpate skull for depressions, protrusions, lacerations Check for drainage from ears, nose, and mouth Test ear and nose drainage for presence of glucose, indicating spinal fluid Examine ears, nose, and hair for foreign objects Notify physician of these abnormalities If signs/symptoms of head injury are present, prepare patient for tests as ordered, which may include Computerized axial tomography (CAT) Arteriography Electroencephalography Echoencephalography

Potential problems	Expected outcomes	Nursing activities
		SEE STANDARD: *Head trauma* If cerebral swelling is suspected and patient is conscious, do not permit patient to further increase intracranial pressure by bearing down during elimination or blowing nose Reevaluate patient's neurological status, including LOC, motor and sensory functions, and pupillary reactions q½-1 hr and prn
■ Skeletal injuries: spinal cord injury, which most commonly occurs at C5, C6, and/or C7; and T12, L1	■ Stabilization of fracture Degree of sensation and movement of extremities remain stable or improve GI function within normal limits Hemodynamic stability, adequate cardiac output	■ Monitor for signs of spinal trauma Sensation to and movement of extremities Sensation of torso Reflexes to extremities, torso If spinal cord injury is suspected, particularly if lesion is high in cord, monitor for signs of decreased sympathetic tone including hypotension, bradycardia, hypothermia Notify physician of any of these abnormalities If spinal cord injury occurs Closely monitor vital signs q¼-1 hr until stable Administer fluids, vasopressor medication as ordered Perform ongoing neurological evaluation, including LOC Sensation, movement of extremities Sensation of torso Reflexes—pupillary size, equality, and reaction Maintain patient in straight alignment Ensure straight alignment of body and head when turning patient (if allowed to turn) Prepare patient for placement of tongs if procedure is necessary Maintain tongs and traction as ordered once applied
■ Skeletal injuries: fracture of extremity	■ Fracture heals with proper alignment of bone Sensation and movement of extremity within normal limits	■ Monitor for Deformity, swelling, or open wounds on admission Pain—location, nature, and severity Reduced movement and range of motion (ROM); marked pain with movement Reduced sensitivity to extremity; note paresis, followed by paresthesia Reduced circulation to any extremity Note pallor, coolness, thready pulses Notify physician of any of these abnormalities If spinal fracture is suspected, keep patient flat and spine in straight, immobile alignment Assist with maintaining immobilization of fractures If casts are applied, monitor circulation to extremities (pulses, warmth, color) and patient's ability to move extremities Maintain sterile dressings on open fracture (nonadherent dressings soaked in saline solution or povidone-iodine may be ordered) Monitor for signs of bleeding associated with the fracture Increasing circumference of extremity, pelvis (lower abdomen) Dropping Hct Signs of developing shock For spinal fracture, see Problem, Skeletal injuries: spinal cord injury For rib fractures where flail chest is suspected, see Problem, Respiratory insufficiency related to flail chest For skull fractures, see Problem, Altered LOC

Potential problems	Expected outcomes	Nursing activities
■ Skeletal injuries with associated fatty micro-emboli and reactive edema of lungs, brain, and kidneys (resulting from fracture of long bones and ribs)	■ Absence or resolution of fatty microemboli Pulmonary, cerebral, and kidney function within normal limits	■ Monitor for signs and symptoms of Pulmonary interstitial edema and hypoxia Delirium Hematuria and fatty droplets in urine Petechiae, which may appear on chest, in axillary folds, in sclera, and under the eyelids Notify physician of these abnormalities If fatty microemboli occur, see Standard: *Embolic phenomena*
■ Trauma to internal organ systems: peritonitis	■ Absence or resolution of peritonitis	■ Monitor for signs and symptoms of peritonitis, particularly in the patient with a history of blunt trauma to the abdomen Increasing abdominal pain Tenderness, rebound tenderness, or rigidity Muscle spasm Abdominal guarding Decreased bowel sounds Tachycardia, fever, leukocytosis Abdominal distention Signs and symptoms of hypovolemia, shock Observe for signs and symptoms of rupture of GI tract or other abdominal organs Radiograph may reveal pneumoperitoneum if an associated rupture of any portion of GI tract occurs If peritonitis occurs, see Standard: *Peritonitis*
■ Esophageal injury; evaluate for in patients with upper to middle chest injury(s) to the aorta, trachea, left main stem bronchus	■ Intact esophagus Normal esophageal function	■ Monitor for Pneumomediastinum on radiograph (occurs in small percentage) Complaints of substernal pain, neck and epigastric discomfort If problem is suspected, a more certain diagnosis can be made by carefully inserting a tube through which a water-soluble opaque material can be passed and visualized by radiograph; assist physician with this procedure as needed If problem is detected, prepare patient for surgery as ordered Assist with insertion of chest tube to drain mediastinum
■ Injury, rupture of bladder	■ Intact bladder Urine output within patient's normal limits	■ Monitor for Urine output through a bladder catheter q2 hr; note presence of gross hematuria and urine in small volumes Suprapubic pain with rebound tenderness Shock from bleeding Presence of large suprapubic mass Large boggy mass above the prostate on rectal examination (usually done by physician) Monitor lab study results, including Urinalysis for presence of red blood cells Kidney, ureter, and bladder for pelvic fracture; increased darkness in vesicular area may indicate extravasation Excretory urograms for injury to the kidney Retrograde cystogram, which is reliable for demonstrating frank extravasation Notify physician of any pertinent findings Prepare patient for and assist with pertinent diagnostic studies as ordered If bladder injury occurs Administer therapy as ordered to treat shock, hemorrhage; closely monitor patient's hemodynamic response Prepare patient for surgery, which may include Drainage of injured site Closure of tear Placement of cystostomy tube (in addition to indwelling urethral catheter)

Potential problems	Expected outcomes	Nursing activities

■ Trauma to kidney(s)	■ Kidney function within normal limits	■ Check for presence of ecchymosis, bruise, contusion, or laceration in mid-lower abdomen
		Monitor for hematuria, flank pain, hypotension, and dropping Hct, which may indicate ongoing bleeding; an abdominal mass in the flank area may be a hematoma associated with trauma to the kidneys
		Monitor lab studies for indices of renal function
		  Urine output
		  BUN
		  Creatinine-serum levels and urinary clearance
		  Uric acid
		Notify physician of notable abnormalities
		Administer therapy aimed at maintaining adequate renal blood flow, maintaining fluid and electrolyte balance, and preventing further renal damage (e.g., avoiding nephrotoxic antibiotics)
		Prepare patient for and assist with certain diagnostic procedures, which may include
		  Kidney, ureter, and bladder (KUB) radiograph
		  Urogram (after treatment for shock)
		  Renal angiography
		Prepare patient for surgery if planned, particularly in the presence of persistent bleeding, when laceration can be sutured; if injury is severe, a nephrectomy may be needed
		Monitor for signs and symptoms of a perinephric infection; if present, notify physician and administer therapy as ordered (surgical drainage may be required)

■ Injuries to the membranous urethra, which often occur in association with fracture of the pubic bone	■ Kidney-bladder function within normal limits, including normal urinary output	■ Monitor for
		  Gross hematuria; hemorrhage
		  Inability to void
		  Lower abdominal or perineal pain
		  Tender suprapubic mass (containing blood and urine)
		Notify physician of any of these abnormalities
		Administer therapy as ordered, including fluids and blood products to maintain blood volume; maintenance of a bladder catheter, which may have a small amount of traction applied
		Closely monitor intake and output, specific gravities of urines, and for continuing signs and symptoms identified before and indices of kidney function

■ Rupture of diaphragm	■ Diaphragm intact
	  Diaphragmatic function within normal limits
	  Absence of respiratory distress
	  Alveolar ventilation within normal limits
		■ Monitor for respiratory distress
		  Presence of tachypnea, dyspnea
		  Serial blood gas results indicating hypoventilation (hypercapnia)
		  Difficulty in delivery of inspiratory volume during mechanical ventilation, e.g., high inspiratory pressures on volume ventilators or low volume delivered on pressure-limited ventilators
		Monitor chest radiograph results for
		  Mediastinal shift
		  Elevated diaphragm and upper abdominal organs
		  Occasionally protrusion of abdominal organs through diaphragm
		  Persistent lower lobe atelectasis
		Notify physician of these abnormalities
		Administer supportive care as ordered, which may include artificial ventilation
		Prepare patient for surgery if planned

Potential problems	**Expected outcomes**	**Nursing activities**
■ Rupture of spleen, which occurs frequently in association with Fractures of the lower ribs In association with childhood trauma (with or without rib fractures) Presence of diseases that make the spleen very friable (malaria, typhoid, sarcoidosis, infectious mononucleosis)	■ Spleen function within normal limits; without signs of internal bleeding	■ Monitor for a ruptured spleen, particularly in patients with a history of blunt abdominal trauma, with fractures of the lower left ribs Monitor for Left flank pain Pain and tenderness in the left upper quadrant of abdomen Left shoulder pain (occurs in about 75% of patients with ruptured spleen and is associated with diaphragmatic irritation; also called *Kehr's sign*) Evidence of blood loss Developing signs of peritoneal irritation Moderate leukocytosis and falling Hct Temperature elevation usually does not occur Radiograph results revealing displacement of the gastric air bubble and loss of splenic outline Assist with diagnostic abdominal tap, which is positive for blood in about 75% of patients with ruptured spleen Notify physician of the aforementioned abnormalities Prepare patient for surgery as planned and ordered
■ Trauma to or rupture of liver Occurs less commonly than rupture of spleen (more force is required) Bleeding may occur and may cease spontaneously Is suspected in the presence of fractures of the lower right ribs or when concurrent laceration of right kidney is present	■ Liver function within normal limits; without signs of internal bleeding	■ Monitor for signs of rupture of the liver, including Right upper quadrant pain and muscle rigidity and tenderness Right shoulder pain (from diaphragmatic irritation) Swelling in right upper quadrant Note presence of concurrent signs of peritonitis indicating possible ongoing hemorrhage Monitor hemodynamic status closely Notify physician of presence of any of these abnormalities If trauma to liver is suspected Monitor vital signs closely (q15-30 min) until stable Note signs of shock Monitor results of serial Hct determinations Measure abdominal girth serially (q1-2 hr) Note increasing size, tension of abdomen If liver trauma or rupture occurs Administer fluids, blood, and blood products as ordered Closely monitor patient's response as before Monitor serial liver function tests; particularly note coagulation studies, protein levels, transaminase levels, etc.
■ Infection related to Local factors Ischemia and devitalization of tissue Reduced blood flow to injured tissue, with deficient delivery of immunoproteins and leukocytes to combat bacterial contamination Hematoma Penetration of contaminated foreign object Puncture of bowel	■ Absence of or resolution of infection Afebrile Wounds, fracture heal without undue necrosis or devitalization of tissue	■ Prevention Provide for adequate systemic oxygenation Administer adequate nutrients to meet calculated metabolic requirements to aid in healing and support immunological activity against infection Sterile dressings to open wounds, as ordered Adhere to careful sterile precautions in handling endotracheal tubes, tracheostomies, bladder catheter, and arterial and IV lines; remove these lines as soon as patient's status allows, as ordered Administer antibiotics if ordered Administer topical antibiotics as ordered Assist with debridement of wounds if needed Prepare patient for surgery for evacuation of hematoma or fluid collections that could be a media for infection Provide for vigorous chest physiotherapy tailored to fit patient's needs See Standard: *Chest physiotherapy* Assist patient with ambulation as soon as possible

Potential problems	Expected outcomes	Nursing activities

with massive fecal soilage of peritoneum
Systemic factors
  Systemic hypoxia
  Hemorrhagic shock
  Severe tissue injury (depletes body of proteins that prepare bacteria for phagocytosis by polymorphonuclear leukocytes)
  History of recent alcohol intake (depresses the phagocytic leukocyte function)
		Monitor
		  Temperature q1-2 hr; note fever
		  For signs of wound infection—redness, swelling, purulent drainage
		  Complete blood count results indicating leukocytosis; elevated erythrocyte sedimentation rate (ESR)
		  For chest radiograph results compatible with atelectasis, subdiaphragmatic abscess
		  C and S results of wound, sputum, blood, and other appropriate sites
		If infection occurs
		  Administer antibiotics as ordered
		  Continue preventive measures identified before
		  Prepare patient for drainage of infected collections and/or debridement of necrotic foci if procedures are necessary

■ Acid-base imbalance	■ Parameters of acid-base balance within normal limits, including
	Arterial pH
	O_2
	CO_2
	Bicarbonate
	Electrolyte levels, particularly
	K^+
	Na^+
	Cl^-
	CO_2
		■ Prevent by
		  Administering electrolyte solutions based on patient's calculated requirements
		  Administering O_2 and supporting ventilation according to patient's needs, as ordered
		Monitor
		  Results of arterial blood gas determinations
		  Serum lactate levels, if determined
		  Serum electrolyte levels
		Notify physician of abnormalities
		Administer therapy as ordered to correct acid-base problem, which may include
		  Correction of electrolyte imbalance, if present
		  Metabolic acidosis
		    Sodium bicarbonate
		    Improvement of blood flows with fluids, blood products
		    Cardiac support with inotropic and/or vasodilating agent
		  Respiratory acidosis
		    Vigorous chest physiotherapy; if necessary, mechanical ventilation may be instituted
		  Respiratory alkalosis
		    Sedation
		    Adjustment of ventilator settings for the intubated patient
		    Decrease in tidal volume, respiratory rate
		  Metabolic alkalosis
		    If pronounced, ammonium chloride may be administered

■ Renal failure, which may result from prolonged low blood flows and ischemia	■ Indices of renal function within normal limits, including
	Urine volume
	Specific gravity
	Urine electrolytes
	Urine osmolality
	Urine-plasma electrolyte, urea, creatinine, and osmolality ratios
		■ Prevent with early resuscitation of trauma patient by administering fluids and blood products as ordered
		Carefully monitor patient's hemodynamic status and daily weights
		Carefully monitor urine output, a good indicator of adequate renal blood flow
		Monitor other indices of renal function including
		  Urine specific gravity
		  Urine electrolyte levels
		  Creatinine clearance*
		  Urine-plasma urea ratio

*Soft tissue, muscle damage results in an increased load of creatinine for kidney clearance. Therefore consider both urine and plasma creatinine levels.

Potential problems	Expected outcomes	Nursing activities
	Free H_2O clearance Serum BUN	Urine-plasma creatinine ratio Urine-plasma osmolality ratio Free H_2O clearance (may fall to 0 in patients with acute renal failure) Serum BUN If problem occurs, see Standard: *Acute renal failure*
■ Stress ulceration, with upper GI bleeding Patients at greatest risk include those with Multisystem trauma Major intracranial injury or surgery Shock Burns Infection/sepsis Renal insufficiency Respiratory insufficiency Corticosteroid therapy Preexisting coagulopathy, GI disorder	■ Absence of or resolution of stress ulceration	■ Prevent stress ulceration with therapy as ordered, which may include An H_2 antagonist (e.g., cimetidine) NG tube Antacids Anticholinergics (particularly for patients with intracranial trauma and for patients who are to undergo surgery) Provision for adequate nutritional intake Prevention with therapy for precipitating causes, including Shock Burns Infection Renal insufficiency Respiratory insufficiency Monitor for Bloody NG drainage Complaints of nausea, epigastric distress Dropping Hct Increasing abdominal girth Melenic, heme-positive stools If stress ulceration occurs, see Standard: *Acute upper gastrointestinal bleeding*
■ Anxiety, which may be associated with Nature of traumatic injuries sustained Inability to move some body parts Loss of sensation Diagnostic tests Therapeutic regimen	■ Reduction in patient/family's anxiety with provision of information, explanations, and encouragement	■ Ongoing assessment of anxiety Assess patient/family's knowledge of disease process including abnormalities in sensation and movement, need for intensive care; diagnostic tests, and therapeutic regimen Explain in simple terms the relationship of the traumatic injury to the rationale for various therapeutic interventions Prepare the patient for and, if appropriate, assist with diagnostic tests Provide opportunity for and encourage patient/family's questions, verbalization of fears and anxieties Provide for and encourage patient/family's participation in care Encourage patient/family with acknowledgement of daily and weekly gains/improvements Provide comfort measures Provide emotional support; administer care in an unhurried manner Assess reduction in level of patient/family's anxiety
■ Insufficient information for compliance with discharge regimen*	■ Before discharge patient/family verbalizes knowledge of discharge regimen, including activity progression	■ Assess patient/family's preliminary knowledge and understanding of discharge regimen Instruct patient/family as needed in activity progression; tailor information to injury and/or surgery patient has experienced Chest surgery with sternotomy and major abdominal surgery Avoid lifting heavy objects (over 5 pounds) for 6 weeks Avoid lifting objects over 15 pounds for 6 months Patient should consult physician before resuming more vigorous activities such as driving a car, lifting stuck windows, etc.

*If responsibility of critical care nurse includes this type of follow-up care.

Potential problems	Expected outcomes	Nursing activities
		Encourage patient that chest movements or use of abdominal muscles with such activities as coughing, housework, driving a car may cause some discomfort for several weeks
		In the first few weeks at home, a mild analgesic may be ordered for use as needed
		Fractures
		In conjunction with physician and physical therapist, instruct patient in extremity movement, muscle-strengthening exercises, weight bearing according to the nature of the fracture and extent of healing
	Patient/family verbalizes knowledge of dietary modifications	Instruct patient in necessary dietary modifications and practices such as
		Eat, chew, and swallow slowly
		For patients with diabetes after severe pancreatitis, see Standard: *Diabetic ketoacidosis*
		If renal failure/dysfunction is present, see Standard: *Acute renal failure*
		See other appropriate standards according to patient's problems and dietary modifications required
	Patient/family is able to perform specific therapeutic measures, such as dressing changes, use of splints, devices	Instruct patient/family in specific therapeutic measures, such as dressings, as appropriate and as ordered
		Provide opportunity for a return demonstration
		Provide for availability of dressings, splints, etc.
	Patient/family verbalizes knowledge of medications	Instruct patient in discharge medications, including
		Purpose and importance
		Identification
		Dosage/number of pills
		Frequency and timing
		Possible adverse effects
		Precautionary measures
		Avoidance of other medications without physician's consent
	Patient/family identifies untoward signs and symptoms requiring medical follow-up	Review untoward signs and symptoms that require medical follow-up; describe possible residual effects that may persist for 3 to 4 months after trauma
		See other appropriate standards according to the patient's priority problems
		Cardiac abnormalities
		Respiratory abnormalities
		Renal abnormalities
	Patient/family's behavior indicates acceptance of any body image change or limitations	Discuss with patient/family importance of successful emotional adjustment to any body image change or limitations in function
		Encourage verbalization of questions, fears, and anxiety regarding any body image change or limitations
		Provide referrals to agencies if appropriate
	Patient/family is able to describe plan for follow-up care	Describe the plan for follow-up care, including purpose for, when and where to go, who to see, and what specimens to bring
		Provide opportunity for and encourage patient/family's questions
		Assess patient's potential compliance with discharge regimen

51 □ Burns

The skin is the largest organ of the body, covering its entire surface. It has two distinct layers, called the *epidermis* and the *derma*. The epidermis, the outer thin avascular layer of stratified squamous epithelial cells, functions as a barrier against environmental hazards. The thicker derma consists of a closely interwoven layer of dense areolar connective tissue, blood vessels, and nerve endings; hair follicles; and sweat and sebaceous glands.

The skin functions as a barrier between the body's internal and external environment and plays an active role in the prevention of infection and trauma. It also protects the body from excessive fluid loss, yet permits elimination of excess water and other waste products. It helps to regulate body temperature, prevents the damaging effects of sunlight (ultraviolet light), secretes oil to soften and lubricate, produces vitamin D with exposure to ultraviolet light, and is an important sense organ with receptor endings for pain, temperature, and touch.

Injury to the skin as in burns will either decrease or eliminate these functions, depending on the amount of skin lost (according to the ''rule of nine'' [Fig. 1] and the depth of damage [Table 8]).

The three most common etiologies of burns are flame (thermal), electrical, and chemical.

Burns cause cellular necrosis, capillary damage, capillary thrombosis, and alteration of collagen and other protein substances of the cells.

The pathophysiology and management of burns can be classified into three periods: (1) emergent period: (2) acute period; and (3) rehabilitation period.

The emergent period includes fluid losses and may involve respiratory distress, which is treated by fluid replacement (Table 9) and respiratory support.*

The acute period includes the formation of eschar (dead skin and proteinaceous exudate) with underlying bacterial growth. To prevent major infections and secondary sepsis, the eschar is therapeutically removed and the burn wound debrided. Treatment of complications and meticulous care of the wound, including grafting, hasten recovery.*

The rehabilitative period actually begins when the patient is admitted and includes prevention of contractures and hypertrophic scarring. Physical therapy helps to prevent contractures and maintain/achieve maximal function of affected body parts.

The patient should be encouraged to assume gradual activities of daily living in preparation for discharge and cosmetic reconstruction. Constant support and encouragement are greatly needed by the patient. Ongoing psychological support and encouragement are needed from the day of admission to assist the patient in coping with the tremendous physiological trauma associated with a burn injury.

ASSESSMENT

1. History that includes
   a. Exact cause of burn
   b. Presence of coincident trauma
      (1) A fall
      (2) Assault
   c. Presence of specific symptoms
      (1) Focal neurological signs
      (2) Headache
      (3) Neck and back pain
      (4) Shortness of breath
      (5) Pain and numbness in the extremities
      (6) Chest and abdominal pain
   d. Presence of underlying conditions including diabetes mellitus, chronic obstructive lung disease, psychological/psychiatric problems, renal and cardiac diseases, alcoholism and drug addiction
2. Physical examination that includes signs and symptoms of
   a. Airway obstruction
   b. Respiratory distress
   c. Adequacy of patient's respirations
   d. Rales, stridor, rhonchi, and wheezes
   e. Adequacy of peripheral circulation
   f. Areas of tenderness on neck, head, and chest
   g. Inhalation injury: bloody or sooty sputum; circumoral or pharyngeal burns; singed nasal hairs, eyebrows, or eyelashes; conjunctivitis and rhinorrhea
   h. Pericardial rub, murmurs, ectopic beats (irregular pulse), tamponade
   i. Abdominal tenderness, rigidity, and/or distention; signs of enlarged spleen or liver
   j. Edema of the extremities; peripheral edema

---

*Feller, I., and Jones, C.: Nursing the burned patient, Ann Arbor, Mich., 1973, Braun-Brumfield, Inc.

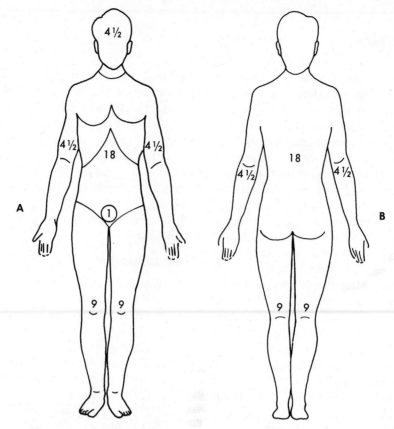

Fig. 1. Estimation of size of burn (percentage of body surface involved) by rule of nine. **A,** Anterior; **B,** posterior. Nines are assigned to specific areas (anterior and posterior) and may be summed as follows:

Head	9
Right upper extremity	9
Left upper extremity	9
Torso	36
Perineum	1
Right lower extremity	18
Left lower extremity	18
TOTAL	100

It is advisable to color code depth of burns for estimating size to give a better picture of the injury to the patient.

    k. Altered mental status
    l. Decreased motor strength, reflexes
3. Burn examination that includes
    a. Age of patient
    b. Time and date of burn
    c. Site, extent, and depth of damage (Fig. 1 and Table 8)
    d. Etiology

    (1) Thermal
      (a) Type (radiant, flame, or heat)
      (b) Duration of exposure
      (c) Closed or open exposure
      (d) Significant exposure to smoke
      (e) Type of burning material (wood, plastic, etc.)
      (f) Presence of explosion

Table 8. Depth of burns

Burn depth	Skin involvement	Sensation	Appearance	Course
First degree	Epidermis	Normal pain Tingling	Erythema Slight edema Blanching on compression	Regeneration within 1 week Peeling
Second degree	Varying depth of epidermis (partial thickness)	Increased sensitivity to pain and temperature; may not be sensitive to contact	Dry or blistered Erythema Edema Moist wound Cherry red or dull white	May spontaneously generate within 2 weeks if infection is prevented Depigmentation and scarring
Third degree	All skin layers (full thickness)	Anesthesia Painless	Wet or dry leathery surface Cherry red to white or black Wet or dry	No chance of regeneration; requires grafting Scarring Decreased function Alteration of appearance

Table 9. Fluid replacement formulas

Baxter formula

First 24 hours — Ringer's lactate 4 ml/kg body weight/percentage of body surface burn + 2000 ml D5W

NOTE: One half of the calculated requirement of the first 24 hours postburn should be administered within 8 hours after injury; the remainder should be administered in the next 16 hours

Second 24 hours

- 40% to 50% burn — 2000 ml D5W + 500 ml colloids
- 50% to 70% burn — 2000 ml D5W + 800 ml colloids
- Greater than 70% burn — 2000 ml D5W + 1200 ml colloids

Brooke Army formula

First 24 hours — Ringer's lactate 1.5 ml/kg body weight/percentage of body surface burn + Colloids 0.5 ml/kg body weight/percentage of body surface burn

Colloids include blood, dextran, or plasma

NOTE: Calculate replacement from time of injury

Give one half of calculated fluid during first 8 hours, one third in second 8 hours, and one fourth in third 8 hours

Second 24 hours — 2000 ml D5W + Colloids

NOTE: Give one half the amount in first 24 hours

(2) Electrical
   (a) Estimation of voltage involved
   (b) Duration of exposure
   (c) If patient was grounded
(3) Chemical
   (a) Name of chemical agent
   (b) Duration of exposure
   (c) Presence of noxious fumes

e. Coincidental injuries: trauma or fracture of the head, neck, chest, abdomen, or extremities
f. Any medications administered
   (1) Tetanus toxoid
   (2) Tetanus immune globulin (Hyper-tet)
   (3) Pain medication and time given
g. Initial wound care if given

4. Lab and diagnostic data, including
   a. Complete blood count for decreased Hct and RBC and leukocytosis
   b. Electrolyte levels for hyponatremia, decreased serum calcium; and elevated alkaline phosphatase
   c. Albuminuria, hemoglobinuria
   d. Head, chest, and abdominal radiograph results for fracture, etc.
   e. ECG for arrhythmias
   f. Results of spinal fluid indicating presence of blood/red blood cells
5. Patient/family's level of anxiety about disease process, diagnostic procedures, and therapy planned
6. Patient/family's understanding of purpose of debridement and surgery, expected prognosis, and psychological reactions
7. Patient's level of anxiety regarding pain, disfigurement, finances, effect on personal life and vocation

GOALS

1. Reduction in patient/family's level of anxiety with provision of information and explanations
2. Respiratory sufficiency
   a. Pa_{O_2} and Pa_{CO_2} within patient's normal limits
   b. Absence of rales, wheezes, and stridor
3. Normovolemia
4. Electrolyte and complete blood count levels within normal limits
5. Hemodynamic stability: absence of arrhythmias; BP, P, and urine output within normal limits
6. Infection free; absence of wound infection
7. Adequate intake of nutrients and vitamins to meet calculated daily requirements; weight stabilization or weight gain; positive nitrogen balance with adequate wound healing
8. Absence or resolution of complications including renal failure, anemia, malnutrition, pulmonary edema or emboli
9. Resolution of burn wound with granulation or skin grafting
10. Restoration to optimal physical, emotional, and psychological functioning
11. Absence of or minimal disability and disfigurement
12. Acceptance of alteration of body image
13. Before discharge patient/family is able to
    a. State ways to prevent burns
    b. Describe specific wound care, with return demonstration as appropriate
    c. Describe the rehabilitation program given by the health care team and demonstrate activities (e.g., exercises) accurately
    d. Describe dietary and medication regimen
    e. Ask questions regarding self-care
    f. State necessary information regarding follow-up visits to physician and/or clinic

Potential problems	Expected outcomes	Nursing activities

■ Patient/family's anxiety related to limited understanding of disease process, diagnostic tests, surgical procedures, and expected outcome	■ Patient/family demonstrates decreased level of anxiety with provision of information and explanations	■ Ongoing assessment of level of anxiety and understanding
		Describe the pathophysiology of the burn process, the signs and symptoms the patient is experiencing, and therapy employed
		Explain the rationale for various diagnostic and therapeutic procedures as they relate to present condition
		Provide time for and encourage questions and verbalization, and discussion of feelings and fears
		Explain diagnostic and therapeutic procedures to patient/family; assist as necessary
		Solicit patient's cooperation and participation in care
		Explain precautionary techniques to prevent infection, including
		  Wear sterile gown, mask, and gloves according to patient's condition
		  Discourage visits by visitors with upper respiratory or skin infections
		Encourage family to participate in care of patient
		Keep patient/family informed of patient's progress
		Provide psychiatric consult to assist patient/family in coping with feelings and situation, if needed

Potential problems	**Expected outcomes**	**Nursing activities**

■ Patient/family's anxiety related to alteration in body image with associated
Disfigurement
Interruption in lifestyle
Unavoidable dependency
Grief and hostility
Pain

■ Resolution and/or adaptation to present body image
Verbalization of fears, grief, and acceptance of body image

■ Assess patient's
  Family interaction
  Religious, ethnic, and cultural background
  Perception of illness
  Values, ideals, and aspirations in life
  Past experiences with stress, illness, and coping mechanisms
  Level of comprehension
Address patient by name and explain all procedures; elicit his/her cooperation and assistance
Allow family visits at frequent intervals
Relate awareness of patient's feelings and encourage verbalization and discussion of fears and anxieties
Provide care in a gentle unhurried manner
Allow use of telephone, outgoing cards, letters, etc.
Approach and administer care in a consistent positive manner with an attitude and desire to help
Set short-term realistic goals with the patient
Express warmth and sincerity in praising patient for accomplishment of goals
Show respect for patient's integrity and self-worth
Support and encourage patient with self-care; readjust environment so that patient is able to reach things
Provide psychiatric consult if needed, as ordered
Provide for physical comfort and emotional support
Administer sedatives and analgesics as ordered and particularly before treatments
  Elevate burned extremities
  Provide diversional activities
Encourage patient to talk about plans for future
Refer patient to appropriate resources for aid in finances, education, and family problems as needed

■ Acute respiratory failure, which may result from
Airway obstruction
Pulmonary edema
Respiratory acidosis
Atelectasis
Pulmonary emboli
Pneumonia
Eschar formation on chest and neck that restricts respiration

■ Patent airway with adequate ventilation and oxygenation
Arterial blood gas results within patient's normal limits
Resolution of respiratory failure
Absence of signs and symptoms of hypoxia

■ Determine history of smoke, fumes, or flame inhalation, including
  Injury occurring in a confined space
  Moist respiration
  Respiratory distress: tachypnea, dyspnea, rales, wheezing, stridorous and harsh breath sounds
  Bloody or black-tinged sputum
  Frank burns of tongue
  Red pharynx
  Cherry red lips
  Hoarseness or voice change
  Burns of head, face, and neck
  Pallor, cyanosis of skin and mucous membrane
  Arterial blood gas results indicating acidosis, hypoxemia
  Diminished breath sounds
For severe burns of the neck and chest that result in eschar formation, prepare for escharotomy
  Prepare scalpel and suture material
  Assist in procedure
Administer antibiotics and steroid therapy if ordered
Notify physician of any abnormality and prepare·for therapy
If problem occurs, see Standard: *Acute respiratory failure*
If intubation and mechanical ventilation are necessary, see Standard: *Mechanical ventilation*

Potential problems	Expected outcomes	Nursing activities
■ Hypovolemia related to Fluid loss from burned areas Hemorrhage from burned area and/or stress ulcers	■ Normovolemia Weight and circulating blood volume within patient's normal limits Hemodynamic stability	■ Monitor for signs and symptoms of hypovolemia, including Hypotension, orthostatic hypotension Tachycardia Decreased CVP and PAP if available Decreased urine output Increased Hct Poor skin turgor Dry mucous membranes Extreme thirst Gross bleeding or fluid loss from wound, NG tube, or other drainage tube Signs of internal bleeding Restlessness and disorientation Notify physician of abnormalities Prepare and administer fluid, including Crystalloid solutions and electrolytes Blood and blood products Use standard Baxter or Brooke Army formula as basis for administering fluid resuscitation as ordered (see Table 9, p. 443) Titrate fluid replacement with hourly urine output and other hemodynamic parameters as ordered Start oral fluids in frequent small amounts as ordered with gradual increase as tolerated Monitor for signs of hypervolemia associated with vigorous fluid administration Increase in BP, tachycardia Increased CVP and PAP Increased urine output Marked weight gain Dyspnea, wheezes, moist rales Chest radiograph results revealing pulmonary congestion Distended neck veins Disorientation Nausea Notify physician of any of these abnormalities Monitor for signs and symptoms of inadequate fluid replacement and continued hypovolemia Monitor for signs and symptoms of renal failure; if renal failure occurs, see Standard: *Acute renal failure*
■ Sepsis secondary to wound infection	■ Absence or resolution of infection Absence of clinical manifestation of infection	■ Use mask, sterile gown, and gloves when caring for the patient Employ strict sterile technique when caring for the wound Administer agents to support immune mechanism including tetanus toxoid, tetanus immune globulin (Hyper-tet), gamma globulin, convalescent plasma, pseudomonas vaccine, and hyperimmune serum if ordered Encourage personnel or visitors with upper respiratory, GI, or skin infections to avoid visiting while infected Employ disinfectant and sterilization technique on equipment or materials used for patient's care Immerse patient in H_2O or rinse with saline solution/H_2O as ordered Assist with debridement if ordered Shave all burned areas, axilla, and perineum Cut scalp hair when patient's burns are severe but scalp is not burned; for burns of neck and above, shave head as appropriate

Potential problems	Expected outcomes	Nursing activities
		Administer prescribed dietary regimen to support defenses against infection and promote wound healing
		Monitor for signs and symptoms of infection, including
		Swollen lymph glands q6 hr
		Leukocytosis; complete blood count daily
		Complaint of headache, chills, malaise
		Anorexia
		Increased respiratory, pulse rate
		Decreased BP, CVP
		Decreased urinary output; accurate intake and output q1 hr
		Sudden rise in temperature
		Cyanosis and/or facial flushing
		Petechiae on skin
		Ileus and decrease in bowel sounds
		Positive culture results from wound, sputum, blood, stool, and/or urine
		Notify physician of any abnormality
		Administer therapy as ordered
■ Malnutrition related to Inadequate intake of nutrients Increased metabolic requirements associated with burn injury	■ Absence and/or resolution of malnutrition Positive nitrogen balance Consumes most of recommended diet/feeding Weight gain if appropriate Wound healing well	■ Assess cultural and social dietary habits, food idiosyncrasies, nutritional status, and food allergies and set nutritional requirement accordingly (usually high in protein with 20 g of nitrogen/square meter of body surface/day and high in calories) in collaboration with the dietitian and physician
		Start with full fluid diet in small frequent feedings and gradually progress to desired diet
		Administer antacid and milk between meals as ordered
		Administer supplementary vitamin therapy as ordered
		Ensure required caloric and fluid intake
		List foods taken daily
		Accurate intake and output
		Daily weights
		Have dietitian plan meals and substitutes with patient
		Allow home-cooked foods within set limits
		Provide supplementary nourishment with snacks
		Provide conditions conducive to eating
		Frequent oral hygiene
		Provide for cleaning dentures as needed
		Assist with eating or feed patient if needed
		Position for comfort, ease in reaching food
		If tube feeding is needed
		Ensure patency and proper location of tube
		Place patient in semi-Fowler's position
		Aspirate feeding tube before each feeding or periodically during continuous infusion
		Notify physician for abnormally large aspirate and heme positive test
		Check feedings for any change of consistency or odor
		Warm feedings before administering
		Start with small amount of feeding, given as continuous drip or intermittent drip/bolus method
		Monitor for adverse effects: abdominal cramping, diarrhea, nausea, vomiting, gastric distention
		Notify physician if occurs; alter feeding program as ordered
		Slowly increase amount of feeding as ordered
		Check for bowel sounds q4-8 hr
		If hyperalimentation is required, see Standard: *Total parenteral nutrition through central venous catheter*

Potential problems	Expected outcomes	Nursing activities

		Ongoing assessment of nutritional status and therapy
		  Weight loss and gain
		  General appearance; note presence of
		    Dry, flaky, and cracked skin
		    Tongue dry and discolored
		    Sunken eyeballs
		    Loss of appetite
		    Lethargy
		    Poor skin turgor, flaccidity
		    Poor wound healing
		    Decreased muscle control, tremors, and twitching

▪ Contractures/deformities	▪ Absence and/or resolution of contractures/deformities
	Adherence to rehabilitation activities
	Restoration of optimal physical function
		▪ Assess for areas liable to develop contractures and deformities
		Collaborate with physician and therapist regarding activities to prevent contractures and deformities
		  Explain to patient all activities and reasons for them
		  Application of splints, traction or functional devices to fingers, limbs; check for improperly applied devices
		  Maintain burned area in position of physiological function
		  Passive and active range-of-motion exercises q2-4 hr
		  If necessary place patient in Stryker or electrocircular bed
		  While patient is in bed, prevent contractures of burn areas as follows
		    Head and anterior aspect of neck—no pillows; a small foam pad may be placed under head
		    Posterior aspect of neck—pillow under upper chest
		    Upper chest, axilla, and arms—arms abducted at 90 degrees and slightly above shoulder level
		    Ankles and feet—feet at 90 degrees; dorsiflexion at ankles using footboard
		  Encourage patient to assist in care, i.e., feeding
		  Ambulate as ordered
		  Gradually increase patient's self-care, graded activities, and social activities as condition permits
		  Use bed cradle to keep sheets off burned areas
		  Maintain heat and humidity in room at comfort level
		Monitor for any increase of alkaline phosphatase and decrease in serum Ca^{2+} levels, which may be associated with Ca^{2+} deposition near joints and tendons
		Prepare patient for corrective/reconstructive surgery as ordered
		Ensure intake of prescribed dietary regimen
		Observe measures to prevent infection

▪ Insufficient knowledge for compliance with discharge regimen*	▪ Sufficient information to comply with discharge regimen
	Patient/family's behavior indicates successful emotional adjustment to situation
	Patient/family correctly performs procedures, use of special equipment devices, exercises, splinting, and activities of daily living
		▪ Assess patient/family's level of understanding, ability to comprehend, and any physical limitations regarding follow-up plan of care or discharge regimen
		Discuss success in rehabilitation program, including the patient's emotional adjustment, with patient/family and the health team
		Encourage verbalization of doubts, fears, and questions
		Explain thoroughly burn care with return demonstration
		  Normal bathing
		  Application of lubricating cream to burn site and grafts (e.g., lanolin base cream)
		  Application of any antibiotics and/or dressings as ordered
		Procure supplies, equipment, and splint for patient's use after discharge

*If responsibility of critical care nurse includes such follow-up care.

Potential problems	Expected outcomes	Nursing activities
	Patient/family identifies signs and symptoms of wound infection and when to notify the physician	Demonstrate with return demonstration ROM exercises, application and use of equipment and devices
		Describe signs and symptoms of wound infection, including
		Redness
		Swelling
		Tenderness, pain, and warmth to touch
		Any sudden bleeding or secretions
	Patient/family describes dietary, medication, and activity regimens	Explain and discuss
		Need for gradual resumption of activities
		Importance of well-balanced diet, particularly a high calorie and high protein diet if wound is not completely healed; stress importance of maintaining prescribed weight
	Patient/family describes plan for follow-up care	Need for medications prescribed and then identification, route, dosage, action, side effects
		Explain importance of ongoing and follow-up care, including
		Keeping appointment for physical therapy if applicable
		Purpose for, when and where to go, who to see, and what specimens to bring
		Provide opportunity for and encourage questions and verbalization of anxiety regarding discharge regimen and any residual disability
		Stress importance of safety measures in preventing burns
		Assess patient/family's potential compliance with discharge regimen

52 □ Disseminated intravascular coagulation

Disseminated intravascular coagulation (DIC) syndrome, also known as the *defibrination syndrome, consumption coagulopathy, intravascular coagulation syndrome,* and *diffuse intravascular clotting,* is one of the most serious of the acquired coagulation disorders, difficult to diagnose and treat. DIC syndrome involves an abnormal activation of the hemostatic mechanism leading to a generalized consumption of platelets and a widespread deposition of platelets and fibrin in the microvasculature. This precipitates the formation of thrombi and emboli producing tissue necrosis, ischemia, depletion of clotting factors, degradation of fibrin products, and generalized hemolysis resulting in a severe hemorrhagic diathesis.

Generally accepted clinical criteria for the diagnosis of DIC include depletion of coagulation Factors V and VIII and fibrinogen (less than 100 mg/100 ml); thrombocytopenia (less than 100,000/mm³); production of excessive amounts of circulating fibrin-split products; and increased fibrinolytic activity of the blood.

In acute DIC hemorrhagic manifestations generally predominate as seen in venipuncture, surgical wounds, cutaneous petechiae, and gastrointestinal bleeding. Other signs and symptoms may include severe abdominal, back, and muscle pain; nausea and vomiting; dyspnea and acrocyanosis (generalized diaphoresis with mottled cold fingers and toes); convulsion, coma, and shock.

DIC has been associated with conditions including overwhelming viral or bacterial sepsis and shock, especially gram-negative septicemia and acute severe hemolysis; abruptio placentae; carcinoma, particularly if metastases are present; components of coagulation disorders of liver failure; and a variety of other circumstances in which thromboplastic materials may enter the circulation or where diffuse endothelial damage is present.

The objective of treatment for patients with DIC is to terminate the accelerated coagulation process for which heparin is the agent of choice. However, the ultimate cure depends on accurate diagnosis and proper treatment of the underlying factor(s) precipitating the activation of the accelerated coagulation process.

Although heparin is the usual agent of choice, it has to be administered early in the course of treatment to be most effective.

Replacement therapy (use of blood, platelets, and fresh frozen plasma) may be required for severe depletion of platelets and coagulation factors. Any replacement therapy should follow initiation of heparin; otherwise the blood and blood products will also be rapidly consumed in the accelerated coagulation process.

The overall therapy for DIC can be very complex and is associated with considerable risk.

ASSESSMENT

1. History, presence, and nature of
   a. Sudden onset of hemorrhage associated with profound circulatory collapse
   b. Underlying conditions precipitating DIC, that is, infections, carcinomas, leukemias, immune complex diseases, obstetrical conditions, etc.
   c. Thromboembolic diathesis as manifested by angina, confusion, convulsions, coma, fever, and azotemia
   d. Coagulation disorders, that is, vitamin K deficiency and deficiency of Factors VIII and IX
   e. Intake of medications that alter the coagulation mechanism, such as, aspirin, coumadin
   f. Hepatic abnormalities with or without hepatomegaly
   g. Hemarthrosis, that is, blood in joint space
   h. Diffuse bleeding from body orifices, venipuncture and incisional sites, respiratory, renal, or upper gastrointestinal tracts
   i. Ecchymosis, hematomas, hematuria, and menorrhagia
   j. Arterial hypotension often associated with shock
2. Lab and diagnostic data, including
   a. Platelet counts indicate thrombocytopenia
   b. Clotting factors depleted in plasma, that is, reduced fibrinogen with increased fibrinogen degradation products and decreased Factors V and VIII
   c. Other coagulation tests: results of PT and APTT tests may be prolonged or normal
   d. Presence of fragmented red cells in peripheral blood
   e. Arterial blood gas results indicating acidosis
   f. ECG for any arrhythmias
   g. Chest radiograph for presence of reactive interstitial edema associated with diffuse deposition of microemboli in the lungs
   h. Results of throat, blood, sputum, urine, and stool cultures
3. Patient/family's knowledge and understanding of disease process, diagnostic procedures, and therapy planned
4. Patient/family's level of anxiety related to disease process, therapy employed, and anticipated prognosis

GOALS

1. Reduction of patient/family's anxiety with provision of information and explanations
2. Hemodynamic stability—adequate perfusion of central and peripheral organ systems
3. Respiratory function sufficient to maintain adequate oxygenation and ventilation; absence of respiratory distress syndrome
4. Rapid resolution or control of impaired coagulation
5. Resolution of the underlying conditions associated with DIC
6. Prevention of complications associated with generalized bleeding diathesis and thrombosis
7. Adequate intake of nutrients, vitamins to meet calculated daily requirements, to maintain weight or to achieve weight gain
8. Sufficient information for compliance with discharge regimen; patient/family is able to
   a. Accurately describe activity, dietary, and medication regimen
   b. Identify signs and symptoms requiring medical attention
   c. Describe plan for follow-up care

Potential problems	Expected outcomes	Nursing activities
■ Patient/family's anxiety related to Insufficient knowledge of disease process, diagnostic procedures, and therapy employed	■ Patient/family's behavior demonstrates decreased level of anxiety with provision of information and explanations Patient/family vebalizes understanding of disease process and its relation to diagnostic procedures and therapy employed Patient/family verbalizes questions, fears, and any anxieties related to the aforementioned Patient/family participates actively in planning and implementing care	■ Ongoing assessment of level of patient/family's anxiety Assess patient/family's knowledge and understanding of disease process, anticipated diagnostic procedures, and therapy employed Describe the nature of the disease syndrome, reasons for the signs and symptoms the patient is experiencing, and the rationale for various diagnostic and therapeutic interventions to be employed Explain and assist in preparing patient for anticipated diagnostic procedures Encourage patient/family's questions, verbalization of fears and anxieties Involve patient/family in planning and assessing care Provide reassurance Evaluate for decrease in level of anxiety with provision of information and explanations Provide appropriate consultation for patient/family with clergy and social service
Pain	Relief of pain Reduction in nonverbal evidence of pain	Assess behavioral response to pain, intensity, location, and associated LOC Offer and/or administer pain medications as ordered Position for utmost comfort with proper body alignment Encourage patient to verbalize fears and anxieties related to pain and the course of disease process Apply warm and cold compresses on joints as ordered; if needed, use bed cradle and immobilized affected joint Plan nursing activities to allow uninterrupted rest periods Support patient/family Evaluate for reduction of pain
■ Impaired coagulation as evidenced by Thrombosis formation with consumption of platelets and coagulation factors Hemorrhage Hypotension Acidosis	■ Early resolution of impaired coagulation Hemodynamic stability Normotensive Arterial blood gas levels within normal limits	■ Prevent by administering immediate therapy for presence of etiological factors, including sepsis, cancer, leukemias, immunological abnormalities, obstetrical complications Monitor for Any bleeding including occult, internal, hemorrhaging from orifices, mild oozing from injection sites; petechiae and ecchymosis Hematest results on all urine, stool, and emesis Signs and symptoms that may indicate DIC without bleeding include fatigue, malaise, weakness, myalgia, peripheral thrombosis, sudden vision changes, hypotension, acrocyanosis (generalized sweating with mottled, cold toes and fingers), nausea and vomiting, severe muscle, back, abdominal, bone, and joint pain; dyspnea and cyanosis, oliguria; convulsions, coma, and shock Lab test results for prolonged APTT and PT; thrombocytopenia; low fibrinogen levels; elevated fibrin-split products, strongly positive protamine sulfate test; reduced factor assay levels particularly II, V, and VII; complete blood count for decreased Hct, Hgb, and leukocytosis; electrolytes for hyperkalemia; and arterial blood gas levels for decreased bicarbonate levels and acidosis Hypotension and hyperthermia/hypothermia, vital signs including temperature q2 hr and prn

Potential problems	Expected outcomes	Nursing activities
		Changes in mental status, i.e., headaches, vertigo, irritability, and confusion
		Chest radiograph results for infiltrate or pleurisy
		Notify physician of any abnormalities
		If problem occurs
		Administer blood products as ordered; observe necessary precautions, which include
		Monitoring vital signs and temperature before, during, and after transfusion, and monitoring for any untoward reaction, i.e., skin reactions
		Double-checking patient's name and product on label before administration
		Using an ultrafilter in transfusing blood and packed cells
		Administer heparin if ordered and monitor lab results, i.e., APTT accordingly
		Estimate blood loss
		Daily weights
		Serial Hgb and Hct results q12-24 hr and prn
		Measure intake and all drainage, i.e., NG drainage, melena
		Administer adequate nutritional intake, as ordered, in small frequent feedings
		Prevent further bleeding
		Mouth care
		Use soft toothbrush or cotton swabs with mild mouthwash
		May use carbonated drinks to break crust in mouth without bleeding
		Apply liquid lubricant on lips
		Medications
		Given preferably by oral, rectal, and IV routes
		Use smallest gauge needle, rotate sites, and apply steady pressure for 3 to 5 minutes whenever injections are given
		Use electric shaver to reduce any incidence of abrasions
		Administer stool softeners as ordered, if needed
		Handle patient gently at all times to protect skin and prevent mucosal trauma
		Elevate head if patient is dyspneic, and administer O_2 if ordered
		Apply cold and/or hot compresses as appropriate for joint and bone pain; use bed cradle and immobilize affected area
		Refer to monitoring activities to detect further signs and symptoms of bleeding
		Notify physician of any abnormalities
■ Insufficient knowledge to comply with discharge regimen*	■ Patient/family has sufficient information to comply with discharge regimen	■ Assess patient/family's level of understanding and ability to comprehend follow-up plan of care and the discharge regimen
		Explain relationship of disease process to prescribed therapy
	Patient/family accurately describes medication, dietary, and activity regimens	Provide required information so that before discharge patient/family is able to
		Describe medication regimen
		Names of drugs and purpose
		Specific dosage schedule
	Patient/family identifies signs and symptoms requiring medical attention	Expected adverse side effects, how to deal with them, and when to notify the physician
		Describe activity regimen
		Describe dietary regimen, i.e., therapeutic diet if ordered

*If responsibility of critical care nurse includes such follow-up care.

Potential problems	Expected outcomes	Nursing activities
	Patient/family accurately describes plans for follow-up care	If recurrence of underlying condition is possible, describe signs and symptoms Describe follow-up visits including purpose for, when and where to go, who to see, and what specimens to bring Provide opportunity for and encourage patient/family's questions and verbalization Assess patient/family's potential compliance with discharge regimen

53 □ Poisoning

Poisoning is one of the most common pediatric medical emergencies among young children. Boys are more frequently involved than girls, and the physically active, mobile, and curious child under 5 years of age is most vulnerable. The younger child has a tendency to ingest common household items, the older child, medicines. Almost one half of all poisonings occur in the kitchen, and one fifth occur in the bathroom. The most frequent causes of poisoning in the under-5 age-group are aspirin, soaps, detergents, cleansers, bleaches, vitamins, minerals, insecticides, plants, polishes and waxes, hormones, tranquilizers and other analgesics, and antipyretics.

The diagnosis of poisoning is made by history, presenting signs and symptoms, and lab data. The signs and symptoms of poisoning are also common to many conditions of childhood, making diagnosis, without a positive history, difficult. The possibility of poisoning should always be considered in children who present with signs and symptoms of questionable etiology.

Signs and symptoms of poisoning by ingestion, inhalation, or skin absorption may include gastrointestinal disturbances with anorexia, vomiting, diarrhea, and abdominal pain. Symptoms of CNS involvement may occur and are usually one of either depression or stimulation. Depression of the CNS can result in lethargy, stupor, and coma. On the other hand, stimulation can result in convulsions, restlessness, and confusion. Further symptoms of poisoning may include shock, cardiac arrhythmias, and cardiac failure. There may be notable gray cyanosis that develops as a result of the conversion of hemoglobin to methemoglobin when specific drugs and chemical poisons are present. The patient may become oxygen depleted and have respiratory symptomatology. Other symptoms may develop as a result of the poisoning.

The lab tests used for diagnosis are those specific for identification of the toxic substance. Specimens from the stomach, blood, and urine are analyzed.

The general method of treatment of acute poisoning is identification and removal of the substance, prevention of further absorption, administration of an antidote, and supportive therapy of the various organ systems related to symptomatology.

In the emergency room, treatment is directed toward identification and removal of the poison. If the substance is not caustic or is not a hydrocarbon, removal by emesis or lavage will be instituted. Vomiting is never induced if the child is comatose or having seizures. The goal here is to remove the substance prior to absorption. To facilitate the removal of the poison, fluid diuresis and, in a few specific instances, dialysis may be used.

Additional measures to prevent further absorption of the substance are often necessary because all gastric contents are not removed by these techniques.

Antidotes may be administered to inactivate the ingested substance. Activated charcoal is a common local antidote. There are some specific antidotes for particular substances ingested; however, these are relatively few. If the ingested substance is caustic, attempts will be made to neutralize it and to prevent its absorption.

Once emergency treatment has been rendered, general supportive therapy becomes the priority. This type of therapy is greatly dependent on the substance involved and its actions on body systems.

The CNS may be affected and control of seizures and treatment of agitation or depression may be required.

Respiratory support for adequate respiratory exchange may be necessary. Treatment of shock with fluids and replacement of electrolyte losses as well as prevention of renal failure may also be part of supportive therapy. Other vital functions may be seriously affected. It is for these reasons that children in an acute poisoning episode are at risk and have need for critical care.

ASSESSMENT

1. Careful history surrounding poisoning incident
   a. Identification of ingested substance
   b. Estimation of how much was ingested
   c. When ingestion occurred
2. Physical signs and symptoms
   a. Neurological
      (1) Agitation
      (2) Depression
      (3) Convulsions
      (4) Delirium
      (5) Headache
      (6) Mental changes
      (7) Disturbances of equilibrium
      (8) Pupil response
      (9) Visual disturbance
   b. Cardiac
      (1) Alteration in heart rate
      (2) Arrhythmia
      (3) Hypotension
   c. Renal
      (1) Anuria
      (2) Hematuria
      (3) Oliguria
      (4) Color of urine
   d. Respiratory
      (1) Hyperventilation
      (2) Respiratory depression
      (3) Coughs
      (4) Wheezes
      (5) Rales
      (6) Abnormal odor on breath
      (7) Alteration in salivation
   e. Gastrointestinal
      (1) Nausea
      (2) Vomiting
      (3) Diarrhea
      (4) Abnormal color of vomitus and stool
   f. Temperature
      (1) Hypothermia
      (2) Hyperthermia
   g. Skin
      (1) Burns
      (2) Interruption of skin integrity
      (3) Edema
      (4) Cyanosis
      (5) Skin staining or discoloration
      (6) Hair loss
      (7) Absence or presence of perspiration
      (8) Abnormal color of tissues
3. Monitor lab data for results of
   a. Complete blood count
   b. Serum electrolytes
   c. Blood glucose
   d. Blood levels of specific ingested substance
   e. Blood gas levels
   f. BUN
   g. Creatinine
   h. Urinalysis
   i. Urine chemistry
4. Developmental level of the child
   a. Effect of incident on child (guilt, punishment)
   b. Effect of hospitalization on child
   c. Developmental tasks according to age
5. Response of parents to child's illness and hospitalization
   a. Level of anxiety
   b. Guilt
   c. Degree of understanding of incident and therapeutic management

GOALS

1. Restoration of normal CNS functioning
2. Normal cardiac function and circulatory perfusion
3. Normal renal function
4. Normal respiratory function
5. Normal fluid and electrolyte function
6. Resolution of gastrointestinal irritation
7. Restoration of normal body temperature–regulating system
8. Absence of infection
9. Supportive therapy for child and family during crisis period
10. Effective parental coping mechanisms
11. Hospitalization as positive developmental experience
12. Discharge planning related to prevention

Potential problems	**Expected outcomes**	**Nursing activities**

■ Alteration of CNS related to toxic action of poison involved	■ Detection of alteration
	Supportive therapy
	Return to optimum level of functioning
		■ Prevent by
		    Administration of specific antidote for ingested substance
		    Early detection of further CNS changes
		Monitor for
		    Stimulation
		        Confusion
		        Restlessness
		        Delirium
		        Convulsions
		    Depression
		        Lethargy
		        Stupor
		        Coma
		NOTE: CNS depression is an ominous complication of poisoning
		Intervention if problem occurs
		    Stimulation
		        Cautious administration of sedatives
		    Convulsions
		        Protect patient from injury
		        Observe seizure
		            1. Activity and progression
		            2. Muscular involvement
		            3. Body parts involved
		            4. Tongue deviation
		            5. Duration of seizure
		        Determine LOC prior to, during, and after seizure
		        Administer anticonvulsants as ordered by physician
		        Maintain adequate ventilation and airway
		            1. Insert airway if possible (only when jaw is relaxed)
		            2. Side-lying position
		            3. Suction
		            4. O_2
		        See Standard: *Seizures*
		    Depression
		        Stimulation of CNS
		        Serial observation of the following
		            1. Vital signs
		            2. State of consciousness
		            3. Orientation
		            4. Pupil size and reaction to light
		            5. Muscle strength of extremities
		            6. Reflexes
		            7. Response to pain

■ Peripheral circulatory collapse related to toxic action of poison	■ Restore and maintain adequate circulatory blood volume and tissue perfusion	■ Prevent by
		    Continuous monitoring of indices of circulatory perfusion
		Monitor for
		    Change in skin temperature
		    Pallor
		    Declining BP
		    Rapid shallow respirations
		    Rapid thready pulse
		    Thirst
		    Restlessness, nervousness, apprehension
		    Change in LOC
		    Change in temperature
		    Declining CVP
		    GI disturbances

Potential problems	Expected outcomes	Nursing activities
		Intervention if problem occurs
		Serial monitoring of vital signs
		Serial measurement of CVP
		Volume expansion through IV administration as indicated and
		as ordered
		Intake and output q1 hr
		Administration of medication as ordered
		Body positioning
		Blood gas analysis
		Administration of O_2
		Respiratory support
		Cardiac monitoring
■ Renal damage related to toxic action of poison involved or renal ischemia produced by shock	■ Indices of renal function within normal limits	■ Prevent by
		Continuous monitoring of parameters of circulatory perfusion
		and renal function
		Monitor for
		Change in lab data
		BUN
		Creatinine
		Urinalysis
		Specific gravity
		Urine electrolytes
		Serum electrolytes
		ECG
		Change in urine output
		Decreased volume
		Presence of edema
		Change in mentation
		Drowsiness
		Disorientation
		Change in cardiac rhythm
		Arrhythmia related to electrolyte imbalance
		Change in weight
		Change in BP
		Intervention if problem occurs
		Management of shock as ordered
		Management of metabolic acidosis as ordered
		IV fluid and electrolyte replacement
		IV fluid and electrolyte maintenance
		Accurate measurement and recording of intake and output
		Administration of medications as ordered
		Mannitol
		Furosemide
		Dialysis
		Peritoneal (see Standard: *Peritoneal dialysis*)
		Hemodialysis (see Standard: *Hemodialysis*)
■ Alteration of respiratory function related to respiratory depression and/or obstruction	■ Respiratory function normal as indicated by arterial blood gas levels	■ Prevent by
		Continuous monitoring of respiratory status
		Implementation of medical and nursing regimen to provide
		and maintain adequate respiratory function
		Monitor for
		Change in arterial blood gas levels
		Change in respiratory status
		Rate
		Depth
		Quality
		Degree of difficulty
		Color

Potential problems	Expected outcomes	Nursing activities

		Intervention if problem occurs
		  Respiratory support
		    O_2 therapy
		    Intubation
		    Mechanical ventilation (see Standard: *Mechanical ventilation*)

■ Fluid and/or electrolyte imbalance related to poisoning episode	■ Weight within normal limits
	Electrolytes within normal parameters
		■ Prevent by
		  Parenteral maintenance
		  Fluid replacement
		  Electrolyte replacement according to serum levels and maintenance requirements
		Monitor for
		  Change in fluid and nutritional intake
		  Change in weight
		  Change in state of hydration
		    Mucous membranes
		    Skin turgor
		    Thirst
		    Tears
		    Behavior
		    Urine specific gravity
		  Change in indices of intravascular volume
		    BP
		    P
		    CVP
		    Urine output and specific gravity
		  Changes in lab data
		    Serum electrolytes
		    Hct
		Intervention if problem occurs
		  Frequent assessment of vital signs
		  Accurate measurement and recording of intake and output
		  Daily weight
		  Accurate parenteral administration of fluids and electrolytes
		    Monitor IV q1 hr for rate of flow and amount infused (use infusion pump if available)
		    Observe IV site q1 hr
		  Monitor lab data

■ GI irritation related to specific action of ingested poison	■ GI system intact and functioning normally	■ Monitor for
		  Nausea
		  Vomiting
		  Diarrhea
		  Bleeding
		  Distention
		  Pain
		Intervention if problem occurs
		  Documentation of symptoms
		  Symptomatic treatment
		  Documentation of patient's response to treatment

Potential problems	Expected outcomes	Nursing activities

■ Alteration in body temperature regulation related to toxic action of poison involved	■ Maintenance of normal body temperature	■ Prevent by
		   Measuring body temperature q1-2 hr
		Monitor for
		   Change in body temperature
		      Hypothermia
		      Hyperthermia
		Intervention if problem occurs
		   Hyperthermia
		      Cooling mattress
		      Tepid sponge
		   Hypothermia
		      Heating mattress
		      Blankets

■ Bacterial superinfection related to increased susceptibility	■ Absence of infection	■ Prevent by
		   Serial monitoring of blood and urine cultures
		   Administration of antibiotics as ordered
		   NOTE: Antibiotic therapy is not instituted routinely as prophylactic treatment
		Monitor for
		   Temperature elevation greater than 101° F (38.2° C)
		   Change in lab values
		      WBC and differential
		      Cultures of blood and urine
		      Chest radiograph
		Intervention if problem occurs
		   Temperature elevation
		      Check temperature q2-4 hr or as indicated
		      Tepid sponge
		      Cooling mattress
		      Encourage fluid intake (as per appropriate route)
		   Institute mode of therapy as per physician's order
		      Antibiotics

■ Family crisis related to
   Poisoning episode
   Need for hospitalization
   Guilt
   Anxiety
	■ Facilitate coping mechanisms within the family	■ Assess degree of stress and ability to cope
		Determine level of understanding of the child's condition, treatment, and need for hospitalization
		   Offer factual information
		   Clarify misconceptions
		Encourage parenteral expression of feelings about incident and hospitalization
		   Establish relationship
		   Plan time for interaction
		   Reassure parents
		   Support parents
		Determine with the parents their degree of involvement in the care of their child
		Maintain parental sense of adequacy to care for their child
		Periodically evaluate effect of interventions on parents' behavior

■ Emotional stress related to trauma of hospitalization	■ Reduced emotional trauma	■ Prevent by
		   Minimal separation of parents and child
		   Continuity of care
		Monitor for
		   Presence of separation anxiety
		   Phase of separation anxiety (if present)
		      Protest
		      Despair
		      Denial

Potential problems	Expected outcomes	Nursing activities
		Presence of fears of
		Bodily harm
		Mutilation
		Loss of body integrity
		Strangers
		Unfamiliar surroundings
		Presence of feelings of
		Guilt
		Wrongdoing
		Loss of love
		Anger
		Intervention if problem occurs
		Separation anxiety
		Presence of parents
		Parent participation
		Presence of security object
		Fears
		Orientation to surroundings
		Consistent nursing personnel
		Correct misconceptions
		Provide accurate information
		Feelings
		Verbalization
		Play
		Drawing
■ Recurrence of poisoning episode related to Insufficient education Environmental conditions Developmental age of child	■ Change in attitude through increased knowledge of developmental influences on poisoning incidence and poisoning prevention	■ Assessment and translation of findings into an educational program, which may include
		Accident prevention
		Risk factors that most often result in injury
		Significant areas in household that cause problems relevant to age of child
		Protective measures helpful in accident avoidance
		Human development
		Gross motor and fine motor coordination for age
		Importance of exploration, investigation for children

NEONATAL-PEDIATRIC

54 □ The unstable premature infant

The term *premature* refers to an infant born before the completion of 37 weeks of gestation. The problems associated with prematurity are primarily related to the relative immaturity of the organ systems. The immature infant is not sufficiently physically or physiologically developed to meet basic needs in extrauterine life. Maturity is determined by actual gestational age.

The premature infant, in addition to immaturity, may also be small for gestational age. This implies poor intra-uterine growth, which may further complicate the postnatal course. The presence of anomalies present further hazards to survival. Moreover, the handicap of immaturity limits the premature infant's ability to cope with illness.

Other factors related to premature delivery frequently cause mechanical disadvantages that can complicate the infant's postnatal outcome, for example, breech presentation, multiple birth, prolapsed cord, abruptio placentae and related abnormalities, premature rupture of membranes, and greater uterine tone and/or contractility.

About 8% of live births in the United States are premature. Etiological factors associated with prematurity include chronic hypertension, limited prenatal care, malnutrition, smoking, and drug use (including alcohol and caffeine). Often these factors overlap and are associated with poor socioeconomic conditions. There is increased likelihood for premature delivery when there is a history of premature delivery(ies). Recent experience indicates a higher incidence of prematurity when there is a history of induced abortion.

Assessment of gestational age is important. As indicated before, the infant's relative immaturity is an index of risk for potential problems. It also presents clues as to what can/should be expected, and it is the basis for specific nursing assessment and interventions. For example, an infant of 34 to 36 weeks gestation may be able to suck at the mother's breast. An infant of less than 32 weeks gestation will probably require tube feedings. An infant of 28 weeks gestation may rely on parenteral feedings for several weeks.

Immaturity is manifested by differences in activity and neurological responses. The more immature infant is less active with a weaker cry and less muscle tone and resistance. Movements are irregular and jerky because the immature muscles cannot sustain contraction. The central nervous system (CNS), lungs, liver, and other organs have not completely developed.

Prematurity accounts for 59% of newborn deaths. Mortality is greater with lesser gestational age and/or lesser birth weight. Those that are both premature and small for gestational age have a poorer outlook.

Morbidity is also considerably higher, as much as 10 times greater for premature infants than for full-term infants. As indicated before, immaturity is not only in itself a handicap but also limits an infant's ability to cope with problems that may evolve. Clinical signs of problems may be less easily identified because of overlapping signs of immaturity.

Respiratory distress syndrome (RDS) is the most frequent cause of death. Necrotizing enterocolitis (NEC) is a most serious complication considering its insidious onset, rapid course, and high mortality. Even slight elevations of serum bilirubin levels are cause for concern because the immature liver is slow to conjugate and excrete bilirubin, thus increasing the risk of kernicterus.

The outlook for later growth and development of surviving premature infants is not yet fully known. In general, current prognoses are optimistic.

Assessment of growth must account for premature birth by subtracting the number of weeks preterm at birth from the infant's age at time of assessment (e.g., a 2-month-old infant born at 32 weeks gestation should in fact be compared to a 3-week-old term infant).

Later developmental lags are probably associated with factors other than prematurity, for example, CNS injuries, nutritional deficiencies in the perinatal period, intrauterine growth retardation, and hypoxia. Regarding these latter, the long-range impact of intensive neonatal care has not been fully evaluated.

A significant sequela to both the immediate separation of infant and mother and the prolonged hospitalization of the high-risk infant who requires intensive care is subsequent child neglect and abuse and other parenting problems including marital discord.

ASSESSMENT

1. Gestation
   a. Gestation is estimated in weeks beginning with mother's first day of last menstrual period; prior to birth, uterine size, ultrasonography, and amniocentesis may be used
   b. Neurological examination
   c. Physical examination
2. Appropriate intrauterine growth (compare infant with standard charts; infants who fall in the ninetieth percentile are considered small or large for gestational age)
   a. Weight (about 50% of low birth weight infants are premature)
   b. Length (length is more closely related to maturity than weight)
   c. Head circumference (head circumference should be determined at weekly intervals in low birth weight infants to assess aberrations from expected growth)
3. Results of serial lab tests
   a. Arterial blood gas levels
   b. Serum glucose, bilirubin, electrolytes

GOALS

1. Premature infant will grow and thrive
2. Family will be able to cope with the unanticipated crises of the birth experience and remain an intact, mutually nurturing dyad or group
3. Successful parent-infant bonding
4. Infant will develop normally, considering gestational age
5. Adequate but not excessive oxygenation
6. Adequate nourishment with weight gain
7. Thermoneutral environment maintained
8. Normal psychosocial and psychomotor growth
9. Parents will develop and have confidence in their parenting skills

Potential problems	Expected outcomes	Nursing activities
▪ Hypoxia secondary to apnea, RDS, cardiac insufficiency, anemia Apnea in the premature infant may be related to CNS immaturity Cold stress Dehydration Electrolyte imbalance Hypoglycemia Hypocalcemia (Apnea may be the presenting symptom of a variety of neonatal problems)	▪ Adequate oxygenation	▪ Assess respiratory status Attach infant to cardiorespiratory monitor and turn on alarm; observe infant's breathing pattern Note and record apneic episodes Include duration and presence or absence of 1. Bradycardia 2. Cyanosis 3. Abdominal distention Note activity and position of infant prior to, during, and after apneic episodes, e.g., feeding, sleeping, prone, supine Note temperature of infant and Isolette Note resumption of respirations 1. Whether spontaneous 2. Whether stimulation is required 3. Note type and amount of stimulation required Monitor and record Respiratory rate Breathing pattern; note 1. Retractions 2. Flaring nostrils 3. Grunting Skin color $F_{I_{O_2}}$ (q2 hr) Airway pressures Assist with intubation if necessary See Standards: *Mechanical ventilation* and *Neonatal respiratory distress* Tracheobronchial suctioning prn Administer chest physiotherapy frequently in the compromised infant

Potential problems	Expected outcomes	Nursing activities
		Gentle percussion may be applied by hand or with fingers (nipples or small masks may be a substitute of more convenient size to adequately rotate over the various lung segments)
		Posturing is important
		Vibration for the small premature infant is controversial
		Either manual or electric vibration can be used
		Administer aminophylline po or IV for intractable frequent apnea if needed, as ordered
		SEE STANDARD: *Neonatal respiratory distress*
		Support infant's respiratory efforts
		Avoid restraining infant (restraints reduce sensory stimulation)
		Change infant's position regularly; prone positions enhance ventilation/perfusion ratios and reduce asynchronous chest wall motion
		Nonnutritive sucking has been found to enhance oxygenation
		Allow infant to suck on soft nipple
		During apneic spells, stimulate infant gently at first
		Stroke feet, hands, face, back
		Then move extremities and trunk
		More vigorous stimulation may be required
		Continuous positive airway pressure (CPAP) may be prescribed
		Administer good skin care around nares when prongs are used; topical steroids may be prescribed
		Monitor for
		1. Gastric distention and aspirate prn
		2. Signs of pneumothorax or pneumomediastinum
		Minimize conditions that increase O_2 consumption
		Hyperthermia
		Cold stress
▪ Hypothermia May be related to hypoglycemia, hypoxia, or sepsis; it may be the presenting sign of infection Cold stress increases metabolism; if hypoglycemia ensues, anaerobic metabolism leads to metabolic acidosis	▪ Body heat will be conserved Alleviation/resolution of underlying causes of fluctuant temperature	▪ Dry infant immediately at birth and place under radiant heat source Do not allow infant to touch metal or other conductive surface Do not place infant in drafts Wrap infant in warmed blanket (remember that radiant heater does not prevent heat loss by convection) Transport infant in an Isolette to maintain the thermoneutral environment Warmers and/or incubators in both delivery room and nursery should be preheated Use warmed linen NOTE: Thermoneutral environment is one in which the oxygen requirement (i.e., O_2 consumption) is lowest for maintaining body temperature Utilize a servocontrolled unit (radiant warmer or Isolette) Position skin probe over liver Use heat reflecting adhesive to prevent the probe sensing environmental heat Set heater output between 37° and 37.5° C Maintain abdominal skin temperatures between 35.8° and 36.5° C Use warmed blankets when holding infant outside Isolette or warmer NOTE: The servocontrol mechanism limits the gradient between skin and environmental air temperature; when the

Potential problems	Expected outcomes	Nursing activities
		infant's temperature goes above or below a desired temperature the mechanism automatically turns off or on accordingly; overheating (abdominal temperatures over 36.5° C) and/or rapid rewarming may cause apnea; the basis for this heat-induced apnea mechanism is not known
		Monitor
		Axillary temperature q30 min until stable, then q2 hr
		Signs and symptoms of cold stress
		Reduced activity
		Flaccid movements
		Pallor
		Cyanosis
		Cold to touch
		Pupils dilate
		Slow, shallow, irregular breathing
		Bradycardia
		Investigate changes in infant's temperature; assess infant's thermal response to hypoxic episodes (oxyhemoglobin may fail to dissociate)
		Warm blood and other infusions to body temperature
		Warm O_2 to ambient temperature
		Monitor O_2 temperature
		Maintain Oxyhood temperature at 31° to 34° C
		Increase infant's temperature gradually; after first week, the larger and/or more stable premature infant should have servo-control discontinued
		Clothe and wrap infant, allowing face to be exposed to cooler temperatures (29° to 30° C)
		Assess stability of core temperature; as the infant grows and becomes stable, temperature is maintained without supplementary heat input and infant may be transferred to bassinet
		Ambient nursery temperature should be about 25° C
■ Hyperthermia related to overheating	■ Normal temperature	■ Monitor environmental temperature
		Maintain thermoneutral environment as described in Problem, Hypothermia
		Note signs and symptoms of hyperthermia
		Flushing
		Tachycardia
		Labored respirations
		Skin moisture
		Seizure activity
		Apneic episodes
■ Delayed parent-infant bonding and/or inhibited attachment due to Separation from infant Prolonged hospitalization of infant Grieving over loss of healthy normal newborn Poor outlook for positive outcome and/or unpreparedness due to early arrival	■ Parents demonstrate nurturant responses to infant Parents communicate their feelings about infant Successful parent-infant bonding	■ As soon as infant has been stabilized in high-risk nursery, allow parents to visit (this may be just the father at first; in this instance, introduction and orientation will have to be repeated for the mother)
		This visit should include the parents touching and examining the baby; parents may need help to initiate contact; relaxation techniques and therapeutic touch may assist parents at this time
		Minimize environmental potentiation of crisis
		Prepare parents for equipment and setting before they enter nursery
		Explain purpose of equipment, particularly tubes and wires attached to the infant; explain that the amount of equipment is not an index to how sick the infant is (remember the technology appears even more overwhelming in comparison to the infant's small size)

Potential problems	Expected outcomes	Nursing activities
		At the end of the visit, clarify parents' perceptions of situation; help them set realistic goals
		Recognize grief and withdrawal due to perceived condition
		Encourage verbalization of feelings of shock, failure, guilt, anger
		Recognize defense mechanisms, e.g., denial, anger, rejection
		Recognize negative comments as an expression of need for support
		Visiting times should be flexible; encourage parents to visit frequently; identify staff members by name; a relationship with a primary nurse is optimal but parents should be acquainted with other staff members also
		If visits decrease or become sporadic or irregular, follow up with phone call
		Point out signs of progress and growth; help parents anticipate a nonlinear course so they are not needlessly overwhelmed by apparent setbacks, e.g., if infant is moved back to radiant warmer from Isolette or if IV therapy is restarted
		Model nurturant behavior; provide opportunities for parents to care for infant; reinforce nurturant behaviors; describe to parents their special value to infant
		Support and reinforce parent-infant attachment (it is important when someone other than parents, e.g., a grandparent, will be a primary caregiver that this person is included in the attachment process from soon after birth)
		Set realistic prognostic expectations for survival; do not hesitate to be optimistic in early period; focus on immediate and day-to-day goals and progress
		Clarify misconceptions with factual information (nurse should be present at conferences with physicians to be better prepared to provide explanations)
		Encourage breast-feeding
		Teach advantages
		Nutrient
		Immunological
		Psychological/interactive
		Teach methods of expression (supply is directly related to the amount and frequency of breast stimulation)
		Stimulation of let-down reflex
		1. Hot moist towels for 10 minutes or warm shower
		2. Relaxation and centering techniques
		3. Breast massage
		Manual
		Electric or hand pump
		Care of pump
		Frequency: q3 hr during day
		Assist mother to breast-feed
		Breast-feeding should be initiated as soon as possible
		Reassure mother as she initiates breast-feeding
		Explain infant's learning needs, weak suck, etc.
		Maximize privacy
		In-between feedings should not be with nipple; use dropper technique
		Position baby for maternal comfort and to allow adequate grasp of nipple; premature infant should be positioned on side on pillows so that mother can support the head while keeping arms and shoulders relaxed
		Support and reassure mother
		Show an interest in how *she* is feeling
		Convey the importance of *her* milk for *her* baby

Potential problems	Expected outcomes	Nursing activities

		Discuss methods of support with husband; explain that the support is for the mother, not for the breast-feeding itself
		Importance of massaging interscapular area
		Importance of mother's nutritional and fluid intake
		Relaxation techniques
		Instruct parents regarding storage of breast milk
		    Label with name, date, and time
		    Refrigerate for 2 to 3 days and then discard (milk may be frozen and kept for 6 months; when removed from freezer, it should be used within 48 hours); refrigeration is preferable to freezing because leukocytes are destroyed when frozen
		    Use plastic containers because leukocytes stick to glass

■ Peripheral cyanosis due to vasomotor instability related to immaturity	■ Adequate oxygenation	■ Monitor breathing pattern
		    Weak, irregular respirations imply CNS involvement
		    Tachypneic or labored respirations may be due to pulmonary or cardiac problems
		Measure axillary temperature
		    Assess gradient between skin and environmental temperatures
		Observe for signs of sepsis, including lethargy, change in feeding pattern

■ Hypoglycemia (less than or equal to 25 mg/100 ml) related to
Delayed feedings
Low liver glycogen stores
Cold stress
Continuous low blood sugar may result in increased risk of cerebral damage; untreated hypoglycemia may be fatal
Immaturity limits the adrenal medullary response to low glucose
	■ Serum glucose within normal limits
	Adverse side effects of low blood sugar will be prevented, and fluid and electrolyte balance will be maintained through appropriate replacement therapy
		■ Assure adequate glucose intake
		    Early feeding is important; monitor intake
		    If infant is not taking oral feedings, parenteral glucose must be given (10% dextrose in water [D10W], 75 ml/kg body weight/day) as prescribed by physician
		Beware of increased metabolic demands of cold stress, hypoxia, etc.
		Monitor blood sugar by Dextrostix at 12 hours of age, then q4-8 hr for 48 hours
		Be alert to signs and symptoms of hypoglycemia
		    Lethargy, either as an isolated finding or with irritability and tremulousness (may be one of first signs)
		    Jittery movements or muscle twitching
		    Apnea
		    Cyanosis or pallor
		    Convulsions
		    Irritability
		    Hypotonia
		    Hypothermia
		    Diaphoresis
		If Dextrostix is below 45%, notify physician and administer therapy as prescribed
		    IV therapy may be increased to 15% dextrose in water (D15W)
		    Steroids may also be prescribed

■ Fluid and electrolyte imbalance related to insensible H_2O loss	■ Fluid and electrolyte balance maintained	■ Monitor intake and output q1 hr Weigh infant daily, at same time each day and prior to feeding Weight may be monitored more frequently (q8 hr) if situation is unstable, e.g., phototherapy, move from incubator to radiant warmer Perform Clinitest* on urine q4-8 hr; monitor urine specific gravity (it should be 1.015 or less) Monitor serum Na^+

*Clinitest, Ames Co., Elkhart, Ind.

Potential problems	Expected outcomes	Nursing activities

■ Malnutrition related to inadequate caloric intake due to small gastric capacity (3 to 5 ml) and poor absorption of fats and vitamins	■ Adequate caloric intake Infant growth	■ Monitor intake and output q1 hr
		   Oral intake record should include type and caloric content of feedings
		Administer hyperalimentation (total parenteral nutrition [TPN]) as ordered (hyperalimentation solutions should be prepared by a pharmacist under an ultraviolet hood)
		Monitor
		   Weights daily
		   Head circumference weekly
		   Urine Clinitest q4 hr if stabilized (q½-1 hr until stable)
		   When TPN is discontinued, monitor Dextrostix q1 hr for 6 to 8 hours
		Administer Intralipid as ordered; this may be infused simultaneously with TPN through a Y connector or intermittently
		Administer intermittent or continuous gavage feedings (gavage feeding may be indicated also when the premature infant is too immature to suck and swallow)
		NG or orogastric feedings
		   Insert No. 5 French feeding tube through nose or mouth, down the esophagus, and into stomach
		   Confirm placement
		      1. Aspirate stomach contents
		      2. Auscultate 2 to 5 cc injection of air into stomach via tube; this may be visualized by gastric distention (remove air immediately)
		   Position infant on right side with head and thorax elevated slightly
		   Allow measured amount of formula to flow by gravity
		   Keep infant on right side with head and thorax elevated or position on abdomen for at least 1 hour
		   Note and record emesis (emesis of 1 to 2 ml is normal in premature infant)
		Nasojejunal feedings*†
		   (This method is indicated when gastric gavage is contraindicated, e.g., recurrent aspiration, persistent respiratory distress, and mechanical ventilation make gastric feedings unsafe)
		   Tube is usually inserted by physician
		   Correct placement is verified by radiograph before feedings are initiated
		      Note radiograph results
		   Restrain upper extremities prn
		   Feeding should be warmed to body temperature
		   Use infusion pump; initial rate is usually 2 to 3 ml/kg body weight/hour and may be increased 1 ml/hour q6-8 hr as tolerated
		   Change infusion catheters q8 hr
		   Do not allow formula or breast milk to remain at room temperature for more than 4 hours
		   Agitate Volutrol at least once q1 hr to mix H$_2$O and soluble components of breast milk
		   Aspirate residual in jejunum q2-4 hr; it should be less than 1 ml; notify physician if residual increases
		   Measure gastric residual if ordered when jejunal/duodenal

*Passage of gastric tube may stimulate vagal response, resulting in serious bradycardia and/or apnea. Gastric distention during and following feeding may also stimulate this reflex.

†Oral medications should be administered through a gastric tube when jejunal or duodenal feedings are used.

Potential problems	Expected outcomes	Nursing activities
		tube is in place; this is not considered routinely necessary by some
		Monitor and record stool consistency and guaiac
		Initial feeding is 3 to 5 ml
		Feeding quantity is gradually increased
		Monitor for complications
		1. Perforation
		2. Intussusception
		3. Catheter blockages
		4. Changes in intestinal flora
		5. Diarrhea
		Nasoduodenal feedings*
		(Some neonatal clinicians have found this method more advantageous than the jejunal route)
		The exact nutrient absorption from the duodenum and jejunum is not certain
		During continuous drip feedings (which are indicated whenever the amount tolerated by bolus is insufficient for nutrition)
		Check catheter position q2 hr
		Note emesis
		Test for guaiac
		Bile may indicate reflux or misplacement of tube
		Notify physician if abnormalities are observed
		Holding the infant is not precluded by either intermittent or continuous tube feedings
		Oral nipple feedings may be used for infant mature enough to suck and swallow
		Feedings should begin with 3 to 5 ml volume
		Guidelines for increasing or withholding feedings may be specified by physician
		Note gastric residuals (residuals may not indicate intolerance of feeding; a residual of as much as 5 ml may persist even when feeding is reduced; meanwhile, it may not increase with increased feedings)
		Rock infant in nurse's or parent's lap for 5- to 20-minute periods at prescribed intervals (at least twice each shift)†
		When infant is 5 days old, temperature stability should be adequate; larger babies may be able to tolerate this sooner (during first few days, a smaller premature infant can be rocked in nurse's hands or arms under heat source or in Isolette)
		Administer therapeutic touch several times a day for 5 to 20 minutes‡
■ Abdominal distention (Stomach may become distended from positive airway pressure—either continuous positive airway pressure or mechanical/manual ventilatory assistance)	■ Diaphragm movement is not inhibited Absence of abdominal distention	■ Measure abdominal circumference just above umbilicus at time of admission; thereafter take this measurement daily (at the same time each day and prior to feeding)
		Note distention in relation to feeding pattern
		Whether abdomen usually becomes distended with feedings; whether this distention is gross or limited to gastric area
		Length of time that distention persists
		If distention persists until subsequent feeding time, aspirate via gastric tube
		Note quantity of air aspirated as well as other stomach con-

---

*Oral medications should be administered through a gastric tube when jejunal or duodenal feedings are used.
†Rocking has been found to stimulate newborn growth. The effects of rocking may be enhanced by interpersonal contact.
‡The exact mechanism of its effect in this situation is not fully understood. It may enhance energy and/or O_2 consumption, thus increasing reserves. The infant's need for proprioceptive stimulation may be involved.

Potential problems	Expected outcomes	Nursing activities
		tents; discard air and mucus and replace partially digested formula
		Note changes in pattern of distention in relation to feeding
		Institute more frequent measurements of abdominal girth
		Report increasing abdominal girth and other abnormal changes to physician
		Remove air from stomach q½-2 hr or prn when infant is receiving ventilatory assistance
		Observe for signs of respiratory distress
		Adjust infant's feeding schedule as tolerated
		Smaller, more frequent feedings may be better tolerated
		Experiment with varied infant positions
		Leave NG tube open and in place to decompress stomach
■ Sensory deprivation and/or bombardment	■ Infant receives appropriate stimulation from environment Infant develops socially responsive behavior Infant learns behaviors that influence subsequent stimuli Parents and staff respond appropriately to infant's cues Infant associates feeding with pleasant social stimuli	■ Provide verbal stimulation
		Soft talk and gentle tactile stimuli should precede other care giving
		Hold one's face within 9 inches of infant and in his line of vision
		Avoid repeated and sudden noise or jerky handling of infant
		Control noise level in unit
		Provide bright and moving visual stimuli
		Provide tactile stimulation
		Rock and stroke infant gently and rhythmically
		Avoid touching infant with cold objects, e.g., stethoscope
		Play music at intervals
		Continuous playing of music or radio talk should be avoided
		Lower lights during night hours
		Provide social stimulation
		Provide continuity of care by primary nurse and same caregiver each shift as much as possible
		Talk to infant whenever he/she is being handled
		Talk to infant whenever near him/her
		Initiate talk in enface position
		Provide stroking and cuddling even when infant cannot be taken from Isolette or warmer
		Assess infant's social responsiveness
		Alertness
		Visual responsiveness
		Inanimate stimuli
		People
		Ability to be consoled
		Muscle tone
		Self-quieting behavior
		Smiling behavior
		Note responses of pleasure, dissatisfaction, or inattention to various interactions
		Signs of attention include
		Head turning
		Staring
		Slowed heart rate and respiratory rate
		Change in motor activity, visual function
		Continuous, repetitious stimuli do not arouse interactive behaviors
		Avoid stimulating infant when he/she is irritable; assure parents that infant can hear and see them; help parents recognize infant's response to various stimuli and when infant is able to receive stimuli

Potential problems	Expected outcomes	Nursing activities
		Support parents' interaction with infant
		Make baby as attractive as possible
		Allow parents to bring in clothes and toys
		Encourage parents to see and touch infant frequently
		Infant should be fully awake when offered feedings
		Stimulate infant, change diaper, etc., before offering feeding
		Provide nonnutritive sucking at regularly scheduled intervals if/when infant is NPO; during these periods, infant should be held for at least 20 minutes
		Stimulates rooting reflex
		Develops proprioception of sucking activity
		If dropper or gavage feedings are necessary, infant should be offered nipple so that sucking becomes associated with food intake and relief of hunger
■ Hyperbilirubinemia related to immaturity, delayed feeding	■ Absence or resolution of hyperbilirubinemia Absence of neurotoxic effects of kernicterus	■ Administer phototherapy as ordered
		Apply eye shields to closed eyes (check eyes for signs of conjunctivitis)
		Uncover infant for maximum exposure
		Change position q2 hr
		Verify regular maintenance checks of phototherapy lights to assure proper wavelength
		Cover ultraviolet light with a plastic shield to protect infant from ultraviolet radiation
		Monitor temperature; prevent overheating
		Replace insensible H_2O loss
		Monitor and record specific gravity; notify physician of increase
		Give supplemental glucose H_2O between feedings if infant is taking po feedings (this will vary with size and gastric capacity of infant)
		Turn lights off when drawing blood specimens
		Assist with exchange transfusion if needed
		The preferred route is umbilical artery and vein (withdrawing from the artery and infusing into vein)
		Place infant under radiant warmer and attach to cardiorespiratory monitor
		Exchanged blood should be less than 1 day old
		Warm exchanged blood to 35° to 37° C
		Before and after transfusion, monitor the following parameters
		Hct and Hgb
		Platelets
		Arterial blood gas levels and pH
		Heart rate, respiratory rate, BP, and temperature
		Serum electrolytes, including Ca^{2+}
		Total serum protein
		Total and direct serum bilirubin
		Reticulocytes
		Dextrostix and serum glocose
		During transfusion observe for signs of
		Hypotension
		Hypoglycemia
		Hypocalcemia
		Bradycardia
		Acidosis
		Hypoxia
		Hypovolemia
		Ca^{2+} may be prescribed per unit volume of blood infused, especially if pretransfusion level is low (less than 7.5 mg/100 ml)

Potential problems	Expected outcomes	Nursing activities
		Postexchange, monitor Dextrostix q15-20 min for 2 hours (hypoglycemia is a frequent after effect)
		Notify physician of abnormalities in the aforementioned, and alter therapy as ordered
		Remember that the premature or low birth weight infant and/or an infant with respiratory distress may require intervention at lower bilirubin levels because associated hypoxia, acidosis, hypoglycemia, or infection makes him/her more susceptible to neurotoxicity
■ Sepsis	■ Absence of infection	■ Prevent exposure to nosocomial infection by the following activities
		Practice strict aseptic technique with all procedures (mask and gloves only when indicated, e.g., umbilical catheterizations)
		Limit visitors
		Allow only parents to handle infant
		(Parents or staff with upper respiratory infection, open wounds, diarrhea, etc., are not permitted in nursery)
		Teach parents proper handwashing technique
		Parents wear long sleeve gowns over clothing when entering nursery
		Allow parents to touch only their own infant
		Instruct parents not to handle other infants' supplies or to move things from one Isolette or crib to another
		Precautions are taken with invasive life-support procedures
		Respiratory therapy equipment should be changed daily
		Humidifiers should be changed daily; fill with sterile H_2O (q8 hr)
		Do not allow condensation in tubing to drain back to humidifier
		Change IV apparatus q24 hr; cover stopcocks at all times
		Continuous NG feeding apparatus should be changed q8 hr
		Feedings (whether formula or breast milk) should be restarted q4 hr
		Date multidose vials when first opened (because of the very small doses used with these patients, they are not consumed quickly)
		Multidose vials should be cultured according to unit policy routines
		Perform bacteriological examination of formulas weekly
		Monitor for signs of infection
		Cultures should be taken at admission as per protocol of unit
		Few signs and symptoms are unique to sepsis; any infant who is regressing should be evaluated for sepsis (repeat cultures)
		Apnea
		Lethargy
		Poor feeding
		Acidosis
		Hypotension
		Hypothermia
		Note local signs of infection related to therapies, e.g., eyes of infant who has been in humidifid Oxyhood, heel stick sites, sites of IVs, umbilical cord stump
		Monitor culture results
		Report any abnormal observations to physician

Potential problems	Expected outcomes	Nursing activities
■ Retrolental fibroplasia (retinopathy of prematurity) due to hyperoxia	■ Absence of effects of retinotoxic O_2 levels	■ Maintain minimal level of inspired O_2 (FI_{O_2}) that is sufficient to maintain Pa_{O_2} at 50 to 70 mm Hg ($FI_{O_2} \leqslant 0.4$ is usually adequate) Monitor FI_{O_2} and record concentration q1-2 hr FI_{O_2} should be prescribed based on arterial blood gas levels Infants who receive O_2 for any period should have optic fundi examined by ophthalmologist during and following O_2 therapy, at discharge, and at 5 months of age or 3 months after discharge Arrange for consultation as per hospital routine Instruct parents regarding discharge follow-up; arrange clinic appointment
■ Intracranial bleeding (occurs in more than 50% of infants born weighing less than 1500 g)	■ Absence of intracranial bleeding Unimpaired neurological function	■ Measure head circumference weekly Note rate of growth Note changes in level of alertness, activity, reflex responses, and behavior Notify physician for abnormalities and administer supportive therapy as ordered
■ Patent ductus arteriosus (PDA) related to immaturity	■ Adequate oxygenation	■ Note signs of pulmonary edema or murmur Notify physician and administer therapy as ordered, which may include fluid restriction, digitalization, and/or diuresis
■ NEC	■ Absence of NEC	■ Monitor for Changes in feeding pattern Poor absorption of feedings Emesis Presence of bilious material in gastric aspirate Hematest positive stools or emesis Increasing abdominal distention SEE STANDARD: *Neonatal necrotizing enterocolitis* Encourage and support breast-feeding
■ Parents lack confidence in their skills to care for infant at home—related to perceived "special needs," dependency on staff, anxiety	■ Infant will thrive and receive appropriate physical and psychological nurturing Parents demonstrate readiness to assume infant's care and enthusiasm for homecoming Appropriate parent-infant attachment	■ Prepare parents for assuming care of baby at home Help parents plan for infant's homecoming Recognize that parents probably were not prepared for early delivery Allow parents to discuss this experience and their feelings; while primary attention is directed to the newborn, mother may feel neglected, inadequate, or guilty Instruct parents in care of baby; fathers should be included in active caregiving participation in the nursery Feeding techniques 1. Infant should be awake and alert 2. Methods to stimulate sucking a. Moving nipple in baby's mouth b. Pressure on chin c. Stroking chin Bathing Normal and individual sleep/wake patterns and other behaviors, e.g., crying Special needs Signs and symptoms of and immediate intervention for aspiration As discharge time nears, assess preparation of home situation Refer to public health nurse or Visiting Nurse Association Discuss specific preparations Assess parents' readiness to assume responsibility for infant's care

Potential problems	Expected outcomes	Nursing activities
		Note visiting patterns
		Frequency
		Regularity
		Whether parents come together
		Assess parent-infant interactions
		Stimulate and reinforce social interaction/dialogue (premature infants take less initiative and give less feedback than full-term infants)
		Point out individual attractive features; assure parents that apparent unattractiveness is typical of premature infants and their baby will grow to look normal
		Note whether parents make positive comments about infant, infant behavior, and impact of infant on them
		Note evidence of parents' self-esteem, emotional exhaustion, support for each other
		Note whether parents demonstrate nurturant behavior
		Note whether parents are attentive to infant's behavior
		Gradually decrease parents' dependence on staff
		Parents should be able to spend time with infant without interference from staff
		Infant's supplies should be at crib so that parents do not have to continually ask questions or seek assistance from staff
		Allow parents to improvise and do things in a comfortable manner; allow them to arrange infant's things
		Infant's schedule (bath, etc.) should be geared to parents' visiting
		Offer approval and reinforce proper techniques
		"Nesting" or live-in arrangements for parents to provide all caregiving prior to discharge of infant has been investigated with significant results
		Arrange for follow-up care and support
		Clinic appointments
		Visiting nurse or public health nurse referrals
		Social service referrals (social service should be actively involved from soon after birth so that social problems can be assessed and appropriate intervention initiated)
		Follow-up phone calls by primary nurse and nursery staff to offer support and identify problems
		Encourage phone calls to ask questions, refer problems, or seek encouragement

55 □ Growth retardation

The term *growth retardation* is applied to infants whose birth weight is below the level expected for gestational age. The terms *intrauterine growth retardation (IUGR), small for gestational age (SGA),* and *small for dates (SFD)* are often used interchangeably when referring to fetal underdevelopment of any etiology.

There is much not known about IUGR. It can result from an insult early in fetal embryological development, resulting in a fewer number of cells, or from an insult later in pregnancy in which the number of fetal cells are normal but the cells are of reduced size. There are two major factors that determine fetal growth: the adequacy of the "supply line" (mother and placenta) and the growth potential of the fetus itself. Therefore, causative factors may be divided into maternal, placental, and fetal. Maternal factors include malnutrition, hypertension, preeclampsia, alcohol and/or drug abuse, cigarette smoking, advanced diabetes, chronic renal disease, and heart disease. Placental factors include premature separation, single umbilical artery, placental infarction, and the twin transfusion syndrome. Fetal factors include chronic intrauterine infection, congenital malformations, multiple gestation, and chromosomal abnormalities.

The assessment of gestational age for all newborns is of paramount importance. Using a system such as described by Dubowitz,* the nurse can quickly assess an infant at birth. Having calculated the infant's gestational age, this can be plotted on the Denver intrauterine growth curve to determine the infant's growth status.

The infant's physical appearance at birth is dependent on a number of factors, including duration of the growth-retarding influence. If the insult occurred within a few days or weeks of birth, the infant will appear wasted. Weight may be the only growth parameter that is less than expected. The infant's skin is often dry, and meconium staining may be evident. The infant may seem alert and even hungry. The hair may be thin and sparse. The infant who has been subject to chronic intrauterine stress will not appear wasted, but all growth parameters will be below normal for gestational age.

Treatment begins by anticipating the birth of a growth-retarded infant and/or identifying the growth-retarded infant at birth. Adequate provisions for warmth and for immediate assessment of the airway must be available in the delivery room. Since growth-retarded infants do not tolerate the stress of labor, asphyxia should be anticipated and resuscitative measures instituted if necessary.

Hypoglycemia may not be present at birth but should be anticipated during the first 48 hours as the infant's already low glycogen stores are exhausted. Although not as accurate as blood glucose measurement, close monitoring by Dextrostix must be part of nursing care. If low, blood sugar determinations should then be ordered.

Treatment by intravenous infusion of glucose is begun after two successive blood glucose levels indicate a blood glucose level below 20 to 25 mg/100 ml in low birth weight infants and 30 to 35 mg/100 ml in full-term infants. Oral formula or breast milk feedings are begun

*Dubowitz, L., Dubowitz, V., and Goldberg, C.: Clinical assessment of gestational age in the newborn infant, J. Pediatr. **77:**1-10, 1970.

as soon as possible. A thorough physical examination should be performed early to recognize congenital anomalies. The hematocrit should be followed closely to detect polycythemia, which is often asymptomatic.

Prognosis for the growth-retarded infant is dependent on a number of factors, including the cause of growth retardation and the gestational age at birth. Much research is being done by following the physical and psychological progress of these infants, and parents must understand the importance of close follow-up.

ASSESSMENT

1. Maternal history of
   a. Infection
   b. Hypertension
   c. Preeclampsia
   d. Alcohol/drug abuse
   e. Smoking
   f. Advanced diabetes
   g. Renal disease
   h. Malnutrition
   i. Multiple gestation
2. Determination of infant's gestational age, using criteria developed by Dubowitz
3. Infant's weight below tenth percentile for gestational age according to Denver intrauterine growth curve
4. Monitor lab data
   a. Hct
   b. Blood sugar
   c. Immune globulin type M (IgM)
5. Signs and symptoms of complications
   a. Seizures
   b. Respiratory distress
   c. Hyperbilirubinemia
   d. Meconium aspiration
   e. Hypothermia
   f. Hypoglycemia

GOALS

1. Blood glucose within normal limits
2. Adequate nutrition for weight gain
3. Thermal stability
4. Before discharge, parents
   a. Verbalize understanding of infant's condition
   b. Demonstrate ability to bathe, feed, and care for infant
   c. State plans for follow-up visits

Potential problems	Expected outcomes	Nursing activities
■ Perinatal asphyxia due to chronic hypoxia and/or hypoxic stress during labor	■ Asphyxiated state will be recognized and appropriate treatment instituted at birth	■ Anticipate growth-retarded infant from maternal history Monitor fetal heart during labor Suction airway immediately at birth Provide O_2 as indicated by infant's condition

■ Hypoglycemia as a result of reduced glycogen stores	■ Blood sugar will be maintained between 45 to 120 mg/100 ml	■ Monitor blood glucose by Dextrostix at birth and q3-4 hr; notify physician if below 45 mg/100 ml
		Observe infant carefully for symptoms of hypoglycemia
		  Jittery movements
		  Apnea
		  Lethargy
		  Seizures
		  Color change
		Begin feedings as soon as possible after birth

■ Hypothermia, as a result of limited subcutaneous insulation	■ Temperature will be maintained in thermoneutral zone (97° to 98° F [36° to 36.5° C])	■ Monitor axillary temperature at least q2-3 hr; if infant is in Isolette, check Isolette temperature
		Observe for symptoms of thermal instability
		  Cold skin temperature
		  Lethargy
		  Grunting respirations
		  Poor feeding
		Avoid placing infant on cold surfaces or in drafty locations
		Institute warming measures
		  Dry off infant
		  Add additional blanket
		  Place infant in Isolette and attach servocontrol mechanism
		  Warm infant slowly (1°/hour) to avoid hyperthermia

■ Polycythemia
  Etiology is unclear, but may be a result of placental insufficiency
	■ Hct will be maintained below 65%	■ Monitor Hct at birth and follow as necessary
		Observe for signs of increased blood viscosity
		  Respiratory distress
		  Cyanosis
		  Seizures
		If indicated, assist physician with partial exchange transfusion; monitor vital signs; keep accurate records of withdrawn blood and infused plasma

■ Congenital anomalies	■ Abnormalities will be recognized and appropriate management instituted	■ Thorough physical assessment at birth or on admission to nursery Notify physician of abnormalities Administer supportive care according to the abnormality present, as ordered

■ Hyperbilirubinemia as a result of hemolysis	■ Indirect bilirubin will be maintained below level acceptable for weight and gestational age	■ Observe and record infant's color q4 hr
		Monitor indirect bilirubin at least q8 hr beginning 48 hours after delivery
		If phototherapy is indicated
		  Keep infant warm by placing in Isolette and recording temperature q4 hr; remove infant only for feedings
		  Apply eye patches over closed lids
		  Remove eye patches for eye care and feeding q4 hr and replace
		  Offer H_2O between feedings to prevent dehydration

■ Late anemia as a result of rapid weight gain and low iron stores	■ Hct will be maintained within normal limits for age	■ Administer iron supplement as ordered Instruct parents in proper administration of iron supplement

Potential problems	Expected outcomes	Nursing activities
■ Parents have insufficient knowledge and/or skills to comply with discharge regimen	■ Parents verbalize understanding of cause(s) and effects of infant's growth retardation Parents demonstrate ability to care for infant Parents state provision for follow-up care	■ Assess parents' knowledge and understanding of infant's condition Teaching program* that includes Cause and effect of underlying problem (should be done by physician and reinforced by nurse) Newborn care—bathing, feeding, diaper care, etc. Follow-up—necessity of timing and where and by whom to be provided

*If responsibility of critical care nurse includes such follow-up care.

56 □ Neonatal respiratory distress

Respiratory distress in the newborn may be caused by conditions of pulmonary and nonpulmonary origin. The most common pulmonary causes are hyaline membrane disease, meconium aspiration syndrome, and transient tachypnea of the newborn. The failure of the newborn to establish respirations at birth is also considered respiratory distress. Congenital heart disease, CNS disorders, and metabolic and hematological disturbances are nonpulmonary causes of respiratory distress.

Hyaline membrane disease (HMD) is a disease of prematurity. Respiratory distress occurs as a result of an inadequate amount of surfactant, a substance that lines the alveoli and prevents alveolar collapse. Insufficient surfactant levels result in atelectasis and increased pulmonary resistance. This, in turn, results in hypoxia and hypercapnia. Infants with HMD exhibit mixed acidosis. Respiratory acidosis is a result of gas exchange difficulties. Metabolic acidosis is a result of hypoxia and anaerobic metabolism. A chest radiograph reveals the typical ''ground glass'' appearance of the lungs.

There is no definitive treatment for HMD. Treatment is aimed at supporting the infant until surfactant is produced in sufficient quantity. This is accomplished by providing or assisting ventilation; correcting acid-base disturbances; providing nutritional support; and maintaining blood pressure and hematocrit levels.

In a vertex presentation, meconium in the amniotic fluid is abnormal. It is associated with the passage of meconium into the amniotic fluid due to hypoxia, and meconium may be aspirated into the lungs as the infant gasps or takes the first breath. It is important to visualize the vocal cords and to carefully suction the meconium before the infant takes the first breath and before resuscitative measures are taken. Once respiration has begun, meconium may be sucked deep into the bronchial tree. The main problem is blockage of the air passages and pneumonia as a result of chemical irritation.

An overdistended chest is characteristic of the infant with meconium aspiration syndrome. The infant is prone to pneumothorax. Treatment is again aimed at supportive measures, including vigorous pulmonary therapy, since the lungs, in time, are capable of removing the foreign material.

Transient tachypnea of the newborn is characterized by rapid respirations without retractions. The etiology of transient tachypnea is unclear, but it may be due to a decreased rate of reabsorption of lung fluid. These term infants may need supplemental oxygen. Spontaneous recovery usually occurs within 4 to 5 days.

Surgical conditions such as tracheoesophageal fistula and diaphragmatic hernia are nonpulmonary causes of respiratory distress. Other nonpulmonary causes are congenital heart disease, hypoglycemia, hypothermia, loss of blood, and CNS disturbances.

A variety of symptoms may be present in infants with respiratory distress (see Assessment). They may be present at birth or they may be delayed for several hours. An expiratory grunt, as the infant attempts to keep alveoli from collapsing by increasing ''back pressure'' in the respiratory system, is characteristic of HMD.

Management of respiratory distress is aimed at identifying the etiology, maximizing pulmonary function, and minimizing oxygen consumption. Respiratory assistance can be provided by the use of supplemental oxygen and by continuous positive airway pressure (CPAP). The monitoring of blood gas levels is essential as is attention to electrolytes, nutrition, and cardiovascular status. Thermoregulation is imperative to minimize oxygen consumption.

The prognosis for these infants is dependent on a number of factors, including the etiology of the respiratory distress. Hypoxia may have an effect on the infant's subsequent development. Careful monitoring of arterial blood gas levels and appropriate adjustment of oxygen levels has reduced the incidence of retrolental fibroplasia. All infants who have received oxygen should have an ophthalmoscopic examination before discharge. Chronic pulmonary disease is becoming more common as a result of intensive respiratory therapy and the use of ventilators and positive pressure therapy. Long-term data is only now becoming available on the consequences of intense respiratory therapy. Infants receiving such treatment will require close follow-up after discharge.

ASSESSMENT

1. Maternal history of
   a. Premature delivery
   b. Bleeding
   c. Meconium-stained amniotic fluid
2. Pulmonary causes leading to respiratory distress
   a. Transient tachypnea of the newborn
   b. Hyaline membrane disease
   c. Aspiration syndrome(s)
   d. Airway obstruction
   e. Pneumothorax
   f. Pneumonia
   g. Pulmonary hemorrhage
3. Nonpulmonary causes leading to respiratory distress
   a. Congenital heart disease
   b. Metabolic factors
      (1) Hypoglycemia
      (2) Hypothermia
      (3) Hyperthermia
   c. CNS factors
      (1) Drug effect
      (2) Cerebral hemorrhage
      (3) Meningitis
   d. Hematological factors
      (1) Polycythemia
      (2) Anemia
      (3) Acute blood loss
   e. Sepsis

4. Signs and symptoms of respiratory distress
   a. Sternal and intercostal retractions
   b. Nasal flaring
   c. Expiratory grunt
   d. Cyanosis in room air
   e. Tachypnea/apnea
   f. Tachycardia/bradycardia
   g. Decreased breath sounds on auscultation
5. Results of lab data
   a. Arterial blood gas levels
   b. Blood glucose
   c. Hct
   d. Electrolytes
6. Chest radiograph findings
7. Signs and symptoms indicating need for assisted ventilation, with criteria for the following modes of assisted ventilation
   a. Oxygen via Oxyhood
      (1) Absent or mild retractions
      (2) Blood gas levels within normal limits in less than 40% oxygen
   b. CPAP
      (1) Spontaneous respirations, grunting, tachypnea
      (2) Recurrent apnea
      (3) Mild to moderate retractions
      (4) Requires 40% to 60% oxygen to maintain blood gases within normal limits
      (5) Rising Pa_{CO_2}
   c. Mechanical ventilation
      (1) Severe retractions
      (2) Apnea
      (3) Requires greater than 60% oxygen to maintain blood gases within normal limits
      (4) Pa_{CO_2} greater than 70 mm Hg
8. Complications of assisted ventilatory therapy
   a. Bronchopulmonary dysplasia
   b. Pneumothorax
   c. Intracranial hemorrhage
   d. Retrolental fibroplasia
9. Parental response to neonatal illness
   a. Understanding of etiology of respiratory distress
   b. Understanding of rationale for and effects of treatment
   c. Guilt associated with failure to produce a "normal" baby
   d. Coping mechanisms and support system

GOALS

1. Absence and/or resolution of respiratory distress
2. Maximum pulmonary function

3. Minimum metabolic requirement and oxygen consumption
4. Nutritional intake supportive for growth
5. Successful weaning from oxygen and/or assisted ventilatory therapy
6. Absence of complications resulting from oxygen and/or assisted ventilatory therapy
7. Absence of infection
8. Successful parent-infant attachment
9. Before discharge, parents
   a. Verbalize understanding of etiology, therapeutic management, and prognosis
   b. Demonstrate ability to bathe, feed, and care for infant
   c. State plans for follow-up care by pediatrician and, if indicated, specialists

Potential problems	Expected outcomes	Nursing activities

■ Respiratory insufficiency related to inadequate ventilation, airway obstruction	■ Maximum pulmonary function
	Absence of respiratory distress
		■ Position infant for maximal lung expansion
		  Extend infant's head by placing small blanket roll under shoulders; *do not hyperextend*
		  Elevate head of bed slightly
		  Keep infant's hands off chest
		  Change position from sides to back at least q2 hr
		Observe and auscultate for bilateral air entry at least q1 hr; possible causes of decreased or unequal air entry
		  Endotracheal tube displaced into nasopharynx
		  Endotracheal tube displaced into right main stem bronchus
		  Airway clogged with secretions
		  Pneumothorax
		Maintain patency of airway
		  Suction at least q2 hr and prn for removal of secretions
		    Oxyhood—suction nasopharynx and oropharynx
		    CPAP—suction nasopharynx and oropharynx
		    Endotracheal tube
		      1. Instill ⅓ to ½ ml sterile saline solution to loosen secretions
		      2. Reattach ventilator and ventilate 30 seconds
		      3. Turn head to one side
		      4. Using gloved hand and sterile catheter, quickly suction
		      5. Replace on ventilator for 30 seconds, then repeat steps 3 and 4 on other side
		Chest physiotherapy via toothbrush method* for infants with poor air exchange and positive radiological findings of atelectasis
		Monitor Hct at least daily; record amount of blood withdrawn for lab analysis

■ Increased metabolism related to increased tissue O_2 consumption	■ Minimum metabolic requirement and adequate tissue oxygenation	■ Avoid excessive stimulation
		Maintain thermoneutral environment
		  Provide care within Isolette or under radiant heater
		  Monitor and record axillary temperature q2-3 hr (thermoneutral zone is 97° to 98° F [36° to 36.5° C])
		  If warming measures are necessary, warm infant slowly (1°/hour) to avoid hyperthermia
		Administer O_2 via heated humidified nebulizer with temperature at same level as ambient air
		Administer gavage feedings to minimize energy expenditure
		  Have formula or breast milk at room temperature
		  Administer slowly, maximum 2 ml/minute

*Curran, C. L., and Kackoyeanos, M. K.: The effects on neonates of two methods of chest physical therapy, MCN **4:**309-313, 1979.

Potential problems	Expected outcomes	Nursing activities
■ Acid-base disturbance	■ Acid-base balance	■ Monitor arterial blood gas levels q2-4 hr according to patient's condition Notify physician of any abnormal results Keep flow sheet for recording blood gas results and interventions as ordered Respiratory acidosis—correct by reducing CO_2 levels by controlled ventilation Metabolic acidosis—correct by slowly infusing $NaHCO_3$ diluted in a one-to-one ratio with sterile H_2O Respiratory alkalosis—correct by reducing breathing rate
■ Nutritional imbalance Fluid and electrolyte imbalance	■ Fluid and electrolyte balance Nutritional intake supportive for growth	■ Monitor results of serial serum Na^+, K^+, and Cl^- determinations Keep bedside flow sheet for recording all intake/output Intake Gavage feedings Insert NG or orogastric feeding tube Verify tube placement in following three ways 1. Absence of bubbles when tip placed under H_2O 2. Aspiration of gastric contents 3. Auscultate while injecting 0.5 to 1 cc of air through feeding tube; listen below xiphoid process for air entry into stomach; remove air Elevate head of bed slightly Administer breast milk or formula at room temperature Administer feeding slowly, maximum 2 ml/minute, to minimize metabolic activity and to reduce pressure on diaphragm Observe for 1. Cyanosis 2. Tachypnea 3. Apnea 4. Bradycardia 5. Abdominal distention 6. Emesis After feeding, place infant on side Record type and amount of feeding as well as infant's response IV infusions Use infusion pump to maintain constant flow rate Keep IV at rate ordered Protect IV site Inspect IV site q1 hr for infiltration or leakage Record q1 hr 1. Type of solution 2. Amount infused 3. Running balance in relation to rate ordered Hyperalimentation (see Standard: *total parenteral nutrition through central venous catheter*) Output Daily weights on same scale Weigh diapers to determine urine output Test urine q4 hr for specific gravity, pH, and presence of sugar and protein Record number, color, and consistency of stools Record amount of blood withdrawn for lab analysis Monitor for signs and symptoms of dehydration Elevated Hct Elevated total protein level Poor skin turgor

Potential problems	Expected outcomes	Nursing activities
		Loss of 5% total body weight within 24 hours
		Elevated Serum Na^+
		Elevated urine specific gravity
		Decreased urine output
		Notify physician of the aforementioned abnormalities, and alter the therapeutic regimen as ordered
■ O_2 toxicity	■ Absence or minimization of O_2 toxicity	■ Measure and record FI_{O_2} q1 hr
		Administer prescribed amount of O_2
		Verify all changes in FI_{O_2} with an O_2 analyzer
		Calibrate O_2 analyzer at least once each shift
		Humidify and warm all O_2
■ Infection	■ Prevention or absence of infection	■ Meticulous handwashing
		Change Isolette weekly; change Isolette sleeves every 2 to 3 days
		Suction with gloved hand and sterile catheter
		Care of ventilatory equipment
		Change tubing and/or Oxyhood and humidifier q24 hr
		Refill humidification source with sterile H_2O each shift
		Check tubing for condensation and drain into basin; do not drain back into humidifier
		Change indwelling feeding tube daily
		Care of IV infusion
		Change IV bottle, tubing, and stopcocks q24 hr
		Cleanse umbilical catheter insertion site daily according to unit protocol
		Observe insertion site for inflammation, discharge, etc.
		Monitor for signs and symptoms of infection
		Thermal instability
		Inflammation of umbilical stump
		Lethargy
		Apnea
		Assist physician in drawing of blood cultures, spinal taps, etc.
		Administer antibiotics as ordered
■ Respiratory insufficiency related to use and function of Oxyhood and assisted ventilatory equipment	■ Maximum therapeutic effects of assisted ventilatory equipment	■ Oxyhood
		Use hood of appropriate size*
		Small: less than 2½ pounds (1134 g)
		Medium: 2½ to 8 pounds (1135 to 3629 g)
		Large: over 8 pounds (3630 g)
		Do not plug holes; they allow for removal of CO_2
		Do not seal space between hood and infant's neck
		CPAP
		Use nasal prongs of size appropriate for nares
		Keep nasal prongs securely in nares; remove q4 hr to give care
		1. Stimulate skin under nares
		2. Cleanse and dry nostril openings and skin thoroughly
		3. Check for redness due to pressure
		4. Replace and anchor securely
		Connections of tubes and gauges must be tight with no air leakage
		Administer prescribed amount of CPAP
		Monitor and record amount of CPAP q1 hr
		Mechanical ventilation
		Monitor pulse and respiration during intubation

*Williams, T. J., and Hill, J. W., editors: Handbook of neonatal respiratory care, Riverside, Calif., Bourns, Inc., p. 55.

Potential problems	Expected outcomes	Nursing activities

		Use appropriate size endotracheal tube*
		   2.5 inside diameter: under 1000 g
		   3.0 inside diameter: 1000 to 1500 g
		   3.5 inside diameter: 1500 to 2200 g
		   4.0 inside diameter: over 2200 g
		 Secure endotracheal tube in proper position; obtain radiographic confirmation of tube position
		 Keep an extra tube of appropriate size at bedside
		 Set alarms at reasonable limits and keep in *on* position
		 Maintain bedside flow sheet for q1 hr recording of
		   All settings (pressures, rate, CPAP, PEEP, O_2, etc.)
		   Changes made and by whom
		 Check tubes for kinking, which can result in blocked airway
		 Keep tubing free of accumulated moisture
		 Place manual resuscitator bag with appropriate size mask at bedside and within reach in case of ventilator failure or extubation

■ Inability to wean from O_2 due to
 Anemia
 Sepsis
 Hypoglycemia
 Inadequate nutritional state
 Pneumothorax
 Severe asphyxia or CNS disturbance
	■ Successful weaning from O_2	■ Monitor infant for signs and symptoms of
		   Anemia
		   Sepsis
		   Hypoglycemia
		   Poor nutritional state
		   Pneumothorax
		   Severe asphyxia or CNS disturbance
		 To lower FI_{O_2}
		   Repeat Pa_{O_2} before each decrease
		   Reduce environmental O_2 in 5% decrements per hour; when below 30%, reduce in 2% decrements
		   Observe infant for
		     Cyanosis
		     Pallor
		     Tachypnea
		     Hypothermia
		   Record all changes and infant's response
		   Notify physician of any difficulty in weaning, and administer corrective therapy as ordered

■ Difficulties in parent-infant bonding due to separation, guilt, and anxiety	■ Resolution of parental guilt feelings and beginning of parent-infant attachment process	■ Encourage parents to verbalize feelings regarding illness of their child; reassure parents as to "normalcy" of guilt feelings
		 Encourage parents to communicate with each other and with other parents
		 Promote parent-infant involvement during hospitalization
		   Refer to the infant by his/her name
		   Encourage early and frequent visitation and phone contact
		   Involve parents in infant's care, i.e., feeding, bathing, diapering
		   Encourage parents to touch and hold infant as much as feasible
		   Ask parents to bring in "something" for infant—clothes, family picture to hang at cribside, new small stuffed animal, music box, etc.

*Avery. G. B.: Neonatology. Philadelphia. 1975. J. B. Lippincott Co.. p. 268.

Potential problems	Expected outcomes	Nursing activities

■ Insufficient parental knowledge and/or skills to successfully care for infant after discharge	■ Parents
	  Verbalize etiology of the respiratory distress, rationale and effects of treatment, and prognosis
	  Demonstrate ability to care for infant at home
	  State provisions for follow-up care by pediatrician and other specialists
		■ Ongoing assessment of parents' knowledge and understanding of condition and treatment
		Explain and clarify when indicated
		Reassure parents of their ability to care for infant after discharge
		Referral to local visiting nurse agency
		Involve parents in infant's care throughout hospitalization
		Teaching plan* to include
		  Etiology, management, and prognosis (should be done initially by physician and nurse and reinforced by nurse)
		  Demonstration of newborn care—bathing, feeding, diapering, etc.; return demonstration by parents
		  Explanation and demonstration of special procedures and/or medication administration; return demonstration by parents
		  Importance and necessity of follow-up care

*If responsibility of critical care nurse includes such follow-up care.

57 □ Hemolytic disease due to Rh/ABO incompatibility

Hemolytic disease of the newborn is most commonly due to Rh or ABO incompatibility. Hemolysis is the result of an antigen-antibody reaction in the fetus or newborn. Incompatible red blood cells leak into the maternal circulation where antibodies are produced and pass back into the fetal circulation, causing hemolysis.

The most serious form of the disease occurs in Rh incompatibility in which the mother is Rh negative and the fetus is Rh positive. Sensitization occurs at the time of placental separation. The first pregnancy is usually not affected. During subsequent pregnancies, the transfer of maternal antibodies into the fetal circulation causes the hemolytic process. This disease begins in utero. Its severity can be gauged by maternal antibody titers and by repeated amniocentesis. Since bilirubin is excreted via the placenta, the main risk to the fetus is anemia. The fetus responds to this anemia by attempting to increase erythropoiesis, which is responsible for the hepatosplenomegaly seen in affected infants. The most severe form of the disease is hydrops fetalis. Progressive anemia leads to hypoxia, heart failure, and generalized edema.

After birth, jaundice usually becomes evident within the first few hours of life. The degree of anemia reflects the severity of the disease. Immediate exchange transfusion at birth is indicated in the presence of hydrops

fetalis or congestive heart failure. The diagnosis can be confirmed by the direct Coombs' test, which demonstrates the presence of maternal antibodies on the infant's red blood cells.

The most effective treatment for Rh disease is prevention. Since the early 1960s it has been possible to prevent maternal sensitization through the administration of a vaccine that destroys fetal antigens before they stimulate the production of antibodies. This vaccine must be administered to the mother within 72 hours after delivery and repeated after each pregnancy.

Hemolytic disease from ABO incompatibility is usually of a much milder form. Most often, the mother is type O and the fetus type A or B. First pregnancies may be affected, since anti-A or anti-B antibodies are already present in maternal blood. Severe forms of the disease are rare. The diagnosis is made in the newborn based on clinical and hematological findings. Jaundice is common, as is mild anemia. Peripheral blood smears reveal the presence of spherocytes. A direct Coombs' test may be weakly positive or negative, but maternal serum analysis reveals the presence of anti-A or anti-B titers. Exchange transfusions are generally not indicated in cases of ABO incompatibility.

When immediate transfusion is not indicated at birth,

the infant's bilirubin and hematocrit levels should be closely followed every 4 to 6 hours. The danger to the infant is that of kernicterus (bilirubin toxicity), which results in CNS damage. Several factors influence this risk, including the concentration of serum bilirubin, albumin-binding capacity, gestational age, acid-base balance, and the use of drugs that may interfere with the ability of albumin to bind bilirubin.

Exchange transfusion is indicated to treat hyperbilirubinemia or severe anemia (see Assessment). A double volume exchange of 170 ml/kg body weight replaces 85% of the infant's blood. Fresh Rh negative blood is used. The use of old blood may cause hyperkalemia. Blood preserved with acid citrate dextrose (ACD) predisposes the infant to hypocalcemia, rebound hypoglycemia, and acidosis. The exchange is done through the umbilical vein, alternately removing and infusing 5 to 20 ml of blood, and usually takes about 1 hour. Several exchange transfusions may be necessary as bilirubin rebounds and hemolysis continue to occur. In some institutions, an exchange transfusion may be preceded by the administration of albumin to increase availability of binding sites.

Phototherapy is of value in mild to moderate cases of hemolytic disease and is usually the only treatment necessary for ABO incompatibility. It should not be used in place of an exchange transfusion when bilirubin levels are rising rapidly, but it may be used following an exchange transfusion. Once phototherapy has begun, skin color is no longer an adequate indicator of bilirubin concentration, since photodecomposition of bilirubin occurs in the capillaries of the skin.

If kernicterus can be prevented, the prognosis for these infants is excellent. Anemia may occur in the second week as remaining antibodies continue to hemolyze the newborn's red blood cells. It is important to explain this to parents as these infants may require blood transfusions after discharge. This form of anemia does not respond to iron therapy.

ASSESSMENT

1. Family history
   a. Rh incompatibility
      (1) Rh negative mother
      (2) Rh positive father
      (3) Rising titer of anti-D antibodies in maternal serum
   b. ABO incompatibility
      (1) Mother's blood type O
      (2) Previous child with ABO disease
2. Results of prenatal amniotic fluid testing
   a. Intrauterine diagnosis of fetal hemolytic disease
   b. Fetal lung maturity
3. Results of lab studies (neonate)
   a. Indirect bilirubin
   b. Hgb and Hct
   c. Peripheral blood smear
   d. Direct and indirect Coombs' test
   e. Blood and Rh type
   f. Reticulocyte count
4. Signs and symptoms of hydrops fetalis
   a. Prematurity
   b. Severe pallor
   c. Subcutaneous edema
   d. Hepatosplenomegaly
   e. Congestive heart failure
   f. Ascites
5. Signs and symptoms of anemia in infant without hydrops fetalis
   a. Mild edema
   b. Pallor
   c. Hepatosplenomegaly
   d. Hypoglycemia
6. Indications for exchange transfusion
   a. At birth
      (1) Hydrops fetalis
      (2) Congestive heart failure
   b. Cord Hgb less than 14 mg in premature infant or 11 mg in full-term infant
   c. Term infant
      (1) Bilirubin greater than 6 mg/100 ml in first 6 hours
      (2) Bilirubin greater than 10 mg/100 ml in first 12 hours
      (3) Bilirubin 20 mg/100 ml at any time
   d. Premature infant—bilirubin level equal to infant's birth weight divided by 100 (e.g., for an infant weighing 1200 g, do an exchange transfusion when bilirubin is 12 mg/100 ml)
   e. Rate of rise of bilirubin 0.5 mg/100 ml/hour
7. Complications of exchange transfusion
   a. Vascular
      (1) Embolization
      (2) Thrombosis of portal vein
      (3) Perforation of vessel
   b. Cardiac
      (1) Volume overload
      (2) Arrhythmias
      (3) Arrest
   c. Metabolic

(1) Hypoglycemia
(2) Hyperkalemia
(3) Hypernatremia
(4) Hypocalcemia
(5) Acidosis
d. Clotting
(1) Thrombocytopenia
(2) Overheparinization
e. Infections
(1) Hepatitis
(2) Bacteremia
f. Other
(1) Perforated intestine
(2) Mechanical injury to donor cells
(3) NEC
8. Parental response to neonatal illness
a. Understanding of hemolytic process
b. Understanding of the course of treatment
c. Guilt related to birth of ''abnormal'' infant
d. Coping mechanism and support system

GOALS

1. Absence of kernicterus
2. Absence of anemia
3. Maximum therapeutic effect of phototherapy and/or exchange transfusion
4. Absence or resolution of complications of exchange transfusion
5. Successful parent-infant attachment
6. Before discharge, parents
   a. Verbalize understanding of etiology and management of infant's hemolytic disease
   b. Demonstrate ability to bathe, feed, and care for infant
   c. Understand need for close monitoring of Hct after discharge
   d. State plans for follow-up care

Potential problems	Expected outcomes	Nursing activities
■ Competition for albumin-binding sites Cold stress Hypoxia Drugs Hypoglycemia	■ Maximum availability of bilirubin-binding sites	■ Monitor temperature q4 hr Observe for respiratory distress (see Standard: *Neonatal respiratory distress*) Read literature regarding each drug infant receives; request alternate drug when indicated Monitor Dextrostix q4 hr Observe for signs and symptoms of hypoglycemia 　Jittery movements 　Apnea 　Lethargy 　Seizures 　Color change Notify physician if any of the aforementioned occurs and alter therapy as ordered
■ Hypoglycemia due to islet cell hyperplasia in Rh disease	■ Normoglycemia (45 to 120 mg/100 ml)	■ Keep IV at rate ordered Monitor Dextrostix q4 hr Observe for signs and symptoms of hypoglycemia 　Jittery movements 　Apnea 　Lethargy 　Seizures 　Color change Notify physician if any of the aforementioned occurs and after therapy as ordered
■ Kernicterus (bilirubin toxicity)	■ Absence of kernicterus	■ Monitor serum bilirubin q4 hr Observe for signs and symptoms of kernicterus 　Decreased sucking ability 　Reduced muscle tone 　High pitched cry 　Opisthotonos 　Muscle rigidity

Potential problems	Expected outcomes	Nursing activities
		Inform physician immediately if any of the aforementioned are present Prepare for immediate exchange transfusion

■ Hyperbilirubinemia; delayed resolution of hyperbilirubinemia related to use and function of phototherapy equipment	■ Maximum therapeutic effect of phototherapy
	Bilirubin level within normal limits
		■ Keep infant nude (can wear diaper)
		Keep eyes covered while under lights
		   Apply eye patches over closed lids
		   Do not apply too tightly
		   Remove q4 hr for eye care, and inspect for conjunctivitis
		Use plastic shield to separate lights from infant
		Assess energy output of lights each shift
		   Measure energy output by spectroradiometer
		   Record number of hours bulbs used
		   Change bulbs according to manufacturer's directions
		Monitor bilirubin and Hct q4 hr
		   Turn lights *off* when drawing blood
		   Skin color not indicative of serum bilirubin once phototherapy begins

■ Side effects of phototherapy
Hyperthermia
Increase H_2O loss
Increase in rate of metabolism
Loose stools
Maculopapular rash
	■ Absence/resolution of side effects and maintenance of fluid balance	■ Weigh infant daily
		Keep infant in Isolette
		Record temperature q4 hr
		Record intake and output
		   Offer H_2O between feedings
		   If IV is present, maintain at rate ordered
		   Measure urine specific gravity
		   Record color, consistency, and number of stools
		Observe skin for
		   Presence of rash
		   Skin color q4 hr (turn off lights to observe)
		Keep diaper area clean and dry
		Notify physician if any side effects occur

■ Complications of exchange transfusion
 	
Air embolus
 	
Cardiac arrhythmias
 	
Metabolic imbalance
	■ Absence or resolution of complications	■ Monitor and record infant's response to procedure
		Observe for and anticipate complications during and after procedure
		   Use stopcock to prevent air from entering umbilical line
		   Flush umbilical catheter before insertion
		   Attach infant to cardiac monitor
		   Have O_2 and suction in working order
		   Monitor and record
		      TPR and BP q10 min during procedure, then q15 min four times, q30 min six times
		      Amount of blood infused and withdrawn
		      Presence of arrhythmias
		Do procedure under radiant warmer
		Obtain baseline electrolytes
		Administer fresh blood as ordered
		Administer blood at room temperature
		Observe for signs and symptoms of hypocalcemia
		   Irritability
		   Tachycardia
		   Twitching
		   Prolonged Q-T interval
		Administer calcium as ordered
		   Infuse slowly
		   Observe for bradycardia
		Hypoglycemia (see aforementioned signs and symptoms)

Potential problems	Expected outcomes	Nursing activities

Sepsis
Aspiration
Perforated intestine
		Maintain strict sterile technique
		Aspirate stomach before procedure
		Keep NPO after procedure
		Observe for signs and symptoms of perforation
		  Abdominal distention
		  Bloody stools
		  Bilious vomiting
		  Hypotension
		  Pallor

Thrombocytopenia		Monitor platelet count
		Observe all puncture sites for bleeding
		No venipuncture or IM injections should be given until plate-
		  let count is known (unless absolutely necessary)
		After transfusion, notify physician of any symptoms of com-
		  plications, and administer corrective therapy as ordered

■ Bilirubin rebound fol- lowing exchange trans- fusion (caused by bind- ing of extravascular tissue bilirubin to fresh albumin)	■ Bilirubin level remains stable and within nor- mal limits	■ Montior serum bilirubin immediately after exchange transfusion and q4 hr Prepare for repeat exchange transfusion

■ Anemia
Vulnerable RBC re-
main in circulation
with phototherapy
In second week af-
ter exchange trans-
fusion as remaining
antibodies destroy
more cells
	■ Hct level is within normal
	limits
		■ Monitor Hct at birth and q4 hr during first 24 hours, then at least
		  q8 hr
		Assist physician with blood transfusion if indicated
		  Administer blood at room temperature
		  Administer at ordered rate
		  Monitor vital signs q15 min during administration
		Instruct parents
		  Explain physiology
		  Stress need for follow-up
		  Tell parents of possible need for transfusion after discharge

■ Difficulties in parent-
infant bonding due to
separation, guilt, and
anxiety
	■ Resolution of guilt feel-
	ings and beginning
	of parent-infant at-
	tachment process
		■ Promote parental involvement during hospitalization
		  Encourage early and frequent visitation and phone contact
		  Allow parents to verbalize feelings; reassure them that guilt
		    feelings are normal
		  If baby is under bililights, remove eye patches and allow par-
		    ents to feed while out from lights

■ Parents have insufficient
knowledge and/or
skills to comply with
discharge regimen
	■ Parents are able to
	Describe mechanism
	of hemolytic disease
	Explain rationale and
	effects of treatment
	Discuss the need for
	close observation
	and follow-up for
	anemia, and recog-
	nize possibility of
	need for future trans-
	fusion
	Demonstrate ability
	to care for infant
	State provisions for
	follow-up care
		■ Assessment of parents' knowledge of hemolytic disease and
		  treatments used
		Involve parents in infant's care
		Referral to local visiting nurse agency
		Teaching program,* including
		  Physiology of hemolytic disease
		  Rationale for and effects of treatment
		  Demonstration of newborn care; return demonstration by par-
		    ents
		  Potential for anemia and possible transfusion after discharge
		  Importance of follow-up care

*If responsibility of critical care nurse includes such follow-up care.

58 □ Neonatal necrotizing enterocolitis

Necrotizing enterocolitis (NEC) is an idiopathic, potentially lethal septic necrosis of the intestines occurring primarily in very immature newborn infants. The incidence of this problem has been increasing despite decreasing birth rates, perhaps because the incidence of prematurity is rising. Improved survival rates of premature and low birth weight infants enlarge the most susceptible population. Full-term infants are also susceptible to NEC (approximately one in five infants who develop this condition is full-term). Most at risk are infants weighing less than 1250 g.

The actual pathology varies. The integrity of the mucosal wall is compromised by a number of factors. The necrosis is diffuse or patchy, occurring most often along the right side within the ileum, ascending colon, or rectosigmoid. The mucosal ulceration may be followed by perforation with gas dissecting under the mucosa, peritonitis, and death. The mortality may be increased by 30% if peritonitis occurs. Disseminated intravascular coagulation (DIC) may result from the release of tissue thromboplastin by damaged bowel, further enhancing the risk of mortality.

Etiology is uncertain. Current theory hypothesizes that the immature infant overshoots the reflexive circulatory redistribution response to hypoxia or hypothermia. In the normal reflex response, blood is shunted from organs that tolerate ischemia comparatively well to those that would suffer irreversible damage if deprived of oxygen. This selective ischemia decreases mesenteric circulation. If extreme or prolonged, this results in reduced mucus secretion, which progresses to proteolysis and autodigestion. The mucosal ischemia provides an ideal situation for bacterial growth. The organisms involved are normal bowel flora; *Escherichia coli,* enterococci, alpha streptococcus, enterobacterium, and *Proteus.* Gas-forming bacteria invade areas damaged by proteolysis and autodigestion. This results in pneumatosis. The damaged bowel releases thromboplastin, promoting DIC and subsequently vascular thrombosis. DIC is a late sequela, and there is rapid clinical deterioration (within hours) when this develops. DIC usually cannot be reversed unless the bowel is resected. The entire clinical course may be as rapid as 4 to 48 hours.

Treatment of NEC is aimed at resting the injured bowel and managing any coagulation disorder and sepsis present. Usually surgery is not required. Exacerbation may occur if feeding is resumed too early. An infant who has recovered from NEC is still at risk for subsequent occurrence.

Surgical removal of all necrotic and acutely inflamed bowel is indicated when there are symptoms of peritonitis; progressive, intractable acidosis; or respiratory insufficiency. A temporary ileostomy or colostomy is created. Mechanical and functional abnormalities of the intestine may occur following surgery. These include stricture and short gut syndrome. Diagnosis of these problems may be made as long as 3 months postoperatively.

With early recognition of NEC, survival is better than 80%. The insidious onset and subtle nature of early symptoms and the rapid course of NEC make astute nursing observation critical in recognition and timely intervention.

ASSESSMENT

1. History of perinatal stress or other predisposing factors (recognizing that NEC may occur when none of these is evident)
   a. Prematurity
   b. Birth asphyxia
   c. Hypotension
   d. Respiratory distress
   e. Premature rupture of membranes
   f. Placenta previa or abruptio placentae
   g. Maternal sepsis
   h. Toxemia of pregnancy
   i. Breech or cesarean delivery
   j. Low birth weight (incidence increases at less than 1500 g)
   k. Umbilical vessel catheterization
   l. Patent ductus arteriosus
2. Abdominal girth measurement on admission and serially before feedings
3. Symptoms of infection, stress, hypoxia, and immunological abnormalities
4. Other nonspecific early symptoms
   a. Thermal instability
   b. Lethargy
   c. Metabolic acidosis
   d. Jaundice

e. Apnea

f. Vomiting

5. Poor absorption of feedings (it should be remembered that a majority of premature infants do not absorb their feedings initially)

6. Gastrointestinal symptoms (usually occur between 2 to 10 days after feeding is initiated and appear 12 to 24 hours after increasing gastric residuals are noted)

 a. Abdominal distention

 b. Vomiting (bilious emesis)

 c. Localized erythema and induration of abdominal wall

 d. Occult blood in stools

 e. Decreased bowel movements

7. Diagnostic radiographic results confirming NEC, including

 a. Nonspecific intestinal dilation appearing as multiple separate dilated loops with air-fluid levels in upright position

 b. Intraperitoneal air

 c. Pneumatosis cystoides intestinalis (linear strip or bubbles of gas alongside gas-filled loop; the bubbles may appear like cysts)

 d. Portal venous gas

8. Lab data results

 a. C and S reports

 b. Complete blood count with differential, prothrombin time (PT) and activated partial thromboplastin time (APTT), platelets

 c. Serum electrolytes

 d. Serum glucose

 e. Blood gas levels

 f. Blood in stools, emesis, nasogastric drainage

9. Advanced symptoms, including

 a. Hyperglycemia

 b. Frank intestinal bleeding

 c. Peritonitis (reddening or shininess of abdominal wall)

 d. Progressive DIC

 e. Metabolic acidosis

GOALS

1. Integrity of bowel

2. Adequate nutrition

3. Parents verbalize understanding of disease and therapeutic regimen

4. Parents demonstrate interest and desire in participating in care of patient

5. Infant thrives

6. Family unit remains functional

Potential problems	Expected outcomes	Nursing activities

■ Poor absorption of feedings (retained gastric contents are usually undigested formula; this progresses from clear formula at first to bile-tinged material)	■ Absorption of po intake adequate for growth	■ Successful therapy relies on early recognition
		  Aspirate gastric contents prior to each feeding, noting quality and quantity
		  Report increasing residuals or bile-stained material immediately
		Encourage and support breast-feeding (breast milk is more easily absorbed by newborn, especially premature infant)
		Parenteral alimentation as ordered by physician and prepared by pharmacist
		Monitor and record
		  Daily weight
		  Hourly intake and output
		  Clinitest q2 hr (less frequently when glucose tolerance has stabilized, usually after 2 days)
		  Serum electrolyte and osmolality per medical routine (usually daily for first week) for any imbalances

Dehydration and electrolyte imbalance resulting from poor absorption	Fluid and electrolyte balance	Monitor serum electrolytes and osmolality; urine output, specific gravity, and osmolality Notify physician of abnormalities and alter therapy as ordered

■ DIC (the onset may be more than 24 hours before the onset of NEC)	■ Absence or resolution of DIC	■ The underlying or associated problems must be ameliorated; e.g., sepsis, hypoxia, shock
		  Be alert to early suggestive signs, e.g., lethargy
		Observe for evidence of progressive bleeding
		  Examine skin; note pallor, ecchymoses, petechiae
		  Observe and test emesis, stools, and gastric residuals for positive Hematest

Potential problems	Expected outcomes	Nursing activities
		Be attentive to venipunctures and capillary heel sticks for prolonged bleeding
		Notify physician of abnormalities
		In the newborn, infections of bacterial and viral origin are the most common stimuli activating the clotting process
		Transfusions may be necessary as indicated by coagulation studies; sometimes exchange transfusions are done; heparin has been found to be less effective in newborns than in adults
		See Standard: *Disseminated intravascular coagulation*
■ Sepsis	■ Maximal protective resources maintained; absence or resolution of sepsis	■ Encourage and support breast-feeding
		Explain importance of breast milk in supplying the protective immunological activity of secretory IgA (IgA is the principal immunoglobulin in intestinal secretions and is lacking for several days in newborns)
	Minimal exposure to nosocomial infection	In addition, colostric leukocytes provide passive immunity against enteric pathogens
		Teach manual and pump expression techniques so that breast milk may be given if infant cannot suck at breast, requires tube feedings, small feedings, or NPO periods; keep breast milk in plastic (not glass) containers because leukocytes adhere to glass
		Use appropriate aseptic technique
		Particularly in relation to feeding and invasive procedures
		Change tubing q24 hr on all IVs and q8 hr on continuous feedings
		Remove NG tubes between intermittent feedings if residuals are not large
		The catheter is not only a potential reservoir for bacteria, but a foreign body that can cause irritability and inflammation in the tissue; such irritated or inflamed tissue may be susceptible to further damage (see description of pathology)
		NG tube should not be left in place for intermittent feedings if infant demonstrates discomfort
		NG tube may be left in place if there is no apparent irritation and if infant does not pull at it, since frequent reinsertion can be traumatic and may injure tissue
		Nasojejunal tubes should be changed q72 hr
		Opened formula should not be kept at room temperature for more than 4 hours; no more than a 4-hour supply of formula or breast milk should be assembled for continuous drip feedings; unfrozen breast milk should not be used after 72 hours in refrigerator
		Be alert to signs of sepsis in neonate to assure early treatment
		Monitor for
		Change in feeding pattern (usually first sign)
		Lethargy
		Irritability
		Temperature elevation in stable thermal environment
		Notify physician of any signs of infection
		Monitor potential infection sources, including culture results

Potential problems	Expected outcomes	Nursing activities
■ Parental anxiety, apprehension and misunderstanding Anxiety and apprehension do not follow continuum of progress; parents' perceptions and feelings may be labile Often both parents will not exhibit the same feelings at the same time	■ Parents' behavior demonstrates Reduced level of anxiety Ability to discuss concerns and fears, ask questions, and verbalize realistic expectations of potential outcomes	■ Assess parents' level of anxiety, perceptions, and depth of understanding Recognize denial and disbelief Appreciate and accept Encourage and strengthen each parent's ability to complement and support the other Allow parents to express feelings of remorse, helplessness, anger, guilt, and pain; encourage validation of feelings Assure parents that such feelings are normal Provide atmosphere that allows convenient and comfortable interaction with staff Provide continuity in assigning nurses to care for patient Provide ongoing explanations of all treatments and routine care, appropriate to parents' level of understanding Encourage questions Provide realistic information and reassurance Prepare parents in advance for potential complications as well as likely outcomes; this helps to ameliorate uncertainty and establish trust Allow parents to participate in infant's care as much as possible During the most critical periods, encourage visits Explain the rationale for minimal handling, and encourage contact such as stroking forehead or fingers
■ Compromised parent-infant attachment	■ Parents visit, call, and express concern	■ Assess parents' interactions with infant Share nuances of infant's behavior with parents; encourage verbal interactions with baby Reinforce appropriate patterns of behavior Talk to infant in front of and with parents Nurses must be aware of surrogate attachment patterns they develop with infant patients (especially those requiring intensive care) and avoid the unconscious exclusion of parents Encourage frequent parental visits Encourage phone calls between visits
■ Respiratory insufficiency related to abdominal distention	■ Adequate oxygenation Diaphragm movement is not inhibited	■ Note subtle changes in breathing pattern; intervene with assistance to minimize work of breathing and assure adequate ventilation; tilt warmer and position infant to minimize abdominal pressure on diaphragm Monitor Arterial blood gas values for any abnormalities Abdominal girth Note distention in relation to feeding Remove air from stomach q30 min and prn Note amount
■ Exacerbation of symptoms following treatment, or recurrence of symptoms	■ Resumption of feeding regimen with adequate absorption Bowel integrity	■ Maintain NPO for 7 to 10 days to rest injured bowel Resume feedings slowly in small amounts Do not continue feedings if residuals persist Avoid formula feedings Substrates in formula contribute to production of H_2 gas, which would augment pathogenic activity of gas-forming bacteria Serial abdominal girth measurements before feedings; note sudden or continuing increase

Potential problems	Expected outcomes	Nursing activities
■ Progressive inflammation and damage to mucosal wall of intestine	■ Integrity of bowel Absence or resolution of enterocolitis	■ Umbilical catheter should be removed, if NEC is suspected Prevent injury of gut wall Avoid excessive handling Do not palpate abdomen unnecessarily Avoid diapering Take axillary temperature Allow bowel to rest by withholding feedings; be attentive to infant's tolerance for po intake; monitor absorption of feedings; monitor for signs of perforation Apnea Shock Sudden drop in temperature Bradycardia Sudden listlessness Rag doll limpness Involuntary rigidity of abdomen Radiograph (radiograph is usually taken q4-6 hr) Notify physician of any abnormalities Administer medications and treatments as ordered
■ Perforation and/or peritonitis	■ Absence or resolution of peritonitis	■ Note increasing reddening or shininess of abdominal wall Monitor abdominal girth Notify physician of any changes Peritonitis is an indication for immediate surgery See following postoperative care

Postoperative care

Potential problems	Expected outcomes	Nursing activities
■ Sepsis and/or wound infection	■ Wound intact, well healed, infection free	■ Keep suture line clean; this may be a challenge due to proximity of stoma on the small abdomen of a premature infant; avoid dressings (may serve as reservoirs for infection) Monitor surgical site and temperature for any abnormalities and notify physician if abnormalities occur If sepsis occurs, administer antibiotics as ordered If wound infection occurs, administer antibiotics and local wound care as ordered
■ Respiratory insufficiency	■ Adequate oxygenation	■ Administer chest physiotherapy prn Assisted ventilation as indicated Monitor arterial blood gas levels; breathing pattern
■ Skin breakdown from enzymes in ileal drainage (The immature infant's skin is less resistant to excoriation than others)	■ Skin will remain clean, dry, and intact	■ Improvise appropriate stoma bags Infant urine collection bags may be cut and shaped for this purpose Plastic medicine cups can be adopted by cutting stoma-size hole in bottom of cup; then aspirate cup contents prn Karaya powder is helpful Monitor skin condition
■ Wound disruption due to catabolism	■ Wound heals Weight gain Closure of colostomy or ileostomy	■ Assure adequate nutrition Feedings will be resumed via NG tube Good skin care Maintain aseptic technique Monitor Daily weights Caloric intake
■ Electrolyte imbalance	■ Fluid and electrolyte balance within normal limits	■ Accurately record intake and output including all drainage q1 hr Maintenance IVs should be augmented with replacement for bowel secretions according to physician's order

Potential problems	Expected outcomes	Nursing activities
■ Dehydration from ileostomy diarrhea especially if more than 50% of small intestine was removed	■ Adequate hydration Adequate absorption of nutrients	■ Accurate monitoring of intake and output to assess fluid balance and determine replacement needs Appropriate IV therapy as ordered, including total parenteral nurition Patient may have to be kept NPO until ileostomy is closed
■ Short gut syndrome may be protracted; this may be due to size of portion that remains or it may be due to disease process	■ Parents verbalize signs and symptoms of short gut syndrome and bowel stricture	■ Teach parents to note and report changes in feeding patterns, bowel patterns, abdominal distention, weight loss, vomiting, diarrhea, etc.
■ Parental anxiety and/or apprehension	■ Parents demonstrate confidence in their own child care abilities relative to this infant's special needs Parents verbalize or demonstrate understanding of discharge management of feeding difficulties	■ Enable parents to continue participating in infant's care after immediate postoperative period, including ostomy care; colostomy is closed before discharge after weight gain improves Help parents become familiar with infant's individuality Give parents appropriate phone numbers, etc. Assure them their calls are welcome any time and that you are interested Suggest some specific times to encourage them to call even if there are no identified problems Arrange appropriate follow-up care Prepare parents for homecoming Explain to parents that it may take several weeks or even months for remaining bowel to function adequately Multiple formula changes may be necessary Parents should be informed that rehospitalization may be necessary for appropriate IV therapy, including hyperalimentation These explanations may have to be repeated often; parents will need encouragement

59 □ Croup syndrome

Acute infections of the larynx and trachea occur in infants and young children. These infections are of great significance because of the small size of the airways in children. An inflammatory process generated by an infection can render these airways even smaller.

The term *croup* is commonly applied to a group of infectious conditions characterized by a brassy cough. Inspiratory stridor is often present. Stridor is a crowing noise that occurs on inspiration as air passes through a narrowed, edematous airway. Stridor is indicative of a high respiratory obstruction. Substernal inspiratory retraction may be present and also indicates upper airway obstruction. Hoarseness or aphonia are variable findings that may or may not be present.

There are a large number of infectious agents that can cause croup. Viral agents have now been identified as the cause of croup in a high percentage of patients. Parainfluenza virus is probably the most common agent. Other viral agents include adenoviruses, respiratory syncytial, and influenza. Croup due to a virus usually has a gradual onset and course, although an influenza virus may cause an abrupt onset and severe course.

Bacterial agents that cause croup are *Haemophilus influenzae* type B, *Corynebacterium diphtheriae,* pneumococci, and group A streptococci. *H. influenzae* croup is usually an extreme emergency. It is usually characterized by supraglottic obstruction with a red, swollen epiglottis and has a rapid course.

Viral croup is seen more frequently in the younger child from age 3 months to 3 years. Bacterial croup is seen more commonly in children from 3 years to 7 years. Males have a higher incidence of croup than females. There is no known reason for this. Croup seems to occur more frequently in cold weather.

Allergic laryngeal edema can be severe and dangerous. Inhaled irritants may produce laryngeal spasm in some children. Croup syndrome may be produced by foreign body aspiration and subsequent subglottic obstruction. Croup is a classical example of a respiratory infection in which the main problem is upper airway obstruction. Laryngeal edema and spasm are the major causes of this obstruction. The significant physiological problem that results from this is hypoxemia. Low arterial PO_2 is frequently seen, whereas PCO_2 retention is unusual. The PCO_2 is low because of the hyperventilation stimulated by the hypoxemia. There are several clinical forms of croup. *Laryngotracheobronchitis,* also known as *viral* or *subglottic croup,* is the most common form. As the name suggests, the infection involves the subglottic area of the larynx, trachea, and bronchi. The onset is gradual with a history of upper respiratory infection prior to the appearance of the croupy cough and stridor. The temperature is not usually elevated. Symptoms of respiratory distress appear as the laryngeal obstruction progresses. Stridor becomes associated with sternal, subcostal, and abdominal retractions. The expiratory phase of respiration is prolonged and may be associated with wheezing. Breath sounds are decreased with rhonchi and scattered rales. Cyanosis is a late sign and is indicative of severe obstruction.

The management of viral croup includes the use of mist to reduce laryngeal edema. Syrup of ipecac has been effective in relieving the symptoms by inducing vomiting. The use of corticosteroids has produced good results as well. Racemic epinephrine has been used recently with success. It is administered by intermittent positive pressure or nebulized mist. If these measures are not successful in reducing the degree of respiratory distress, an artificial airway must be considered.

The majority of children with laryngotracheobronchitis usually do not progress beyond the cough, stridor, and mild distress stage. The condition runs its course within 3 to 7 days with complete recovery. Of all the children with laryngotracheobronchitis, only a small percentage will need to be cared for in an intensive care unit.

The most severe form is *acute epiglottitis,* also referred to as *bacterial* or *supraglottic croup.* As previously mentioned, it is most commonly caused by *H. influenzae* type B. It has a rapid, progressive, and fulminant course. The onset is abrupt. The younger child usually presents with high fever and respiratory distress. The older child complains of a severe sore throat and difficulty in swallowing. Pooling of secretions in the pharynx and drooling are common signs because of the dysphagia. This child usually assumes a sitting position with chin thrust forward, mouth open and tongue slightly protruding. The voice may be absent, hoarse, or muffled. Temperature is elevated. Within hours after onset, the child may be in marked respiratory distress with stridor, retractions, and nasal flaring. The diagnosis is made by visualizing the large, edematous, cherry red epiglottis. This should *only* be done in a controlled setting with a team ready to perform an immediate tracheostomy. Stimulation of the epiglottis while attempting to visualize it has produced complete obstruction and death. Lateral radiographs of the larynx may be of value in confirming the enlarged epiglottis without resorting to direct visualization. Leukocytosis of more than 15,000/ mm^3 is usually present. Blood cultures will identify *H. influenzae* type B (or other causative organisms).

When the diagnosis of epiglottitis is suspected, the approach should be to provide an artificial airway. If an airway is not provided promptly, the mortality may be quite high. Preparation should be for controlled intubation or tracheostomy. Corticosteroids have not proven to be of any significant value. Parenteral antibiotics are indicated. Ampicillin is the drug of choice.

The child wth epiglottitis usually responds rapidly to antibiotics and may be extubated or decannulated in 48 to 72 hours.

The nurse in the critical care area will most certainly be involved in the care of all children with acute epiglottitis.

ASSESSMENT

1. Recent history of minor upper respiratory infection
2. Physical signs and symptoms
   a. Laryngotracheobronchitis
      (1) Characteristic brassy cough

(2) Inspiratory stridor (crowing noise)

(3) Retraction

(4) Prolongation of exhalation with wheezing

(5) Diminished breath sounds

(6) Rhonchi and scattered rales

(7) Hypoxemia

  b. Acute epiglottitis

    (1) High fever

    (2) Brassy cough

    (3) Inspiratory stridor

    (4) Dysphagia

    (5) Retractions

    (6) Nasal flaring

    (7) Irritability

    (8) Restlessness

    (9) Tripod position—sitting up, arms in front, chin thrust forward, mouth open and drooling

    (10) Hypoxemia

3. Monitor lab data for results of

  a. Lateral neck and chest radiographs

  b. WBC and differential

  c. Throat culture

  d. Blood culture

  e. Serum *H. influenzae* antigen

  f. Arterial blood gas levels

4. Developmental level of the child

a. Effect of illness on child (guilt, punishment)

b. Effect of hospitalization on child

  (1) Fear of strangers

  (2) Fear of bodily harm

  (3) Fear of separation and abandonment

c. Developmental tasks according to age

5. Response of parents to child's illness and hospitalization

  a. Level of anxiety

  b. Degree of understanding of illness and therapeutic management

  c. Guilt

GOALS

1. Resolution of acute respiratory distress
2. Relief of upper airway obstruction
3. Absence of infection
4. Normal cardiac function
5. Normal fluid and electrolyte balance
6. Normal sleep/wake pattern
7. Child's and parent's behavior indicates a reduction in anxiety
8. Hospitalization as a positive developmental experience for the child
9. Parent's behavior demonstrates effective coping mechanisms

Potential problems	Expected outcomes	Nursing activities

▪ Acute respiratory failure related to laryngeal obstruction	▪ Respiratory function normal as indicated by arterial blood gas levels	▪ Prevent by
		  Continuous monitoring of respiratory status
		  Implementation of medical and nursing regimen to provide and maintain adequate respiratory function
		Monitor for
		  Change in arterial blood gas levels
		  Change in degree of respiratory distress
		    Tachypnea
		    Tachycardia
		    Retractions
		    Nasal flaring
		    Color
		    Stridor
		    Breath sounds
		    Posture
		    Mentation
		NOTE: A decrease in stridor, increase in heart rate, and decrease in respiratory rate are indicative of an emergency
		Intervention if problem occurs
		  Pediatric emergency procedure
		  Intubation
		  Tracheostomy
		  Mechanical ventilation (see Standard: *Mechanical ventilation*)
		NOTE: Epiglottitis of acute onset represents one of the few true pediatric emergencies

Potential problems	Expected outcomes	Nursing activities

■ Fluid and/or electrolyte imbalance related to degree of respiratory distress	■ Weight within normal limits
	Electrolytes within normal parameters
		■ Prevent by
		  Parenteral maintenance
		  Fluid replacement
		  Electrolyte replacement according to serum levels and maintenance requirements
		Monitor for
		  Change in fluid and nutritional intake
		  Change in weight
		  Change in state of hydration
		    Mucous membranes
		    Skin turgor
		    Thirst
		    Tears
		    Behavior
		    Urine specific gravity
		  Change in indices of intravascular volume
		    BP
		    P
		    CVP
		    Urine output and specific gravity
		  Changes in lab data
		    Serum electrolytes
		    Hct
		Intervention if problem occurs
		  Frequent assessment of vital signs
		  Accurate measurement and recording of intake and output
		  Daily weights
		  Accurate parenteral administration of fluids and electrolytes
		    Monitor IV q1 hr for rate of flow and amount infused (use infusion pump if available)
		    Observe IV site q1 hr
		  Monitor lab data

■ Infection related to presence of parainfluenza virus, *H. influenzae,* group A streptococcus, or pneumococci	■ Infection free
	Complication free
		■ Prevent by
		  Proper handwashing techniques
		  Administration of antibiotics as ordered
		Monitor for
		  Temperature elevation greater than 101° F (38.2° C)
		  Extension of infectious process to other regions of the respiratory tract such as the middle ear and the lungs
		  Lab values
		    WBC count and differential
		    Cultures—throat and blood
		    Chest radiograph
		Intervention if problem occurs
		  Temperature elevation
		    Check temperature q2-4 hr or as indicated
		    Administer antipyretics as ordered
		    Tepid sponge
		    Cooling mattress
		    Encourage fluids (as per appropriate route)
		  Extension of infectious process
		    Assess respiratory status as indicated
		    Institute mode of therapy as per physician's orders
		      1. Antibiotics
		      2. Mist tent
		      3. Chest physiotherapy

Potential problems	**Expected outcomes**	**Nursing activities**

■ Congestive heart failure related to degree of respiratory failure	■ Cardiac function within normal limits	■ Prevent by
		  Following medical and nursing regimen in the management of respiratory distress and failure (see Problem, Acute respiratory failure)
		Monitor for
		  Tachycardia
		  Tachypnea
		  Dyspnea—grunting, nasal flaring, coughing
		  Weight increase
		  Urinary output decrease
		  Feeding difficulty
		Intervention if problem occurs
		  Frequent assessment of vital signs
		  Fluid restriction as ordered
		  Daily weights
		  Accurate measurement and recording of intake and output
		  Sitting position
		  Careful feeding to avoid aspiration
		  Administration of (as ordered by physician)
		    Digoxin
		    Furosemide
		    O_2
		    Chest physiotherapy

■ Sleep deprivation related to respiratory distress	■ Sleep/wake pattern restored to pre-illness state	■ Prevent by
		  Decreased amount of sensory stimulation
		  Minimal disturbance of patient by nursing and other health team members
		  Proper body positioning to ease the work of breathing and provide for maximum comfort
		  Decreased amount of emotional stress; allow parents to remain with child
		Monitor for
		  Change in level of consciousness
		    Difficult to arouse
		    Responds to verbal stimuli
		    Responds to painful stimuli
		  Change in level of mentation
		    Confusion
		    Disorientation
		  Change in mood
		    Passive
		    Aggressive
		    Crying
		    Irritable
		  Change in work of breathing
		    Degree of difficulty
		    Degree of comfort
		  NOTE: Changes in any or all of the aforementioned may indicate hypoxemia
		Intervention if problem occurs
		  Plan a sleep/wake pattern by
		    Decreasing the amount of stimuli (noise) and limiting time when nursing and medical team activities take place
		    Utilizing sleep-promoting activities (stroking, rubbing, gentle soft voices)
		    Providing for maximal comfort by adjusting body position to ease the work of breathing (head elevated)
		    Sedatives are contraindicated

Potential problems	Expected outcomes	Nursing activities

■ Emotional stress related to trauma of hospitalization	■ Reduced emotional trauma	■ Prevent by
		   Minimal separation of parents and child
		   Continuity of care
		Monitor for
		   Presence of separation anxiety
		   Phase of separation anxiety (if present)
		      Protest
		      Despair
		      Denial
		   Presence of fears
		      Bodily harm
		      Mutilation
		      Loss of body integrity
		      Strangers
		      Unfamiliar surroundings
		   Presence of feelings of
		      Guilt
		      Wrongdoing
		      Loss of love
		      Anger
		Intervention if problem occurs
		   Separation anxiety
		      Presence of parents
		      Parent participation
		      Presence of security object
		   Fears
		      Orientation to surroundings
		      Consistent nursing personnel
		      Correct misconceptions
		      Provide accurate information
		   Feelings
		      Verbalization
		      Play
		      Drawing

■ Family crisis related to
   Illness of child
   Need for hospitalization
   Lack of knowledge about condition
   Guilt
   Anxiety
	■ Facilitate coping mechanisms within the family	■ Assess degree of stress and ability to cope
		Determine level of understanding of the child's condition, treatment, and need for hospitalization
		   Offer factual information
		   Clarify misconceptions
		Encourage parental expression of feelings about illness and hospitalization
		   Establish relationship
		   Plan time for interaction
		   Reassure parents
		   Support parents
		Determine, with the parents, their degree of involvement in the care of their child
		Maintain parental sense of adequacy to care for their child
		Periodically evaluate the effect of the interventions on the parents' behavior

60 □ Asthma/status asthmaticus

Asthma is a reversible, episodic, obstructive condition affecting the lower respiratory tract. It is characterized by wheezing and various degrees of dyspnea. The wheezing is caused as airway flow is restricted by bronchospasm, edema, and increased mucus production.

The onset of asthma is usually in early childhood, between the ages of 3 and 8 years. Boys are affected more than girls in the early years. During adolescence and thereafter, both are affected equally. Asthma may be controlled but not cured.

All children with asthma have a hypersensitivity of the smooth muscle of the airways to a variety of factors. Bronchospasm may occur in response to inhalants such as dust, molds, animal hair, and airborne pollens. Cold air and rapid changes of temperature may provoke an asthmatic attack. Foods, as a source of allergy, also may precipitate an attack. Such foods include egg white, cow's milk, fish, chocolate, and nuts.

It is well-documented that asthma is a complex disorder with biochemical, infectious, immunological, endocrine, and psychological factors playing roles of varying degrees of importance.

Episodes of asthma may be insidious or abrupt in onset. Those associated with infections are frequently insidious and prolonged, whereas those associated with specific allergens are abrupt and brief once the allergen is removed.

The asthmatic episode is characterized by increasing dyspnea, coughing, wheezing, and a prolongation of the expiratory phase of respiration. Coarse and fine rales are present. The episode is progressive, and as pulmonary ventilation becomes more limited, the heart and respiratory rates increase along with retractions, nasal flaring, and cyanosis. The skin may be flushed and moist with sweating prominent. The child becomes restless and fatigued. Abdominal pain may be present if coughing is severe. Very often the child will vomit, and this will somewhat relieve the symptoms. This is only temporary, however.

Diagnosis is made by family history of atopic disease, child's history of episodes of coughing and wheezing, clinical signs and symptoms, lab data, and response to previous therapy.

The conventional mode of therapy during an asthmatic episode is primarily pharmacological. The medications used are those specific for bronchodilatation, relief of mucosal edema, liquefaction, and expectoration of mucus. These medications include epinephrine, phenylephrine, ephedrine, aminophylline, and theophylline. Isoproterenol by inhalation is also used. Other therapy includes moisturized oxygen and intravenous fluid administration.

If the child fails to respond clinically to the administration of the aforementioned medications, the diagnosis of *status asthmaticus* is generally made. There is no precise definition for status asthmaticus. It is said to exist when the asthmatic episode is severe and unresponsive to conventional therapy.

Status asthmaticus is a pediatric medical emergency. Therapy is directed toward maintaining adequate ventilation. Arterial blood gas levels are monitored closely. Moisturized oxygen is administered because these children are usually hypoxemic. The usual pharmacological agents are administered and, in addition, corticosteroids. Intravenous fluid replacement and maintenance is important to ensure adequate hydration. Measures are taken to correct the associated metabolic acidosis in the form of administration of sodium bicarbonate. Antibiotics are given as indicated.

If respiratory failure ensues, assisted ventilation by a mechanical respirator may be required.

The nurse in the critical care area will be involved in the care of those children with a severe episode of asthma and, of course, of those with status asthmaticus.

ASSESSMENT

1. Family history of allergy
2. History of eczema or food intolerance
3. History of episodes of coughing and wheezing
4. Recent history of infection
5. Physical signs and symptoms
   a. Dyspnea
   b. Wheezing
   c. Productive cough
   d. Prolonged expiratory phase of respiration
   e. Coarse and fine rales
   f. Tachypnea
   g. Retractions
   h. Nasal flaring
   i. Tachycardia

497

j. Cyanosis
k. Perspiration
l. Apprehension
m. Restlessness
n. Fatigue
6. Response to conventional pharmacological therapy
   a. Sympathomimetics
   b. Theophyllines
7. Monitor lab data for results of
   a. Arterial blood gas levels
   b. Throat and sputum smear and culture (eosinophilia is common)
   c. Chest radiograph
   d. WBC count
   e. Pulmonary function studies

GOALS

1. Resolution of acute respiratory distress
   a. Relief of bronchospasm
   b. Relief of mucosal edema
   c. Removal of secretions
2. Normal fluid and electrolyte balance
3. Absence of infection
4. Normal sleep/wake pattern
5. Supportive therapy for child and parents during asthmatic crisis
6. Discharge planning for the control of chronic asthma

Potential problems	Expected outcomes	Nursing activities

■ Acute respiratory failure related to
Bronchospasm
Mucosal edema
Mucus production
	■ Respiratory function within normal limits	■ Prevent by
		  Continuous monitoring of child's respiratory status
		  Implementation of medical regimen
		    Bronchodilating adrenergic drugs
		    Vasoconstrictive adrenergic drugs
		    Corticosteroids
		    Moisturized O_2
		    Hydration
		  Implementation of nursing regimen
		    Percussion and vibration
		    Postural drainage
		    Suctioning
		    Body positioning to enhance respiratory effort and to facilitate removal of secretions
		Monitor for
		  Change in arterial blood gas levels
		  Change in response to pharmacological agents
		  Change in degree of the following parameters
		    Respiratory rate and quality
		    Heart rate
		    Wheeze
		    Cough
		    Breath sounds
		    Color
		    Mentation
		NOTE: Significant decrease in or absence of inspiratory breath sounds, severe retractions during inspiration, use of accessory muscles, diminished level of consciousness, and cyanosis despite administration of O_2 are signs of acute respiratory failure and are considered a medical emergency
		Intervention if problem occurs
		  Intubation
		  Mechanical ventilation (see Standard: *Mechanical ventilation*)

Potential problems	Expected outcomes	Nursing activities

■ Acidosis related to respiratory insufficiency	■ Serum pH within normal limits	■ Prevent by
		  Continuous monitoring of respiratory status
		  Monitoring of serial arterial blood gas levels
		  Respiratory support
		Monitor for
		  Change in arterial blood gas levels
		Intervention if problem occurs
		  Respiratory support
		  Drug therapy
		NOTE: Acidosis must be corrected for pharmacological agents to be effective

■ Fluid and/or electrolyte imbalance related to degree of respiratory distress	■ Weight within normal limits
	  Electrolytes within normal parameters
		■ Prevent by
		  Parenteral maintenance
		  Fluid replacement
		  Electrolyte replacement according to serum levels and maintenance requirements as ordered
		Monitor for
		  Change in fluid and nutritional intake
		  Change in weight
		  Change in state of hydration
		    Mucous membranes
		    Skin turgor
		    Thirst
		    Tears
		    Behavior
		    Urine specific gravity
		  Change in indices of intravascular volume
		    BP
		    P
		    CVP
		    Urine output and specific gravity
		  Changes in lab data
		    Serum electrolytes
		    Hct
		Intervention if problem occurs
		  Frequent assessment of vital signs
		  Accurate measurement and recording of intake and output
		  Daily weights
		  Accurate parenteral administration of fluids and electrolytes
		    Monitor IV q1 hr for rate of flow and amount infused (use infusion pump if available)
		    Observe IV site q1 hr
		  Monitor lab data

■ Respiratory infection related to asthmatic episode	■ Infection free
	  Complication free
		■ Prevent by
		  Administration of antibiotics and sulfonamides to which invading organisms are sensitive as ordered by physician
		NOTE: Penicillin and related semisynthetic derivatives (i.e., ampicillin and oxacillin) are used cautiously because of known possible serious reactions when used with asthmatics
		Monitor for
		  Temperature elevation greater than 101° F (38.2° C)
		  Change in color of sputum
		  Extension of infectious process to further areas of respiratory tract
		  Lab values
		    WBC count and differential
		    Cultures—throat, sputum, blood
		    Chest radiograph

Potential problems	Expected outcomes	Nursing activities

		Intervention if problem occurs
		  Temperature elevation
		    Check temperature q2-4 hr or as indicated
		    Administer antipyretics as ordered
		    Tepid sponge
		    Cooling mattress
		    Encourage fluid intake (as per appropriate route)
		  Extension of infectious process
		    Assess respiratory status as indicated
		    Institute mode of therapy as per physician's orders
		      1. Antibiotics, sulfonamides
		      2. Humidified O_2
		      3. Chest physiotherapy

■ Sleep deprivation related to respiratory distress	■ Sleep/wake pattern restored to preillness state	■ Prevent by
		  Decreased amount of sensory stimulation
		  Minimal disturbance of patient by nurse and other health team members
		  Proper body positioning to ease the work of breathing and to provide for maximum comfort
		  Decreased emotional stress; allow parents to remain with child
		Monitor for
		  Change in level of consciousness
		    Difficult to arouse
		    Responds to verbal stimuli
		    Responds to painful stimuli
		  Change in level of mentation
		    Confusion
		    Disorientation
		  Change in mood
		    Passive
		    Aggressive
		    Crying
		    Irritable
		  Change in work of breathing
		    Degree of difficulty
		    Degree of comfort
		NOTE: Changes in any or all of the aforementioned may indicate hypoxemia
		Intervention if problem occurs
		  Plan a sleep/wake pattern by
		    Decreasing the amount of stimuli (noise) and limiting time when nursing and medical team activities take place
		    Utilizing sleep-promoting activities (stroking, rubbing, gentle soft voices)
		    Providing for maximal comfort by adjusting body position to ease the work of breathing (head elevated)
		    Sedative contraindicated

■ Increased anxiety level of child and parents related to severity of asthmatic episode	■ Reduced anxiety level as demonstrated by behavior of child and parents	■ Prevent by
		  Therapeutic intervention to relieve symptoms
		  Accurate information as to physical status
		  Establish a trusting relationship; provide reassurance
		Monitor for
		  Change in facial expression
		  Change in body posture
		  Change in mood
		  Change in behavior

Potential problems	Expected outcomes	Nursing activities

		Intervention if problem occurs
		  Establish a trusting relationship
		  Encourage verbalization related to asthma and asthmatic episodes
		  Convey accurate information
		  Reassure child and parents as to positive outcome
		  Do not leave child or parents alone during crisis
		  Evaluate effectiveness of nursing interventions as demonstrated by level of anxiety of child and parents

■ Family crisis related to
  Illness of child
  Need for hospitalization
  Lack of knowledge about condition
  Guilt
  Anxiety
	■ Coping mechanisms within the family facilitated	■ Assess degree of stress and ability to cope
		Determine level of understanding of the child's condition, treatment, and need for hospitalization
		Offer factual information
		Clarify misconceptions
		Encourage parental expression of feelings about illness and hospitalization
		  Establish relationship
		  Plan time for interaction
		  Reassure parents
		  Support parents
		Determine with the parents their degree of involvement in the care of their child
		Maintain parental sense of adequacy to care for their child
		Periodically evaluate the effect of the interventions on the parents' behavior

■ Insufficient control of asthma related to increasing frequency of episodes	■ Control of chronic asthma	■ Assess level of understanding of disease process and implications on child and family
		Establish teaching plan to include
		  Explanation of disease
		  Signs and symptoms of impending asthmatic attack
		  Factors influencing asthma
		    Allergens
		    Respiratory irritants
		    Upper respiratory infection
		    Exercise
		    Emotional upset
		  Home management
		    Medication (purpose, dosage, and time taken)
		    Medical follow-up
		    Breathing exercises
		    Supportive therapy
		Evaluate parents' and child's knowledge of home health routine by having them verbalize information

61 □ Reye's syndrome

Reye's syndrome is an acute toxic encephalopathy and fatty degeneration of viscera affecting mainly the liver, brain, and kidney. The encephalopathy consists of cerebral swelling without evidence of inflammation. Its pathogenesis is not understood.

Reye's syndrome occurs in children from infancy through adolescence as a sequela to acute or mild febrile infections, usually involving the upper respiratory tract and accompanied by anorexia. This prodrome may last from 1 day to 2 weeks, and the child usually demonstrates spontaneous improvement until severe sudden vomiting occurs. This vomiting characterizes the onset of Reye's syndrome.

Deterioration is rapid with fever, hyperventilation, irritability, lethargy, confusion, and hypertonia progressing to convulsions and coma. Decorticate/decerebrate movement and respiratory arrest ensue if there is no intervention. This course has been classified into five stages* (see Assessment).

The duration of the entire course may be less than 24 hours, or it may last 1 week or more. The outcome is usually apparent within 3 to 4 days. Prognosis seems to be related to the rate of progress through the disease stages and the stage at which supportive therapy is initiated. Neurological impairment is a frequent sequela. Mortality is 50% to 75%. Death is usually attributed to increasing intracranial pressure secondary to cerebral edema.

Hypotheses regarding the etiology of Reye's syndrome have suggested that susceptibility is related to exposure to viruses or toxins, whereas others suggest that these factors precipitate the syndrome in already susceptible individuals. There may be an interaction between a virus and a toxin. Or the biochemical response to such an interaction may be due to an enzymatic deficiency or a Krebs cycle defect. The syndrome may actually represent the similar clinical and pathological manifestations of a variety of etiologically unrelated conditions.

Reye's syndrome is a multisystem disease affecting the respiratory, central nervous, renal, metabolic, and cardiovascular systems. Therapy consists of empirically based, supportive regimens. The focus of treatment is on maintaining homeostatic function through the acute phase and preserving neurological integrity. Most symptoms seem to be reversible, provided there is no brain damage from hypoxia.

ASSESSMENT

1. Prodromal upper respiratory infection and/or viral syndrome
2. Signs and symptoms
   a. Severe vomiting
   b. High fever
   c. Tachypnea with respiratory alkalosis and marked dyspnea
   d. Confusion/delirium/agitation
   e. Hypertonus
   f. Convulsions
   g. Coma
   Deterioration is rapid
3. Results of lab and diagnostic procedures, including
   a. Serum glucose, electrolytes, and urea
   b. Increased serum ammonia
   c. Complete blood count with differential
   d. Acid-base status
   e. Prolonged prothrombin time
   f. Liver function tests (note elevated SGPT, SGOT)
   g. Arterial blood gas levels
   h. Cerebrospinal fluid
      (1) C and S
      (2) Chemistry (note low glucose level in cerebrospinal fluid)
   i. Liver biopsy (note microvesicular fat droplets)
   j. EEG
   k. A typical pattern may be observed, but this is not in itself diagnostic
4. Presence of specific disease stage
   a. Stage 1
      (1) Vomiting, lethargy, sleepiness
      (2) Abnormal liver function tests
      (3) Type 1 EEG
   b. Stage 2
      (1) Disorientation, delirium, combativeness, hyperventilation, hyperactive reflexes
      (2) Type 2 EEG

*Lovejoy, F. H., et al.: Clinical staging of Reye's syndrome, Am. J. Dis. Child. **128:**36-41, 1974.

c. Stage 3
   (1) Hyperventilation, decorticate rigidity, and obtunded state
   (2) Type 2 EEG
d. Stage 4
   (1) Deepening coma, decerebrate rigidity, loss of oculocephalic reflexes, fixed pupils with hippus, dysconjugate eye movements
   (2) Improved liver function
   (3) Type 3 or 4 EEG
e. Stage 5
   (1) Seizures, loss of deep tendon reflexes, respiratory arrest, flaccidity
   (2) Liver function may be normal
   (3) Type 4 EEG

5. Patient/family's level of anxiety related to disease condition, signs and symptoms, and therapeutic interventions

GOALS

1. Reduction of parents' anxiety and feelings of inadequacy in coping with sudden acute life-threatening situation
2. Adequate oxygenation and tissue perfusion
3. Adequate hydration and electrolyte balance
4. Intracranial pressure readings within normal limits
5. Cardiac, renal, hepatic, and respiratory function within normal limits
6. Absence of neurological deficit or mental impairment
7. Resumption of preillness activity level

Potential problems	Expected outcomes	Nursing activities

■ Parents' anxiety related to disease condition and therapy; they may feel confused, frightened, and guilty	■ Reduction of parents' anxiety and feelings of guilt and inadequacy
	
	Parents will be able to describe events in the course of child's disease without assigning inappropriate correlations
		■ Provide support to parents
		   Reassure parents that they gave appropriate care, took correct action, and sought help in a timely manner
		   Describe what is known about Reye's syndrome
		   Explain procedures
		   Explain the child's status and anticipated course
		   Assure parents that it is not common for siblings to contract the same disease
		   Allow parents to express their feelings
		   Time and attention must be given to help parents cope with the suddenness of the situation (and possibly rapid deterioration) and the sense of helplessness in the face of a problem that has incomplete medical answers
		   Allow parents to be at patient's bedside and to touch and stroke the child

■ Dehydration and electrolyte imbalance
 	
Shock related to dehydration, reduced cardiac output, neurogenic factors, or coagulation disorder
 	
Cardiac arrhythmias secondary to hypokalemia associated with increased aldosterone secretion, which accompanies dehydration
	■ Fluid and electrolyte balance
	
	Hemodynamic stability
	
	Absence of cardiac arrhythmias
		■ Monitor strictly the hourly intake and output and record; include medications given and blood specimens taken
		Replace NG drainage according to physician's orders
		Monitor and record
		   Peripheral pulses
		   Skin temperature of hands and feet
		   Skin color
		   CVP, BP, and P (CVP should be maintained at 3 to 8 cm H_2O or as ordered)
		   Hct should be maintained at 40% (this index is falsely elevated due to fluid restriction)
		   Hematest results of stools and gastric drainage
		   Lab data q4 hr
		      Serum osmolality; BUN (these values will be altered not only by hydration, but also by therapeutic administration of urea and osmotic diuretics)
		      Serum electrolytes, creatinine, and glucose q4-8 hr
		   Cardiac rate and rhythm continuously by oscilloscope
		Notify physician of abnormalities and initiate appropriate intervention, according to unit protocol or as ordered; this may include administration of
		Fluids
		Cardiotonic, vasopressor, or antiarrhythmic medications
		Diuretics
		Blood products

Potential problems	Expected outcomes	Nursing activities
■ Respiratory distress Alkalosis secondary to hyperventilation	■ Absence/resolution of respiratory distress Acid-base balance	■ Administer chest physiotherapy q1 hr, and reposition patient unless contraindicated; administer O_2 therapy with humidification if ordered (monitor arterial blood gas results) Observe respirations and assess breath sounds Notify physician of abnormalities, and alter therapy as ordered Assist in intubation and mechanical ventilation if needed, as ordered Hyperventilation is used to maintain Pco_2 at 20 to 25 mm Hg See Standard: *Mechanical ventilation*
■ Rapidly progressive neurological deficit due to cerebral edema Cerebral perfusion is decreased due to increased intracranial pressure; the resulting hypoxia may be exacerbated by hypoxemic condition	■ Neurological function within normal limits Cerebral perfusion pressure at or greater than 50 mm Hg Resolution of cerebral edema	■ Assess neurological status q1 hr Check reflexes: Babinski's, deep tendon, doll's eye, pupillary Note posturing Assess level of consciousness NOTE: If pancuronium bromide is being used to paralyze patient for mechanical ventilation, only the pupils can be checked; posturing may be noted as a dose wears off Note seizure activity; record Type Foci Frequency Duration Position patient with head elevated 30 degrees Avoid sudden position changes Take seizure precautions, including restraints and padded siderails; see Standard: *Seizures* Monitor and record q1 hr BP Arterial blood gas levels and pH Intake and output Fluid intake is restricted to one half to two thirds the daily maintenance needs Monitor intracranial pressure continuously Direct measurement of intracranial pressure is indicated in patients with Stage 2 signs and symptoms (see Assessment) Calculate and record cerebral perfusion pressure q1-2 hr, depending on fluctuation* Intracranial pressure monitoring is discontinued when recovery is apparent (after 3 to 4 days), and extubation is achieved *or* there is no recovery and pressure remains stable for about 1 week (4 to 6 days) *Sequence for discontinuing intracranial pressure monitoring* as ordered (this process will take 36 to 72 hours; there should be a 6- to 12-hour equilibration between each step) 1. Decrease mechanical ventilation slowly so Pco_2 rises gradually (5 mm Hg q4-8 hr) 2. Discontinue muscle relaxants 3. Taper drug therapy 4. Discontinue mechanical ventilation 5. Discontinue sedation 6. Discontinue intracranial pressure monitoring Administer O_2 therapy as ordered Keep Pco_2 at 20 to 25 mm Hg by hyperventilation (to maintain decreased cerebral blood flow) Modify respiratory therapy to avoid increases in intracranial pressure

*Cerebral perfusion pressure = Mean arterial pressure − Intracranial pressure.

Potential problems	Expected outcomes	Nursing activities
		Observe intracranial pressure fluctuation related to respiratory therapy
		Administer physiotherapy gently
		Hyperventilate for 1 minute prior to suctioning (frequent suctioning may require sedation)
		Administer minimal positive end expiratory pressure to prevent increased intrathoracic pressure
		Positive end expiratory pressure should be less than or equal to 2 cm H_2O
		Temperature monitoring is an important concomitant of intracranial pressure monitoring
		Administer osmotic diuretic as prescribed
		Hypothermia may be ordered to reduce cerebral blood flow through decreased cerebral metabolism
■ Inappropriate secretion of antidiuretic hormone	■ Fluid and electrolyte balance	■ Monitor Urine osmolality Urine specific gravity Urine Na^+ Serum electrolytes and osmolality Intake and output; restrict fluids as ordered Signs and symptoms of H_2O intoxication—(confusion, stupor, coma, seizures) May be masked because they are consistent with Reye's syndrome Notify physician of abnormalities
■ Diabetes insipidus	■ Normal circulatory volume	■ Monitor BP, intake and output, and urine specific gravity q15-30 min Replace urinary output q30 min or q1 hr as ordered until specific gravity is greater than or equal to 1.010 Administer vasopressor infusion as ordered Maintain NPO
■ Hyperammonemia related to renal failure	■ Reduction of serum levels of ammonia	■ Administer neomycin as ordered Administer peritoneal dialysis if ordered; see Standard: *Peritoneal dialysis* (this mode of therapy in Reye's syndrome is controversial) Assist with exchange transfusions if prescribed Monitor Heart rate and rhythm BP Respiratory rate Temperature Glucose (Dextrostix) Arterial blood gas levels and pH Electrolytes, including Ca^{2+} Serum ammonia Hct Hgb Administer calcium gluconate before and during procedure as ordered Continue monitoring aforementioned parameters after transfusion Hypoglycemia and hypotension are risks during immediate posttransfusion period

Potential problems	Expected outcomes	Nursing activities
■ Hepatic failure	■ Absence of hepatic decompensation	■ Monitor Prothrombin time and activated partial thromboplastin time q12 hr Ammonia, SGOT, SGPT, total serum protein, bilirubin, alkaline phosphatase, and amylase Dextrostix q4 hr Serum glucose every day Administer fresh frozen plasma prior to liver biopsy as ordered; assist with liver biopsy
■ Infection	■ Absence of infection	■ Maintain asepsis with all invasive monitoring procedures, IVs, etc. Culture all catheter tips when removed Monitor for signs of local infection and sepsis Monitor temperature q1-2 hr and prn Notify physician if these abnormalities occur, and alter therapy as ordered
■ Hyperpyrexia	■ Afebrile	■ Monitor temperature q1 hr or more frequently if unstable Administer tepid sponge baths Apply hypothermia as ordered Use servocontrol mechanism or monitor temperature q15 min when patient is on hypothermia blanket Antipyretics are contraindicated
■ Impending death	■ Family prepared for impending death	■ Reassure parents that they are not to blame for death Review medical facts Allow parents to review history of illness, their response to symptoms, and the events prior to and during hospitalization Assure parents that they did all that they should have done and that their actions were appropriate Encourage parents to verbalize their feelings Recognize steps in grieving process Accept expressions of anger, denial, etc. Include siblings' needs when discussing situation with parents Help parents understand children's age-related perceptions of death so that they may give appropriate explanations and consolation
■ Fear and anxiety related to separation from family, sensory bombardment of intensive care unit environment, etc. (The waking child who was obtunded on admission is not familiar with all the procedures he/she has been experiencing)	■ Reduction of anxiety Behavior appropriate to prehospitalization level of psychosocial development	■ Explain all procedures to child Include those events he/she may observe occurring with other patients Describe environment to child to reduce fear and to answer questions about machinery Orient child to time, place, and the multiple people who come and go in the unit Provide social stimulation by talking to the patient; do not approach patient, manipulate tubing, etc. without conversing with him/her; allow choices when possible Encourage and promote the parents' participation in care Allow child to verbalize feelings about hospital experiences

62 □ Diaphragmatic hernia

Diaphragmatic hernia in the newborn consists of incomplete embryonic formation of the diaphragm, which allows displacement of abdominal viscera into the thorax, displacing the lungs and heart and causing severe respiratory distress.

This defect occurs in about 1 in 5000 births. The left side is involved in over 80% of cases. The herniation may occur in the posterolateral segment, in the anterior portion directly beneath the sternum (foramen of Morgagni), or at the esophageal hiatus.

The most common diaphragmatic hernia (and the most serious) is posterolateral, known as *Bochdalek hernia*. It results when the triangular pleuroperitoneal canal fails to close. In the majority of cases, a sac covers the abdominal contents. If the abdominal viscera migrate into the thorax early in gestation, left lung development is affected, resulting in hypoplasia. The heart is displaced to the right, and the right lung is smaller than normal. If the migration of abdominal organs occurs later, there is less hypoplasia of the left lung. When the left side is involved, the intestine, stomach, and spleen compress the lung and displace the mediastinum to the right; when the lesion is on the right side, the liver and/or intestine are involved.

The less common Morgagni hernia usually results from incomplete muscularization of the diaphragm.

The severity of symptoms is related to the amount of lung compressed and the relative hypoplasia of lung tissue. Hypoplastic lungs are associated with small pulmonary vascular beds, a decreased number of pulmonary resistance vessels per unit of lung tissue, and increased pulmonary vascular smooth muscle. Pulmonary vascular resistance is increased by hypoxemia and hypercapnia. A right to left shunting through the ductus arteriosus results and persists following surgical repair.

The presenting sign is severe respiratory distress, usually immediately at birth. This quickly worsens. Immediate surgical intervention is indicated. Surgical repair may be via thorax or abdomen. The latter is usually preferred because of the difficulty in finding appropriate space in the abdomen for all the organs. Frequently, a temporary ventral hernia must be left to accommodate the viscera. A chest tube is placed postoperatively, regardless of the approach used.

Management of these patients focuses on maintenance of adequate oxygenation and ventilation. Postoperatively, respiratory support and scrupulous management of fluid, electrolyte, and acid-base balance are essential.

The high mortality of patients with this problem (over 50%) is related to the severity of the pulmonary hypoplasia, which prevents adequate gas exchange.

ASSESSMENT

1. Presence of signs and symptoms of diaphragmatic hernia, including
   a. Birth asphyxia
   b. Progressive respiratory distress and increasing cyanosis following clamping of umbilical cord
   c. Scaphoid (concave) abdomen (indicates displacement of a considerable amount of intestine)
2. Auscultation
   a. Displacement of cardiac impulse to one side of chest
   b. Diminished breath sounds in the involved hemithorax
   c. Bowel sounds in thorax
3. Diagnostic radiograph results confirming diaphragmatic hernia (a chest radiograph is always indicated as soon as possible in the presence of respiratory distress)
   a. Absence of diaphragmatic margin on affected side
   b. Presence of inappropriate thoracic structures
   c. Mediastinal displacement
4. Results of lab tests,* including
   a. Arterial blood gas levels
   b. Serum electrolytes

GOALS

1. Adequate oxygenation
2. Adequate nourishment with weight gain
3. Successful parent-infant bonding
4. Normal psychosocial and psychomotor growth
5. Family will be able to cope with crisis and remain an intact, mutually nurturing dyad or group
6. Parents will develop and have confidence in their parenting skills

---

*Usually there is marked acidosis with accompanying hyperkalemia.

Potential problems	Expected outcomes	Nursing activities

■ Respiratory insufficiency	■ Adequate oxygenation	■ Assess respiratory status; note
		   Respiratory rate, breathing pattern, color
		   Notify physician of abnormalities
		  Insert large NG tube to decompress air-filled intestines
		   Apply suction
		  Position infant so that lung on unaffected side is allowed to fully expand
		  Assist with intubation and mechanical ventilation as ordered to maintain PO_2 at 50 to 60 mm Hg
		   Administer O_2 immediately if cyanosis of mucous membranes is present
		   Resuscitator bag is contraindicated to prevent overinflation of unaffected lung
		   See Standard: *Mechanical ventilation*

■ Acidosis related to anaerobic metabolism	■ Acid-base parameters within normal limits, including Pa_{O_2}, Pa_{CO_2}, bicarbonate, base excess, lactate	■ Maintain rapid respiratory rate 50 to 60/minute
		  Administer curare or pancuronium if needed, as ordered
		  Administer sodium bicarbonate infusion as ordered
		  Monitor
		   Arterial blood gas levels q1 hr
		   Respiratory status
		   Heart rate and rhythm
		   Level of activity
		  Notify physician of changes, and alter therapy as ordered

■ Delayed bonding because mother does not see baby at delivery and/or baby is rushed away for emergency treatment
  This initial separation during the immediate postnatal period can be exacerbated by prolonged hospitalization and parental grief because newborn is sick and/or dying
	■ Parents interact with infant as soon as possible
	  Successful parent-infant bonding
	  Parents communicate their feelings about infant
		■ Explain disease process and need for therapy prescribed
		  Explain procedures, their purpose, etc. to parents
		   Allow repetitive questions
		  Allow and encourage frequent visits
		   Give parents telephone number of unit and name of primary nurse; encourage them to call to check on baby, ask questions, etc.
		  Encourage parents to touch and stroke infant; encourage parents to participate in infant's care to whatever extent possible
		  Assess parent-infant interactions
		   Stimulate and reinforce social interaction/dialogue
		  Encourage verbalization of both positive and negative feelings
		  Assure parents that feelings of failure, guilt, frustration, bitterness, anger, sorrow, and disappointment are normal, i.e., shared by others in similar circumstances
		  Reassure parents that they are not to blame for the problem
		   Allow them to review history of pregnancy, labor, and delivery
		   Review medical facts
		  Point out infant's responsive behaviors
		  Point out infant's individual characteristics
		  Educate parents regarding infant's special needs and problems
		  Encourage questions
		  Prepare parents for prolonged hospitalization and follow-up
		   Tell them what to expect
		   Assure them that they will be able to see and handle infant to a greater extent after initial acute period
		  If/when situation appears grave, give honest explanations to parents
		  Recognize denial, anger, and withdrawal as steps in the grieving process and mechanisms of defense
		   Encourage parents to observe infant and repeat explanations; this will help parents to formulate and accept "real" situation

Potential problems	Expected outcomes	Nursing activities
		Allow parents to verbalize feelings
		Discuss siblings at home so that parents may verbalize impact of situation on family interaction
		Recognize parents as individuals

Postoperative

Potential problems	Expected outcomes	Nursing activities
■ Respiratory insufficiency related to	■ Absence or resolution of respiratory insufficiency	■ Prevention
Pneumothorax	Full lung expansion Intact contralateral lung	Use low peak inspiratory and end expiratory pressure as ordered Maintain patency of chest tubing Milk q1-2 hr as necessary Monitor drainage q1-2 hr (chest tubes are connected to straight drainage without suction)
Mediastinal shift	Absence or resolution of mediastinal shift	Monitor Chest radiograph q2-4 hr Breath sounds q½-1 hr Breathing pattern
Hypoxia due to reduced lung expansion*	Adequate oxygenation and ventilation	Administer mechanical ventilation via endotracheal tube as ordered Maintain inspiratory pressure at less than or equal to 20 cm H_2O Monitor arterial blood gas levels Notify physician of any changes in respiratory status and alter therapy as prescribed
■ Hypotension	■ Adequate tissue perfusion maintained through hemodynamic stability BP within normal limits for newborn	■ Monitor BP, P Urine output, including specific gravity (minimum output should be 1 ml/kg/hour) Color Temperature Level of activity Notify physician of abnormalities in the aforementioned, and alter therapy as ordered
■ Malrotation of abdominal organs (This is usually assessed and corrected at the time of surgery)	■ Intake of nutrients sufficient to achieve weight gain	■ Accurately measure and record intake and output Observe for distention and poor absorption following feeding Weigh infant daily Administer feedings as ordered Gastrostomy tube is in place postoperatively
■ Infection	■ Absence of infection	■ Use appropriate aseptic techniques Change respiratory therapy tubing daily Place fresh sterile H_2O in humidifiers q8 hr Change IV tubing q24 hr Refrigerate breast milk or formula after it has been opened; discard after 4 hours at room temperature Teach parents proper handwashing technique Monitor for signs of infection Apnea Lethargy Change in absorption of feeding Acidosis Hypotension Hypothermia Monitor culture results Report any abnormal observation to physician

*Improvement of respiratory status postoperatively depends on the degree of hypoplasia.

Potential problems	Expected outcomes	Nursing activities
■ Retrolental fibroplasia (retinopathy of prematurity) due to hyperoxia	■ Absence of effects of retinotoxic O_2 levels	■ Maintain inspired O_2 concentrations at minimum level necessary to achieve adequate oxygenation Monitor FI_{O_2} and record concentration q1-2 hr FI_{O_2} should be prescribed based on arterial blood gas levels Monitor Pa_{O_2} q4 hr if FI_{O_2} is less than 40% q2 hr if FI_{O_2} is greater than 40% Arrange for consultation by ophthalmologist as per hospital routine* Instruct parents regarding discharge follow-up; arrange clinic appointment
■ Delayed wound healing, infection	■ Wound intact and heals without infection	■ Monitor incision site for Drainage Erythema Edema Notify physician of any abnormalities Keep area dry and clean Dressing is not necessary
■ Parental anxiety related to lack of confidence in their parenting skills, their perception of infant's special needs, etc.	■ Reduction of anxiety Infant receives appropriate physical and psychological nurturing Parents demonstrate readiness to assume care of infant	■ Prepare parents for assuming care at home Allow parents to discuss their experiences and feelings Instruct parents in care of baby (include father) Feeding techniques Bathing Signs and symptoms of and intervention for respiratory distress Arrange public health nurse or Visiting Nurse Association referral Assess parent-infant interactions See Problem, Lack of confidence in parenting skills, in Standard: *Unstable premature infant*

*Infants who receive O_2 for any period should have optic fundi examined by ophthalmologist during and following O_2 therapy, at discharge, and at 5 months of age or 3 months after discharge.

63 □ Tracheoesophageal fistula

Tracheoesophageal fistula (TEF) is an abnormal congenital or acquired communication between the trachea and esophagus.

In most cases of congenital TEF, there is also an associated esophageal interruption, or atresia (Fig. 2, *A*). In this case, swallowed fluid enters the proximal esophageal pouch, then is aspirated into the trachea, causing a chemical pneumonia (most often the right upper lobe). Gastric contents are regurgitated through the distal esophagus and fistula into the lungs, and air travels from the lungs into the stomach (causing gastric distention). TEF should be suspected in an infant with excessive

drooling, respiratory distress (particularly choking or cyanosis during feeding), frequent pneumonia, and excessive gastric air.

Occasionally, the infant may have congenital TEF without esophageal atresia (Fig. 2, *B* and *C*). In these cases, the child may not demonstrate excessive drooling or gastric air but will have frequent aspiration pneumonia, coughing spells, and cyanosis.

Acquired TEF may occur following trauma, penetrating wounds, prolonged tracheal and esophageal intubation, and with carcinoma.

The diagnosis of congenital TEF with esophageal atre-

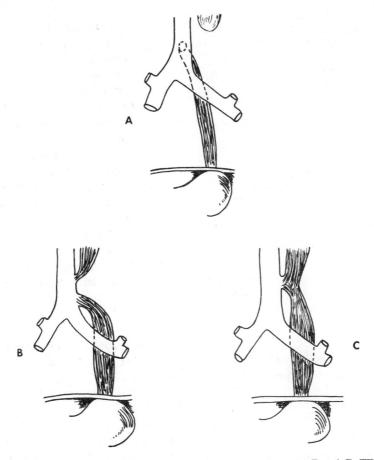

Fig. 2. A, Most common form of congenital TEF with esophageal atresia. **B** and **C,** TEF without esophageal atresia.

sia should be confirmed by inability to pass a catheter from the esophagus into the stomach of an infant with excessive gastric air revealed on the radiograph. To detect congenital or acquired TEF without esophageal atresia, contrast studies with esophagogram or bronchoscopy may be performed. Contrast radiography is *extremely* hazardous in newborns, however, since aspiration of even small amounts of contrast medium causes severe chemical pneumonitis; therefore, these studies are avoided in the small infant if the diagnosis can be made another way. Any patient should be monitored for signs of aspiration during contrast radiography, with emergency suction and intubation equipment readily available.

Once the diagnosis is established, catheterization of the blind esophageal pouch (with associated esophageal atresia) or stomach (with simple fistula) and gastrostomy are performed to prevent further aspiration and gastric reflux. Surgical intervention is necessary once the patient's respiratory status is acceptable.

If associated esophageal atresia is present, the surgeon will attempt primary anastomosis of proximal and distal esophageal segments with closure of the TEF. If esophageal segments are too short to join directly, the fistula is closed using a retropleural approach, and an esophagostomy (for emptying of the blind pouch) and gastrostomy (for feeding) are created. Several months later, esophageal reanastomosis or reconstruction is then performed. If an uncomplicated TEF is present, it is closed through a cervical or thoracotomy incision. Local resection of lung tissue is performed as needed.

Following surgery, the patient is kept NPO with gastrostomy or parenteral nutrition for 3 to 14 days. The most common postoperative complications include leakage from the esophageal anastomosis, esophageal stricture, continued respiratory infection, recurrent fistulas, and dysphagia.

Children with congenital TEF have increased incidence of associated congenital heart disease, renal anomalies, gastrointestinal anomalies (especially imperforate anus), skeletal and neurological problems, and thrombocytopenia.

ASSESSMENT

1. Gestational history (gestational age, perinatal distress, cyanosis at birth or during feeding, excessive drooling)
2. Congenital fistula
   a. Respiratory distress: cyanosis, tachypnea, nasal flaring, copious secretions, retractions, decreased lung aeration, evidence of pneumonia or pneumonitis by radiograph or clinical examination
   b. Cardiovascular status: evidence of cyanotic heart disease or heart failure (see introduction to Standard: *Cardiac surgery*)
   c. Level of hydration: fontanelle in infants less than 18 months old, mucous membranes, skin turgor, tearing in patients over 3 months old
   d. Nutritional status: amount of subcutaneous fat, recent daily caloric intake, wound healing, and serum glucose in infants
   e. Temperature: presence of fever or hypothermia (in infants)
   f. Hematological status: leukocytosis or thrombocytopenia
   g. Associated anomalies: imperforate anus or other gastrointestinal anomalies; skeletal, renal, or neurological disorders
3. Acquired fistula
   a. Cause of fistula (wound, trauma, prolonged intubation, carcinoma)
   b. Respiratory status: evidence of pneumonia or pneumonitis by radiograph or clinical examination, excessive sputum production, cyanosis, dyspnea, tachypnea, nasal flaring, retractions, orthopnea
   c. Evidence of infection: leukocytosis, fever, sputum production, wound inflammation
   d. Presence of other complications of penetrating tracheoesophageal injury
   e. Presence of complications of carcinoma and necessary therapy
4. Patient/family's anxiety about and comprehension of disorder and therapy

GOALS

1. Adequate respiratory status, including absence of further aspiration and resolution of current pneumonia
2. Adequate nutritional status and fluid and electrolyte balance
3. Absence of respiratory or wound infection
4. Patient/family's comprehension of disease, treatment plan, and prognosis, with manageable stress levels
5. Patient/family's comprehension of necessary home health care and medical follow-up
6. Patient/family's demonstration of appropriate skills in performing home health care

Potential problems	Expected outcomes	Nursing activities
■ Respiratory distress related to aspiration pneumonia, gastric reflux, chemical pneumonitis, and postoperative atelectasis, pneumothorax, or anastomosis dehiscence	■ Stable respiratory status as measured by Normal respiratory rate Minimal respiratory effort (no use of accessory muscles) Absence of pulmonary infection on radiograph and clinical examination Absence of further aspiration pneumonia and resolution of existing pneumonia	■ Monitor respiratory rate and lung aeration, and notify physician if increased distress is present Normal adult's respiratory rate: 10 to 18/minute Normal newborn's respiratory rate: 30 to 50/minute Normal 6- to 18-month-old child's respiratory rate: 20 to 30/minute Normal 2- to 10-year-old child's respiratory rate: 18 to 30/minute Normal adolescent's respiratory rate: 12 to 20/minute NOTE: Consider your patient's individual normal range Monitor for signs of increased respiratory effort, and notify physician if present Adults and children: use of accessory muscles, nasal flaring, cyanosis, diaphoresis, increased pulmonary congestion on radiograph and/or clinical examination Infants will demonstrate the aforementioned with more severe retractions, head bobbing (up to the age of 4 months), grunting, and mottling or pallor instead of (or in addition to) cyanosis

Potential problems	**Expected outcomes**	**Nursing activities**
		Maintain NPO as soon as diagnosis is suspected and for 3 to 14 days postoperatively as ordered

Have suction equipment, O_2, and resuscitator bag at bedside

Suction oropharynx frequently to prevent aspiration of secretions (after surgery, do not allow suction catheter to extend to area of tracheal or esophageal suture lines—may need to use marked catheter for comparison when suctioning)

If patient is intubated and mechanically ventilated following surgery, see Standard: *Mechanical ventilation*

Insert Raplogle tube into proximal pouch of esophagus (if esophageal atresia is present) to provide continuous removal of secretions

Record tube output as part of patient's daily output

Irrigate and aspirate tube to ensure patency, using small amounts of sterile saline solution or air (0.5 to 1 cc) q1-2 hr

Elevate head of bed 20 to 30 degrees, and keep patient on side or prone as much as possible prior to surgical repair (to prevent aspiration and to reduce gastric reflux)

If patient has pharyngostomy or esophagostomy, patient should be turned to side of "ostomy" to facilitate drainage

If gastric tube or gastrostomy is inserted to remove gastric contents (to prevent gastric reflux), check its placement and function by irrigating with small amounts of normal saline solution or air (1 to 5 cc) q2 hr (reaspirate irrigation material after each check)

Prepare patient for and monitor patient during any diagnostic radiographic studies (bring emergency equipment—resuscitator bag, endotracheal tube, etc.—to radiology, and do not leave patient unattended at any time during studies)

Collect sputum specimen for C and S and Gram stain studies if patient demonstrates any evidence of respiratory infection

Administer appropriate antibiotics as ordered; check dosage and patient allergies prior to administration

Administer steroids as ordered; check dosage and monitor wound healing (and observe for evidence of GI bleeding) during course of administration

During gastrostomy feedings and once oral feedings are resumed, put small amount of food coloring into food and monitor for any evidence of aspiration; be prepared to discontinue feedings and institute emergency measures quickly (have suction equipment close at hand)

Provide chest physiotherapy

Do not place patient in Trendelenburg position for drainage as it may promote gastric reflux

Use rib-springing exercises and innovative games with children to promote deep breathing

Provide care of thoracotomy pleural drainage tubes (with water seal drainage) following surgical repair as needed

Maintain water seal

Monitor for evidence of pneumothorax (decreased breath sounds, tachypnea, increased respiratory effort, and hyperresonance to percussion) or hemothorax (decreased breath sounds and dullness to percussion, tachypnea, increased respiratory effort, increased chest tube drainage of 100 ml/hour in adults or greater than 3 ml/kg/hour in children); notify physician if these occur

Potential problems	Expected outcomes	Nursing activities

■ Poor nutrition related to inability to maintain oral feedings, severe illness, and stress	■ Adequate nutritional status as measured by
	  Appropriate weight gain
	  Adequate subcutaneous tissue
	  Moist mucous membranes
	  Good skin turgor
	  Adequate wound healing
		■ Calculate patient's daily caloric requirements; ensure adequate caloric intake via parenteral alimentation or gastrostomy feedings
		
		Monitor infant's serum glucose or Dextrostix as needed; notify physician of any evidence of hypoglycemia (glucose storage in infants is minimal)
		
		If gastrostomy feedings are ordered
		  Secure tube carefully once appropriate placement is determined
		  Begin gastrostomy feedings with small, dilute amounts and advance volume and osmolarity slowly, as patient's tolerance permits
		  Prior to each feeding, aspirate tube and measure any residual formula; do not advance feedings if residual is greater than 5 ml in the infant and 20 ml in the adult (or as hospital policy dictates)
		  Monitor for abdominal distention (measure abdominal girth q2 hr) and diarrhea when feedings are increased in volume or osmolarity; if either occur, notify physician and reduce feeding
		  Gastrostomy feedings *should be accomplished through gravity drainage only and never through pressure* (gastric perforation can occur)
		  Provide oral stimulation with pacifier for infant during feeding
		  Follow feedings with 5 to 10 ml normal saline solution or sterile H_2O to flush tubing; then leave tube unclamped but elevated (so air and regurgitant matter can reflux up tubing instead of into esophagus) for several minutes (30 to 40) after each feeding
		
		If parenteral alimentation is begun, see Standard: *Total parenteral nutrition through central venous catheter*
		
		NOTE: These neonates are especially prone to the development of NEC; monitor for evidence of Hematest positive stools and abdominal distention; see Standard: *Neonatal necrotizing enterocolitis*
		
		Provide gastrostomy and esophagostomy stomal care; monitor for peristomal excoriation, and notify physician of any stomal breakdown
		
		Turn patient frequently; keep skin warm and dry; massage any bony prominences to stimulate circulation
		
		Monitor Hgb and Hct; notify physician of significant changes
		Weigh patient daily, and notify physician of any significant weight gain or loss (greater than 1 kg/24 hours in adults, greater than 200 g/24 hours in children, and greater than 50 g/24 hours in neonates)
		
		Monitor fluid intake and output; calculate patient's daily fluid requirements, and discuss with physician if patient is not receiving them
		
		Monitor level of hydration
		  Palpate fontanelle in infants under 18 months—will be sunken if dehydration is present
		  Mucous membranes should be moist, and tearing should be present in infant beyond the age of 3 months
		  Skin should not "tent" when pinched
		  Urine output should be adequate (1 to 2 ml/kg/hour) with normal specific gravity (1.005 to 1.020)
		  Notify physician if there is evidence of dehydration

Potential problems	Expected outcomes	Nursing activities
		Once oral feedings are resumed, monitor closely for dysphagia and/or aspiration; notify physician immediately if either occurs, and be prepared to institute emergency measures if respiratory distress occurs May wish to add food coloring to initial fluid intake and stop feedings if color appears in respiratory secretions
■ Patient/family's anxiety regarding diagnosis, surgery, prognosis, hospitalization, and change in appearance (due to scarring or stoma)	■ Patient/family (as appropriate) demonstrates comprehension of diagnosis, surgical and medical plan of care, and prognosis Patient/family's stress levels do not interfere with their ability to support one another and function appropriately	■ Prepare patient/family for any diagnostic or surgical procedures (for children, play or art may be utilized to provide information in a less threatening manner); focus on what the patient will see, feel, or hear Orient patient/family to the nursing care unit, staff, and policies Provide patient/family with sufficient opportunity to discuss fears, concerns, and questions (if gastrostomy or esophagostomy is necessary, patient/family will need assistance in coping with patient's change in appearance) Frequently orient patient to time and place following any surgical intervention or sedation Frequently explain care regimen to patient/family; include description of and explanation for tubes and NPO Provide child with frequent reassurances that he or she is a "good boy" or "good girl," and be able to tell patient when parents or other significant family members will return Assist parents of newborn in mourning for the loss of a healthy, perfect child and adjustment to the fact that their child has a congenital defect; parents will need reassurances that they could not have prevented their child's congenital lesion Make sure that patient/family is given consistent explanations
■ Infection related to aspiration pneumonia, surgical anastomosis dehiscence, and poor nutritional status NOTE: If acquired fistula has been caused by penetrating injury, infection can result	■ Absence of infection with no evidence of pneumonia on radiograph or clinical examination, wound infection, (erythema, heat, drainage), leukocytosis, fever (or hypothermia in infants), or sepsis	■ Monitor temperature: notify physician and obtain blood cultures if fever occurs (greater than 38° C); since an infant can become hypothermic with infection, monitor also for temperature instability Auscultate lungs and report any evidence of congestion NOTE: Empyema may ocur with dehiscence of esophageal anastomosis if a retropleural approach was not used for surgical correction Monitor blood counts for evidence of infection Note wound appearance; report any heat, erythema, or drainage, and obtain culture of wound if these occur Administer any ordered antibiotics—check patient's dosage and allergies prior to administration If patient is receiving steroids or chemotherapy, observe patient closely for evidence of infection and be particularly cautious with assignments of patient's roommates (to prevent introduction of other sources of infection or contamination) Provide care of any existing stoma and prevent peristomal excoriation

Potential problems	Expected outcomes	Nursing activities
■ Patient/family may have inadequate information to comply with home health care regimen and health maintenance*	■ Patient/family demonstrates comprehension of and ability to perform home health care Patient/family demonstrates knowledge of planned physician follow-up and future surgical and medical intervention	■ Provide adequate time for teaching and return demonstration of home health care regimen; include medications, "ostomy" or wound care, return checkup visits, and signs of emergency requiring immediate medical intervention Provide patient/family with list of appropriate physicians and why, how, and where to contact them Parents of infant will require information on timing of immunizations—usually immunizations should be delayed until several weeks after child has recovered from surgery Provide reinforcement of home health care teaching by all members of the health team (all should use the same terminology when communicating with patient/family) If needed, provide ongoing therapy with family to help them deal with patient's altered appearance and health care needs Initiate appropriate community health referrals

*If responsibility of critical care nurse includes such follow-up care.

BIBLIOGRAPHY

RESPIRATORY

Abels, L. F.: Acute respiratory failure, Critical Care Quarterly **1:**1-82, 1979.

Abels, L. F.: Mosby's manual of critical care, St. Louis, 1979, The C. V. Mosby Co.

Adams, Maj. N. R.: The nurses' role in systematic weaning from a ventilator, Nurs. '79 **9:**34-41, 1979.

Beatrous, W. P.: Tracheostomy (tracheotomy). Its expanded indications and its present status. Based on an analysis of 1,000 consecutive operations and a review of the recent literature, Laryngoscope **78:**3-55, 1968.

Bendixen, H. H., et al.: Respiratory care, St. Louis, 1965, The C. V. Mosby Co.

Berk, J. L., et al., editors: Handbook of critical care, Boston, 1976, Little, Brown & Co.

Brunner, L., and Suddarth, D.: Textbook of medical surgical nursing, ed. 3, Philadelphia, 1975, J. B. Lippincott Co.

Burrell, Z. L., and Burrell, L. O.: Critical care, ed. 3, St. Louis, 1977, The C. V. Mosby Co.

Bushnell, S. S.: Respiratory intensive care nursing, Boston, 1973, Little, Brown & Co.

Cameron, M. I.: What patients need most before and after thoracotomy, Nurs. '78 **8:**28-36, 1978.

Chusid, E., et al.: When your patient is on respiratory therapy, Nursing Digest **4:**43-46, 1976.

Clarke, E. B., and Niggeman, E. H.: Near-drowning, Heart Lung **4:**946-955, 1975.

Clutario, B. C., and Holzman, B. H.: Uncommon diseases, extrapulmonary diseases, systemic diseases, and toxins. In Scarpelli, E. M., et al., editors: Pulmonary disease of the fetus, newborn and child, Philadelphia, 1978, Lea & Febiger.

Conn, A. W., Edmonds, J. F., and Barker, G. A.: Cerebral resuscitation in near-drowning, Pediatr. Clin. North Am. **26:**691-701, 1979.

Cunningham, J. H., et al.: Interstitial pulmonary edema, Heart Lung **6:**617-623, 1977.

Dammert, W., and Mast, C. P.: Tracheostomy. In Levin, D. L., Morris, F. C., and Moore, G. C., editors: A practical guide to pediatric intensive care, St. Louis, 1979, The C. V. Mosby Co.

Dunphy, J. E., and Way, L. W.: Current surgical diagnosis and treatment, ed. 2, Los Altos, Calif., 1975, Lange Medical Publications.

Egan, D. F.: Fundamentals of respiratory therapy, ed. 3, St. Louis, 1977, The C. V. Mosby Co.

Gallagher, T. J., et al.: Terminology update: optimal PEEP, Crit. Care Med. **6:**323-326, 1978.

Martz, K. V., Joiner, J., and Shepherd, R. M.: Management of the patient-ventilator system—a team approach, St. Louis, 1979, The C. V. Mosby Co.

Mathewson, H. S. Respiratory therapy in critical care, St. Louis, 1976, The C. V. Mosby Co.

Modell, J. H., et al.: Clinical course of 91 consecutive near-drowning victims, Chest **70:**231-238, 1976.

Peterson, B.: Morbidity of childhood near-drowning, Pediatrics **59:**364-370, 1977.

Rachow, E., and Fein, I. A.: Fulminant noncardiogenic pulmonary edema in the critically ill, Crit. Care Med. **6:**360-363, 1978.

Scarpelli, E. M., et al., editors: Pulmonary disease of the fetus, newborn and child, Philadelphia, 1978, Lea & Febiger.

Shapiro, B. A., et al.: Clinical application of respiratory care, ed. 2, Chicago, 1979, Year Book Medical Publishers, Inc.

Sweetwood, H.: Acute respiratory insufficiency, Nurs. '77 **7:**24-31, 1977.

Tecklin, J. S.: Positioning, percussing and vibrating patients for effective bronchial drainage, Nurs. '79 **9:**64-71, 1979.

Van Haeringen, J. R., et al.: Treatment of the respiratory distress syndrome following nondirect pulmonary trauma with positive end-expiratory pressure with special emphasis on near-drowning, Chest **66**(suppl.):30S-34S, 1974.

CARDIOVASCULAR

Abels, L. F.: Mosby's manual of critical care, St. Louis, 1979, The C. V. Mosby Co.

Adams, N.: Reducing the perils of intra-cardiac monitoring, Nurs. '76 **6:**66-74, 1976.

Adams, N.: Hemodynamic monitoring, Critical Care Quarterly **2:**1-86, 1979.

Andreoli, K., et al.: Comprehensive cardiac care, ed. 4, St. Louis, 1979, The C. V. Mosby Co.

Aspinall, M. J.: Nursing the open-heart surgery patient, New York, 1973, McGraw-Hill Book Co.

Bailen, M. T.: Intra-aortic balloon pumping, lectures presented at the Cardiovascular Laboratory, College of Physicians and Surgeons, Columbia Presbyterian Medical Center, New York, 1976-1979.

Barash, P. G., et al.: Intra-operative use and interpretation of Swan-Ganz catheter data, New Haven, Conn., 1978, Department of Anesthesia, Yale School of Medicine.

Berk, J. L., et al., editors: Handbook of critical care, Boston, 1976, Little, Brown & Co.

Boedeker, E., and Dauber, J.: Manual of medical therapeutics, Boston, 1974, Little, Brown & Co.

Bregman, D.: Medical and surgical management during clinical dual-chambered intra-aortic balloon pumping in conjunction with the Datascope System 80. Practical guidelines for the physician, Paramus, N.J., 1972, Datascope Corp.

Bregman, D.: Mechanical support of the failing heart, Curr. Probl. Surg. **13**(12):1-84, 1976.

Brunner, L., and Suddarth, D.: Textbook of medical surgical nursing, ed. 3, Philadelphia, 1975, J. B. Lippincott Co.

Brunner, L., and Suddarth, D.: The Lippincott manual of nursing practice, ed. 2, Philadelphia, 1978, J. B. Lippincott Co.

Burrell, Z. L., and Burrell, L. O.: Critical care, ed. 3, St. Louis, 1977, The C. V. Mosby Co.

Caprini, J. A., et al.: Heparin therapy. I, Cardiovasc. Nurs. **13**:13-16, 1977.

Caprini, J. A., et al.: Heparin therapy. II, Cardiovasc. Nurs. **13**:17-20, 1977.

Chung, E.: Cardiac emergency care, Philadelphia, 1975, Lea & Febiger.

Chung, E.: Quick reference to cardio-vascular diseases, Philadelphia, 1977, J. B. Lippincott Co.

Cromwell, R., et al.: Acute myocardial infarction: reaction and recovery, St. Louis, 1977, The C. V. Mosby Co.

Cudkowicz, L., and Sherry, S.: Current status of thrombolytic therapy, Heart Lung **7**:97-100, 1978.

Daily, E. K., and Schroeder, J. S.: Techniques in bedside hemodynamic monitoring, ed. 2, St. Louis, 1980, The C. V. Mosby Co.

Davidson, S. V. S., et al.: Nursing care evaluation: concurrent and retrospective review criteria, St. Louis, 1977, The C. V. Mosby Co.

Durie, M. E.: Use of an intra-aortic balloon pump following postoperative pump failure and cardiac arrest: case presentation and discussion, Heart Lung **3**:971-975, 1974.

Edwards Laboratories: Understanding hemodynamic measurements made with the Swan Ganz catheter, Santa Ana, Calif., 1977, Edwards Laboratories.

Fink, B. W.: Congenital heart disease: a deductive approach to its diagnosis, Chicago, 1975, Year Book Medical Publishers, Inc.

Fitzmaurice, J. B.: Venous thromboembolic disease: current thoughts, Cardiovasc. Nurs. **14**:1-4, 1978.

Ford, P., and Weintraub, M.: Intra-aortic balloon pumping manual, Boston, 1975, Beth Israel Hospital.

Foxworth, G. D.: Rehabilitation for hospitalized adults after open-heart procedures: the team approach, Heart Lung **7**:834-839, 1978.

Gazes, G.: Clinical cardiology, Chicago, 1975, Year Book Medical Publishers, Inc.

Gildae, J. H., et al.: Congenital cardiac defects, Am. J. Nurs. **78**:255-278, 1978.

Goldman, M. J.: Principles of clinical electrocardiography, ed. 9, Los Altos, Calif., 1976, Lange Medical Publications.

Guide to physiological pressure monitoring, Waltham, Mass., 1977, Hewlett Packard Co.

Hallman, G. L., and Cooley, D. A.: Surgical treatment of congenital heart disease, ed. 2, Philadelphia, 1975, Lea & Febiger.

Harrington, D.: Disparities between direct and indirect arterial systolic blood pressure measurements, CVP **6**:40-44, Aug.-Sept., 1978.

Hart, L. K., and Frantz, R. A.: Characteristics of postoperative patient—education programs for open-heart surgery patients in the United States, Heart Lung **6**:137-142, 1977.

Hazinski, M. G.: Congenital heart lesions, Chicago, 1978, Bio-Services Corp.

Hazinski, M. G.: The cardiovascular system. In Armstrong, M. E., et al., editors: McGraw-Hill handbook of clinical nursing, New York, 1979, McGraw-Hill Book Co.

Ho, C. S., et al.: Major complications of cardiac catheterization and angiocardiography in infants and children, Johns Hopkins Med. J. **131**:247, 1972.

Hurst, J. W., et al.: The heart, ed. 4, New York, 1978, McGraw-Hill Book Co.

King, O. M.: Congenital heart disease, In King, O. M.: Care of the cardiac surgical patient, St. Louis, 1975, The C. V. Mosby Co.

Jahre, J., et al.: Medical approach to the hypotensive patient and the patient in shock, Heart Lung **4**:577-587, 1975.

Lalli, S.: The complete Swan-Ganz, R. N. Magazine **41**:65-77, 1978.

Long, G. D.: Managing the patient with abdominal aortic aneurysm, Nurs. '78 **8**:20-27, 1978.

Meltzer, L., et al., editors: Concepts and practices of intensive care for nurse specialists, Bowie, Md., 1976, Charles Press Publications, Inc.

Miller, S. P., and Shada, E. A.: Preoperative information and recovery of open heart surgery patients, Heart Lung **7**:486-493, 1978.

Monson, D. O., et al.: Management of the pediatric cardiac surgical patient. In Golden, M. D., editor: Intensive care of the surgical patient, ed. 2, Chicago, 1980, Year Book Medical Publishers, Inc.

Moss, A. J., et al.: Heart disease in infants, children and adolescents, ed. 2, Baltimore, 1977, The Williams & Wilkins Co.

Neu, H.: Early treatment of infection of unknown origin, Indianapolis, 1976, Eli Lilly & Co.

Pastellopoulos, A. E., and Cullum, J.: Intra-aortic balloon assist for cardiogenic shock, J. Cardiovasc. Technol. **16**:21-30, 1974.

Prakash, O., et al.: Cardiorespiratory and metabolic effects of profound hypothermia, Crit. Care Med. **6**:165-171, 1978.

Prakash, O., et al.: Erratum: cardiorespiratory and metabolic effects of profound hypothermia, Crit. Care Med. **6**:339-346, 1978.

Rakoczy, M.: The thoughts and feelings of patients in the waiting period prior to cardiac surgery: a descriptive study, Heart Lung **6**:280-287, 1977.

Robbins, S. L.: Pathologic basis of disease, ed. 2, Philadelphia, 1979, W. B. Saunders Co.

Rodman, M.: Drugs for treating shock, RN **39**:77-86, 1976.

Rudolph, A. M.: Cardiac catheterization and angiography. In Congenital diseases of the heart, Chicago, 1974, Year Book Medical Publishers, Inc.

Sadler, P. D.: Nursing assessment of postcardiotomy delirium, Heart Lung **8**:745-750, 1979.

Schwartz, S. I., et al., editors: Principles of surgery, ed. 3, New York, 1979, McGraw-Hill Book Co.

Shearer, J. K., and Caldwell, M.: Use of sodium nitroprusside and dopamine hydrochloride in the postoperative cardiac patient, Heart Lung **8**:302-307, 1979.

Shoemaker, W.: Hemodynamic and oxygen transport patterns of common shock syndromes. In the proceedings of a Symposium on Recent and Current Clinical Practice in Shock, Kalamazoo, Mich., 1975, Upjohn Co.

Sokolow, M., and McIlroy, M. B.: Clinical cardiology, Los Altos, Calif., 1977, Lange Medical Publications.

Sørensen, M. B., et al.: Cardiac output measurement by thermal dilution, Ann. Surg. **183**:67-72, 1976.

Thompson, W. L.: The patient in shock. In the proceedings of a Symposium on Recent Research Developments and Current Clinical Practice in Shock, Kalamazoo, Mich., 1976, Upjohn Co.

Tucker, S. M., et al.: Patient care standards, ed. 2, St. Louis, 1980, The C. V. Mosby Co.

Vinocur, B., et al.: Application of a critical care monitoring program in the diagnosis and management of critically ill patients, presented at the Forty-first Annual Scientific Assembly, American College of Chest Physicians, 1975.

Wells, S., Stokes, S., and Mahoney, K.: Manual of cardiovascular assessment, Reston, Va., Reston Publishing Co., Inc. (In press).

Woods, S.: Monitoring pulmonary artery pressures, Am. J. Nurs. **76**:1765-1771, 1976.

Zschoche, D. A.: Mosby's comprehensive review of critical care, ed. 2, St. Louis, 1980, The C. V. Mosby Co.

NEUROLOGICAL

Adams, R. D., and Victor, M.: Principles of neurology, New York, 1977, McGraw-Hill Book Co.

Baker, A. B., and Baker, L. H., editors: Clinical neurology, vol. I, New York, 1973, Harper & Row, Publishers, Inc.

Bannister, R., editor: Brain's clinical neurology, ed. 3, London, 1974, Oxford University Press.

Bickerstaff, E.: Neurology for nurses, ed. 2, London, 1973, English Universities Press Ltd.

Carini, E., and Owens, G.: Neurological and neurosurgical nursing, St. Louis, 1970, The C. V. Mosby Co.

Chusid, J. C.: Correlative neuroanatomy and functional neurology, Los Altos, Calif., 1975, Lange Medical Publ.

Ciba Pharmaceutical Co.: Clinical symposia of nervous system, vols. 15, 18, 19, 26, and 29, New Jersey, 1963, 1966, 1967, 1974, 1977, Ciba-Geigy Corp.

Forster, F. M.: Clinical neurology, ed. 4, St. Louis, 1978, The C. V. Mosby Co.

Gatz, A. J.: Manter's essentials of clinical neuroanatomy and neurophysiology, ed. 4, Philadelphia, 1971, F. A. Davis Co.

Howe, J. R.: Patient care in neurosurgery, Boston, 1977, Little, Brown & Co.

Kahn, E. A., et al.: Correlative neurosurgery, ed. 2, Springfield, Ill., 1969, Charles C Thomas, Publisher.

Lewis, A. J.: Mechanisms of neurological disease, Boston, 1976, Little, Brown & Co.

Merritt, H. H.: A textbook of neurology, Philadelphia, 1967, Lea & Febiger.

Noback, C., and Demarest, R.: The nervous system: introduction and review, New York, 1972, McGraw-Hill Book Co.

Noback, C., and Demarest, R.: The human nervous system, ed. 2, New York, 1975, McGraw-Hill Book Co.

Peele, T. L.: The neuroanatomic basis for clinical neurology, ed. 3, New York, 1977, McGraw-Hill Book Co.

Plum, F., and Posner, J. B.: Diagnosis of stupor and coma, Philadelphia, 1972, F. A. Davis Co.

Simpson, J. F., and Magee, K.: Clinical evaluation of the nervous system, Boston, 1973, Little, Brown & Co.

Wehrmaker, S., and Wintermute, J.: Case studies in neurological nursing, Boston, 1978, Little, Brown & Co.

GASTROINTESTINAL

Boedeker, E., and Dauber, J.: Manual of medical therapeutics, ed. 21, Boston, 1974, Little, Brown & Co.

Brunner, L., and Suddarth, D.: The Lippincott manual of nursing practice, ed. 2, Philadelphia, 1978, J. B. Lippincott Co.

Boyer, C. A., and Oehlberg, S. M., editors: Symposium on diseases of the liver, Nurs. Clin. North Am. **12**:257-356, 1977.

Brunner, L., and Suddarth, D.: Textbook of medical surgical nursing, ed. 3, Philadelphia, 1975, J. B. Lippincott, Co.

Burrell, Z. L., and Burrell, L. O.: Critical care, ed. 3, St. Louis, 1977, The C. V. Mosby Co.

Castle, M.: Wound care, Nurs. '75 **5**:40-44, 1975.

Cimetidine-warfarin interaction may cause hemorrhage, Nurses' Drug Alert **3**:9-16, 1979.

Condon, R., and Nyhus, L., editors: Manual of surgical therapeutics, ed. 4, Boston, 1978, Little, Brown & Co.

Conn, H. O.: A rational approach to the hepatorenal syndrome, Gastroenterology **65**:321-340, 1973.

Croushore, T. M.: Postoperative assessment: the key to avoiding most common nursing mistakes, Nurs. '79 **9**:47-51, 1979.

Dunphy, J. E., and Way, L. W.: Current surgical diagnosis and treatment, ed. 2, Los Altos, Calif., 1975, Lange Medical Publications.

Durham, N.: Looking out for complications of abdominal surgery, Nurs. '75 **5**:24-31, 1975.

Ellis, P. D.: Portal hypertension and bleeding esophageal and gastric varicees: a surgical approach to treatment, Heart Lung **6**:791-798, 1977.

Galambos, J. T., et al.: Selective and total shunts in the treatment of bleeding varicees, N. Engl. J. Med. **295**:1089-1095, 1976.

Kinney, J. M., et al., editors: Manual of preoperative and postoperative care, ed. 2, Philadelphia, 1971, W. B. Saunders Co.

Kinney, J. M., et al., editors: Manual of surgical intensive care, Philadelphia, 1977, W. B. Saunders Co.

Kratzer, J. B., and Rauschenberger, D. S.: What to teach your patient about his duodenal ulcer, Nurs. '78 **8**:54-56, 1978.

Long, G. D.: G.I. bleeding: what to do and when, Nurs. '78 **8**:44-50, 1978.

McConnell, E. A.: After surgery: how you can avert the obvious hazards and the not-so-obvious ones, too, Nurs. '77 **7**:32-39, 1977.

McDermott, W., Jr.: Surgery of the liver and portal circulation, Philadelphia, 1974, Lea & Febiger.

Papper, S., editor: Manual of medical care of the surgical patient, Boston, 1976, Little, Brown & Co.

Steinheber, F.: Bleeding from the upper gastrointestinal tract, Hosp. Med. **15**:47-64, 1979.

Tucker, S. M., et al.: Patient care standards, ed. 2, St. Louis, 1980, The C. V. Mosby Co.

Wapnick, S., et al.: La Veen continuous peritoneal-jugular shunt, J.A.M.A. **237**:131-133, 1977.

Warren, W. D., et al.: The metabolic basis of portasystemic encephalopathy and the effect of selective versus non-selective shunts, Ann. Surg. **180**:573-579, 1974.

RENAL

Berk, J. L., et al., editors: Handbook of critical care, Boston, 1976, Little, Brown & Co.

Brundage, D. J.: Nursing management of renal problems, ed. 2, St. Louis, 1980, The C. V. Mosby Co.

Burrell, Z. L., and Burrell, L. O.: Critical care, ed. 3, St. Louis, 1977, The C. V. Mosby Co.

Davidson, S. V., et al.: Nursing care evaluation: concurrent and retrospective review criteria, St. Louis, 1977, The C. V. Mosby Co.

Dolan, P. O., and Greene, H. L.: Renal failure and peritoneal dialysis, Nurs. '75 **5**:40-49, 1975.

Flamenbaum, W., and Leslie, B. R.: Diagnosis and management of renal failure in surgical patients, Orthop. Clin. North Am. **9**:845-857, 1978.

Gutch, C. F., and Stoner, M. H.: Review of hemodialysis for nurses and dialysis personnel, ed. 3, St. Louis, 1979, The C. V. Mosby Co.

Juliani, L., and Reamer, B.: Kidney transplant: your role in aftercare, Nurs. '77 **7**:46-53, 1977.

Richard, C.: Nursing implications in prevention of complications in peritoneal dialysis, Heart Lung **4**:890-893, 1975.

Simon, N. M., et al.: Chronic renal failure. I. Pathophysiology and medical management, Cardiovasc. Nurs. **12**:7-16, 1976.

Smith, E. C., and Freedman, P.: Dialysis—current status and future trends, Heart Lung **4**:879-883, 1975.

Tucker, S. M., et al.: Patient care standards, ed. 2, St. Louis, 1980, The C. V. Mosby Co.

Zschoche, D. A.: Mosby's comprehensive review of critical care, ed. 2, St. Louis, 1980, The C. V. Mosby Co.

METABOLIC

Abels, L. F.: Mosby's manual of critical care, St. Louis, 1979, The C. V. Mosby Co.

Blackburn, G. L.: Hyperalimentation in the critically ill patient, Heart Lung **8**:67-70, 1979.

Boedeker, E.: Manual of medical therapeutics, ed. 21, Boston, 1974, Little, Brown & Co.

Brunner, L., and Suddarth, D.: Textbook of medical surgical nursing, ed. 3, Philadelphia, 1975, J. B. Lippincott Co.

Brunner, L., and Suddarth, D.: The Lippincott manual of nursing practice, ed. 2, Philadelphia, 1978, J. B. Lippincott Co.

Campbell, C.: Nursing diagnosis and intervention in nursing practice, New York, 1978, John Wiley & Sons.

Cataland, S.: Hypoglycemia: a spectrum of problems, Heart Lung **7**:455-462, 1978.

Colley, R., and Wilson, J.: Meeting patients' nutritional needs with hyperalimentation: how to begin hyperalimentation therapy, Nurs. '79 **9**(5):76-83, 1979.

Colley, R., and Wilson, J.: Meeting patients' nutritional needs with hyperalimentation: managing the patient on hyperalimentation, Nurs. '79 **9**(6):57-61, 1979.

Colley, R., and Wilson, J.: Meeting patients' nutritional needs with hyperalimentation: providing hyperalimentation for infants and children, Nurs. '79 **9**(7):50-63, 1979.

Guthrie, D., and Guthrie, R.: Coping with diabetic ketoacidosis, Nurs. '73 **3**:16-23, 1973.

Guthrie, D., and Guthrie, R.: DKA—breaking a vicious cycle, Nurs. '78 **8**:54-61, 1978.

Huang, S.: Nursing assessment in planning care for a diabetic patient, Nurs. Clin. North Am. **6**:135-143, 1971.

Isselbacher, K. J., et al., editors: Harrison's principles of internal medicine, ed. 9, New York, 1980, McGraw-Hill Book Co.

Lumb, P. D., et al.: Aggressive approach to intravenous feeding of the critically ill patient, Heart Lung **8**:71-80, 1979.

Manfredi, C., et al.: Developing a teaching program for diabetic patients, Continuing Education in Nursing **8**:46-52, 1977.

Mayers, M., et al.: Quality assurance for patient care, New York, 1977, Appleton-Century-Crofts.

Meltzer, L., et al., editors: Concepts and practices of intensive care for nurse specialists, Philadelphia, 1975, Charles Press Publications, Inc.

Nurses' Drug Alert **2:**145-160, Dec., 1978.

Skillman, T. G.: Diabetic ketoacidosis, Heart Lung **7:**594-602, 1978.

Tucker, S., et al.: Patient care standards, ed. 2, St. Louis, 1980, The C. V. Mosby Co.

Weil, M. H., and Henning, R. J.: Handbook of critical care medicine, Miami, 1978, Symposia Specialists, Inc.

Williams, S. R.: Essentials of nutrition and diet therapy, ed. 2, St. Louis, 1978, The C. V. Mosby Co.

Wilson, J., and Colley, R.: Meeting patients' nutritional needs with hyperalimentation: administering peripheral and enteral feedings, Nurs. '79 **9**(9):62-69, 1979.

GENERAL
Multiple trauma

Berk, J. L., et al., editors: Handbook of critical care, Boston, 1976, Little, Brown & Co.

Civetta, J. M.: Assessment of the patient following multi-systemic trauma, lecture presented at the Seventeenth Annual Symposium on Critical Care Medicine, Las Vegas, 1979, University of Southern California School of Medicine, Postgraduate Division, and Institute of Critical Care Medicine.

Flint, L. M.: Intraperitoneal injuries, Heart Lung **7:**273-277, 1978.

Horovitz, J. H., and Luterman, A.: Post-operative monitoring following critical trauma, Heart Lung **4:**269-277, 1975.

Lance, E., and Sweetwood, H.: Chest trauma, Nurs. '78 **8:**28-33, 1978.

Molyneux-Luick, M.: The ABC's of multiple trauma, Nurs. '77 **7:**30-36, 1977.

Richardson, J. D.: Management of non-cardiac thoracic trauma, Heart Lung **7:**286-292, 1978.

Burns

Brunner, L., and Suddarth, D.: Textbook of medical surgical nursing, ed. 3, Philadelphia, 1975, J. B. Lippincott Co.

Brunner, L., and Suddarth, D.: The Lippincott manual of nursing practice, ed. 2, Philadelphia, 1978, J. B. Lippincott Co.

Burrell, Z. L., and Burrell, L. O.: Critical care, ed. 3, St. Louis, 1977, The C. V. Mosby Co.

Dawson, H.: Basic human anatomy, ed. 2, New York, 1974, Appleton-Century-Crofts.

Feller, I., and Jones, C.: Nursing the burned patient, Ann Arbor, Mich., 1973, Braun-Brumfield, Inc.

Hayter, J.: Emergency nursing care of the burned patient, Nurs. Clin. North Am. **13:**223-234, 1978.

Mathewson, H. S.: Respiratory therapy in critical care, St. Louis, 1976, The C. V. Mosby Co.

McCrady, V.: Burn management, Critical Care Quarterly **1:**1-111, 1978.

Meltzer, L., et al., editors: Concepts and practices of intensive care for nurse specialists, Bowie, Md., 1976, Charles Press Publications, Inc.

Murray, R.: The concept of body image, Nurs. Clin. North Am. **7:**593-707, 1972.

Tucker, S., et al.: Patient care standards, ed. 2, St. Louis, 1980, The C. V. Mosby Co.

Disseminated intravascular coagulation

Boedeker, E., and Dauber, J.: Manual of medical therapeutics, ed. 21, Boston, 1974, Little, Brown & Co.

Burrell, Z. L., and Burrell, L. O.: Critical care, ed. 3, St. Louis, 1977, The C. V. Mosby Co.

Colman, R. W., Robboy, S. J., and Minna, J. D.: Disseminated intravascular coagulation (DIC): an approach, Am. J. Med. **52:**679-689, 1972.

Colman, R., et al.: Disseminated intravascular coagulation: a problem in critical care medicine, Heart Lung **3:**789-796, 1974.

Condon, R., and Nyhus, L., editors: Manual of surgical therapeutics, ed. 4, Boston, 1978, Little, Brown & Co.

Hudak, C., et al.: Critical care nursing, ed. 2, Philadelphia, 1977, J. B. Lippincott Co.

Isselbacher, K. J., et al., editors: Harrison's principles of internal medicine, ed. 9, New York, 1980, McGraw-Hill Book Co.

Jennings, B.: Improving your management of DIC, Nurs. '79 **9:**60-67, 1979.

Mayer, G.: DIC, Am. J. Nurs. **73:**2067-2069, 1973.

Nursing grand rounds: DIC—disseminated intravascular coagulation, Nurs. '74 **4:**66-71, 1974.

Picklesimer, L.: The nurse-challenging syndrome, RN **37:**46-47, 1974.

Zschoche, D. A.: Mosby's comprehensive review of critical care, ed. 2, St. Louis, 1980, The C. V. Mosby Co.

Poisoning

Arena, J. M.: Poisoning—toxicology—symptoms—treatments, ed. 4, Springfield, Ill., 1970, Charles C Thomas, Publisher.

Dreisbach, R. H.: Handbook of poisoning—diagnosis and treatment, ed. 9, Los Altos, Calif., 1977, Lange Medical Publications.

Graef, J. W., and Cone, T. E., Jr., editors: Manual of pediatric therapeutics, Boston, 1974, Little, Brown & Co.

Kempe, H. C., Silver, H. K., and O'Brien, D.: Current pediatric diagnosis and treatment, ed. 4, Los Altos, Calif, 1976, Lange Medical Publications.

Vaughan, V. C., et al.: Nelson textbook of pediatrics, ed. 11, Philadelphia, 1979, W. B. Saunders Co.

NEONATAL-PEDIATRIC

Alfonso: Newborn's potential for interaction, JOGN Nurs. **7:**9, 1978.

Aladjem, S., and Brown, A. K., editors: Perinatal intensive care, St. Louis, 1977, The C. V. Mosby Co.

Arena, J. M.: Poisoning—toxicology—symptoms—treatments, ed. 2, Springfield, Ill., 1970, Charles C Thomas, Publisher.

Avery, G. B.: Neonatology, Philadelphia, 1975, J. B. Lippincott Co.

Chinn, P. L.: Issues in lowering infant mortality: a call for ethical action, Advances in Nursing Science **1**:63-78, 1979.

Coran, A. G., et al.: Esophageal atresia. In Surgery of the neonate, Boston, 1978, Little, Brown & Co.

Clark, L. J. H., and Godfrey, S.: Asthma, Philadelphia, 1977, W. B. Saunders Co.

Curran, C. L., and Kachoyeanos, M. K.: The effects on neonates of two methods of chest physical therapy, MCN **4**:309-313, 1979.

Dreisbach, R. H.: Handbook of poisoning—diagnosis and treatment, ed. 9, Los Altos, Calif., 1977, Lange Medical Publications.

Dubowitz, L., Dubowitz, V., and Goldberg, C.: Clinical assessment of gestational age in the newborn infant, J. Pediatr. **77**:1-10, 1970.

Edwards, M.: Nursing case study: Reye's syndrome, Nursing Times **93**:1039-1040, 1977.

Evans, H. E., and Glass, L.: Perinatal medicine, Hagerstown, Md., 1976, Harper & Row, Publishers, Inc.

Fomon, S. J.: Human milk in premature feeding, Am. J. Public Health **67**:361-363, 1977.

Graef, J. W., and Cone, T. E., Jr., editors: Manual of pediatric therapeutics, Boston, 1974, Little, Brown & Co.

Greenberg, M., and Morris, N.: Engrossment: the newborn's impact upon the father, Am. J. Orthopsychiatry **44**:520-531, 1974.

Greenwood, R. D., and Rosenthal, A.: Cardiovascular malformations associated with tracheoesophageal fistula and esophageal atresia, Pediatrics **57**:87-91, 1976.

Haller, J., and Talbert, J.: Surgical emergencies in the newborn, Philadelphia, 1972, Lea & Febiger.

Hendren, W. H., and Kim, S. H.: Pediatric thoracic surgery. In Scarpelli, E. M., et al., editors: Pulmonary disease of the fetus, newborn and child, Philadelphia, 1978, Lea & Febiger.

Johnson, S. H.: High risk parenting: nursing assessment and strategies for the family at risk, New York, 1979, J. B. Lippincott Co.

Kattan, M.: Long-term sequelae of respiratory illness in infancy and childhood, Pediatr. Clin. North Am. **26**:525-535, 1979.

Kempe, H. C., Silver, H. K., and O'Brien, D.: Current pediatric diagnosis and treatment, ed. 4, Los Altos, Calif., 1976, Lange Medical Publications.

Kinsey, V. E., et al.: Pa$_{O_2}$ levels and retrolental fibroplasia: a report of the cooperative study, Pediatrics **60**:655-668, 1977.

Klaus, D., editor: Parent to infant attachment: special issue, Birth and the Family Journal **5**:183-253, 1978.

Klaus, M. H., and Fanaroff, A.: Care of the high risk neonate, Philadelphia, 1973, W. B. Saunders Co.

Klaus, M. H., and Kennell, J. H.: Maternal-infant bonding: the impact of early separation or loss on family development, St. Louis, 1976, The C. V. Mosby Co.

Korones, S. B.: High-risk newborn infants: the basis for intensive nursing care, ed. 2, St. Louis, 1976, The C. V. Mosby Co.

Laugh, M. D., Doershuk, C. F., and Stern, R. C.: Pediatric respiratory therapy, Chicago, 1974, Year Book Medical Publishers, Inc.

La Salle, A. J., et al.: Congenital tracheoesophageal fistula without esophageal atresia, J. Thorac. Cardiovasc. Surg. **78**:583-588, 1979.

Lovejoy, F. H., et al.: Clinical staging of Reye's syndrome, Am. J. Dis. Child. **128**:36-41, 1974.

Measel, C. P., and Anderson, S.: Non-nutritive sucking during tube feedings: effect on clinical course in premature infants, JOGN Nurs. **8**:265-272, 1979.

Miner, H.: Problems and prognosis for the small-for-gestational-age and the premature infant, MCN **3**:221-226, 1978.

Moffett, H. L.: Pediatric infectious diseases: a problem oriented approach, Philadelphia, 1975, J. B. Lippincott Co.

Nalepka, C. D.: Understanding thermoregulation in newborns, JOGN Nurs. **5**:17-19, 1976.

Neifert, M. R.: Medical management of breastfeeding, Keeping Abreast Journal of Human Nuturing **3**:274-282, 1978.

Patton, B., editor: Symposium on neonatal care, Nurs. Clin. North Am. **13**:1-84, 1978.

Pollack, D. J.: Reye's syndrome, New York, 1975, Grune & Stratton, Inc.

Priestley, B. L.: Low birthweight: born too early or too small, Nursing Mirror **148**:38-40, 1979.

Problems in neonatal intensive care, Briefs **43**:25-27, 1979.

Reye, R. D., et al.: Encephalopathy and fatty degeneration of the viscera: a disease entity in childhood, Lancet **2**:749-752, 1963.

Roberts, F. B.: Perinatal nursing, New York, 1977, McGraw-Hill Book Co.

Rothfeder, B.: Feeding the low birthweight neonate, Nurs. '77 **7**:58-59, 1977.

Slade, C. L.: Working with parents of high risk newborns, JOGN Nurs. **6**:21-26, 1977.

Thaler, M. M.: Pathogenesis of Reye's syndrome, Pediatrics **56**:1081-1084, 1975.

Vaughan, V. C., et al.: Nelson textbook of pediatrics, ed. 11, Philadelphia, 1979, W. B. Saunders Co.

Weeks, Holly, L.: What every ICU nurse should known about Reye's syndrome, Journal of Maternal Child Nursing **1**:231-238, 1976.

Williams, J. K., et al.: Thermoregulation of the newborn, MCN **1**:355-360, 1976.

Williams, T. J., and Hill, J. W., editors: Handbook of neonatal respiratory care, Riverside, Calif., Bourns, Inc.

Zamansky, H. A., et al.: Care of the critically ill newborn in an infant care center, Am. J. Nurs. **76**:566-581, 1976.

APPENDICES

A ☐ Abbreviations

ABO blood types A, B, and O
ADH antidiuretic hormone
ADL activities of daily living
AMI acute myocardial infarction
APTT activated partial thromboplastin time
AV atrioventricular (cardiovascular); arteriovenous (renal)
BP blood pressure
BUN blood urea nitrogen
°C degree(s) Celsius
C and S culture and sensitivity
Ca²⁺ calcium ion
CABG coronary artery bypass grafting
CAT computerized axial tomography
CBC complete blood count (including hematocrit, hemoglobin, white blood cell count)
cc cubic centimeters
CHF congestive heart failure
Cl⁻ chloride anion
CNS central nervous system
CO₂ carbon dioxide
COPD chronic obstructive pulmonary disease
CPAP continuous positive airway pressure
CPB cardiopulmonary bypass
CPR cardiopulmonary resuscitation
CSF cerebrospinal fluid
CVA cerebrovascular accident
CVP central venous pressure
DIC disseminated intravascular coagulation
ECG electrocardiogram
EEG electroencephalogram
ESR erythrocyte sedimentation rate
°F degree(s) Fahrenheit
FEV₁ fraction of air (volume) expired in 1 minute
FEV (FEVC) forced expiratory volume (capacity)
FI₀₂ fraction of inspired oxygen
FRC functional residual capacity
g gram
GAD glucose and acetone determination
GI gastrointestinal

Hct hematocrit
Hgb hemoglobin
HMD hyalin membrane disease
hr hour
ICP intracranial pressure
IgA immune globulin type A
IgM immune globulin type M
IM intramuscular
IPPB intermittent positive pressure breathing
IUGR intrauterine growth retardation
IV intravenous
K⁺ potassium ion
KUB kidney, ureter, and bladder
LAP left arterial pressure
LOC level of consciousness
LUQ left upper quadrant
LV left ventricular
MAP mean arterial pressure
mg milligram
MI myocardial infarction
min minute(s)
mm Hg millimeters of mercury
Na⁺ sodium ion
NaHCO₃ sodium bicarbonate
NEC necrotizing enterocolitis (neonatal)
NG nasogastric
NPO nothing per os (nothing by mouth)
O₂ oxygen
P pulse
Pa₀₂ partial arterial pressure of oxygen
Pa_{CO₂} partial arterial pressure of carbon dioxide
PAP pulmonary artery pressure
PCWP pulmonary capillary wedge pressure
PEEP positive end expiratory pressure
% percent
pH symbol for the logarithm of the reciprocal of the hydrogen ion concentration, thus reflecting hydrogen ion concentrations. High hydrogen ion concentration is reflected by low pH level; low hydrogen ion concentration is reflected by high pH level.

523

po per os (by mouth)
P$_{O_2}$ partial pressure of oxygen
PP perfusion pressure
PPN peripheral parenteral nutrition
prn as needed
PT prothrombin time
q every
RBC red blood cells
Rh the Rh antigen in the blood (coined when human blood tested with blood of Rhesus monkeys and the Rh antigen found)
ROM range of motion
SAH subarachnoid hemorrhage
SB Sengstaken-Blakemore (tube)

SFD small for dates
SGA small for gestational age
SGOT serum glutamic oxaloacetic transaminase
SGPT serum glutamic pyruvic transaminase
stat immediately
TEF tracheoesophageal fistula
TIA transient ischemic attack
TLC total lung capacity
TPN total parenteral nutrition
TPR temperature, pulse, and respirations
VC vital capacity
VSD ventricular septal defect
V$_T$ tidal volume
WBC white blood cells

B □ Surgical procedures: assessment

1. Patient/family's knowledge and level of understanding regarding operative therapy
   a. What they have been told
   b. Expectations
   c. Fears regarding surgery and outcome
   d. Previous surgical experiences
2. Significant intraoperative data
   a. Type of anesthesia; amount and reversal given
   b. Type, time, and amount of narcotic agents and muscle relaxants; amount and reversal given
   c. Medications administered during procedure; amount, time, frequency
   d. Any problems encountered during procedure: type, time, treatment, duration, effects, and side effects
   e. Any elective special techniques used such as hypotension, hypothermia
      (1) Medication used for control: amount, length of time, effects and side effects; level systolic blood pressure reduced to
      (2) If hypothermia: period and length of time induced, temperature reading, effects and side effects, rewarming regimen
   f. Blood loss and replacement
   g. Intake and output during procedure
   h. Blood determinations including serum electro-lytes, hemoglobin, hematocrit, arterial blood gas levels (monitored intraoperatively)
   i. Diuretics administered during procedure (e.g., furosemide, mannitol, or urea)
   j. Length of surgery
3. Significant operative procedure data
   a. Procedure performed
      (1) Thoracic
         (a) Biopsy
         (b) Nature and extent of tissue excised
         (c) Nature of repair
      (2) Cardiac
         (a) Number, type, and location of coronary artery bypass grafts
         (b) Site of valvular replacement and type of valve used
         (c) Defect repaired; type of graft material used
         (d) Length of surgery and time on cardiopulmonary bypass
      (3) Vascular: aneurysms; decompressive portovenous shunting procedures
         (a) Location, type, and extent of vessel repair
         (b) Presence and type of graft
      (4) Neurological
         (a) Biopsy

(b) Partial or total tumor removal

(c) Aneurysm wrapping or clipping

(d) Clot evacuation

(e) Type of shunt insertion; pressure valve placed

(5) Gastrointestinal (including jejunal-ileal bypass surgery)

(a) Nature of gastrointestinal tract repair (e.g., plication of ulcer, amount of tissue resected)

(b) Type of anastomosis

(6) Renal transplantation

(a) Type of transplant (e.g., cadaver, living related donor)

(b) Placement of transplanted kidney and type of anastomosis

b. Pathology apparent at surgery

(1) Thoracic

(a) Appearance of abnormal tissue (e.g., traumatized tissue; fibrotic, emphysematous changes; degree of tracheal stenosis)

(b) Extent of tumors, cysts, abscesses, etc.

(c) Extent of tissue resected

(2) Cardiac

(a) Location and extent of coronary artery disease, including distal arterial blood flows and myocardial dysfunction (as revealed by preoperative and intraoperative assessment)

(b) Graft blood flows

(c) Location and extent of valvular stenosis and/or insufficiency; vegetations present

(d) Presence and extent of ventricular aneurysm; the estimated proportion of ventricle involved; and the amount of ventricle resected

(e) Presence and extent of a septal defect; the type and size of patch used

(3) Vascular: aneurysms

(a) Size, type, and location of aneurysm

(b) Visible areas of ischemia, necrosis

(c) Vessel "clamp" time (absence of blood flow through artery while repair is being accomplished)

(4) Neurological

(a) Benign versus malignant tumor

(b) Tumor type and extent

(c) Degree of carotid artery stenosis if carotid endarterectomy performed

(d) Nature of malfunction requiring shunt revision

(e) Other significant operative findings such as increased intracranial pressure, cerebral edema, fluid accumulation, cranial nerve involvement

(5) Gastrointestinal

(a) Decompressive portovenous shunting procedures

(i) Type of vessel anastomosis

(ii) Portal pressures before and after anastomosis is made

(b) Pancreatic and gastrointestinal surgery—presence and extent of (as appropriate)

(i) Tumor

(ii) Ulcer

(iii) Ulcerative colitis

(iv) Adhesions

(v) Obstruction—partial or total

(vi) Ischemic bowel

(vii) Necrotic debris

(viii) Cyst, abscess(es)

(ix) Peritonitis

(x) Fluid inside or outside peritoneum

(6) Renal transplantation—appearance of patient's diseased kidneys (e.g., atrophy, polycystic biopsy)

c. Presence of drains: number, type, and location; suction or gravity

d. Presence of any operative factors requiring special precautions

(1) Maintenance of blood pressure in a prescribed range

(2) Positioning

(3) Observation for dysfunction of certain organs such as occurs after prolonged clamping of a major vessel, with organ dysfunction related to the disease process, or associated with operative trauma

e. Any complications of surgical procedure: treatment, effects, side effects, anticipated course/prognosis

f. Information and detail surgeon has provided patient/family regarding operative therapy and pathology

C ☐ Neonatal-pediatric data

Normal blood pressures (systolic)

Newborn: 60 to 90 mm Hg
1 to 12 months: 74 to 100 mm Hg
1 to 2 years: 80 to 110 mm Hg
2 to 6 years: 82 to 112 mm Hg
6 to 8 years: 84 to 116 mm Hg
8 to 10 years: 88 to 120 mm Hg
10 to 12 years: 94 to 130 mm Hg
12 to 14 years: 100 to 134 mm Hg
14 to 16 years: 104 to 140 mm Hg
16 to 18 years: 108 to 142 mm Hg

Normal heart rates*

Infant: 110 to 160/minute
Toddler: 90 to 130/minute
Preschooler: 90 to 120/minute
School-age child: 80 to 110/minute
Adolescent: 60 to 90/minute

Normal respiratory rates*

Newborn: 30 to 50/minute
6 to 18 months: 20 to 30/minute
2 to 10 years: 18 to 30/minute
Adolescent: 12 to 20/minute

Calculation of maintenance fluids

Weight	Formula
0 to 10 kg	100 ml/kg (neonates may tolerate up to 150 ml/kg if renal and cardiac functions are adequate)
11 to 20 kg	1000 ml for the first 10 kg + 50 ml/kg for each kilogram over 10 kg
21 to 30 kg	1500 ml for the first 20 kg + 25 ml/kg for each kilogram over 20 kg

Average daily caloric requirements

High-risk neonate: 120 to 150 calories/kg
Normal neonate: 100 to 120 calories/kg
1 to 2 years: 90 to 100 calories/kg
2 to 6 years: 80 to 90 calories/kg
7 to 9 years: 70 to 80 calories/kg
10 to 12 years: 50 to 60 calories/kg

*Increased heart and respiratory rates are expected in the distressed child.

INDEX

A

Abducens nerve dysfunction in Guillain Barré syndrome, 313

ABO incompatibility, hemolytic disease due to, 481-485; *see also* Hemolytic disease due to Rh/ABO incompatibility

Acidosis
  in cardiogenic shock, 83
  in hyaline membrane disease, 475

Adenohypophysis, 266

Air emboli, 181

Airway obstruction, 6-7

Akinetic seizures, signs and presentation of, 273t

Alcohol abuse
  ketoacidosis due to, 411
  pancreatitis and, 336

Allergic laryngeal edema, 492

Amniotic emboli, 181

Anaphylactic shock, 93

Anemia in hemolytic disease of newborn, 481, 482

Aneurysm(s)
  aortic, types of, 171
  definition of, 171
  dissecting, 171
  medical management of, 171
  mortality rates from, 171-172
  signs of, 171
  surgery for, 171
    assessment for, 172-173
    critical care plan for, 173-180
    goals of critical care in, 173
  ventricular, cardiac surgery for, 147

Angina pectoris, 55-59
  assessment of, 55-56
  critical care plan for, 56-59
  differential diagnosis of, 55
  goals of critical care in, 56
  management of, 55

Angiograms
  cardiac catheterization for, 141
  indications for, 141

Anticholinesterases for myasthenia gravis, 292

Antidiuretic hormone (ADH), function and release of, 266

Antidotes in poisoning management, 453

Aorta
  aneurysms of, types of, 171
  coarctation of, cardiac surgery for, 149t

Arrhythmias, 107-114
  assessment of, 108-109
  clinical significance of, 108

Arrhythmias—cont'd
  critical care plan for, 109-114
  etiologies of, 108
  goals of critical care in, 109
  hemodynamic significance of, 108
  management of, 108

Arteriovenous (AV) shunts for hemodialysis, 389

Artery(ies)
  cerebral, transient ischemic attacks in, signs and symptoms of, 259t
  coronary, left, anomalous, cardiac surgery for, 155t
  emboli in, 181
  plaques in, removal of, carotid endarterectomy for, 258-265; *see also* Endarterectomy, carotid
  superior mesenteric, embolus in, surgery for, 353

Aspiration
  of meconium, respiratory distress due to, 475
  of water in near drowning, 27-28

Asthma, 7
  in children, 497-501
    assessment of, 479-498
    characteristics of, 497
    critical care plan for, 498-501
    diagnosis of, 497
    goals of critical care in, 498
    therapy of, 497

Atherosclerosis
  aneurysms due to, 171
  myocardial infarction caused by, 60

Atresia
  esophageal, tracheoesophageal fistula with, 510-511
  pulmonary valvular, cardiac surgery for, 152t
  tricuspid, cardiac surgery for, 153t

Atrial septal defect, cardiac surgery for, 150t

Automaticity, 107-108

Autoregulation in increased intracranial pressure with decreased perfusion pressure, 193

B

Bacteremic shock, 93

Bacterial croup, 492

Bacterial meningitis, 281-282

Balloon pumping, intra-aortic, 122-132; *see also* Intra-aortic balloon pumping

Baxter formula for fluid replacement in burns, 443t

Bilirubin, serum levels of, elevated, in premature infant, 460

Blood pressure of infants and children, normal, 526

Blood vessels
  aneurysms of; *see* Aneurysm(s)
  surgery on, for aneurysm, 171-180; *see also* Aneurysm(s), surgery for

Page numbers in *italics* indicate illustrations.
Page numbers followed by *t* indicate tables.

Bochdalek hernia, 507
Brain
  concussion of, 204*t*
  contusion of, 204*t*
  injury to, in head trauma, 203, 204*t*
Brain stem
  cranial nerve nuclei in, 238
  lesions of, symptoms of, 239*t*
Bronchitis, 7
Bronchoscopy in diagnosis of tracheoesophageal fistula, 511
Bronchospasm in asthma, 497
Brooke Army formula for fluid replacement in burns, 443*t*
Brudzinski's sign in bacterial meningitis, 282
Bullectomy, indications for, 17
Burns, 441-449
  assessment of, 441-444
  critical care plan for, 444-449
  depth of, 443*t*
  estimating size of, *442*
  etiologies of, 441
  fluid replacement formulas for, 443*t*
  goals of critical care in, 444
  management of, periods of, 441
  pathophysiology of, periods of, 441

C

Caloric requirements for infants and children, average daily, 526
Cardiac output, monitoring of, 134
Cardiogenic shock, 83-92, 93
  assessment of, 84
  critical care plan for, 85-92
  early recognition of, 83-84
  goals of critical care in, 84
  hypotension in, 83
  symptoms of, 83
Carotid arterial system, transient ischemic attacks in, signs and symptoms of, 259*t*
Carotid endarterectomy, 258-265; *see also* Endarterectomy, carotid
Catheter(s)
  central venous, total parenteral nutrition through, 417-423; *see also* Total parenteral nutrition (TPN)
  pulmonary artery, types and functions of, 133
  Swan-Ganz, functions of, 133
Catheterization, cardiac, 141-146
  assessment for, 142-143
  critical care plan for, 143-146
  goals of, 143
  procedures accompanying, 141-142
  purposes of, 141
  risks with, 142
Central nervous system (CNS), involvement of, in poisoning, symptoms and treatment of, 453
Central venous catheter, total parenteral nutrition through, 417-423; *see also* Total parenteral nutrition (TPN)
Central venous pressure (CVP), measurement of, purpose of, 133
Cerebellopontine angle, lesions of, symptoms of, 239*t*
Cerebellum, lesions of, signs of, 238
Cerebral arteries, transient ischemic attacks in, signs and symptoms of, 259*t*
Cerebral cortex, lobes of, pathology of, focal neurological signs of, 229-230

Cerebral perfusion pressure, 193
Cerebrospinal fluid (CSF)
  in bacterial meningitis diagnosis, 282
  changes in, in subarachnoid hemorrhage, 215
  impaired absorption of, in hydrocephalus, 250
  obstructed outflow of, in hydrocephalus, 249, 250
  overproduction of, in hydrocephalus, 249, 250
  protein content of, elevated, in Guillain Barré syndrome diagnosis, 313
Charcoal, activated, in poisoning management, 453
Chest physiotherapy, 52-54
  assessment of, 53
  critical care plan for, 54
  goals of critical care in, 53
  sequence of, 53
Children
  blood pressure of, normal, 526
  caloric requirements for, average daily, 526
  heart rate of, normal, 526
  maintenance fluids for, calculation of, 526
  respiratory rate of, normal, 526
Chronic obstructive pulmonary disease (COPD), acute deterioration of, 6-7
Coagulation, disseminated intravascular, 449-453; *see also* Disseminated intravascular coagulation (DIC)
Coagulopathy, consumption, 449-453; *see also* Disseminated intravascular coagulation (DIC)
Coarctation of aorta, cardiac surgery for, 149*t*
Concussion, cerebral, 204*t*
Consumption coagulopathy, 449-453; *see also* Disseminated intravascular coagulation (DIC)
Contralateral signs of cerebral lobe pathology, 229
Contusion, cerebral, 204*t*
Cor pulmonale, 7
Coronary artery, left, anomalous, cardiac surgery for, 155*t*
Coronary artery bypass grafting, 147
Corticosteroids for myasthenia gravis, 292
Coughing in chest physiotherapy, 53
Counterpulsation, 122-132; *see also* Intra-aortic balloon pumping
Cranial nerves
  dysfunction of, in Guillain Barré syndrome, 313
  nuclei of, in brain stem, 238
Craniotomy
  infratentorial, 238-249; *see also* Infratentorial craniotomy
  supratentorial, 229-237; *see also* Supratentorial craniotomy
Crescendo angina, 55
Crohn's disease, gastrointestinal surgery for, 353
Croup syndrome, 491-496
  assessment of, 492-493
  causes of, 491-492
  characteristics of, 491
  clinical forms of, 492
  critical care plan for, 493-496
  goals of critical care in, 493
Cyanotic heart disease, systemic complications of, 148

D

Decompressive portovenous shunting procedures for liver failure, 326-327
  critical care plan for, 333-335
Decubitus angina, 55

Defibrination syndrome, 449-453; *see also* Disseminated intravascular coagulation (DIC)

Dehydration in hyperglycemia, 411

Depolarization of myocardium, 107-108

Derma, 441

Diabetic ketoacidosis, 411-417
    assessment of, 411-412
    critical care plan for, 413-417
    goals of critical care for, 412
    precipitating factors for, 411
    therapeutic goals of, 411

Dialysis, peritoneal, 378-388; *see also* Peritoneal dialysis

Diaphragmatic hernia, 507-510
    assessment of, 507
    critical care plan for, 508-510
    goals of critical care in, 507
    signs and symptoms of, 507
    surgery for, 507

Diffuse intravascular clotting, 449-453; *see also* Disseminated intravascular coagulation (DIC)

Disseminated intravascular coagulation (DIC), 449-453
    assessment of, 450
    conditions associated with, 449
    critical care plan for, 451-453
    diagnosis of, 449
    goals of critical care in, 450
    in neonatal necrotizing enterocolitis, 486
    signs and symptoms of, 449
    therapeutic goals in, 449-450

Diuretic phase of acute renal failure, 373

Diverticulitis, gastrointestinal surgery for, 353-354

Diverticulosis, gastrointestinal surgery for, 353-354

Drainage, postural, in chest physiotherapy, 53

Drowning, near, 27-35
    assessment of, 28-29
    critical care plan for, 29-35
    fresh water aspiration in, 27-28
    goals of critical care in, 29
    hypoxia complicating, 28
    neurological sequelae of, 28
    salt water aspiration in, 28

Duodenum, ulcers of, surgery for, 353

Dyspnea in asthma, 497

E

Edema
    laryngeal, allergic, 492
    pulmonary, of cardiac origin, 1-5; *see also* Pulmonary edema

Electrocardiogram in diagnosis of myocardial infarction, 60-61

Embolus(i)
    air, 181
    amniotic, 181
    assessment of, 181-182
    critical care plan for, 183-192
    definition of, 181
    fat, 181
    goals of critical care in, 182
    superior mesenteric artery, surgery for, 353
    therapeutic goals for, 181

Emphysema, 7

Encephalitis, 282

Encephalitis—cont'd
    assessment of, 283
    causes of, 282
    critical care plan for, 284-291
    goals of critical care in, 283-284

Endarterectomy, carotid, 258-265
    assessment for, 258
    critical care plan for, 259-265
    goals for critical care in, 258-259

Endocardial cushion defect, cardiac surgery for, 150-151*t*

Endocarditis, 102-107
    assessment of, 103
    critical care plan for, 104-107
    diagnosis of, 103
    goals of critical care in, 103
    management of, 103
    predisposition to, 102

Endotracheal tube, patient with, chest physiotherapy for, sequence of, 53

Enteritis, regional, gastrointestinal surgery for, 353

Enterocolitis
    necrotizing, in premature infant, 460, 486-491; *see also* Necrotizing enterocolitis (NEC) in premature infant
    regional, gastrointestinal surgery for, 353

Enzymes in myocardial infarction, 61

Epicardium, 97

Epidermis, 441

Epiglottitis, acute, 492

Epilepsy
    definition of, 272
    idiopathic, 272

Esophagogram in diagnosis of tracheoesophageal fistula, 511

Esophagus
    atresia of, tracheoesophageal fistula with, 510-511
    varices of, upper gastrointestinal hemorrhage due to, 347

Exchange transfusion for hemolytic disease of newborn, 482

F

Facial nerve dysfunction in Guillain Barré syndrome, 313

Fat emboli, 181

Fat emulsions for total parenteral nutrition, 417-418

Fetus, growth of, retardation of, 472-475; *see also* Growth retardation, intrauterine

Fistula(s)
    pancreatic, surgery for, 341
    tracheoesophageal, 510-516

Fluids, maintenance, for infants and children, calculation of, 526

Fracture, skull, 204*t*

Frontal lobe, damage to, focal neurological signs of, 230*t*

G

Gastritis, upper gastrointestinal hemorrhage due to, 347

Gastrointestinal tract
    obstruction of, surgery for, 353
    surgery on, 353-365
        assessment for, 354-355
        care following, 354
        critical care plan for, 355-365
        goals of critical care for, 355
        indications for, 353-354
    upper, bleeding from, acute, 347-353

Gastrointestinal tract—cont'd
  upper, bleeding from, acute—cont'd 347-353
    assessment of, 347-348
    causes of, 347
    clinical manifestations of, 347
    critical care plan for, 348-353
    goals of critical care in, 348
    therapy for, 347
Gland(s)
  pituitary; *see* Pituitary gland
  thymus, removal of, for myasthenia gravis, 292-293
    critical care plan for, 304-312
Glossopharyngeal nerve dysfunction in Guillain Barré syndrome, 313
Grafting, coronary artery bypass, 147
Grand mal seizures, signs and presentation of, 273*t*
Great vessels, transposition of, cardiac surgery for, 154-155*t*
Growth retardation, intrauterine, 372-375
  assessment of, 473
  causes of, 472-473
  critical care plan for, 474-475
  goals of critical care in, 473
  prognosis in, 473
  treatment of, 473
Guillain Barré syndrome, 312-320
  assessment of, 313
  critical care plan for, 314-320
  diagnosis of, 313
  etiological theories of, 312
  goals of critical care in, 313-314
  signs and symptoms of, 312-313

H

Head, trauma to, 203-215
  assessment of, 205-207
  complications of, 203
  critical care plan for, 207-215
  goals of critical care in, 207
  treatment of, 203-204
    priorities of, 203
Heart
  arrhythmias of, 107-114; *see also* Arrhythmias
  catheterization of, 141-146; *see also* Catheterization, cardiac
  conduction velocity in, 108
  defects of, congenital, cardiac surgery for, 148, 149-155*t*
  disease of, cardiogenic shock in, 83; *see also* Cardiogenic shock
  excitability of, 108
  failure of, 74-83
    assessment of, 74-75
    cardiogenic shock in, 83; *see also* Cardiogenic shock
    critical care plan for, 76-83
    etiologies of, 74
    goals of critical care in, 75
  output of, low, 74-83; *see also* Heart, failure of
  rate of, in infants and children, normal, 526
  refractoriness of, 108
  surgery on, 147-170
    assessment for, 156-157
    critical care plan for, 157-170
    goals for critical care in, 157
    indications for, 147
    postoperative care and problems in, 147

Heart—cont'd
  valves of
    insufficiency of, valvular repair or replacement for, 147
    replacement or revision of, indications for, 147
    stenosis of, valvular repair or replacement for, 147
Hematemesis in acute upper gastrointestinal bleeding, 347
Hematochezia in acute upper gastrointestinal bleeding, 347
Hematoma, subdural, 222-229
  acute, 222
  assessment of, 222-223
  causes of, 222
  chronic, 222
  critical care plan for, 223-229
  diagnosis of, 222
  goals of critical care in, 223
  symptoms of, 222
  treatment of, 222
Hemodialysis, 388-401
  assessment for, 389-390
  critical care plan for, 390-401
  goals of critical care in, 390
  monitoring of, 389
  principles of, 388-389
  vascular access for, 389
Hemodynamic monitoring, 132-141
  assessment of, 134-135
  critical care plan for, 135-141
  goals of critical care in, 135
  intra-arterial, 132-133
Hemolytic disease due to Rh/ABO incompatibility, 481-485
  assessment of, 482-483
  critical care plan for, 483-485
  exchange transfusion for, 482
  goals of critical care in, 483
  treatment of, 482
Hemorrhage
  subarachnoid, 215-221
    assessment of, 216
    critical care plan for, 216-221
    diagnosis of, 215
    etiologies of, 215
    goals of critical care in, 216
    signs and symptoms of, 215
    therapeutic goals in, 215
  subdural, 222; *see also* Hematoma, subdural
  upper gastrointestinal, 347-353; *see also* Gastrointestinal tract, upper, bleeding from, acute
Heparin
  for disseminated intravascular coagulation, 449, 450
  in hemodialysis, 389
  in peritoneal dialysis, 379
Hernia
  Bochdalek, 507
  diaphragmatic, 507-510; *see also* Diaphragmatic hernia
  Morgagni, 507
Herpes simplex, encephalitis due to, signs of, 282
Herpes zoster, encephalitis due to, signs of, 282
Hormone(s)
  antidiuretic, function and release of, 266
  secreted by adenohypophysis, 266
  secreted by neurohypophysis, 266

Hyaline membrane disease (HMD) in infants, respiratory distress in, 475

Hydrocephalus
  communicating, 250
  etiologies of, 250
  in fourth venticle pathology, 238
  internalized shunting procedures for, 249-257; *see also* Shunting procedures, internalized
  noncommunicating, 250
  normal pressure, 250
Hyperglycemia, diabetic ketoacidosis and, 411
Hypertension, aneurysm formation and, 171
Hypoglossal nerve dysfunction in Guillain Barré syndrome, 313
Hypoglycemia in intrauterine growth retardation, monitoring for, 473
Hypophysectomy, transphenoidal, 266-272
  assessment for, 267-268
  critical care plan for, 268-272
  goals of critical care in, 268
Hypophysis; *see* Pituitary gland
Hypotension in cardiogenic shock, 83
Hypoventilation, acute respiratory failure and, 6
Hypovolemic shock, 92-93
Hypoxemia
  in cardiogenic shock, 83
  in croup syndrome, 492
Hypoxia complicating near drowning, 28

I

Ileitis, regional, gastrointestinal surgery for, 353
Immunosuppressive agents in renal transplantation, 402
Infant
  blood pressure of, normal, 526
  caloric requirements for, average daily, 526
  croup in, 491-496; *see also* Croup syndrome
  diaphragmatic hernia in, 507-510; *see also* Diaphragmatic hernia
  gestational age of, in assessment of prematurity, 460
  heart rate of, normal, 526
  hemolytic disease of, due to Rh/ABO incompatibility, 481-485; *see also* Hemolytic disease due to Rh/ABO incompatibility
  maintenance fluids for, calculation of, 526
  premature
    characteristics of, 460
    complicating conditions in, 460
    definition of, 460
    etiological factors associated with, 460
    morbidity and mortality of, 460
    prognosis for, 460-461
    unstable, 460-472
      assessment of, 461
      critical care plan for, 461-472
      goals of critical care for, 461
  respiratory rate of, normal, 526
  small for dates, 472-475; *see also* Growth retardation, intrauterine
  small for gestational age, 472-475; *see also* Growth retardation, intrauterine
Infarction, myocardial; *see* Myocardial infarction
Infections, pulmonary, in near drowning, 28
Infratentorial craniotomy, 238-249
  assessment for, 239-240
  critical care plan for, 240-249
  goals of critical care in, 240

Infratentorial craniotomy—cont'd
  indications for, 238
Insulin, function of, 411
Intra-aortic balloon pumping, 122-132
  assessment of, 122-123
  contraindications to, 122
  critical care plan for, 124-132
  device for, 122
  goals of critical care in, 123
  indications for, 122
  monitoring of, 123
Intracranial pressure (ICP)
  compensatory mechanisms in, 193
  components of, 193
  increased, 193-203
    assessment of, 194
    causes of, 193
    critical care plan for, 195-203
    with decreased perfusion pressure, compensatory mechanisms for, 193
    in fourth ventricle pathology, 238
    goals of critical care in, 194-195
    symptoms of, 193-194
  monitoring of, 134
Intravascular coagulation syndrome, 449-453; *see also* Disseminated intravascular coagulation (DIC)
Ipsilateral signs of cerebral lobe pathology, 229-230
Ischemia
  mucosal, in neonatal necrotizing enterocolitis, 486
  transient attacks of, 258, 259; *see also* Transient ischemic attacks (TIA)

J

Jacksonian seizures, signs and presentation of, 273*t*
Jaundice in hemolytic disease of newborn, 481
Jejunal-ileal bypass surgery, 365-372
  assessment for, 365-366
  care following, 365
  critical care plan for, 366-372
  goals of critical care in, 366
  indications for, 365
  psychosocial evaluation for, 365
  side effects of, 365

K

Kernicterus in hemolytic disease of newborn, 482
Kernig's sign in bacterial meningitis, 282
Ketoacidosis
  diabetic, 411-417; *see also* Diabetic ketoacidosis
  in hyperglycemia, 411
Kidney(s)
  failure of
    acute, 373-378
      assessment of, 373-374
      critical care plan for, 375-378
      diagnosis of, 373
      etiology of, 373
      goals of critical care in, 374
      phases of, 373
      signs of, 373
    dialysis during, 378-388; *see also* Peritoneal dialysis

Kidney(s)—cont'd
  failure of—cont'd
    renal transplantation for, 401-410; *see also* Kidney(s), transplantation of
  problems with, after cardiac surgery, 147
  transplantation of, 401-410
    assessment for, 402-403
    critical care plan for, 403-410
    goals of critical care in, 403
    indications for, 401-402
    rejection following, prevention of, 402

L

Laryngotracheobronchitis, 492
Larynx, edema of, allergic, 492
Lavage, peritoneal, in diagnosis of peritonitis, 321
Leptomeningitis, 281
Liver
  failure of, 326-335
    assessment of, 327-328
    critical care plan for, 328-335
    decompressive portovenous shunting procedures for, 326-327
      critical care plan for, 333-335
    diseases producing, 326
    goals of critical care in, 328
    hepatotoxins causing, 326
    manifestations of, 326
    medical management of, critical care plan for, 328-332
    prognosis in, 326
  functions of, 326
Lung(s)
  diffusion in, impairment of, acute respiratory failure and, 6
  disease of, chronic obstructive, acute deterioration of, 6-7
  infections in, in near drowning, 28
  problems with, after cardiac surgery, 147

M

Mallory-Weiss syndrome, upper gastrointestinal hemorrhage due to, 347
Meconium aspiration syndrome, respiratory distress in, 475
Medulla, lesions of, symptoms of, 239*t*
Melena in acute upper gastrointestinal bleeding, 347
Meningitis, 281-282
  aseptic, 282
  assessment of, 283
  bacterial, 281-282
    clinical manifestations of, 282
  critical care plan for, 284-291
  goals of critical care in, 283-284
  viral, 282
Midbrain, lesions of, symptoms of, 239*t*
Monitoring, hemodynamic, 132-141; *see also* Hemodynamic monitoring
Morgagni hernia, 507
Myasthenia gravis, 292-312
  assessment of, 293
  clinical manifestations of, 292
  critical care plan for, 294
  diagnosis of, 292
  etiology of, 292

Myasthenia gravis—cont'd
  goals of critical care in, 294
  medical management of, 292
    critical care plan for, 294-304
  muscles involved in, 292
  thymectomy for, 292-293
    critical care plan for, 304-312
Myocardial infarction
  acute, 60-73
    assessment of, 61-62
    cardiogenic shock in, 83; *see also* Cardiogenic shock
    critical care plan for, 62-73
    goals of critical care in, 62
  angina and, 55
  diagnosis of, 60
  ECG changes in, 60-61
  healing of, 60
  hemodynamic consequences of, 60
  site of, 60
  subendocardial, 60
  transmural, 60
Myocardium, depolarization of, 107-108
Myoclonic seizures, signs and presentation of, 273*t*

N

Necrotizing enterocolitis (NEC) in premature infant, 460, 486-491
  assessment of, 486-487
  critical care plan for, 487-491
  etiological theories of, 486
  goals of critical care for, 487
  pathology of, 486
  treatment of, 486
Neonate; *see* Infant
Nerve(s), cranial
  dysfunction of, in Guillain Barré syndrome, 313
  nuclei of, in brain stem, 238
Neurogenic shock, 93
Neurohypophysis, 266
Neurological sequelae of near drowning, 28
Neurological signs of lobe pathology, 229-230
Newborn; *see* Infant
Nutrition, parenteral
  peripheral, 418
    critical care plan for, 419-423
  total, 417-423; *see also* Total parenteral nutrition (TPN)

O

Obesity, morbid, jejunal-ileal bypass for, 365; *see also* Jejunal-ileal bypass surgery
Occipital lobe, damage to, focal neurological signs of, 230*t*
Oculomotor nerve dysfunction in Guillain Barré syndrome, 313
Oligemic shock, 92-93
Oliguric phase of acute renal failure, 373
Optic chiasm, effect of pituitary tumors on, 266
Oxygen for respiratory distress in infants, complications of, 476

P

Pacemakers
  artificial, 114-121
    asynchronous, 114

Pacemakers—cont'd
  artificial—cont'd
    demand, 114
    functions of, 114
    implantation of, approaches to, 114-115
    indications for, 115
    permanent
      assessment of, 119
      critical care plan for, 120-121
      goals of critical care in, 119
      synchronous, 114
    temporary
      assessment of, 115
      critical care plan for, 116-119
      goals of critical care in, 115
  of heart, 107
Pancreas
  functions of, 336
  inflammation of, 336-340; *see also* Pancreatitis
  surgery on, 341-346
    assessment for, 341
    critical care plan for, 342-346
    goals of critical care in, 342
    indications for, 341
Pancreatitis, 336-340
  acute edematous, 336
  alcohol abuse and, 336
  assessment of, 336-337
  causes of, 336
  critical care plan for, 337-340
  goals of critical care in, 337
  hemorrhagic, 336
  surgery for, 341
Paralysis in Guillain Barré syndrome, 312-313
Parenteral nutrition
  peripheral, 418
    critical care plan for, 419-423
  total, 417-423; *see also* Total parenteral nutrition (TPN)
Paresthesias in Guillain Barré syndrome, 312
Parietal lobe, damage to, focal neurological signs of, 230*t*
Patent ductus arteriosus, cardiac surgery for, 149*t*
Percussion in chest physiotherapy, 52
Pericarditis, 97-102
  assessment of, 98
  critical care plan for, 98-102
  etiologies of, 97
  goals of critical care in, 98
  hemodynamic consequences of, 98
  management of, 98
  mechanisms of, 97-98
  signs and symptoms of, 97
Pericardium
  parietal, 97
  visceral, 97
Peripheral parenteral nutrition (PPN), 418
  critical care plan for, 419-423
Peritoneal dialysis, 378-388
  advantages and disadvantages of, 379
  assessment for, 379-380
  critical care plan for, 380-388

Peritoneal dialysis—cont'd
  equipment for, 379
  goals of critical care in, 380
  principle of, 378-379
Peritonitis, 321-326
  assessment of, 322
  critical care plan for, 322-326
  diagnosis of, 321
  goals of critical care in, 322
  medical therapy for, 321
  surgery for, 321-322
  symptoms of, 321
Petit mal seizures, signs and presentation of, 273*t*
Phototherapy for hemolytic disease due to ABO incompatibility, 482
Physiotherapy, chest, 52-54; *see also* Chest physiotherapy
Pituitary gland
  anatomy and function of, 266
  tumors of, 266-267
    signs and symptoms of, 267
    transphenoidal hypophysectomy for, 266-272; *see also* Hypophysectomy, transphenoidal
    treatment of, 267
Plasma-electrophoresis for myasthenia gravis, 292
Pneumonia, aspiration, in near drowning, 28
Pneumothorax in meconium aspiration syndrome, 475
Poisoning, 453-459
  assessment of, 454
  critical care plan for, 455-459
  diagnosis of, 453
  goals of critical care in, 454
  signs and symptoms of, 453
  treatment of, 453-454
Pons, lesions of, symptoms of, 239*t*
Positive end expiratory pressure (PEEP), 48-52
  assessment of, 49
  critical care plan for, 49-52
  goals of critical care in, 49
Postural drainage in chest physiotherapy, 53
Potassium, decreased, in diabetic ketoacidosis, 411
Premature infant, unstable, 460-472; *see also* Infant, premature, unstable
Pressure, intracranial; *see* Intracranial pressure (ICP)
Prinzmetal's angina, 55
Pseudocyst, pancreatic, surgery for, 341
Psychological problems after cardiac surgery, 147
Psychomotor seizures, signs and presentation of, 273*t*
Pulmonary artery pressure (PAP), monitoring of, 133-134
Pulmonary capillary wedge pressure (PCWP), monitoring of, 133
Pulmonary edema
  of cardiac origin, 1-5
    assessment of, 1
    critical care plan for, 2-5
    goals of critical care in, 1-2
  causes of, 1
  definition of, 1
Pulmonary valve
  atresia of, cardiac surgery for, 152*t*
  stenosis of, cardiac surgery for, 152*t*
Pulmonary venous return, anomalous, total, cardiac surgery for, 155*t*

R

Respiratory distress syndrome (RDS)
adult, 7-8
in infant, 475-481
assessment of, 476
causes of, 475
critical care plan for, 477-481
goals of critical care in, 476-477
management of, 475-476
prematurity and, 460, 475
prognosis in, 476
Respiratory failure, acute, 6-17
assessment of, 8-9
critical care plan for, 9-17
etiology of, 6
goals of critical care in, 9
pathological mechanisms in, 6
signs and symptoms of, 6
Respiratory rates of infants and children, normal, 526
Retardation of growth, intrauterine, 472-475; *see also* Growth retardation, intrauterine
Reye's syndrome, 502-506
assessment of, 502-503
characteristics of, 502
course of, 502
critical care plan for, 503-506
etiological theories of, 502
goals of critical care in, 503
treatment of, 502
Rh incompatibility, hemolytic disease due to, 481-485; *see also* Hemolytic disease due to Rh/ABO incompatibility

S

Salicylate intoxication, ketoacidosis due to, 411
Seizures, 272-281
assessment of, 272-274
causes of, 272
classification of, 272, 273*t*
critical care plan for, 275-281
goals of critical care in, 274
treatment of, 272
Septal defect
atrial, cardiac surgery for, 150*t*
ventricular, cardiac surgery for, 147, 150*t*
Shock, 92-97
anaphylactic, 93
assessment of, 93-94
bacteremic, 93
cardiogenic, 83-92; *see also* Cardiogenic shock
critical care plan for, 94-97
findings in, 92
goals of critical care in, 94
hypovolemic, 92-93
neurogenic, 93
oligemic, 92-93
types of, 92-93
vasogenic, 93
Shunt, arteriovenous, for hemodialysis, 389
Shunting, intrapulmonary, acute respiratory failure and, 6

Shunting procedures
decompressive portovenous, for liver failure, 326-327
critical care plan for, 333-335
internalized, 249-257
assessment for, 250-251
critical care plan for, 251-257
devices for, 249-250
goals of critical care in, 251
Skin
burns of 441-449; *see also* Burns
functions of, 441
Skull, fracture of, 204*t*
Sodium, decreased, in diabetic ketoacidosis, 411
Somatic sensory seizures, signs and presentation of, 273*t*
Spinal accessory nerve dysfunction in Guillain Barré syndrome, 313
Status asthmaticus, 7
in children, 497-501
assessment of, 497-498
critical care plan for, 498-501
goals of critical care in, 498
therapy of, 497
Stenosis, valvular
pulmonary, cardiac surgery for, 152*t*
valve repair and replacement for, 147
Stomach
ulcers of, surgery for, 353
varices of, upper gastrointestinal hemorrhage due to, 347
Subarachnoid hemorrhage, 215-221; *see also* Hemorrhage, subarachnoid
Subdural hematoma, 222-229; *see also* Hematoma, subdural
Subglottic croup, 492
Supraglottic croup, 492
Supratentorial craniotomy, 229-237
assessment for, 230-231
critical care plan for, 231-237
goals of critical care in, 231
indications for, 229
pathological conditions warranting, neurological symptoms of, 229
Surgical procedures, assessment for, 524-525
Swan-Ganz catheter, functions of, 133

T

Tachypnea, transient, of newborn, respiratory distress in, 475
Temporal lobe, damage to, focal neurological signs of, 230*t*
Tetralogy of Fallot, cardiac surgery for, 152-153*t*
Thoracotomy, indications for, 17
Thorax, surgery on, 17-27
assessment for, 17-18
critical care plan for
postoperative, 20-27
preoperative, 18-20
goals of critical care in, 18
Thrombus, 181
Thymectomy for myasthenia gravis, 292-293
critical care plan for, 304-312
Thymus gland, removal of, for myasthenia gravis, 292-293
critical care plan for, 304-312
Total anomalous pulmonary venous return, cardiac surgery for, 155*t*

Total parenteral nutrition (TPN), 417-423
  assessment for, 418
  critical care plan for, 419-423
  goals of critical care in, 418-419
  indications for, 417
  monitoring of, 418
  solution for, composition of, 417-418
  team approach to, 418
Tracheoesophageal fistula (TEF), 510-516
  acquired, 510, 511
  assessment of, 512
  congenital, 510-511, 512
    conditions associated with, 512
  critical care plan for, 512-516
  diagnosis of, 510-511
  goals of critical care in, 512
  postoperative complications of, 511-512
  surgery for, 511
Tracheostomy
  complications of, 36
  indications for, 36
  patient with, 36-42
    assessment of, 36
    critical care plan for, 37-42
    goals of critical care for, 36
Transducer in hemodynamic monitoring, 132
Transfusion, exchange, for hemolytic disease of newborn, 482
Transient ischemic attacks (TIA)
  carotid endarterectomy for, 258-265; *see also* Endarterectomy, carotid
  signs and symptoms of, 259*t*
Transient tachypnea of newborn, respiratory distress in, 475
Transphenoidal hypophysectomy, 266-272; *see also* Hypophysectomy, transphenoidal
Transplantation, renal, 401-410; *see also* Kidney(s), transplantation of
Transposition of great vessels, cardiac surgery for, 154-155*t*
Trauma, multiple, 424-440
  assessment of, 425-426
  critical care plan for, 427-440
  goals of critical care in, 426-427
  hemodynamic monitoring in, 424-425
  immediate management of, 424
Triage in assessment of multiple trauma, 424
Tricuspid atresia, cardiac surgery for, 153*t*
Truncus arteriosus, cardiac surgery for, 151*t*

Tumor(s)
  gastric, surgery for, 353
  pancreatic, management of, 341
  pituitary, 266-272; *see also* Pituitary gland, tumors of

U
Ulcers
  gastrointestinal surgery for, 353
  upper gastrointestinal hemorrhage due to, 347

V
Vagus nerve dysfunction in Guillain Barré syndrome, 313
Vasogenic shock, 93
Vasomotor control in increased intracranial pressure with decreased perfusion pressure, 193
Veins, emboli in, 181
Ventilation, mechanical, 42-48
  assessment of, 42-43
  after cardiac surgery, 147
  critical care plan for, 44-48
  goals of critical care in, 43
  indications for, 42
  ventilators for, 42
Ventilation/perfusion mismatch, acute respiratory failure and, 6
Ventricle(s)
  fourth, lesions of, hydrocephalus in, 238
  heart, failure of, 74; *see also* Heart, failure of
Ventricular aneurysm, cardiac surgery for, 147
Ventricular septal defect, cardiac surgery for, 147, 150*t*
Vertebrobasilar artery system, transient ischemic attacks in, signs and symptoms of, 259*t*
Vibration in chest physiotherapy, 52-53
Viral croup, 491-492
Viral meningitis, 282
Vision, effect of pituitary tumors on, 266, 267
Visual seizures, signs and presentation of, 273*t*
Vomiting in Reye's syndrome, 502

W
Water
  fresh, aspiration of, 27-28
  salt, aspiration of, 28
Wheezing in asthma, 497
Whipple, description and indications for, 341